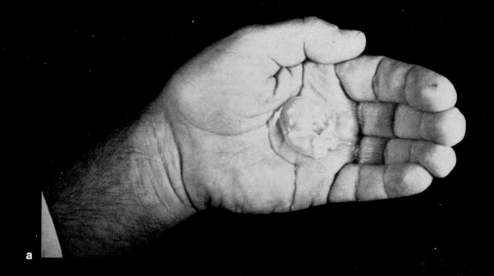

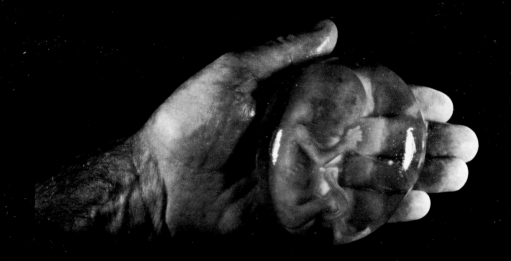

Plate 2
(a) Fetus in sac 8 weeks old. *(Courtesy of Roberts Rugh.)* (b) Fetus in sac. 12 weeks old. *(Courtesy of Roberts Rugh.)*

maternal and infant care

maternal and infant care

SECOND EDITION

edited by

ELIZABETH J. DICKASON, R.N., M.A.
Associate Professor of Nursing
Queensborough Community College

MARTHA OLSEN SCHULT, R.N., M.A.
Associate Professor of Nursing
Queensborough Community College

McGRAW-HILL BOOK COMPANY

New York St. Louis San Francisco Auckland Bogotá
Düsseldorf Johannesburg London Madrid
Mexico Montreal New Delhi Panama
Paris São Paulo Singapore
Sydney Tokyo
Toronto

maternal and infant care

notice

Medicine is an ever-changing science. As new research and clinical experience broaden our knowledge, changes in treatment and drug therapy are required. The editors and the publisher of this work have made every effort to ensure that the drug dosage schedules herein are accurate and in accord with the standards accepted at the time of publication. Readers are advised, however, to check the product information sheet included in the package of each drug they plan to administer to be certain that changes have not been made in the recommended dose or in the contraindications for administration. This recommendation is of particular importance in regard to new or infrequently used drugs.

Copyright © 1979, 1975 by McGraw-Hill, Inc. All rights reserved. Printed in the United States of America. No part of this publication may be reproduced, stored in a retrieval system, or transmitted, in any form or by any means, electronic, mechanical, photocopying, recording, or otherwise, without the prior written permission of the publisher.

1 2 3 4 5 6 7 8 9 0 D O D O 7 8 3 2 1 0 9

This book was set in Helvetica Light by Monotype Composition Company, Inc.
The editors were David P. Carroll, Mary Ann Richter, and Irene Curran;
the designer was Ben Kann;
the production supervisor was Milton J. Heiberg.
New drawings were done by J & R Services, Inc.
R. R. Donnelley & Sons Company was printer and binder.

Library of Congress Cataloging in Publication Data

Dickason, Elizabeth J
    Maternal and infant care.

    Bibliography: p.
    Includes index.
    1. Obstetrical nursing. 2. Pediatric nursing.
I. Schult, Martha Olsen, joint author. II. Title.
[DNLM: 1. Obstetrical nursing. 2. Pediatric nursing. WY157 M423]
RG951.D52 1979   610.73'678   78-14904
ISBN 0-07-016796-6

to our parents

CONTENTS

LIST OF CONTRIBUTORS

Susan E. Anderson, R.N., M.S.
Assistant Professor
School of Nursing
Boston University

Nancy T. Block, M.D.
Clinical Assistant Professor
Department of Psychiatry
College of Medicine and Dentistry
and Assistant Chief for Children's Services
New Jersey Medical College
Community Mental Health Center
Newark, New Jersey

Marvin L. Blumberg, M.D., F.A.A.P.
Chairman, Department of Pediatrics
The Jamaica Hospital
Jamaica, New York

Märretje Jelles Bührer, R.N.
Childbirth Education Instructor
Booth Memorial Hospital Center
Flushing, New York

Constance R. Castor, R.N., B.S.
Childbirth Education Specialist
and Associate Director
Council of Childbirth Education Specialists
Bedford, New York

Elizabeth J. Dickason, R.N., M.A.
Associate Professor
Department of Nursing
Queensborough Community College
Bayside, New York

Joyce Hanna-Nave, R.N., B.S.
Formerly Public Health Nurse
Visiting Nurse Service
New York, New York

Herbert S. Heineman, M.D.
Clinical Professor of Medicine
Thomas Jefferson University Medical College;
Director, Clinical Microbiology Laboratories
Mercy Catholic Medical Center; and
Director, Public Health Laboratory
Philadelphia, Pennsylvania

Beatrice Lau Kee, R.D., M.P.H.
Assistant Professor
Department of Nursing
Queensborough Community College
Bayside, New York

Hilda Koehler, C.N.M., M.S.
Parent Educator
St. Luke's Hospital Center
New York, New York

Dorothea M. Lang, C.N.M., M.P.H.
Director, Nurse-Midwifery Service Program
Maternal and Infant Care and
Family Planning Projects
New York City Department of Health
New York, New York

Jane Corwin Reeves, R.N., P.N.P.
Pediatric Nurse Practitioner
Ocean Springs, Mississippi

**Janet S. Reinbrecht, R.N., M.Ed.
C.N.M.**
Education Director for Parent Education
The Childbearing Center
Maternity Center Association
New York, New York

Arlene Ritz, R.N., M.A.
Professor, Department of Nursing
Queensborough Community College
Bayside, New York

Martha Olsen Schult, R.N., M.A.
Associate Professor
Department of Nursing
Queensborough Community College
Bayside, New York

Bonnie Silverman, R.N., B.S.N., P.N.C.
Perinatal Nurse Clinician
Booth Memorial Hospital Center
Flushing, New York

Christine D. Southall, R.N., M.A.
Assistant Education Coordinator
Community and Social Pediatrics
Harlem Hospital Center
New York, New York

**Francine Heineman Stier, R.N.,
B.S.N., M.A.**
Assistant Professor
Department of Nursing
Greater Hartford Community College
Hartford, Connecticut

Dolores Lake Taylor, R.N., M.S.N.
Senior Associate Professor
Bucks County Community College
Newtown, Pennsylvania

Jane Wilson, R.N.
Nurse Practitioner
Hypertension Control Program
Cornell University Medical College
New York, New York

Philip E. Wilson, C.S.W.
Director, South Brooklyn Human Services
Catholic Charities
and
Coordinator, Social Welfare Certificate Program
Long Island University
Brooklyn, New York

Lois D. Young, R.N., M.A.
Learning Disability Consultant
and
Associate Director
The Grange School
Princeton, New Jersey

PREFACE

A number of new practices that were included in the first edition of *Maternal and Infant Care* have now become thoroughly incorporated into maternity nursing. This second edition has been published during a period when parental-infant bonding and the importance of including both parents in the process of education for childbirth and parenting have been established without question. In addition, the adverse effects of many drugs have been acknowledged, and precautions are being taken to reduce drug intake during pregnancy and the numbers of heavily medicated births. During the four-year period since the publication of the first edition, the technical ability to assess and monitor the fetus during pregnancy and delivery has become widely available. It is now possible to determine the condition of the fetus fairly accurately at each phase of pregnancy. Intervention resulting from this increased knowledge has reduced the numbers of unexpected perinatal deaths, while regionalization of care for the compromised infant has positively affected neonatal mortality.

Preventive health care is the key to achieving the lowest possible rate of maternal and infant morbidity and mortality. Technical advances contribute much to such a reduction, but further progress remains impossible until the adverse social factors which affect health are ameliorated. At every level of society, parents need to know about the factors that contribute to the achievement of a healthy outcome to pregnancy. Therefore, education and support of parents remains a major activity for nurses practicing in this field.

It is essential for the nurse to have not only a grasp of the psychologic and physiologic bases of maternity care but also expert technical skill as well. As role dimensions expand to include more complex functions, the nurse will need to upgrade her or his skills to meet the challenge. A text such as this balances all areas as well as providing a readable, sound foundation for nursing practice.

In this edition, Part 1 again presents the care of the healthy mother and infant. A thorough grasp of the processes of growth and development, physiologic factors, and of the family's need for support during this period is necessary before variations from the normal can be recognized. Care of healthy persons during a specific crisis can be discussed within the childbearing context. Using assessment and intervention, even a beginning student can contribute significantly to a satisfying experience for each involved family member.

The organization of the material in Part 2 is unique. Complications are grouped by body systems rather than separated by trimester of first occurrence because complications during pregnancy often extend throughout the whole time period. This approach will be particularly helpful to students who do not yet have a background in medical-surgical nursing. It is also useful in an integrated curriculum. It is possible to add instruction on obstetric complications to the lecture content when cardiovascular, metabolic, infectious, hematologic, or surgical problems are taught.

A separate unit deals with complications which affect high-risk infants. Because students may not have experience in neonatal intensive care centers, the editors have used the preterm infant to illustrate the complex problems of compromised babies. If it is desired, high-risk infant problems can also be integrated into a pediatric course.

For this new edition, each chapter has been revised. Extensive new material has been added for pharmacology, infant assessment and psychologic development, and the family and family planning. All the material reflects the greater initiative being taken by nurses in planning patient care. The nursing process has been integrated throughout and specifically identified in practice areas which may be new to students, for example, home and clinic care.

The physiologic bases for the changes in pregnancy, recovery from birth, and the newborn are presented in Part 1. Later, complications during pregnancy and in the newborn period are related to the processes underlying those problems. Using this strong foundation, a nurse should be able to reason through a plan of care for most situations in maternity nursing. It is not possible to include every problem, but it is expected that the instructor will guide the student to select the major health problems encountered in a particular setting.

There always will be a challenge to acquire knowledge and to apply that knowledge in a clinical situation. Because of the difficulty in finding appropriate clinical experiences for students, an *instructor's guide* has been made available for this edition. It includes suggestions for teaching maternal and infant care by supplementing the clinical situation with simulation and laboratory experiences. Overhead projections for classroom visual aids can be made using the graphics in the instructor's guide.

Sometimes students feel overwhelmed by the mass of material such a text contains. They need to recognize that not every fact can be retained. Rather, they must learn where to go for information and how to decide which information is essential. With their instructor, students can set goals for learning and practice formulating questions from lead sentences in each chapter. By studying the answers to those self-made questions study skills will be promoted. In addition, study questions are given at the end of each chapter to facilitate students' use of the text.

acknowledgments

When a new edition of a text is prepared, there are many who participate. The editors wish to acknowledge their deep appreciation to those students and friends who shared their evaluations of the first edition and thus became a vital part of the renewal process. Next, we wish to thank those couples who used the text during their own childbearing periods and who freely interacted with us concerning their needs for support and information. The contributors' part in formulating a multiauthored text is essential, and we especially thank our authors for the enthusiasm with which they undertook revision. Finally, those physicians and nurses who reviewed chapters and offered suggestions were another vital part of the revision process.

Special thanks is expressed to our editor, David P. Carroll, to our editing supervisor, Irene Curran, and to Sylvia Rockness, Deena Ryan, and Elsie Downey, who provided generous help with manuscript preparation. Finally, we remember, with love, Mary Ann Richter.

Elizabeth J. Dickason
Martha Olsen Schult

maternal and infant care

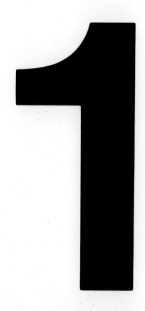

1

THE HEALTHY
MOTHER AND
INFANT

1

PREPARATION FOR PARENTHOOD

LOIS D. YOUNG

1

THE HEALTHY FAMILY

THE FAMILY IN TRANSITION

Traditions are currently being examined and challenged. The role of what could be considered the oldest institution, the family, is being questioned and redefined. In the traditional sense the family usually referred to either the *nuclear family* (husband, wife, and children) or the *extended family,* which might include grandparents, great-grandparents, uncles, aunts, and cousins. Although these two types of family arrangement still may be the most common, today the family may be defined much more loosely.

One description of a family could be *two or more persons living together (or in separate facilities) who feel bound to each other for mutual sharing, caring, comforting, companionship, and pleasure.* Another description of a family could be *almost any group of persons who care about one another, have a commitment to one another, and think of themselves as a family.* Obviously, we all have our own ideas about what constitutes a family.

Both young people and older people today are questioning the established customs in marriage, child rearing, and male-female roles. When so many couples divorce or separate, young people are doubtful about the need, value, and purpose of marriage as their parents and grandparents experienced it. As a result, they may decide that they want neither the finality of marriage nor the trauma of divorce should the marriage bonds disintegrate. Many alternative styles and forms of "togetherness" are being tried and tested.

Some men and women live together without marrying. They desire the closeness of a relationship with a member of the opposite sex without the limitations and finality of ties and bonds. Children may or may not be involved. Some older, widowed people live together without marrying lest they lose pensions and social security benefits from former mates; thus, for both economic reasons and companionship, they choose to live together without marrying.

Many couples or groups of the same sex may live together for a variety of economic, social, and sexual reasons, as well as for companionship. People are gathering together in single or multiple dwellings to share chores and the tasks of rearing and educating children and to find support systems for companionship, fellowship, and development of mutual goals.

For many, communal living is an attempt to get back to basic living off the land, returning to the extended family structure of past history. This way of living may be an attempt to simplify life, to gain peace and serenity of body and soul, and to counteract a materialistic society that fosters competition and the gaining of more and more material possessions.

Another family arrangement, that of the single parent with children, is a result of separation, divorce, widowhood, welfare, or in a few cases, the desire of a single person to raise a child without being married or having a mate.[1] Today single men and women who may or may not have been previously married are also able to adopt or care for foster children.

how things got this way

It may be useful to take a brief look at the history of the family over the last century to find clues to its present variations. We find the history of the American family tied closely to the history of the nation. Families who made their living from farming tended to stay in one place. Parents, grandparents, aunts, uncles, and cousins often worked together. They relied on each other for nurture, teaching, social activity, and economic survival. Families coming from other countries to the United States brought with them the customs of the old country and worked hard to continue these customs in the new country. Families whose main source of support was a small business trained their children to work in that business. Children were usually essential to the economic survival of these families.

As the nation turned to more centralized and larger industry, and as more efficient transportation developed, family patterns began to change as well. Mobility caused scattering. Men and women were drawn to cities, leaving the extended family behind. Especially after two world wars and the development of mass communication, urbanization of the country contributed in large measure to the shift to smaller, isolated family units.

For some, economic pressures and ambitions for upward mobility may have delayed plans for early marriage. Housing, education, and social problems, combined with numerous other factors, led many families to have fewer children in a period when children no longer were an economic asset.

The gradual liberation of women from household tasks, which allowed the rapid increase in numbers of working women, has produced a shift in many child care tasks to outside agencies. Health care agencies, schools, after-school recreation programs, television, and more recently nursery and day-care centers compete with parents in providing primary influences on children. All the demands for the parents' time outside the home, plus the development of strong non-parental influences on the child, have changed the structure of what is needed from parents in order to bring up children.

family purposes

What then are the purposes and functions of the family? Historically the family was established for the continuation of the human race. Childbearing and child rearing were among its primary functions. Passing on traditions and beliefs, establishing discipline, instilling morals and values, providing affection and security, and tending to the physical, emotional, and economic needs of its members were its functions.

Many of these traditional functions have been modified or changed over the years. New or modified functions are being considered. Duvall states, "The new image of family life is that of the nurturing center for human development," and then goes on to describe six emergent major functions: (1) giving and receiving affection; (2) establishing personal security and acceptance of each family member for the unique individual he or she is; (3) providing satisfaction and a sense of purpose; (4) providing continuity of companionship and maintaining association; (5) identifying or providing social placement and socialization; (6) establishing limits and a sense of what is right.[2]

Salerno and Blair identify a more sociologic purpose for the family: "The purpose of the family is to meet the needs of its members and to mediate between the needs and demands of its members and the expectation obligations and demands placed upon them by society."[3]

Such a definition acknowledges what has been described as the coordinating task that parents have, albeit without much power, to obtain the best possible assistance for their children from schools, health care agencies, and other institutional agencies. It also defines the protection, preparation, and support provided by the family for the "world out there."

trends in factors affecting family function

Far from being on the brink of collapse, the American family appears to be in a period of adjustment. The nurse should be aware of significant trends which influence the directions the family may take.[4]

1 Many more married women will work outside the home as economic needs make it desirable for women to enter the work force. Currently about 54 percent already work, including 34 percent who are mothers of preschool or school children.
2 One out of three marriages already ends in divorce. Although the remarriage rate is high, 4 out of 10 children born in the 1970s will spend part of their childhood in a one-parent family, usually with their mother as head of the household.
3 Eleven percent of first births are to women without marriage partners. A higher percentage of these women are choosing to bear a child.
4 An increasing number of women are postponing a first baby until they are in their late twenties or early thirties, after career and financial goals have been sought.

5 The family will remain small, perhaps averaging 2.1 children, as compared with the current rate of 1.8 children. The 2.1 average is considered the minimum level at which the population replaces itself (Fig. 1-1).
6 There will be a continued variety of life-styles, but marriage will still be the choice of the majority. Ways of rebuilding an extended group of supportive relationships will be sought by increasing numbers of people
7 Legal rights of children will become more clearly defined, as will parenting responsibilities. Hopefully, accompanying this will be an increased sense of society's responsibility in supporting parenting.

In this time of shifting, no matter its economic level, the family needs help from society. Certainly it needs more recognition of the vital role it must continue to play in nurturing children. The Carnegie report on the status of the nation's families suggests at least four ways that families could receive supportive help.[5]

fig. 1-1 Live births per 1000 women, age 15 to 44. (From *U.S. Department of Health Education and Welfare*.)

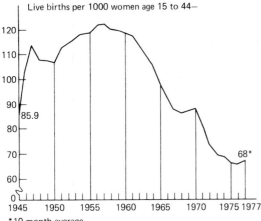

Live births per 1000 women age 15 to 44—

85.9

68*

1945 1950 1955 1960 1965 1970 1975 1977

*10-month average

1 Perhaps the simplest way is to encourage and provide better education for future parents, including the opportunity for adolescent parents to have experience with children, learning growth and development and methods of child care.
2 Day-care facilities are needed which encourage the participation of parents and other family members so that they can continue to be primary in the upbringing of their children.
3 A wider recognition by society of the important role of parenting must underlie any regulatory changes in institutions supporting the family. This would hopefully bring more supports to ease the child care problems of working parents by allowing for tax breaks, child allowances, and more flexible working hours. It would also allow for the "mother" to stay at home to be a full-time parent if she or he chose to do so.
4 New family income and health care programs need to replace the current welfare payments. The stability of the poor family is in the greatest jeopardy, and such families may need dramatic supports to allow survival.

While the family structure is influenced by societal changes, at the same time couples are placing greater demands on the marriage relationship than was true in the past. The traditional task-oriented functions that were done by husband or wife can now often be handled by individuals or organizations outside the home. As we see the decline of function, we also see the increased importance of affection and companionship in marriage. Balswick and Peek have stated: "As American society has become increasingly mechanized and depersonalized, the family remains as one of the few social groups where what sociologists call the primary relationship has still managed to survive. As such, a greater and greater demand has been placed on the modern marriage to provide for this affection and companionship."[6]

The problems of finding support in only one or two other persons must be recognized. When one member of the small family is under stress, it seriously affects the functioning of the whole. For this reason, a number of people are seeking support systems that are wider than the nuclear family because they have understood that a small family cannot always meet its' human needs.

PREPARATION FOR PARENTHOOD

No one can assume that parenting is a natural skill, developed through instinct. Family educators agree that families teach parenting by how they parent. When there have not been adequate role models, parents may be in conflict between societal expectations, their own needs, and their memories of "how to do it," gained from their childhood experience. It is important for the professional involved with families to recognize that feelings of judgment and blame can arise because of one's own cherished myth of what a parent should do or how a "good parent" would cope. Parents do not need accusations about their inadequacy, their dependence upon outside resources, or their struggles to survive in an economically stressful environment. What all parents need, regardless of situation, is the sense that they are being supported in this struggle to raise children and that something is being done to criticize and reform the institutions which complicate their lives.[7]

developmental tasks

Developmental tasks have been identified for critical times in person's life. If these are achieved the individual can progress to the next growth task and to maturity with some degree of competence in living in society. Application of the concept of developmental tasks to parenthood has allowed an understanding of the ways in which the crisis of parenthood can conflict with other crises in a person's life. Where possible, then, the professional involved in supporting the family can assist in resolving those crises that arise through gaps in information or misconceptions. In addition, support services in many areas are available, although these services are often unknown to the parents or unavailable to them because of financial restrictions.

The health professional can detect clues to difficulties in a family's parenting functions and work together with the family to achieve a more satisfactory level of the following factors:

1 Identification of the parent role and responsibility, with recognition of how functions change as the child grows and becomes more independent.
2 Recognition of the stages of growth and development, with some attempt to structure care giving about these changing stages.
3 Utilization of effective communication skills.
4 Ability to provide structure and to set limits.
5 Ability to share love and affection.
6 Recognition of parent's life goals, while being supportive of the child's own potential.

Intervention should always be governed by the acknowledgment that families are the primary units in which children are raised. Every effort should therefore be made to support this vital unit of society. Parents must be enabled to parent. For, as Smoyak states:

Children do not become normal adults unless nurtured in some type of close, continuing social unit, where norms are clearly set, where self-esteem is fostered and where separateness/connectedness issues are worked on openly and directly. The most important work of parents as socializing agents is to get each succeeding generation to want to go on. Parents, in one way or another, have to accomplish getting their children "hooked" on the idea of continuity. Simply put, they have to make it pleasant to be alive, and further, to suggest that one's "debt" for such pleasure is to pass it on to the next person or generation.[8]

the role of the nurse

The maternity nurse is in a position to communicate and interact with families at a very crucial time. It will take a warm and knowledgeable educator who listens well to be accepting of people as individuals as well as to convey information that will be useful in each unique situation. It is also important to recognize that the complexity of the family's social and economic situation is not resolved by information alone.

What must be avoided is the assumption that there is one acceptable pattern of family function. In a pluralistic society, basic needs can be identified, but the methods to achieve satisfaction of those needs may not seem effective to a professional who is accustomed to another set of methods. What is needed is sensitization, or "consciousness raising," of medical personnel about the varieties of adaptive styles of family living. To date, there is no one accepted set of criteria for good parenting, nor is there a validated family assessment tool for use by nurses. There is, however, a great deal of interest in what is happening in the family and what can be done to provide support to the parents as they carry out the basic tasks of parenting.

adaptation to pregnancy

Pregnancy for many is a time of crisis in which the parents will require much support from outside the family. Every expectant mother, whether the pregnancy is her first or her tenth, has an experience special to the context of her own life and family. The relationships among mother, father, siblings, and grandparents affect this experience, as does the family's social, religious, and ethnic background. The mother, of course, is vitally important in the childbearing process, but so are the other members of the family, because they supply the needed support for the mother and infant.

Just as there is a medical diagnosis of pregnancy, there should be a determination of the factual and emotional understanding of the pregnancy and the meaning it has for the mother and her family.

Each pregnant woman who comes for medical care brings with her various concepts, formed by a variety of her own experiences while growing up, about sex, motherhood, the birth process, family relations, and child care. Some of her concepts may be incorrect, mixed with fantasy or anxiety, and highly colored by her prior experiences.

How can we discover the specific questions, fears, and misconceptions of each mother? How do we learn the context that an individual person represents? Where would assessment have to be done in order to provide her with supportive, clarifying information for pregnancy, infant care, or family planning between pregnancies? Table 1-1 provides some questions that can elicit facts on which to base information and support at the level of the particular person's concerns or needs.

It would also help the educator to know how the patient was mothered—whether she was neglected or deprived in childhood or grew

table 1-1 Initial questions to elicit family status regarding pregnancy

questions	factors influencing nursing planning
support available	
1 Length of time living in this location?	An isolated couple will need encouragement to seek support.

2 Support system in this locality?
  a Who is available to help with siblings or during the early postpartum period?
  b What emotional supports are available for each partner?
	Referrals must be considered. Exploration with family about resources is important.
	Parenting classes need, as a major component, to foster sharing about these issues.

3 Financial plans to cover costs of pregnancy?
  a What are their needs for assistance?
  b Are there needs which will keep the pregnant woman working throughout pregnancy?
	Location and type of medical service will influence available referrals.
	Working may be beneficial or harmful depending on risk status.

response to pregnancy	

4 What are the most direct concerns about the idea of being pregnant at this time?
  a What interruptions in life goals?
  b What sense of "this is the right time"?
	Ambivalence about pregnancy is usual in first months but may be a clue to difficulty if still present toward the end of pregnancy.
	Father's responses need to be elicited. Highly recommend his attendance at one prenatal visit and at parenting classes.

5 What reactions of other family members to the pregnancy now?	Single mother will need extra support, as will those in a hostile environment.
6 Are there strong desires to bear only a son or only a daughter? Has there been exploration about acceptance of either sex in infant?	Fixation on sex of infant may hinder bonding after delivery; some opportunity to talk about this aspect is important.
process	

7 What needs for information do the future parents have?
  a Fetal growth and development?
  b Sexuality during pregnancy?
  c Care of woman to promote health?
  d Other questions?
	Information giving must always be preceded by a determination of what the person already knows.

8 What plans for or fears of delivery are present?
  a Which questions need to be asked of physician? (anesthesia, type of delivery)
  b What fears can be identified?
  c How do they feel information can help?
	Fears are not easily elicited. Sharing common misconceptions that other mothers have had may prompt a person to recognize her own fears.
	Fearful women need special assistance and perhaps some group discussions before they can openly admit fears.

9 What interest in parenting classes is expressed?	Encourage attendance whenever possible if classes are supportive. Provide several options for differing approaches and needs.

Remember: "Parents who are secure, supported, valued, and in control of their lives are more effective parents than those who feel unsure and who are not in control."[4]

up in a warm, intact family. Supporting this need is a study which showed that women deprived of adequate parenting before age 11 had greater difficulty assuming the maternal role with their own infants.[9]

Although the pregnant woman needs the understanding support of the maternal health professionals whom she encounters, assessment of her situation is not often adequately included in prenatal care. Sometimes it is done within a formal series of classes in a prenatal clinic as general questions are asked to elicit the concerns of the group. Many times it is not planned for in a regularly scheduled checkup. If the mother can see the same physician for each pregnancy, she may develop a good rapport and be able to discuss problems and questions. Many women, however, go through clinics where a different person sees them at each visit and someone else cares for them at the time of delivery. Often, then, the only place where a woman may verbalize her concerns is in the hospital when she is ready to deliver. By then the task of teaching and assessment is difficult and arbitrary. Consequently, much attention is currently being given to formalizing education on family life and human sexuality so that people will face childbearing with more adequate preparation in the biologic, social, and psychologic aspects of parenting.

ASPECTS OF FAMILY LIFE AND SEX EDUCATION BASED ON DEVELOPMENTAL LEVELS

The most natural and effective place for beginning and continuing preparation for parenthood is within the family itself. The attitudes of parents are most influential in a child's understanding of his or her sexual identity, the basic foundation underlying the child's future ability to parent.

As Wilbur and Aug state: "The most important aspect of sex education is preparing the child to receive sexual knowledge. Planning formal sexual education for children is a secondary force in the development of the sexual life: parental attitudes remain the primary one.[10]

Unfortunately for many in our population, basic education to assume adult parental roles with confidence and pleasure is not adequately taking place in the family context. In some situations, schools, churches, community centers, medical and adolescent pediatric services, and maternal and infant care services are trying, with difficulty, to bridge the gap for children and teenagers. However, questions arise about the value of introducing such external agencies as being yet another way of reducing the parents' authority and responsibility. Some recommend, instead, that parents themselves receive the supportive education so that they are strengthened to do their tasks. McAbee's article on parenting classes in a rural community emphasizes just this point (see Bibliography).

Because the need for education in family life and human sexuality appears to be so widespread, the task of educating parents and helping them to communicate more freely with their children on these subjects has become part of the role of maternal and child health workers. A nursing curriculum emphasizes certain aspects of the basic content needed for teaching parents and children. Other related courses, such as human growth and development and child psychology, contribute to the development of a comprehensive viewpoint of the nurse-teacher.

A recognition of some of the basic concepts about development in young children would help parents to have a much greater understanding and provide for a more open relationship with their own children in the area of family relationships and sex education. Following are some concepts to keep in mind when working with parents or children.

1 Development is a process, and every variable changes with age. The growth tasks of the first years of life are repeated in adolescence on a different level. The child's needs, awareness, and struggles will change as the child develops physically and psychologically.
2 Readiness to learn is a guiding principle in all education. Children retain only what they are ready for at a given age. Children are very open, when allowed to be, with their questions and feelings. Their own understandings should be explored before information or explanations are given. Children's questions about sex need to be answered openly in a matter-of-fact manner as any other questions are answered, simply and without long, complex explanations.
3 Sexuality is more than sex. All human beings from infancy have sexual responses that should be recognized. Some of the ways these responses are demonstrated are by loving and receiving love, by being able to perceive and enjoy sensations, touch, smell, color and taste, and by enjoying exploring and being playful.
4 Sex education for young children deals with sex not as eroticism but as a normal body function. Early direction is in establishing masculine and feminine identity as the child works through the struggle of "Who am I?"

When parents are aware of the developmental stages of their children, their own communication may become more meaningful, since the children give clear signals as to where they are in their growth (see Table 1-2). Parents may need reassurance that there is no danger in a child's learning more than he or she is ready for.

Generally, children will not show interest in or retain what is beyond their level. If there is, however, covert anxiety about giving information, children will retain the anxiety that is engendered in them and will become secretive and noncommunicative with their parents. Anxiety may be reduced by treating the subject as normally as if one were discussing the weather. In dealing with normal fantasies, it is especially helpful to the child to elicit his or her thoughts first. A simple factual explanation can then follow.

The facts are the same at each interest level, but the detail of presentation varies with the growth process. At each level there can be emphasis appropriate to the developmental stage of the child.

Whatever is done in education for parents or children must be guided by the principles stated by Fraiberg:

> Sex instruction per se is successful whenever it has served the purpose of strengthening the child's satisfaction in his own sexual role and his destiny in this sexual role, and when it has dealt with the facts of procreation, of anatomy, of sexual feelings in such a way that the child's guilt and anxiety are reduced, and his confidence and love of his parents are deepened.[11]

infancy

From birth to 3 or 3½ years, children move toward independence from being totally dependent on the parent for all their basic needs. They work through three basic developmental tasks, first establishing basic *trust* in a completely dependent, symbiotic relationship with one or more mothering persons. The second major step in development, *autonomy,* is learning to survive independently of these key persons. This is a gradual process, with the child separating from the parent first for short moments and later for longer periods.

table 1-2 Tool for teaching parents basic developmental concepts and appropriate parenting

age	stage of development	behavior	methods of handling behavior
Birth to 18 months	Basic Trust vs. Basic Mistrust Relationship with mother emphasized Understands own needs Characterized by dependency and a need for consistency	Dependent Cries when mother leaves Demands attention Learns to feel secure Displays needs emotionally Fussy Impatient Will not entertain self Has not learned concept of discipline	If you know child is safe, it does not hurt him to cry Mother needs to teach some separation Meet infant's basic needs Use television for stimulation and/or consolation but not to replace mother Introduce infant to others Spend time with infant, hold, cuddle
18 months to 3 years	Autonomy vs. Shame and Doubt Learns individualization Begins potty training (physical muscle development should be adequate) Feels separate and apart from mother Test limits; forces issues of discipline	Puts everything in mouth Exhibits potty training problems Says "no!" constantly Has tantrums, expressing anger Not able to verbalize Knows when he or she is taking advantage of parent; really wants limits Pulls out furniture drawers and explores	Try not to make potty training a forced issue Check own reactions to messes Set limits and be consistent For safety, put locks on doors Training takes consistent effort for a period of time Consider permissive versus strict discipline Isolate child in room as method of handling behavior
3 to 6 years	Initiative vs. Guilt Learning acceptable behavior Learns concept of discipline, yes and no Exhibits closeness to parent of the opposite sex Organizes activities on own Exhibits guilt; realizes when he or she makes a mistake Forming a sexual identity	Blames mistakes and misbehavior on others Lies to cover mistakes Has imaginary friend(s) Developing vocabulary, sassy Asks questions about sex	Teach that it is okay to make a mistake Differentiate between fantasy and lying Check parent reaction to language and responses Try to identify imaginary "friend" and need for it Answer questions simply to meet needs Have the punishment fit the crime
6 to 18 years	Industry vs. Inferiority Attends school Reaches plateau period of learning personality Develops interests and explores hobbies Develops ego	Views peer group as important Catches self and changes behavior to "yes" instead of "no" behavior (good) Finds things out for self Asks "why?"	Child needs to have efforts noticed and praised Parent as teacher is very important If you do not know, say so Give the child responsibility Show acceptance of child at home Show interest in child's hobbies

Source: Copyright September/October 1977, the American Journal of Nursing Company. Reproduced with permission from *MCN, The American Journal of Maternal Child Nursing* vol. 2, no. 5.

Negative behavior begins at about age 2, when development of the child's own strengths leads to the realization, "I can do it myself!" Toilet training is another step in independent functioning at this age.

During this period, parents can learn to foster healthy attitudes in their children, particularly through accepting a child's exploration of his or her body and environment, through accepting and responding naturally to bowel movements, urinary functions, and food, by using correct names for body parts, by setting limits of behavior, and by encouraging their children to express their feelings about themselves.

childhood

Between the ages of 3 and 6, a child will continue working on the third task, *individuation,* exploring roles to decide who he or she will be. Children at this age find it hard to distinguish between thoughts, feelings, and actions. They move easily from one "play role" to another at home. Many children begin to have preschool experience by 3½ to 4 years of age in preschool programs. They will act out many of their concerns in everyday play situations: a great deal of time is spent in the doll corner playing mommy and daddy (usually taking interchangeable roles), imitating whatever they have seen at home.

some aspects of teaching emphasis for preschoolers Since a difference between sexes is recognized during this period, any preschool education in family life and sex is directed toward focusing on and reinforcing an awareness of relationships within the family. Recognition of the composition of families, understanding the immediate and extended family, and seeing how families differ within the group may be focal points of teacher-child discussions. Simple concepts of life, death, growth, and learning are introduced by realistic examples from families. Most birth- and sex-related questions are answered within the framework of simple factual answers without elaboration. It is important to give proper names to body parts and to realize that there is considerable curiosity, and some anxiety, at this age about why a boy has a penis and a girl does not.

Children 3 to 4 years old are unable to conceptualize how a baby got inside the mother. Like the child who asked his mother to open her mouth and called down her throat, "Hi, baby," they may fantasize that the baby is in the stomach and can hear them. Thus, when asked where the baby grows, it is not helpful to say, "In mommy's stomach." An adequate factual answer would be, "The baby grows inside the mother," holding more explanation until the child asks further questions.

Between the ages of 5 and 6, there is a keen desire to be "big." There is more clear identification with the parent of the same sex, as well as a diminishing of the rivalry that has been experienced in attachment to the parent of the opposite sex.

some aspects of teaching emphasis for primary school From the ages of 6 to 12, the child has no additional psychologic steps to master. Children are in a rest period psychologically, and if development has been successful, they can concentrate on school and play. They will acquire a great deal of their knowledge of concepts and skills during this time. Children will have many questions about all subjects as they go about acquiring knowledge. Questions pour forth, interest flowing from animals to plants to human beings: how things come from seeds or cells, why human beings are mammals, how human mammals and other mammals feed and protect their young, what babies look like inside the mother. What about multiple births, hospitals, doctors? Curiosity about abnormalities, monsters, Siamese twins, and cross-species fertilization might mislead parents or teachers into thinking that children are more sophisticated in their knowledge than they really are. The child may be merely checking out his or her own fantasies or clearing up misinformation.

GRADES 1 TO 3 (AGES 6 TO 9) Teaching objectives at the level of grades 1 to 3 are related to reducing anxieties and fantasies of the prepubertal child. Giving factual information can help to correct misconceptions from peer information. The exchange of sex information among children goes on and is the child's chief source of information and anxiety when families or schools do not assume their responsibilities.

All children have to learn self-control and discipline. These tasks can be emphasized in the first three grades as the child learns the responsibilities of being a family member, helping with household chores, looking out for younger children, and contributing to the smooth functioning of his or her own home (Fig. 1-2).

Emphasis is on developing wholesome attitudes toward the body, use of correct terms, and an active vocabulary in reference to the body. Children learn to speak openly in an appropriate setting. Their curiosity about how things work predominates. They learn avidly, like to start and complete projects and to have a sense of accomplishment. A strong motive is the need to excel: to be the wittiest or the fastest, to exaggerate knowledge—all in order to ward off failure. Conversations are full of comparative adjectives.

GRADES 4 TO 6 (AGES 10 TO 12) Each year the child shows more distinct needs than in earlier years. In the fourth grade, objectives are directed toward preparation for puberty, and the teacher can start giving basic information on menstruation on a co-ed basis. Personal

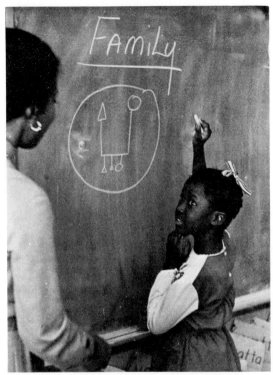

fig. 1-2 Family education in the classroom. *(From C.D. Southall, "Family Life and Sex Education," American Journal of Nursing, **77**(9):14, September 1977; photo by Harvey Shaman.)*

hygiene, friendship, and family relationships continue to be discussed as questions arise.

The beginning of secondary sexual characteristics precedes the start of *menstruation* (menarche) in the adolescent by at least 2 years. Breast budding and pubic hair will have begun to develop before the puberty growth spurt which takes place about 1 year before menarche. The growth spurt results in unfamiliarity with body movements, size, and shape and makes some girls appear awkward and uncoordinated. Others appear to bloom suddenly, surprising everyone around them, as did one teenager who grew 9 in and 25 lb in the 7 months after her eleventh birthday. This growth spurt varies as to when it occurs, of course, but invariably as it slows, menstruation occurs.[12]

Semmens has suggested a timetable to alert physicians and those who work with children.[13] Puberty preparation can be made interesting and nonthreatening for the child if puberty is presented as a biologic time clock that follows a regular normal pattern. Girls can anticipate puberty as the sign of growing up with the same pleasure and anticipation as the 5- and 6-year-old looks forward to "being big enough to go to school."

In the United States, a recent study showed that menarche occurs at 12.7 ± 1.2 (SD) years. Better nutrition appears to be associated with an earlier menarche.[14] Boys mature at an average of 6 to 12 months later than girls.[15]

By the fifth grade, because the body gets ready physically for parenthood long before emotional readiness occurs, there should be discussion of the principle that sexual experimentation carries with it a responsibility which a child may not be able to handle. Human reproduction is taught in more detail. Discussion of the normality of friendships between the same sex at this age is important, because peer group anxieties, produced by pressure from older children (or parents), often move 10- to 12-year-olds into precocious heterosexuality. The objective is to make the child aware of and comfortable with the developmental tasks of his or her own age group.

adolescence

Beginning at about 12 years of age, children are thrown into a tremendous whirl as they face physical and psychologic changes. "The rapid growth in height and weight creates an unfamiliarity with his body. Development of secondary sexual characteristics not only adds to this unfamiliarity but also forces adulthood on him."[16]

Adolescents, in a sense, retrace all their earlier psychologic steps, needing to estab-

lish basic trust, autonomy, and individuation again. This is a replay of infancy and early childhood development in a new way which will allow the individual to operate as a person in the world. Parents need to understand that rejection at this age is part of the struggle for autonomy.

Much has been written about the developmental tasks and needs during adolescence. The nurse working with this age group should become familiar with the classic literature.[13,17]

some aspects of teaching emphasis for junior high school (ages 13 to 14) At this age level, all information given earlier in relation to sexual development and sexuality is reiterated with more complex explanations. Problems specific to this group include inherent tensions in the early teen years, rapid uneven growth, and heterosexual urges without enough emotional security and maturity to deal with all the changes that occur. Some discussion is needed of appropriate defenses against unhealthy sexual approaches from adults to teenagers.

Teenagers begin to realize that their decisions and behavior will always have results. Some suggested areas for discussion in keeping with their interests are the meaning of peer approval, self-image, choices of friends, and choices of recreation. Parent-child relationships are being strained by the changes of these years; frequently children in the early teens welcome adult, nonparental counsel.

Discussions should anticipate and emphasize positive explanations rather than give negative warnings regarding pubertal changes. The discussion leader needs to be careful not to get too deeply into the "feelings" to be anticipated, thus cutting off the spontaneous and discovering quality of personal experiences in this stage of adolescent development.

At this level, teenagers are also curious about details of sex, including conception, the meaning of family planning, fetal development, and homosexuality. Social issues in which they may have intense interest are drug addiction, abortion, pornography in films and literature, marriage and divorce, and communal living. Their interest is not in the detailed aspects, as it will be later, but in the moral aspects.

The important question is, "What is right for me?" Children during these years seem to be asking for leadership from adults on "which way to go," yet they often reject parental guidance. Indecision or ambivalence seems to typify the age. Coupled with indecision might be marked anxiety centered around how masculine or feminine they appear. The changing body image is often reflected in popularity; those who develop earlier look on those who are slower to mature with some pity. Popularity is extremely important, peer approval critical, and failure devastating.

Emphasis in family life and sex education would be well placed on developmental expectations and moral issues, with discussion about choices and their results. Some understanding can be imparted of independence vs. dependency needs to the extent that the struggle is part of the difficulty with parents. Seeking parental guidance somehow implies to the adolescent, "I am still a child," yet the adolescent needs and wants guidance. Adults who understand this dilemma can be supportive role models.

some aspects of teaching emphasis for high school (ages 15 and over) Emphasis in family life and sex education on the high school level is placed on preparation for adult tasks and roles. Sexual identity is completed during this period. Discussions now become far more sophisticated in relation to cultural, religious, and socioeconomic problems. Education is continued toward making choices for specific careers, family structures, and methods of child spac-

ing. Toward the end of this period, parental relationships take on new meaning, and exchanges may begin again, with opinions from both sides beginning to emerge more positively.

Consideration of sex, sexuality, and sensuality takes on new dimensions. Discussion of these topics perhaps is preparation for the next task of finding a partner for adult relationships. Preparation, then, for the next step reflects more sophisticated interest in discussion related to the political aspects of issues such as ecology, population, housing, and implications of the changing roles in society.

By the time this age level is reached there should be thorough knowledge of human reproduction. Interest may now be focused on specific health aspects and ways of obtaining health care, with some discussion of the rights of patients. The task of beginning a family may be anticipated, as well as the more complex tasks of maintaining family responsibilities and relationships. Preparation for pregnancy, delivery, and child care can be included in discussions at this level. Now the teenager's own family situation is viewed more objectively and can be used in general discussions that are freer of the earlier fears of disapproval.

By the end of high school, the task of individuation has progressed. The adolescent's problems have become more personalized, and counseling is increasingly sought on a more individualized basis. Discussions remain a lively source of exploring, testing, and defining personal values as the adolescent's own philosophy emerges.

For many adolescents, graduation from high school marks the end of their formal education. Many women, or couples, attending clinics for prenatal care will have reached this point in their education, but many schools in the country give much less attention to preparation for the future than is discussed above. Therefore it becomes the responsibility of the medical personnel in community education, family crises clinics, and pediatric and maternal care services to continue what seems to be essential preparation for parenting.

Today, thorough preparation for parenthood includes knowledge of the reproductive functions, conception and contraception, and the process of growth and development of children. All the information in the chapters to follow is available to help the nurse who becomes involved in the education of the family during the time of preparation for or during the childbearing years.

study questions

1 Identify at least four pressures which cause stress on a family in your locality.
2 Can you identify at least four different family groupings among those in your immediate circle of friends?
3 In what ways does your own family find a support system?
4 Look at the list of parenting functions on page 7. Evaluate whether all are essential. Note the ways that a nurse can work together with the family to facilitate these parenting abilities.
5 Study the questions in Table 1.1. Think through various answers that will influence the adjustment to pregnancy. Use these questions as an interview tool with a woman who is currently pregnant or with one who has just delivered.
6 For each stage of early development, identify three positive parenting behaviors which would foster a positive sense of self and sexual identity.
7 Plan a short outline of the points you would cover in a class of girls who are approaching puberty.
8 Evaluate the family life and sex education you received in school. In which ways was it beneficial? List at least three suggestions you would have for a person engaged in teaching such information.

references

1 S. Dresden, "The Young Adult Adjusting to Single Parenting," *American Journal of Nursing,* **76**(8):1286, August 1976.
2 E. M. Duvall, *Family Development,* 4th ed., Lippincott, Philadelphia, 1971, pp. 4–7.
3 C. L. Blair and E. M. Salerno, *The Expanding Family: Childbearing,* Little, Brown, Boston, 1976, p. 37.
4 K. Keniston and the Carnegie Council on Children, *All Our Children: The American Family Under Pressure,* Harcourt Brace Jovanovich, New York, 1977, p. 23.
5 Ibid. pp. 75–80.
6 J. D. Balswick and C. W. Peek, "The Inexpressive Male: A Tragedy of American Society," in Skolnick A. S. (ed.), *Intimacy, Family and Society,* Little, Brown, Boston, 1974, p. 240.
7 Keniston, op. cit., p. 23.
8 S. A. Smoyak (ed.), "Symposium on Parenting," *Nursing Clinics of North America,* **12**(3):4, September 19, 1977.
9 E. Siegal and M. Morris, "Family Planning: Its Health Rationale," *American Journal of Obstetrics and Gynecology,* **118**(7):995, 1974.
10 C. Wilbur and R. Aug, "Sex Education," *American Journal of Nursing,* **73**(1):88, 1973.
11 S. H. Fraiberg, *The Magic Years,* Scribner, New York, 1959, p. 211.
12 E. O. Reiter and E. Kulin, "Sexual Maturation in the Female," *Pediatric Clinics of North America,* **19**(3): 583, 1972.
13 J. P. Semmens and K. E. Krantz, *The Adolescent Experience, a Counseling Guide to Social and Sexual Behavior,* Macmillan, New York, 1970.
14 R. E. Frisch and R. Revelle, "Height and Weight at Menarche," *Archives of Diseases in Childhood,* **46**: 695, 1971.
15 W. A. Marshall and J. M. Tanner, "Variations in the Pattern of Pubertal Changes in Boys," *Archives of Diseases in Childhood,* **45**:13, 1970.
16 J. P. Semmens and H. Semmens, "Sex Education of the Adolescent Female," *Pediatric Clinics of North America,* **19**(3):769, 1972.
17 H. S. Arnstein, *Your Growing Child and Sex: A Parent's Guide to the Sexual Development, Education, Attitudes and Behavior of the Child from Infancy through Adolescence,* Bobbs-Merrill, New York, 1967.

bibliography

American Academy of Pediatrics: "Counseling Opportunities in Human Reproduction," *Report of the Committee on Youth, Pediatrics,* **50**:492, 1972.

ACSAA Book Review Committee: *Sex Education: Recommended Reading, Annotated Bibliography,* Child Study Association of America, New York, 1972.

Child Study Association of America: *What to Tell Your Child About Sex,* Child Study Association of America—Wel-Met, Inc., Child Study Press, New York, 1974.

Clausen, J. P., M. H. Flook, and B. Ford (eds.): *Maternity Nursing Today,* McGraw-Hill, New York, 1977, chaps. 4–6.

Edelman, S. K.: "Sex and Life Education in a Rural School," *American Journal of Maternal Child Nursing,* **2**(4):233, July/August 1977.

Hymovich, D. P., and M. U. Barnard: *Family Health Care,* McGraw-Hill, New York, 1974.

Kogut, M. D.: "Growth and Development in Adolescence," *Pediatric Clinics of North America,* **20**(4):789, 1973.

Maier, H. W.: *Three Theories of Child Development,* Harper & Row, New York, 1965.

McAbee, R.: "Rural Parenting Classes: Beginning to Meet the Need," *American Journal of Maternal Child Nursing,* **2**(5):315, September/October 1977.

Rauh, J. L., L. B. Johnson, and R. L. Burket: "The Reproductive Adolescent," *Pediatric Clinics of North America,* **20**(4):1005, 1973.

Roberts, S. O.: "Some Mental and Emotional Health Needs of Negro Children and Youth," in R. Wilcox (ed.), *The Psychological Consequences of Being a Black American,* Wiley, New York, 1971.

Skolnick, A. S. and S. Skolnick: *The Family in Transition,* Little, Brown, Boston, 1974.

Wueger, M. K.: "The Young Adult Stepping into Parenthood," *American Journal of Nursing,* **76**(8):1283, August 1976.

2

FAMILY PLANNING*

FRANCINE HEINEMAN STIER

Family planning is not a new concept; in fact, various methods of birth control have been in existence throughout history. In ancient Egypt, women formed domes with hollowed-out lemon halves to cover the cervix. Other cultures employed various tampons soaked in different solutions or followed elaborate rituals to ward off pregnancy.[1]

The trend today in the United States is toward smaller families, and the concept of the nuclear family† in our society has influenced people to limit family size. In addition, more women in our society are attaining personal fulfillment through a career and/or education instead of through early motherhood. As many middle-class women wait to begin their families, the number of years available for childbearing are considerably shortened.

*The author acknowledges the editorial assistance of Mrs. Norma Helmreich in reviewing the manuscript of this chapter.

†A household consisting only of the mother, the father, and children.

There are also many couples who are committed to help prevent world overpopulation by having smaller families of their own, e.g., Zero Population Growth movements.

The birth control needs of a large part of our society have contributed to the search for newer and more effective means of conception control. Not only have measures of preventing pregnancy improved in the last 30 years, but postconception control measures such as voluntary abortion, menstrual extraction, "morning-after" pills, and sterilization have broadened the contraceptive alternatives for many people.

An ideal method of birth control would have to include the following criteria: it would have to be easy to use, coitus-independent, safe, inexpensive, and 100 percent effective, and have no side effects. Currently, no one method meets all of these criteria. Acceptance and proper use of the measures that are available often depend on several factors: the motivation of the user, the availability of the contraceptive service and method, the expense of the method, religious beliefs, cultural traditions, internalized sexual mores, and personal value systems.[2] Therefore, it is understandable that contraceptive failure, misuse, and nonuse exist within the American Society and are especially high among the less educated. Moreover, the less educated tend to rely on ineffective measures based on hearsay (e.g., douching with Coca-Cola) or measures which are cheaper and more readily available to them (e.g., withdrawal, foam, condom) rather than incur the expense of physician-related methods (e.g., oral contraceptives, intrauterine devices, or diaphragms). It follows, then, that a great deal of work is needed to provide the *total* fertile population with contraception suited to their needs. This chapter provides background data on the various contraceptive measures so that nursing care can be based on knowledge of the existing measures.

METHODS OF FAMILY PLANNING

the rhythm or ovulation method

The rhythm method of birth control is based upon the knowledge that ovulation occurs once a month at a more or less predictable interval. In most women, the menstrual cycle ranges from 22 to 35 days, but cycles may be shorter or longer for some individuals. The time from menstruation until ovulation is called the preovulatory phase. The greatest variation in the length of a cycle takes place during this phase, because menstruation occurs 14 days ± 2 days after ovulation. (Menstruation occurs when the corpus luteum of the ovary degenerates if the ovum has not been fertilized; this takes 14 to 16 days. See Chapter 3 for a more complete discussion of the menstrual cycle and ovulation.)

Because each woman's hormonal production varies in response to stress, infection, and time of life (e.g., premenopause, adolescence), there are times when a cycle may be anovulatory (no ovum released) or lengths of time when amenorrhea occurs. The average adult female between 22 and 45 years of age experiences the least anovulatory cycles (about 15 percent each year), whereas the younger teenager between 12 and 14 years of age may ovulate only during 15 percent of her cycles.[3] The egg, or ovum, is viable for approximately 24 hours after it is released from the ovary. The sperm are able to fertilize the ovum for approximately 48 to 72 hours after being deposited in the vagina. Theoretically, then, the "unsafe" time during each month is 2 days prior to and 2 days after ovulation (4 to 5 days total); thus, if the woman abstains from intercourse during this time, she is less likely to conceive. However, calculating the fertile, "unsafe," or abstinence period can at best, provide only an approximation. There are several ways of determining the fertile time of the month, some of which involve teaching the woman to become more aware of her body's cyclical rhythms.

The first way of determining the "unsafe" time of the month is by the *calendar method,* which is based on a record of the woman's previous 6 to 12 menstrual cycles. The number of days in the shortest and the longest cycles are noted. The woman then calculates as follows:

day A = the number of days
in the shortest cycle *minus* 18
day Z = the number of days
in the longest cycle *minus* 11

For example, if a woman's cycle varies from 27 to 32 days, day A = 27 minus 18, or day 9; and day Z = 32 minus 11, or day 21 of her cycle. For this woman, the fertile period is calculated from day A through day Z, or day 9 through day 21.

Using the calendar method alone, this woman must abstain from sexual intercourse for longer than she may desire. In order to shorten the abstinence period, she may use the *basal body temperature (BBT)* method in conjunction with the calendar. With this method, the temperature is taken every day upon awakening, before getting out of bed or doing any physical or emotional activity. A basal thermometer is measured in 0.1 calibrations rather than in 0.2 increments, so that small changes are easily noted. Prior to ovulation, the basal temperature remains more or less the same. On the day of ovulation, the temperature drops slightly and then rises sharply by the next day. The rise of approximately 1°F is then maintained for 8 to 12 days. The shift in temperature results from the thermogenic influences of progesterone, which is secreted by the corpus luteum after ovulation.

A temperature elevation lasting 3 days signifies an *end* to the period of abstinence even if the calendar count has not ended. (See Fig. 2-1 for an illustration of a "normal" cycle, Fig. 2-2 for an illustration of an anovulatory cycle, and Fig. 2-3 for an illustration of a cycle in which conception has occurred.)

Another method is to have the woman learn to recognize changes in the mucus secretions from her cervix in order to estimate her fertile time.[4] She is taught to observe the degree of wetness of her vaginal discharges. When the discharge appears yellowish and viscid, it can be considered a signal of approaching ovulation. Two to three days prior to ovulation, the wetness changes to a clear, colorless, watery liquid which has the ability to stretch approximately 6 to 15 cm in length into a fine threadlike consistency without separating.[5] When a sample is spread onto a slide and viewed under a microscope, this mucus takes on a "fern pattern." These characteristics of ovulatory mucus are termed *spinnbarkeit,* indicating that the mucus properties will "welcome" sperm. It signifies that a more alkaline environment exists in the vagina and cervix, making it more favorable for sperm survival and motility. To prevent conception, sexual contact is avoided on "wet" days (days of the clear, watery discharge).

Certain physiological sensations can also be indicative of ovulation. For instance, there are some women who experience *mittelschmerz,* or midcycle abdominal or pelvic pain at the time of ovulation. Breast tenderness and spotting of blood may also signify ovulation. However, awareness of these physiological sensations must accompany vaginal mucus, temperature, or calendar monitoring in order to increase the effectiveness of this birth control method.

ADVANTAGES OF RHYTHM   There is no cost involved in the rhythm method, except for the

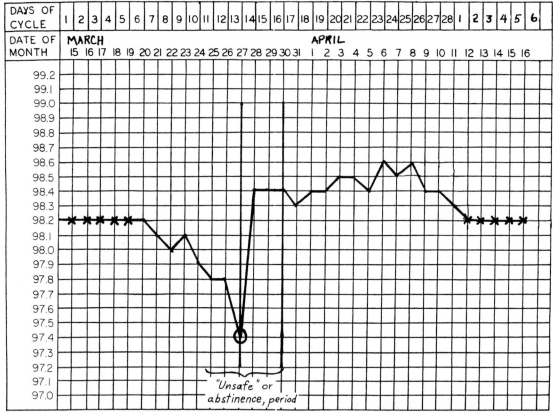

DAYS OF CYCLE	1	2	3	4	5	6	7	8	9	10	11	12	13	14	15	16	17	18	19	20	21	22	23	24	25	26	27	28	1	2	3	4	5	6
DATE OF MONTH	MARCH 15 16 17 18 19 20 21 22 23 24 25 26 27 28 29 30 31																	APRIL 1 2 3 4 5 6 7 8 9 10 11 12 13 14 15 16																		

fig. 2-1 Basal body temperature in a normal cycle; O = ovulation, X = menstruation. (*From C. Mitchell, "Infertility," in McGraw-Hill Handbook of Clinical Nursing, McGraw-Hill, New York, 1979, Chap. 5.*)

purchase of a basal thermometer if desired (the BBT chart is available from Planned Parenthood World Population in New York). There is no need for a physician's prescription. There are no potential side effects resulting from chemical or mechanical interference with bodily functions. The rhythm method is easy to learn for motivated couples. Both husband and wife can share in the choice and decisions involved. The rhythm method is the only type of contraception approved by the Roman Catholic Church. It can be very effective if two or three of the rhythm procedures are followed. Should the woman decide to become pregnant, the rhythm method can

easily be used to pinpoint the time of ovulation.

DISADVANTAGES OF RHYTHM   Very few women have perfectly regular menstrual cycles, and they therefore must keep a record of the cycles. In relying on the calendar method alone, both the time for ovulation (which cannot be pinpointed to the exact day) and the predicted viability of the ovum and sperm may be inaccurate in some people. Thus, individual variation may lower the predictive value of the calendar method alone. The failure rate of the calendar method alone is between 12 and 19 pregnancies per 100

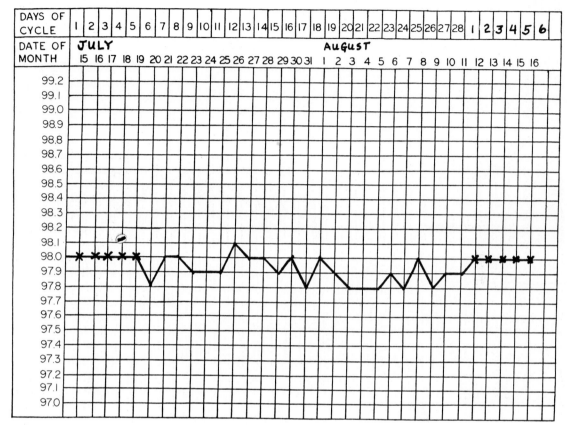

DAYS OF CYCLE	1	2	3	4	5	6	7	8	9	10	11	12	13	14	15	16	17	18	19	20	21	22	23	24	25	26	27	28	1	2	3	4	5	6
DATE OF MONTH	JULY																												AUGUST					
	15	16	17	18	19	20	21	22	23	24	25	26	27	28	29	30	31	1	2	3	4	5	6	7	8	9	10	11	12	13	14	15	16	

fig. 2-2 Basal body temperature during an anovulatory (nonphasic) cycle. X = menstruation. (*From C. Mitchell, "Infertility," in McGraw-Hill Handbook of Clinical Nursing, McGraw-Hill, New York, 1979, Chap. 5.*)

women-years of use.* (One hundred women-years of use = 50 women using a method for 2 years, or 100 women using a method for 1 year). If basal body temperature is used in conjunction with the calendar method, the effectiveness improves to 2 to 3 pregnancies per 100 women-years of use. The couple must be highly motivated to abstain from sexual intercourse during the fertile period. Some

* All rates of effectiveness are from Barbara Vaughan et al., "Contraceptive Failure Among Married Women in the U.S. 1970–1973," *Family Planning Perspectives*, **9** (6): 251–258, November/December 1977, and Planned Parenthood, New York, 1972, unless otherwise indicated.

couples find it difficult to have such premeditated rather than spontaneous intercourse.

coitus interruptus (withdrawal)

Coitus interruptus is an ancient method which requires the male to withdraw his penis from the vagina immediately before ejaculation. As a result, semen is not deposited in or near the vagina.

ADVANTAGES OF COITUS INTERRUPTUS The withdrawal method is useful to those who have no

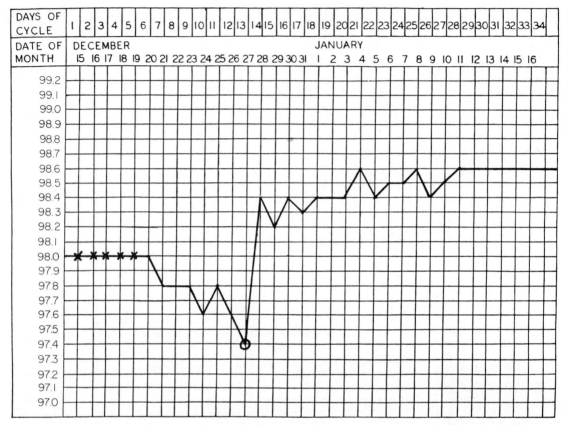

fig. 2-3 Basal body temperature after conception; X = menstruation, O = ovulation. (From C. Mitchell, "Infertility," in McGraw-Hill Handbook of Clinical Nursing, McGraw-Hill, New York, 1978, Chap. 5)

other method available. Withdrawal involves no cost.

DISADVANTAGES OF COITUS INTERRUPTUS   Great skill and self-control are required for the withdrawal method, since approaching orgasm causes an impulse in the male to penetrate as deeply as possible into the vagina. The woman must also hold back activity so as not to threaten her partner's loss of control. Consequently, this method may be extremely frustrating.

Because a small drop of semen may contain thousands of sperm and ejaculation may occur in stages, this method is quite ineffective, resulting in 10 to 40 pregnancies per 100 women-years of use.

chemical barriers

Chemical barriers are usually spermicidal in action and also prevent the sperm from moving rapidly into the cervix. These barriers are available in different forms: jellies, foams, creams, or suppositories. Sperm are known to thrive and move most effectively in an environmental pH of 8.5 to 9.0, which is highly alkaline. The vagina is normally acidic, with a pH of 4 to 5 as a result of the lactic acid produced by the resident Döderlein's bacillus. Sperm motility is reduced by a pH of 6 and destroyed by a pH of 4 or less (see Fig. 2-4). As the ovulatory phase approaches, the vaginal pH gradually rises toward a more alkaline state, thus "welcoming" the sperm. Chemical barriers coat the cervix and vaginal lining with a substance designed to lower the vaginal pH toward 4.

The chemical barriers are inserted deep into the vagina with a plastic applicator (see Fig. 2-5). The most popular and most effective chemical barrier is the foam, which comes in an aerosol container and is less likely to drip. All the chemical agents must be used immediately before intercourse, e.g., 10 to 30 min, and therefore cannot be isolated from the act of intercourse. Repeated intercourse requires reapplication of the chemical. Douching is not necessary and in fact should not be done for 6 h following intercourse, since it will remove the chemical and allow sperm to enter the uterus. If used just after a baby is born, a double application is necessary until the stretched vaginal tissue returns to prepregnant size.

There is a product on the market called Encare Oval, a capsule which is inserted into the vagina 10 min prior to intercourse. It quickly disperses at body temperature and coats the vagina and cervix with a viscous barrier of spermicide. It is only effective for 2 h, however. The package insert claims a

fig. 2-4 Insemination, ovulation, fertilization. Chemical and mechanical barrier techniques of contraception would prevent sperm from entering the cervical opening. (*Reproduced with permission from A Baby Is Born, published by the Maternity Center Association, New York.*)

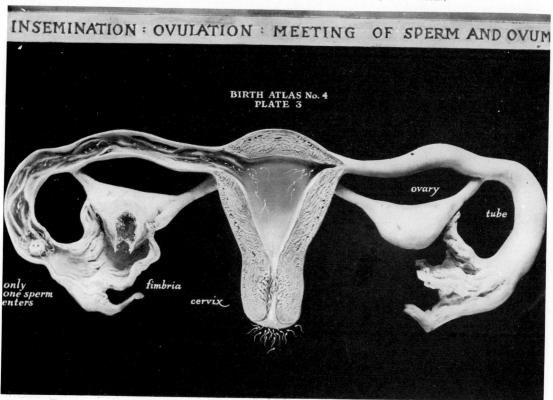

INSEMINATION : OVULATION : MEETING OF SPERM AND OVUM

BIRTH ATLAS No. 4
PLATE 3

ovary

tube

only one sperm enters

fimbria

cervix

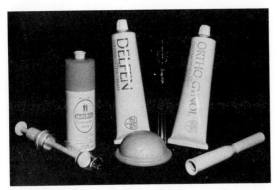

fig. 2-5 Types of foam, jelly, and cream for use in conjunction with the diaphragm or condom.

very high effectiveness rate of 1 pregnancy per 100 women-years if used properly. Because the product is new and has not yet been tested for effectiveness in the United States, this high rate is still open to question. Planned Parenthood categorizes Encare Oval as a vaginal suppository with the same effectiveness rate as that of a chemical barrier.*

ADVANTAGES OF CHEMICAL BARRIERS Chemical barriers are readily available in any drugstore and need no prescription. They are inexpensive and simple to use and thus are used more often by adolescents who seek anonymity. For the woman who forgets her pill for 2 days or who has infrequent intercourse, a chemical barrier may be especially useful as a temporary measure. When used alone, chemical barriers require no special manipulative skills; insertion is much like that of a tampon. The chemical agents do not alter body physiology.

DISADVANTAGES OF CHEMICAL BARRIERS Failure rates range from 15 to 30 pregnancies per 100 women-years of use, depending upon the preparation. The Margaret Sanger Research

Bureau has compiled test results of a varied number of agents and can recommend certain brands.*

A small percentage of women experience burning discomfort from the chemical agent. Since the method must be used immediately before intercourse, planning and forethought are involved, which to some is a disadvantage. Some women are repelled by the genital manipulation involved, however minimal it may be.

mechanical barriers

Mechanical barriers prevent sperm from entering the cervical canal by sealing off an exit (as with the condom) or the cervical entrance (as with the diaphragm). Before the advent of hormonal contraception and intrauterine devices, mechanical barriers were widely used in the United States.

diaphragm The diaphragm (Fig. 2-5) is a curved rubber dome covering a flexible metal ring. Designed to fit snugly over the cervix, it is inserted through the vagina and placed between the posterior fornix and the symphysis pubis (Fig. 2-6). Diaphragms are available in many sizes and must be expertly fitted by a physician or qualified nurse for each woman. Spermicidal jelly or cream must be placed in the cup portion and on the rim of the diaphragm prior to insertion so as to maintain cervical contact with the jelly and maximize protection (see Fig. 2.6a).

The woman may require one or two clinic visits in order to practice proper placement of the diaphragm. It is stretched longitudinally either with a plastic applicator or with the thumb and forefinger and inserted into the vagina toward the spine. The anterior edge must then be pushed gently upward, under-

* Planned Parenthood World Population, Nurse Educator, Miriam Manisoff. Personal communication, December 1977.

* A list of these is available from Planned Parenthood, 810 Seventh Avenue, New York, New York 10019.

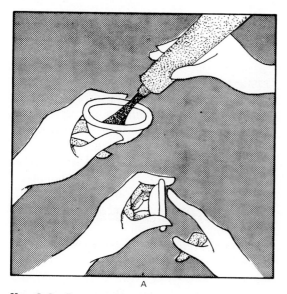
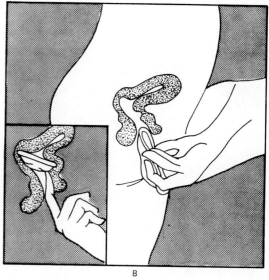

A   B

fig. 2-6 Proper placement of a diaphragm between the posterior fornix and the symphysis pubis. (a) Applying the spermicidal jelly to the cup and rim of the diaphragm. (b) Inserting the diaphragm properly. The diaphragm is stretched longitudinally between the fingers and inserted into the vagina toward the spine. It is then gently pushed upward underneath the symphysis pubis. (*Adapted from the Ortho Pharmaceutical Corp., Raritan, N,J. by Patricia Rodriguez-Lovink.*)

neath the symphysis pubis, so that the rubber cup completely covers the cervix (see Fig. 2-6b). The woman is then taught to check for proper placement by feeling for her cervix (which feels like a rounded knob or the tip of the nose). Once in place, the diaphragm cannot be felt by either partner during intercourse.

The woman should be encouraged to insert the diaphragm and jelly every night before retiring, whether or not intercourse is expected. This ensures protection should intercourse take place within a couple of hours and may seem more spontaneous to the woman. If no coitus occurs, the diaphragm can be removed the next morning. The diaphragm and jelly *must remain* in place for at least 6 h after intercourse. Should coitus occur again within the 6 h, an additional application of jelly is required. Douching is not necessary.

The diaphragm itself is functional for ap-

proximately 2 years, at which time the size should be rechecked. Any excessive weight gain or loss, delivery of a baby, or vaginal surgery requires a change in diaphragm size. Care of the diaphragm requires that it be thoroughly washed with mild soap after use, thoroughly rinsed and dried, inspected for holes, and dusted with talcum powder.

ADVANTAGES OF THE DIAPHRAGM   If used properly and consistently, the diaphragm can have an effectiveness rate of 2 to 3 pregnancies per 100 women-years of use.[6] The woman in a stable environment with some degree of privacy is usually a good candidate for the diaphragm. Manipulation is required but, once learned, becomes matter of fact. It does not interfere with physiologic functioning and does not alter sexual sensation. The expense of the jelly is minimal, but some cost may be involved in the clinic appointment or office visit that is required for proper fit and for a prescription.

DISADVANTAGES OF THE DIAPHRAGM When used inconsistently or without jelly, the diaphragm's failure rate is relatively high—12 to 14 pregnancies per 100 women-years of use.[7] A great deal of motivation and preplanning is required. The expense and time of the office visits may be more than some women can afford. The vaginal self-manipulation may be highly distasteful to some women. Finally, with unusual coital positions, the diaphragm may move out of place.

cervical cap The cervical cap, which is used more often in Europe than in the United States, acts in much the same manner as does the diaphragm. Cervical caps are made of rubber or plastic and are thicker, smaller, and less flexible than the diaphragm. The plastic version may be left in place between menses, which provides coitus independence. It must be left in place 6 h after intercourse. Spermicidal jelly is usually required, and the position of the cap should be checked periodically.
    Advantages and disadvantages are similar to those of the diaphragm.

condom The condom is a very old method of protection and has been in use since the sixteenth century. Originally designed to protect against venereal disease, it was found that the condom also prevented pregnancy. Used by the male, this rubber sheath is placed over the erect penis prior to intercourse to prevent semen from entering the vagina. Many types of condoms contain a small pouch at the tip to receive the semen. If the pouch is not present the man must leave about 1 in loose at the tip after applying the condom. All the air must be released from the tip, since air may cause it to burst or cause the ejaculate to leak out of the base of the condom. After ejaculation, the penis must be withdrawn from the vagina while still erect, and care must be taken to prevent the condom from slipping off so that no semen enters the vagina.

ADVANTAGES OF THE CONDOM The condom's effectiveness can be as high as 2 to 3 pregnancies per 100 women-years if utilized in conjunction with vaginal foam. It is effective in preventing venereal disease and also protects against reinfection from such vaginal infections as trichomoniasis or candidiasis when one partner is under treatment. Condoms are inexpensive and readily available in any drugstore. In addition, some of the responsibility for contraception is placed with the male partner.

DISADVANTAGES OF THE CONDOM Failure rates of the condom used alone range from 10 to 15 pregnancies per 100 women-years of use, depending upon the study cited.[8,9] Many men feel that the condom curtails much of the pleasurable sensation. In order to use the condom, it must be applied prior to vaginal penetration, and foreplay may be interrupted if difficulty is encountered.

intrauterine device (IUD)

The IUD is an old birth control method that was refined in the 1960s so that it is now one of the most effective low-cost methods available. Many developing countries have fostered its use because of its low cost and long action. In the United States, the IUD is ranked second after the pill among choices of birth control methods.[10]

mode of action of the IUD Although the IUD's exact method of preventing pregnancy is unclear, there are certain local effects which seem to create a uterine environment hostile to implantation. Current theories concerning the mechanism of change within the uterus are as follows:

1 The IUD acts as a foreign body [11] in the uterus, generating an inflammatory response of leukocytes and macrophages in the endometrium.
   a A hostile environment exists because the inflammatory process influences hormonal changes.
   b The inflammatory cells may be spermicidal or blastocidal (i.e., destroys the conceptus).
2 The IUD acts to keep the endometrium "out of phase" in the menstrual cycle, e.g., the spongy tissue does not acquire the blood-filled edematous properties required for implantation, and the ovum is lost. Thus the IUD may be said to cause an abortion ("abortifacient").

Recently, certain metals (e.g., copper—the Copper T or the Copper 7) and medications (particularly progesterone—the Progestasert or the Alza T) have been added to IUDs made of flexible polyethylene (see Figs. 2-7 and 2-8). These devices provide timed-release chemicals (copper ions or minute amounts of progesterone) which may induce changes in the endometrium that are unfavorable for implantation.[12] However, implantation can occur despite the presence of the IUD. Those women who do become pregnant with an IUD have an extremely high rate of spontaneous abortions (40 percent). Should the pregnancy continue to term, the IUD usually becomes embedded in the maternal side of the placenta and is rarely found inside the membranes. (The surviving fetus is usually unharmed by the presence of the IUD.)

insertion The IUD must be inserted by a properly trained health professional. The

fig. 2-7 Copper T (300L) and the Lippes Loop T Cu (300L) appears to have an effectiveness rating of 2.0 pregnancies per 100 women years of use, an expulsion rate of 10 percent, a removal rate of 16 percent, and a continuation rate of 71.4 percent. (*From Population Council, August 1973.*) The Lippes Loop has an effectiveness rating of about 2 pregnancies per 100 women years of use, with a continuation rate of 75 percent (*From Family Planning Digest, March 1973.*)

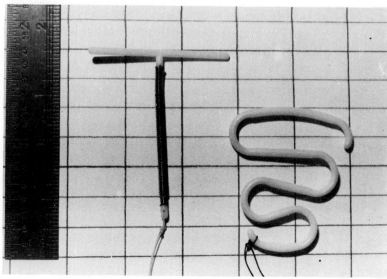

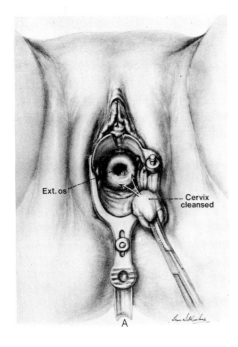

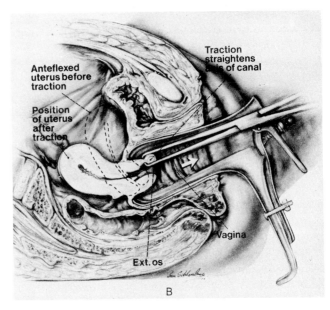

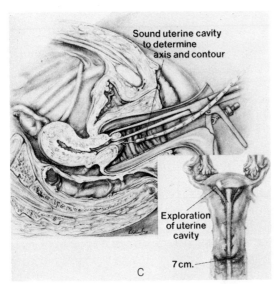

fig. 2-8 Preparation for IUD insertion. (a) Speculum in the vagina. (b) Traction on the cervix to straighten the uterus. (c) Sounding the uterus, a most critical step prior to insertion to check on the dimensions of the endometrial cavity. (*Courtesy of A. H. Robbins Co.*)

woman usually has a Papanicolaou (Pap) test for cancer and a culture for gonorrhea at the time of her examination. Preexisting inflammatory disease of the uterus, suspected pregnancy, cervical or uterine cancer, or large fibroids are all conditions which contraindicate the insertion of the IUD. Insertion is done during the latter part of the menses when the cervix is slightly dilated. After delivery and abortion, the IUD can be inserted, but it is expelled more frequently.

ADVANTAGES OF THE IUD   The IUD generally remains in place after it has been inserted, but in some instances, it is lost (passed out of the cervix). Therefore, overlapping contraception is recommended in some cases for a few months after insertion (foam is usually sufficient). The IUD does not require forethought or preparation prior to intercourse and thus does not interfere with sexual pleasure. The cost is quite minimal (Pap test, insertion, and revisits) if done at a clinic or a

Planned Parenthood center. Effectiveness varies with the type of IUD and with the age and parity (number of pregnancies) of the woman. It ranges from 1 pregnancy per 100 women-years of use for the medicated devices[13] to 5 pregnancies per 100 women-years of use for the nonmedicated devices.[14]

Although IUDs which release progesterone are quite new, the data thus far suggests that the progesterone decreases uterine motility. Thus the medicated IUD is more likely to be retained, since less cramping and blood flow occur during menses. In addition, the quantity of natural progesterone released by this IUD is so minimal (65 μg) that there is virtually no systemic absorption. Thus far, the Progestasert or Alza T seems to be highly acceptable.

The Copper 7 device also has a high retention rate and can be used successfully in nulliparous (never pregnant) women.[15] The Copper 7 device has recently been approved by the U.S. Food and Drug Administration (FDA) for 3-year retention rather than the 2-year limit that previously existed.[16]

Approximately 75 to 85 percent of the IUDs inserted in clinic patients remain in place a year or more, which indicates that the IUD seems to be a highly acceptable form of birth control in this population.[17]

DISADVANTAGES OF THE IUD   The inflammatory process which theoretically serves to prevent pregnancy may also serve to increase uterine contractility after insertion, thus causing many of the devices to be expelled.[18] The possibility of expulsion may continue for three or more menstrual cycles. During her menses, the woman may experience cramping, heavy bleeding, and pelvic pain, all resulting from the highly contractile state of the uterus. Occasionally, the IUD may have to be removed if symptoms remain severe. Following menstruation and about once a week thereafter, the woman must check with her finger for the nylon threads which protrude into the vagina through the cervix. This may be distasteful to some women.

The main disadvantage of the progesterone-releasing IUD is that it must be replaced annually because of the dissolution of the medication.

Ectopic pregnancies have been found to occur more commonly with nonmedicated IUDs than with medicated ones.[19] A serious but rare complication is perforation of the uterus, which may occur during insertion of the IUD.

The IUD is usually an unacceptable method for those couples who have strong feelings against abortion, because it can cause abortion of the conceptus in those cases where the sperm survives the assault of phagocytes and does fertilize the ovum.

oral contraceptives

Oral contraceptives which suppress ovulation are the most effective and popular means of preventing pregnancy. The failure rate is extremely low, ranging from 0.2 to 2 pregnancies per 100 women-years of use, depending upon the type of pill used and the study quoted.[20,21] Two types of pills are currently on the market in the United States: (1) varied combinations of estrogens and progesterones in synthetic form, and (2) minute doses of progesterones alone in synthetic form (which do not suppress ovulation but do lower fertility).

combined regimen pills   The combination pills contain synthetic estrogen and progesterone (progestogens) and are available in 20-, 21-, or 28-day pill packages. There are many products available; differences usually exist in the dosages and strengths of the estrogens. The package containing 20 or 21 pills is taken as follows:

1 For the first cycle on the pill the woman waits until the fifth day of her menses (she counts the start of menstruation as day 1) and begins the first pill.
2 The pill is taken for the next 20 or 21 days, finishing the package.
3 The woman waits 7 days and then begins to take a new package of pills, whether or not menses has occurred.

The 20- or 21-day pill packages are the so-called 3 weeks on, 1 week off schedule. Menses will usually occur during the 7 days off the pill. If bleeding does not occur after the second cycle on the pill, the woman should consult her physician. Actually, the bleeding is not a menses per se but rather withdrawal bleeding resulting from an abrupt cessation of estrogens and progesterones.

The 28-day pill packages have 21 pills which contain hormones; the last 7 pills are either placebos or iron supplements and are a different color. This type of pill schedule means that the woman does not stop taking a pill. While she takes the placebo, however, she will experience withdrawal bleeding. One nurse educator [22] teaches patients who are on the 21- or 28-day pills to use the "Sunday schedule," which requires the woman to begin each new package of pills on a Sunday. In this way, menses are usually over by the weekend.

Should the woman forget a pill, two should be taken the following day. If two pills are missed the woman should finish the cycle of pills and use an alternate method of birth control for that month.

MODE OF ACTION OF THE COMBINED REGIMEN PILL The combined regimen pill suppresses ovulation by inhibiting the hypothalamus, the pituitary, and the ovarian release of hormones. Follicle-stimulating hormones (FSH) and luteinizing hormones (LH) are suppressed; thus the two hormones required to stimulate ovulation are drastically reduced by the influence of the estrogens and progesterones in the pills. (See Chapter 3 for a more complete discussion of the hormonal aspects of ovulation.) The estrogens and progesterones in the pill produce endometrial changes which cause some sloughing of tissue and bleeding when the pill is stopped. Changes in the endometrium which inhibit implantation are secondary effects of this pill. Cervical mucus also becomes more viscous and maintains a pH environment that is hostile to sperm throughout the cycle.

If taken correctly, the combination pill is almost 100 percent effective; human error may account for the 2 pregnancies per 100 women-years of use which is frequently cited.[23] The cost of the pills range from $2 to $5 monthly, but the initial physician visits and checkups may be costly.

SIDE EFFECTS OF THE COMBINED REGIMEN PILL The main disadvantage of the combination pill lies in the myriad side effects it produces. Because the ingestion of hormones tends to alter the woman's own physiological hormonal state, the physician needs to be alert to the subtle differences in dosage requirements for each woman. Many of the side effects may be eliminated by carefully selecting the ratio of estrogens to progesterones. If the appropriate balance is achieved, the woman should experience few side effects.

An "estrogen profile" provides data on each woman's estrogen levels so that the appropriate pill may be chosen. This profile provides a picture of a woman's body type, since it is based on the woman's body build, history of menstrual cycles, libido levels, energy levels, and age. Table 2-1 compares a balanced profile (76 to 80 percent of all women) with a *hypo*estrogenic state. In the hypoestrogenic woman, the physician may prescribe an estrogen-dominant pill. Progestogen-dom-

table 2-1 Estrogen levels

hyperestrogenic, 10 to 12%	balanced, 76 to 80%	hypoestrogenic, 10 to 12%
Heavy menstrual flow	Normal menses	Scanty menses at longer intervals
Large breasts	Normal contours	Small breasts
Tendency to gain weight	Normal weight	Boyish look
Premenstrual syndrome:		
Fluid retention		
Emotional lability		
Increased libido		Lower libido
Increased vaginal secretion	Normal vaginal cytology	Thinner vaginal lining
Mastalgia	and secretions	More vaginitis, pruritus
Tendency toward fibroids		

Source: Adapted from J. Nelson, "Clinical Evaluation of Side Effects of Current Contraceptives—Oral: Combined, Sequential," *Journal of Reproductive Medicine*, **6**:2, 1971.

inant pills (considered as an antiestrogen) are prescribed for the *hyper*estrogenic woman.

Side effects that are related to estrogen tend to mimic the unpleasant sensations in early pregnancy: nausea, vomiting, fluid retention, headaches, chloasma, breast enlargement, and the like. (See Table 2-2 for results of estrogen excess.) If the woman experiences these symptoms, her physician may change the pill to one containing a lower dosage of estrogen, such as Loestrin, LoOvral, or Brevicon, or to a pill with more antiestrogenic progesterones, such as Ovral, Norlestrin, or Zorane. Dosages as low as 25 μg of estrogen are available in some pills.

Progesterone-related side effects include fatigue, depression, acne, oily scalp, and weight gain. (See Table 2-2 for results of progestogen excess). Breakthrough bleeding may also be a problem, occurring more often during the first two cycles of pill use. This signifies the endometrial adjustment to the new hormone level, but if spotting continues the woman should see her physician so that the pill may be reevaluated. Frequently, the physician may prescribe a pill with a larger amount of estrogen to suppress the breakthrough bleeding. Spotting may also occur if the woman misses a couple of pills.

Hypomenorrhea (scanty bleeding) may oc-

cur with the lower estrogen pills and those which have potent antiestrogenic progesterones. Hypomenorrhea is not necessarily a problem, however, unless the woman is not informed that it frequently occurs, in which case she may think that she is pregnant and stop taking the pill.

Oral contraceptives have recently been under intensive study to determine the incidence of benign breast disease, nonmalignant liver tumors, cervical carcinoma, myocardial infarction, thromboemboli, amenorrhea, and hypertension among pill users. At this time, women with a history of embolism, thrombosis, hypertension, liver diseases, migraine related to pill use, undiagnosed breast masses and estrogen-dependent tumors should *not* be on the pill because a causal relationship has not yet been ruled out. Women need extremely careful monitoring while on the pill if diabetes mellitus, gallbladder disease, mental depression, deep vein varicosities, or frequent vaginal yeast infections are present.[24-26]

Postpill amenorrhea is a complication which may occur more often in the female who begins the pill close to her menarche or who has a late menarche. No relationship has been demonstrated between length of time on the pill or type of pill and postpill amenorrhea.[27] The amenorrhea which may occur is

table 2-2 Results of an excess of estrogen and progestogen

estrogen	progestogen
gastrointestinal	
Nausea, bloated feeling	Increased appetite, real weight gain
vascular and renal systems	
Fluid retention, venous capillary engorgement	
Occasional occurrence of spider nevi	
Headaches [migraine] and perhaps some elevation of blood pressure (?)	Depression, nervousness, fatigue
A slight chance of thromboembolism in high-risk patients	
uterus	
Hypermenorrhea, myoma growth	Scanty menses
	Dysmenorrhea usually improved; sometimes break-through bleeding
vagina	
Mucorrhea, excess secretion	Reduction in lining thickness and secretions; more *Candida*, pruritus
breasts	
Mastalgia; possible enlargement of benign cysts	Regression of breast tissue
skin	
Chloasma (darkening of skin over nose and cheeks)	Possible occurrence of acne
glucose metabolism	
Increased levels in fasting state	
Decreased glucose tolerance, increased insulin response to glucose	

Source: Adapted from J. Nelson, "Clinical Evaluation of Side Effects of Current Contraceptives—Oral: Combined, Sequential," *Journal of Reproductive Medicine*, **6**:2, 1971.

temporary; menses usually returns within 6 months.

There are some popular misconceptions among pill users, such as that it is more difficult to become pregnant after discontinuing the pill or that the body needs a "rest" from taking the pill. Both of these theories have been discredited. However, it is widely recommended that oral contraceptives not be taken for 3 months before trying to become pregnant in order to avoid potential birth defects. This theory is still unsubstantiated. If the woman suspects that she is pregnant the pill should be discontinued because the effects on the developing gonads of the fetus may be serious. The pill should always be avoided by nursing mothers, since the effects of progesterone and estrogen tend to suppress prolactin production and milk supply. Long-range effects on infants who ingest the hormones via the milk are not known. The pill has not yet been found to cause cancer,[28] but careful monitoring is necessary for susceptible women, e.g., those women whose mothers or sisters have had breast or uterine cancer.

Although there have been deaths reported which relate to pill use, e.g., pulmonary or cerebral emboli, the risk of death as a result of pregnancy-related illnesses is much higher in all age groups. Consequently, the pill remains quite a popular form of birth control and safer than the possible physiological side effects of pregnancy. It is recommended, however, that women over 40 who are obese and who smoke should not take the pill because of the increased risk of myocardial infarction, hypertension, and thromboemboli.[29] Of course, each woman needs to be carefully evaluated with regard to her medical history to determine whether she is a candidate for the pill.

BENEFICIAL EFFECTS OF THE COMBINED REGIMEN PILL   In order to present a balanced picture of the combination pill, it should be known that combined regimen oral contraceptives are reported to have beneficial side effects; the premenstrual syndrome, endometriosis, menorrhagia, ovarian cysts, and iron deficiency anemia may all be decreased while on the pill.[30]

progesterone only   The progesterone-only oral contraceptives are also called "mini-pills" because of their low dosages of synthetic progesterones. Unlike the combined regimen pills, the mini-pill is taken every day whether bleeding occurs or not. Progesterone-only pills have an effectiveness rate of 3 pregnancies per 100 woman-years use when taken at the same time every day. Dosages of

progesterone range from a low of 0.075 mg. (Ovrette) to 0.35 mg. (Micronor).

MODE OF ACTION OF PROGESTERONE-ONLY PILLS   The progesterone induces physiological changes which interfere with the endometrial phase and the cervical mucus. Thus the uterine environment is hostile to sperm motility and implantation should fertilization occur. The small doses of progesterone do not suppress ovulation except in the progesterone-sensitive woman.

SIDE EFFECTS   The major side effects of this type of oral contraceptive are the unpredictability of menses, the lack of cycle control, and the lower effectiveness rate. Yet, women who cannot take estrogens or in whom the diaphragm or IUD is unacceptable may benefit by using the progesterone-only pill.

In December 1976, the Food and Drug Administration mandated that detailed information about the risks and benefits of various oral contraceptives be included in the package inserts of the pills. In this manner, the woman will be receiving "informed consent" data and will be able to make the final decision about the pill knowledgeably.[31]

postcoital contraception

The so-called morning-after pills are highly effective when used within 72 hours after midcycle unprotected intercourse. Usually used in an emergency, e.g., cases of rape, the pills consist of synthetic estrogen (diethylstilbestrol, or DES). The FDA does not approve DES for repeated or routine use because large doses of estrogen are not considered physiologically safe. The pills are given in 25-mg doses for 5 days and usually produce adverse effects such as nausea and vomiting. The estrogen creates tubal and endometrial changes which hinder implantation.

If pregnancy does occur despite the use of DES, the FDA strongly recommends a therapeutic abortion as a result of the substantial evidence linking DES to predisposition to vaginal cancer and genital malformations in the offspring.

Menstrual extraction may also be performed to induce menstruation when it is overdue. However, this method is very similar to the vacuum aspiration type of abortion. It is a method of suctioning out the uterine contents to cause bleeding.

surgical sterilization

For the most part, surgical sterilization is a permanent measure and should be undertaken only after a great deal of consideration. Sterilization requires informed consent of the patient, which means that all the implications of the procedure must be fully explained prior to obtaining written permission. It is most desirable if both partners sign the consent; however, it is legal in most states when only the patient signs.

The psychological implications involved in losing one's reproductive ability can be far-reaching. Reproductive prowess is often equated with degree of "maleness" or "femaleness," and loss of reproductive ability may serve to lower one's self-esteem. However, the majority of men and women who undergo surgical sterilization are not adversely affected. With fear of unwanted pregnancy gone, many couples report improvement in their sex lives and more frequent intercourse.

The ideal surgical sterilization procedure would be simple enough to be done in a physician's office, inexpensive, 100 percent effective, 100 percent safe, 100 percent reversible, and have few side effects. To date, no method meets these criteria.[32]

female sterilization At present, various surgical techniques exist for sterilizing women. Tubal ligation, tubal removal, tubal cauterization, injection of solutions which sclerose or block the tubes, removal of the fimbriated ends of the tubes, and hysterectomy are some of the measures used. Hysterectomy is not commonly done for sterilization purposes alone because the complications are far greater than those for the other measures, since it is major surgery. Vaginal (culdoscopic) or abdominal (laparascopic) approaches can be used to visualize the tubes and ligate, crush, or remove them. The most popular current methods are laparascopic ("Band-aid" surgery) tubal ligation, which leaves a small abdominal incision and can be done on an outpatient basis. The best time for tubal ligation is immediately after delivery when the tubes have been displaced toward the anterior part of the abdomen and are easily visualized. Side effects are minimal, and uterine function is not altered. Ovulation occurs, but the ovum is absorbed into the peritoneal cavity.

male sterilization Vas ligation, or vasectomy, is a popular form of surgical sterilization in the male. It can be performed in a physician's office with little pain or side effects. For the most part it is permanent, although about 25 percent of the vasectomies performed can be reversed. (However, fertility rates may remain low even if the vas deferens can be rejoined. Many people are recommending storing sperm in a frozen sperm bank should the person have any doubts.)

The vas deferens is severed, making passage of the sperm from the testes to the urethra impossible (see Fig. 2-9). Abstinence from sexual intercourse is required only until the incisions heal (approximately 3 days). It is essential to inform the man that sperm may still be present in the area beyond the ligation and that he is not considered sterile for 8 weeks after the surgery (or until 10 ejaculations have occurred). In addition, the man should bring a specimen of ejaculate for a

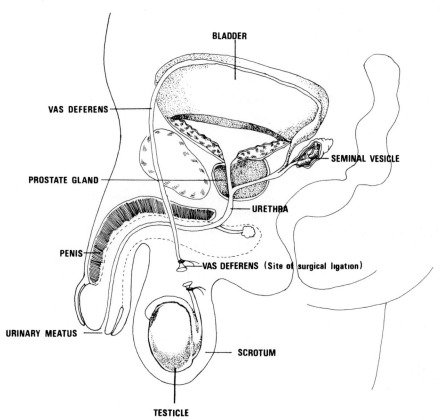

BLADDER

VAS DEFERENS

SEMINAL VESICLE

PROSTATE GLAND

URETHRA

PENIS

VAS DEFERENS (Site of surgical ligation)

URINARY MEATUS

SCROTUM

TESTICLE

fig. 2-9 Illustration of a vasectomy. The vas deferens has been tied off and severed. Sperm cannot enter the ejaculatory duct. (*Courtesy of Patricia Rodriguez-Lovink.*)

sperm count about 2 to 3 months after surgery.

Side effects are rare but can include infection, hematomas at the site, or small spermatic granulomas. These complications are not serious and are easily treated by the physician.

research methods

Research into new contraceptive measures is continually being pursued. The more promising studies are listed below:

Long-acting hormonal interruption of the ovarian cycle by means of injection, subdermal capsules, pills, or vaginal rings

are under investigation. All these hormonal methods involve the use of synthetic progesterones and can potentially cause the side effects of progesterone excess (see Table 2.2).

The use of prostaglandin $F_{2\alpha}$ seems promising. Prostaglandins are found normally in the menstrual fluid and tend to increase right before labor begins in the pregnant woman. Because it is felt that prostaglandins play some role in stimulating uterine activity or in destroying the corpus luteum to induce menstruation or labor, they may be very effective if taken at the time menstruation is expected. The prostaglandins would be absorbed vaginally, acting as an abortifacient.[33]

Luteolytic agents are being actively researched. These compounds either suppress or destroy the corpus luteum, which is essential to maintain pregnancy. The corpus luteum of the ovary produces progesterone after ovulation and provides the proper uterine environment for implantation and nourishment of the conceptus. Should the corpus luteum cease functioning, the fertilized ovum cannot implant or, once implanted, cannot continue.

Male contraceptive measures are currently being researched. New advances are being made in influencing the maturation and fertility capacity of sperm. Techniques for reversibly blocking sperm transport, such as a vas deferens valve, are being sought. As yet, these studies are too new to determine any long-range effects on the male.[34]

The World Health Organization is sponsoring research on a birth control vaccine which may be available within 3 to 10 years. Current testing is being done using synthetic chorionic gonadotropin (the hormone produced by the chorion of pregnancy) as the vaccine.[35]

Intracervical devices which may be simpler and have fewer side effects than IUDs are being studied.

Testing is being done with manipulation of the menstrual cycle to mimic the state existing prepubertally or to mimic the amenorrhea occurring during lactation.[36]

NURSING CARE

Dissemination of birth control information should be an integral part of nursing intervention. Many studies have been done to determine whether availability of birth control information and health services decreases the unwanted pregnancies among the disadvantaged. Thus far, results seem to support wide distribution of birth control information. In New York City, for instance, the birth rate among welfare mothers has gradually declined since 1965 until it now approximates that of middle- and upper-income women. This decline is due in part to family planning clinics and to widespread availability of birth control information. Recent research has indicated a convergence of birth control usage among various racial, socioeconomic, and religious groups, and yet important differences still exist in the *continuity* of use within these groups.[37] This demonstrates the need for special attention to high-risk groups on a continuing basis.

Even with free availability of all birth control methods and information, an alarming number of sexually active adolescents *never* use contraception.[38] Sexual attitudes, manner of upbringing, peer pressures, approach to sexual matters, and self-esteem seem to influence the use or nonuse of contraception among many adolescents.

It follows, then, that provision of information alone is insufficient in helping people to choose, use, and succeed with contraception. The nurse needs the ability to "step inside the shoes" of the client, to "feel" the cultural, traditional, and socioeconomic constraints that govern the choice and use of birth control. It is within this context that the nurse may then incorporate empathy with knowledge of human behavior, knowledge of the different methods of birth control, theories of interviewing, and familiarity with the nursing process in order to work with the individual to choose the appropriate method of birth control. It has been demonstrated that adolescents have fewer unwanted pregnancies after becoming an integral part of the decision-making process in the use of contraceptive measures.[39,40] In order to begin to effect change, the nurse needs to encourage healthy, joyful attitudes toward human sexuality in all child-rearing, educational, and health practices. Once guilt and anxiety concerning sex are reduced, a more active and conscious choice for controlling one's reproductive ability may become commonplace.

The nurse is in a unique position to foster healthy feelings about sex and to provide information, because opportunities exist in all facets of care: postpartum, Pap test exams, postabortion, high school or college classes, Girl or Boy Scout meetings, and the like. Often counseling occurs at a time when birth control failure is apparent, e.g., following abortion, or when the person is highly motivated to prevent pregnancy, e.g., following delivery.

nursing process

Nurses actively involved in family planning usually utilize the nursing process in order to provide effective care. *Assessment* of the individual's needs involves several steps:

1 *Data gathering:* Observing the person's behavior, obtaining a sexual history to identify sexual dysfunction, determining whether the person desires to delay or to prevent pregnancy, and obtaining a marital and family history and other pertinent information may be important in creating an accurate picture of the individual's needs. For instance, extreme discomfort in talking about sex may mean that the person has difficulty planning for sex and may require a coitus-independent type of method which could then be recommended to the physician.

   Factors to be considered whenever gathering data are as follows:
   a Educational level of the contraceptive user,
   b Socioeconomic level,
   c Size of existing family,
   d Cultural beliefs and mores,
   e General physical health of the person,
   f Amount of stress on the person, e.g., economic, social (drug abuse, alcoholism, abuse or neglect of any children in the family),
   g Age of the contraceptive user,
   h Place in life, e.g., career-oriented young woman or older housewife reentering the work force,
   i Motivation level,
   j Pregnancy rate, e.g., date of last pregnancy and number of children in the past 5 years,
   k Active or passive demeanor in seeking birth control.

2 *Identifying the problem* or establishing a *nursing diagnosis:* This involves sifting through the information obtained and determining that contraception is indeed desirable for the person. The nursing diagnosis could be, for instance, "birth control teaching necessary" or "past contraceptive failure."

3 *Validation* that the person actually does need birth control and to what extent teaching is required. For instance, it may be necessary to provide information on male and female reproductive function before detailing the specific method. Or the person may have used the method for the past 2 years and may only need updating.

Accurate assessment, although initially time-consuming, may be more helpful by providing the "right" method and information for the person the first time rather than using the trial-and-error approach. It may also prevent contraceptive failure.

Once the need for birth control is established, the next step of the nursing process is to decide, with the person, on *short- and long-term goals.* Does the person prefer to prevent pregnancy permanently or merely to space the interval between the children in the family? At what stage of life is the person (e.g., age 23 with 4 children or age 30 and newly married?) How motivated to prevent pregnancy does the person seem? Answering these questions may actually help the person make a decision and delineate a birth control goal.

Planning nursing care after setting goals should also involve the person; e.g., teaching sessions should be scheduled at the convenience of both the person and the nurse. Respect for the person enhances any receptivity to nursing intervention.

Implementing the nursing care plan usually involves a great deal of teaching about the birth control method. Information that is provided in a respectful, nonauthoritarian manner usually encourages participation. Active participation in meaningful discussions not only lowers anxiety but also facilitates learning about the methods pertinent to the person. This contributes to successful avoidance of pregnancy.[41-43] Implementation may also involve intensive use of referral systems, e.g., if the nurse determines economic, family, or other problems.

The final step in the nursing process is the *evaluation* of the nursing care given. Any birth control method given to a person requires that some follow-up be done to determine whether the method is used consistently, whether it is used properly, how the person likes the method (convenient, messy, etc.), and finally whether the method is successfully preventing pregnancy. Obviously, long-term follow-up is needed in order to determine prevention of pregnancy.

study questions

1 Mrs. C., a 28-year-old Catholic housewife is interested in using the rhythm method of birth control. She asks you to describe it in simple terms. Explain the various rhythm methods, along with the advantages and disadvantages.
2 Tina is 15 years old and sexually active because "it's the thing to do." She is not eager to use birth control because she is embarrassed to talk about it with someone. If you were the nurse in the clinic, how would you begin to intervene so that Tina might accept a method? What approach would you use? How would you arrange discussion of the matter? How would you encourage follow-up?
3 Discuss the IUD and chemical and mechanical barriers as choices for contraception with Mrs. J., who is a clinic patient on welfare with four children. Include advantages and disadvantages of each.
4 You are asked to teach a high school hygiene class for 1 h about family planning. Which methods are best to discuss in this short time span with this group of people? Plan an approach, choosing only three methods that you feel the students should know.
5 Describe the action, usage, effectiveness, contraindications, and major side effects of both types of oral contraceptives with Mrs. Q, a 28-year-old housewife and mother of two.
6 Mary S., 22, is being seen in the ER after being raped. She has received some pills to prevent pregnancy and looks bewildered. Utilizing the nursing process, formulate a nursing care plan for her.

references

1 R. W. Kistner, *The Pill*, Delacorte, New York, 1968.
2 J. L. Tanis, "Recognizing the Reasons for Contraceptive Non-Use and Abuse," *Maternal Child Nursing*, **2**(6):364–369, November/December 1977.
3 H. W. Rudel et al., *Birth Control*, Macmillan, New York, 1973, p. 79.
4 B. K. Timby, "Ovulation Method of Birth Control," *American Journal of Nursing*, **76**(6):928–929, June 1976.
5 M. R. Cohen, "Methods of Determining Ovulation," *Journal of Reproductive Medicine*, **1**(2):182, 1968.
6 M. R. Cohen, "Methods of Birth Control in the United States," *The Medical Committee of Planned Parenthood*, New York, 1972, p. 23.
7 B. Vaughan et al., "Contraceptive Failure Among Married Women in the U.S. 1970–1973." *Family Planning Perspectives*, **9**(6):251–258, November/December 1977.
8 Ibid., pp. 251–258.
9 D. P. Swartz et al., "Choosing Methods of Family Planning," *American Family Physician*, **13**(4):138, April 1976.
10 Ibid., pp. 138–146.
11 Rudel et al., op. cit., p. 180.
12 K. Hagenfeldt, "The Modes of Action of Medicated Intrauterine Devices," *Journal of Reproduction and Fertility, Supplement*, **25**:123, 1976.
13 Ibid., p. 117.

14   Swartz et al., op. cit., p. 138.

15   J. E. Morganthau et al., "Adolescent Contraception: Follow-Up Study." *New York State Journal of Medicine,* **77**(6):928–931, May 1977.

16   "FDA Approves Use of CU-7 IUD for Up to Three Years," *Family Planning Perspectives,* **9**(4):183, July/August 1977.

17   Swartz et al., op. cit., p. 142.

18   A. R. Measham and A. Villegas, "Comparison of Continuation Rates of Intrauterine Devices." *Obstetrics and Gynecology,* **48**(3):336–340, September 1976.

19   "Ectopics Are Least Common with Combination Pills; Are Most Common with Non-Medicated IUD's." *Family Planning Perspectives,* **9**(2):80, March–April 1977.

20   Swartz et al., op. cit., p. 140.

21   Vaughan, op. cit., p. 251.

22   L. Huxall, "Today's Pill and the Individual Woman," *Maternal Child Nursing,* **2**(6):362, November/December 1977.

23   Vaughan, op. cit., p. 258.

24   S. Back et al., "Benign Liver Cell Adenoma Associated with Use of Oral Contraceptive Agents," *Annals of Surgery,* **183**(3):239, March 1976.

25   L. J. Bennion et al., "Effects Of Oral Contraceptives on the Gall Bladder Bile of Normal Women." *New England Journal of Medicine,* **294**(4):189–192, January 22, 1976.

26   J. G. Boyce et al., "Oral Contraceptives and Cervical Carcinoma. *American Journal of Obstetrics and Gynecology,* **128**(7):761–766, August 1, 1977.

27   J. R. Evrard et al., "Amenorrhea Following Oral Contraceptives," *American Journal of Obstetrics and Gynecology,* **124**(1):88–91, January 1, 1976.

28   "Breast Cancer Found Less Frequently Among Pill Users," *Family Planning Perspectives,* **8**(2):79–80, March/April 1976.

29   C. H. Hennekens and B. MacMahon, "Oral Contraceptives and Myocardial Infarction," *New England Journal of Medicine,* **296**(20):1166–1167, May 19, 1977.

30   L. Fleckenstein et al., "Oral Contraceptive Patient Information," *Journal of the American Medical Association,* **235**(13):1335, March 29, 1976.

31   Huxall, op. cit., p. 361.

32   R. A. Erb et al., "Device and Technique for Blocking the Fallopian Tubes. *Obstetrics and Gynecology,* **3**(2):92, 1974.

33   N. Lauersen and K. H. Wilson, "The Abortifacient Effectiveness and Plasma Prostaglandin Concentrations with 15(s)-15 Methylprostaglandin $F_{2\alpha}$ Methylester-containing Vaginal Silastic Devices." *Fertility and Sterility,* **27**(12):1366–1373, December 1976.

34   R. M. Lewy, "Male Contraceptives." *American Family Physician,* **15**(6):107–109, June 1977.

35   J. P. Hearn, "Immunization Against Pregnancy," in R. V. Short and D. T. Baird (eds.), *Contraception of the Future,* The Royal Society, London, 1976, pp. 149–159.

36   D. T. Baird, "Manipulation of the Menstrual Cycle," in ibid., pp. 137–148.

37   Vaughan, op. cit., pp. 251–258.

38   D. Byrne, "A Pregnant Pause in the Sexual Revolution," *Psychology Today,* July 1977, p. 67.

39   D. Taylor, "A New Way to Teach Teens about Contraceptives," *Maternal Child Nursing,* **1**(6):378–383, November/December 1976.

40   S. W. Andrews, "A College Contraceptive Clinic," *American Journal of Nursing,* **76**(4):592, April 1976.

41   S. B. Gusberg et al., "Therapeutic Listening: An Adolescent Guidance Program in Motivation for Contraception," *Mount Sinai Journal of Medicine, New York,* **42**(5):439–444, September/October 1975.

42   J. Haskin et al., "Project Teen Concern: An Educational Approach to the Prevention of V.D. and Premature Parenthood," *Journal of School Health,* **46**(4):231–234, April 1976.

43   Morganthau et al., op. cit., p. 931.

bibliography

Cabliner, W. G. et al.: "Patterns of Contraceptive Failures: The Role of Motivation Reexamined," *Journal of Biosocial Science,* **7**:307, 1975.

Goldzieher, Joseph W. and Tazewell S. Dazier: "Oral Contraceptives and Thromboembolism: A Reassessment," *American Journal of Obstetrics and Gynecology,* **123**(8):878–914, December 15, 1975.

Hatcher, Robert A. et al.: *Contraceptive Technology 1976–1977,* 8th ed., Halsted, New York, 1976.

Hellman, Louis M. and Jack A. Pritchard: *Williams' Obstetrics,* 14th ed., Appleton-Century-Crofts, New York, 1971.

Manisoff, Miriam: *Family Planning: A Teaching Guide For Nurses,* 4th ed., Planned Parenthood World Population, New York, 1973.

———: "Family Planning Democratized," *American Journal of Nursing,* **75**(10):1660–1666, October 1975.

Newton, John et al.: "Nurse Specialist in Family Planning," *British Medical Journal,* **1**(6015):950–952, April 17, 1976.

Taylor, Howard C. (ed.): *Human Reproduction,* M.I.T., Cambridge, Mass., 1976.

Westoff, Charles and Norman B. Ryder: *The Contraceptive Revolution.* Princeton, Princeton, N.J., 1977.

3

CONCEPTION AND FETAL GROWTH AND DEVELOPMENT

FRANCINE H. STIER

2

THE HEALTHY MOTHER

ORIGIN OF EMBRYOLOGY

Although the science of embryology is a relatively new one, curiosity about the beginnings of life existed as early as 2000 years ago. In the fifteenth century, it was believed that the embryo lived fully formed as a miniature person and was encased in a shell formed by the uterus (Fig. 3-1). In the seventeenth century, the cell was discovered, as were the sperm and the egg of the mammal. During the eighteenth century, a new theory emerged—humans were preformed on the head of a sperm cell and sat with head and body flexed. The uterus was its "home" for 9 months (Fig. 3-2). Darwin's theory of evolution in 1859 proposed embryonic resemblance between human beings and other species. This sparked intense study of the embryo by scientists eager to prove or refute his theory. The twentieth century has heralded the most fascinating and accurate study of the begin-

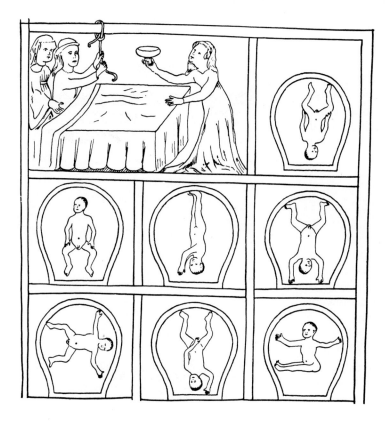

fig. 3-1 Fifteenth-century illustration purporting to show fetal positions within the uterus. (*From Clark Edward Corliss, Patten's Human Embryology, McGraw-Hill, New York, 1976, p. 2.*)

nings of life. As you will see in this chapter, the embryo has been scrutinized, photographed, and filmed from the moment of conception through birth, thus making its study more real than descriptive.

REPRODUCTIVE ANATOMY

In order to understand the nature of pregnancy, it is important to know how the female provides for and sustains the life of the fetus and how the male contributes to the beginning of the new life.

fig. 3-2 Reproduction of Hartsoeker's drawing of a sperm, showing a preformed individual (homonuclus) in the head. (*From Clark Edward Corliss, Patten's Human Embryology, McGraw-Hill, New York, 1976, p. 2.*)

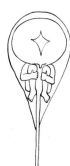

female reproductive anatomy

The ovaries are paired gonads located in the female pelvis closely situated to the *fimbriae* or fingerlike openings of the *fallopian tubes* (uterine tubes). The ovaries are suspended in the pelvic cavity by ligaments. When an *ovum* (egg) is released from the surface of the ovary, it is propelled toward the fimbriated ends of the fallopian tube by continuous motion of cilia in the fimbriae pulling it into the 10.5-cm-long tube. It passes along the tube into the *uterus* (Fig. 3-3).

The uterus is a pear-shaped organ which has very thick smooth muscle walls. It is approximately 8 cm long and 5 cm wide at the uppermost end and is located between the bladder and the rectum. The *anterior* (upper) portion of the uterus is called the *fundus*. The *uterine cavity*, located in the body of the uterus, is continuous with the *internal cervical os*, or the tapered end of the uterus. The *external cervical os* opens into the *vagina*.

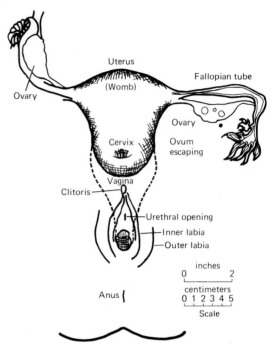

fig. 3-4 External view of perineal structures in relation to internal organs. (*Courtesy of Jane Margolin.*)

fig. 3-3 Uterus, fallopian tubes, and ovaries. (*Courtesy of Jane Margolin.*)

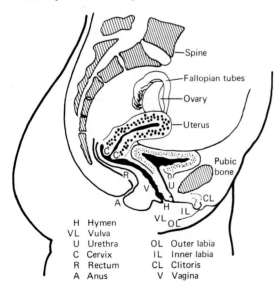

H	Hymen		
VL	Vulva		
U	Urethra	OL	Outer labia
C	Cervix	IL	Inner labia
R	Rectum	CL	Clitoris
A	Anus	V	Vagina

The vagina extends approximately 10.5 cm in length and encloses the lower end of the cervix. The vagina has a single orifice, or *introitus*, to the outside and is surrounded externally by the *labia minora* and the *labia majora* (small and large "lips") (Fig. 3-4).

male reproductive anatomy

Unlike the female ovarian structure, the male gonads or *testes* do not lie in the abdominal cavity but are suspended in a sac called the *scrotum* directly behind the penis. During the fetal development of the male, however, the gonads develop within the peritoneal cavity until approximately the third month of gestation, when they begin to descend toward the scrotum. The scrotum is divided by a *septum* (partition) of connective tissue, so that each testis eventually has its own separate compartment. The *sperm* or male cells produced in the testes must travel through a long series of ducts before leaving the body. *Convoluted* or *seminiferous* tubules are located within the testes. From these seminiferous tubules, where sperm form, the sperm move through several ducts and converge on the *rete testes* which empties into the ducts leading to the epididymus. The mature sperm collect in the epididymis, awaiting expulsion into the *ductus* or *vas deferens* (see Fig. 3-5).

The *seminal vescicle* (or gland) forms the fluid medium for the sperm during ejaculation. The fluid allows the sperm to become mobile and provides for its nourishment. During ejaculation, the sperm travel through the vas deferens and become lubricated with the fluid secreted by the seminal vescicle, the prostate gland, and the bulbourethral or *Cowper's glands*. This fluid is now called *semen* and is passed through the urethra and out of the body by forcible, rhythmic muscular contractions during ejaculation.

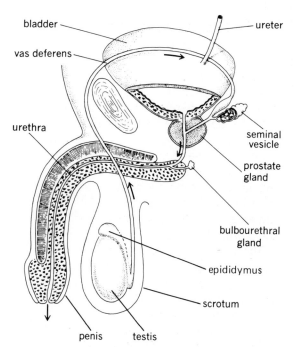

fig. 3-5 Anatomic organization of the male reproductive tract. (*From A. J. Vander, J. H. Sherman, and D. Luciano, Human Physiology, McGraw-Hill, New York, 1970.*)

REPRODUCTIVE PHYSIOLOGY

menstrual cycle

It takes approximately 1 month to complete the female reproductive cycle. The monthly discharge of blood, cellular material, and mucus is called *menstruation* and lasts 3 to 6 days. The events of the menstrual cycle occur in order to prepare the uterus, specifically the *endometrium* (internal uterine lining), to receive a fertilized ovum. Periodic changes of growth and sloughing of the endometrial tissue can be described by phases, which are named for the dominant hormone or activity of the phase. The *follicular* phase begins immediately after menses starts, and *ovulation* (the release of the ovum) occurs approximately 14 days prior to the onset of the next menses. The *luteal* or *progestational phase* ends as menses begins.

The follicular phase of the menstrual cycle is delineated by the rapid growth and repair of the endometrial tissue following the previous menses. This regeneration of tissue is thought to be activated by the hormonal control of *estrogen*, which produces its maximum effect until ovulation occurs. The luteal or progestational phase begins with ovulation and is characterized by the maintenance of thick endometrial tissue resulting from the hormonal influence of *progesterone*. If the ovum is not fertilized, the spongy edematous layer of endometrial tissue begins to slough off. It is thought that this sloughing process occurs because the hormone levels of estrogen and progesterone are withdrawn and the corpus luteum (the tissue in the ovary from which the ovum was released) degenerates (Fig. 3-6).

ovarian cycle

The ovary also goes through rhythmic, cyclical changes. Proliferation of *oocytes* (female cells) and the process of ovulation continues on approximately a monthly schedule.

The ovaries of a female approaching puberty contain all the cells necessary for sexual reproduction. Each *primary oocyte* within the ovaries is surrounded by several layers of cells which will become a *follicle*. Surrounding the follicle as it matures are cells which produce estrogens. In each cycle, only a single follicle matures enough to be called a *graafian follicle*, which ruptures to liberate the ovum inside. On approximately a monthly basis, a primary oocyte (about 40,000 of which

fig. 3-6 Mature human ovum entirely surrounded by follicle cells. *(Courtesy of Landrum B. Shettles, from R. Rugh, and L. B. Shettles, From Conception to Birth: The Drama of Life's Beginnings, Harper & Row, New York, 1971.)*

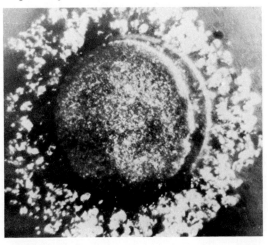

are in the ovaries) will mature to become ova within the graafian follicle, while others atrophy in various stages of maturation.

the process of ovulation

Ovulation is the process of the rupture of the graafian follicle and the release of the ovum into the abdominal cavity. The precise mechanism which causes the follicle to rupture is not known, but several factors contribute: (1) the increased pressure of fluid within the graafian follicle, (2) compression of the surrounding blood vessels due to the size of the follicle and decreased nutrition to the cells, and (3) hormonal stimulation of a surge of LH from the anterior pituitary gland.

The follicle ruptures and, with an explosive force, releases the ovum, which is promptly swept into the fimbriated end of the fallopian tube. (See front inside cover, Plate A.) At the same time, the walls of the graafian follicle collapse, turn yellow, and form what is known as the *corpus luteum.*

The life of the corpus luteum depends upon whether or not the ovum becomes fertilized (see Fig. 3-8). If fertilization occurs, the corpus luteum continues to develop. It produces the hormone progesterone which promotes the growth of the endometrium in the menstrual cycle or maintains the pregnancy until about the fourth month of gestation. If the ovum is not fertilized the corpus luteum develops for 8 to 10 days and then begins to degenerate. Because of this limited life-span, menstruation almost always occurs 14 ± 2 days after ovulation, regardless of the total length of the menstrual cycle. Variation in the time span of the menstrual cycle may be caused by the inconsistent degree of development of the ovarian follicles at the start of each menstrual cycle (Fig. 3-7).

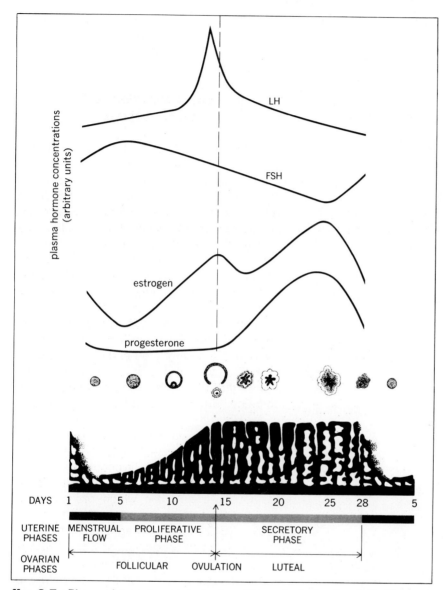

fig. 3-7 Plasma hormone concentration. (*From A. J. Vander, J. H. Sherman, and D. Luciano, Human Physiology, McGraw-Hill, New York, 1970.*)

hormonal regulation of the reproductive cycle

The cyclical rhythm of the female reproductive mechanism is a result of complex coordination of hormones and is influenced by the hypothalamus, which controls the release of hormones from the anterior lobe of the pituitary gland. Three *gonadotropic* hormones (hormones which act on the gonads) from the anterior pituitary gland come into play: (1) the follicle-stimulating hormone (FSH), (2) the luteinizing hormone (LH), and (3) the luteotropic hormone (LTH) or prolactin (Fig. 3-8).

The FSH activates the ovarian follicle to grow and mature. As the follicle matures, it begins producing the estrogenic hormones necessary to complete the cycle of events. These estrogenic hormones cause physiologic changes in the breasts, uterus, fallopian tubes, and vagina in preparation for their reproductive work. The luteinizing hormone is primary, along with FSH for inducing the ovarian follicle to grow, mature, and finally rupture, releasing the mature ovum. After ovulation occurs, LH stimulates the formation of the corpus luteum, which then begins to secrete progesterone. In order for the corpus luteum to continue secreting progesterone, LTH is necessary. Progesterone, along with estrogen and LTH, prepares the uterine lining for the implantation of the fertilized ovum by thickening its mucous membrane and increasing its blood supply. Progesterone also has an inhibitory effect on FSH levels—essentially suppressing the maturation of another follicle while the body is preparing to receive a fertilized ovum. (The higher levels of progesterone during pregnancy also suppress ovulation.)

Hormonal regulation of the male reproductive system is very similar to that of the female. At puberty, the hypothalamus stimulates the anterior pituitary to secrete FSH and LH which activate the testes to secrete *testosterone*. This male hormone begins the process of maturation of the male reproductive cells—the sperm (see Fig. 3-9).

It is important to note that the entire hormonal interplay functions on what is known as a "feedback" mechanism; i.e., the hormone levels and glandular activities are interdependent and reciprocal. The feedback mechanism can be seen in the relationships between the pituitary and ovarian hormones (see Fig. 3-10). When FSH and LH are at their peak, they stimulate the secretion of estrogen and progesterone, respectively. After ovulation, estrogen and progesterone rise and the levels of FSH and LH fall correspondingly.

CELLULAR REPRODUCTION

In discussing ovulation, the maturation of the follicle and ovum was mentioned. In order to mature, the ovum must undergo a complex mechanism of cellular division. Prior to an explanation of the maturation of the ovum and sperm, it is necessary to review briefly how all cells, other than sex cells, divide.

mitosis

In all somatic tissue, the parent cells divide by duplicating each chromosome, along with its DNA, so that each daughter cell receives an exact replica of the genetic material in the parent cell. This type of reproduction assures that all the resultant cells will be exactly like the original cell in chromosomal content.

fig. 3-8 Menstrual cycle influences. (*Courtesy of Wyeth Laboratories.*)

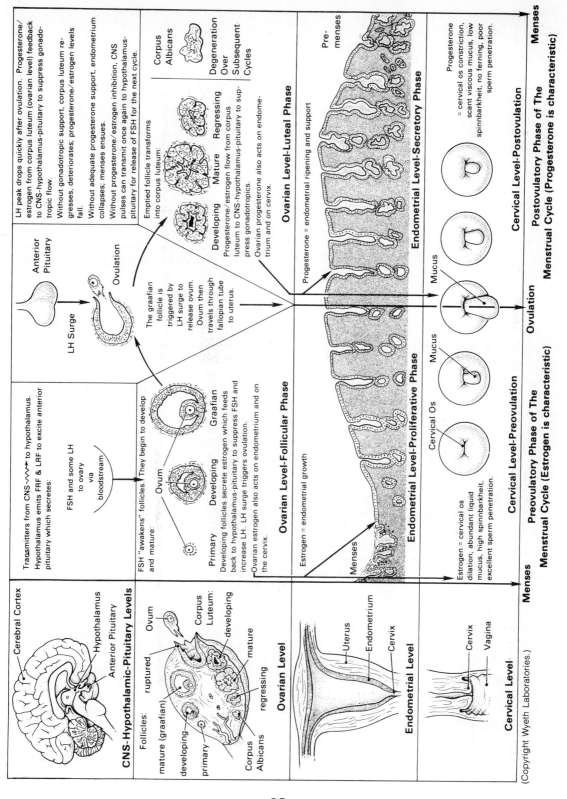

(Copyright Wyeth Laboratories.)

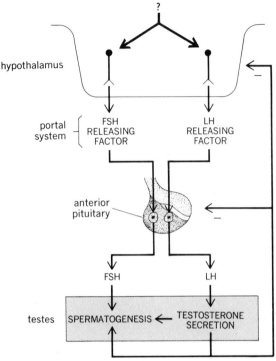

fig. 3-9 Summary of male hormonal control. (*From A. J. Vander, J. H. Sherman, and D. Luciano, Human Physiology, McGraw-Hill, New York, 1970.*)

meiosis or reduction division

The process of *maturation* or *reduction division* assures that when ova and sperm unite, the number of chromosomes remains at 23 pairs or 46 from generation to generation. Therefore, before joining, each gamete must contain half the original number of chromosomes.

The formation of gametes and the reduction in chromosome number is accomplished in two highly unique cell divisions. The first is called the *first meiotic division,* in which both male and female *primitive germ cells* (the primary oocyte and the primary spermatocyte) replicate their DNA and double their chro-

mosomes. These cells undergoing meiosis have a prolonged first phase, in which members of alike or *homologous* chromosomes pair and begin an interchange of similar genetic material from one chromosome to its pair. This interchange is also called *crossing-over.* It provides for a variety of recombinations of hereditary features. Then, the intimately paired chromosomes separate so that one member of each pair of chromosomes goes to a different daughter cell. After the first meiotic division, each daughter cell contains the *haploid* (half) number of chromosomes— 23. (However, each chromosome still contains double the amount of DNA.) (See Fig. 3-11.)

In the *second meiotic division*, the double-

fig. 3-10 Summary of hormonal control of follicle and ovum development. (*From A. J. Vander, J. H. Sherman, and D. Luciano, Human Physiology, McGraw-Hill, New York, 1970.*)

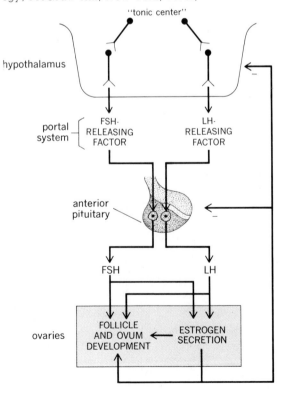

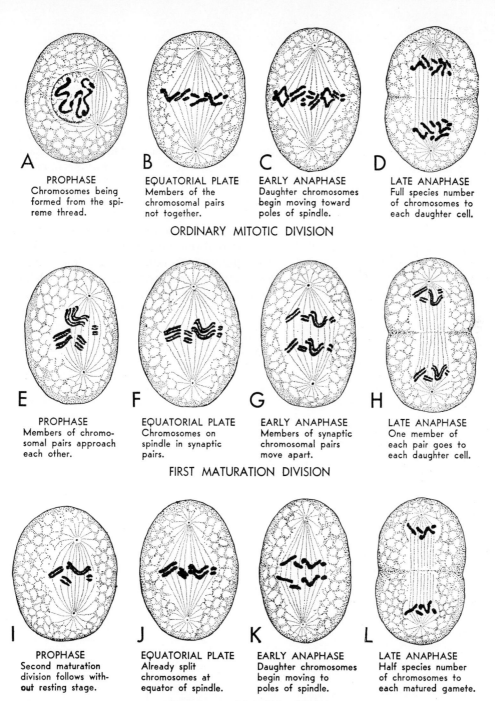

A PROPHASE
Chromosomes being formed from the spireme thread.

B EQUATORIAL PLATE
Members of the chromosomal pairs not together.

C EARLY ANAPHASE
Daughter chromosomes begin moving toward poles of spindle.

D LATE ANAPHASE
Full species number of chromosomes to each daughter cell.

ORDINARY MITOTIC DIVISION

E PROPHASE
Members of chromosomal pairs approach each other.

F EQUATORIAL PLATE
Chromosomes on spindle in synaptic pairs.

G EARLY ANAPHASE
Members of synaptic chromosomal pairs move apart.

H LATE ANAPHASE
One member of each pair goes to each daughter cell.

FIRST MATURATION DIVISION

I PROPHASE
Second maturation division follows without resting stage.

J EQUATORIAL PLATE
Already split chromosomes at equator of spindle.

K EARLY ANAPHASE
Daughter chromosomes begin moving to poles of spindle.

L LATE ANAPHASE
Half species number of chromosomes to each matured gamete.

SECOND MATURATION DIVISION

fig. 3-11 Diagrams showing schematically the differences between the chromosomal behavior in an ordinary mitotic division and in maturation divisions. (*From C. E. Corliss, Patten's Human Embryology, McGraw-Hill, New York, 1976, p. 19.*)

structured chromosomes divide, thus completing the division which began in the first meiotic division. Each resultant cell contains now 23 single strands of chromosomes, so that the amount of DNA is half that of a somatic cell. The purpose of two meiotic divisions, then, is to enable each original pair of chromosomes to exchange their genetic material (the first division) and to provide each germ cell with half the number of chromosomes and half the amount of DNA (the second division).

Each of the four cells resulting from the oocyte meiotic divisions contain 22 autosomes and one X chromosome. One of the four cells will develop into a mature oocyte; the other three cells become *polar bodies,* which receive little cytoplasm for nourishment and eventually degenerate. In contrast, two of

the male gametes will each contain 22 autosomes and one X chromosome, while the other two each contain 22 autosomes and one Y chromosome (see Fig. 3-12).

oogenesis The origin of the germ cells can be traced back to the embryo where primitive germ cells form and grow between the third and fifth week of embryonic life. The primitive germ cells migrate to the gonads during embryonic life, and once there, they begin to differentiate into *oogonia* (early ova). They undergo rapid mitosis and develop into *primary oocytes* and then enter the first meiotic division. By the seventh month of fetal life, the primary oocytes become surrounded by tissue which becomes follicle cells.

At birth, the primary oocytes have finished

fig. 3-12 Summary of ovum and sperm maturation.

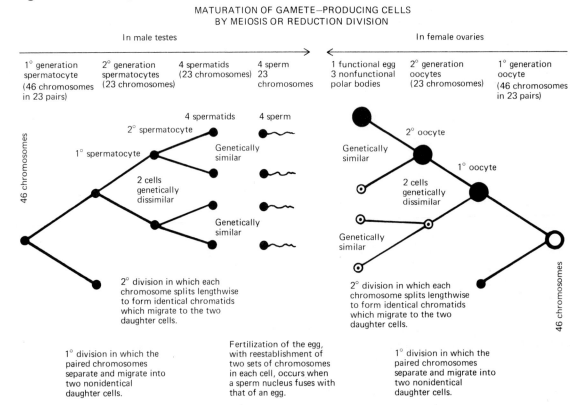

MATURATION OF GAMETE—PRODUCING CELLS
BY MEIOSIS OR REDUCTION DIVISION

In male testes

In female ovaries

| 1° generation spermatocyte (46 chromosomes in 23 pairs) | 2° generation spermatocytes (23 chromosomes) | 4 spermatids (23 chromosomes) | 4 sperm 23 chromosomes | 1 functional egg 3 nonfunctional polar bodies | 2° generation oocytes (23 chromosomes) | 1° generation oocyte (46 chromosomes in 23 pairs) |

46 chromosomes

4 spermatids   4 sperm

2° spermatocyte

1° spermatocyte

Genetically similar

2 cells genetically dissimilar

Genetically similar

2° oocyte

Genetically similar

1° oocyte

2 cells genetically dissimilar

Genetically similar

46 chromosomes

2° division in which each chromosome splits lengthwise to form identical chromatids which migrate to the two daughter cells.

2° division in which each chromosome splits lengthwise to form identical chromatids which migrate to the two daughter cells.

1° division in which the paired chromosomes separate and migrate into two nonidentical daughter cells.

Fertilization of the egg, with reestablishment of two sets of chromosomes in each cell, occurs when a sperm nucleus fuses with that of an egg.

1° division in which the paired chromosomes separate and migrate into two nonidentical daughter cells.

part of the first meiotic division and enter a resting phase until puberty. The total number of primary oocytes at birth is between 700,000 and 2 million, but the number will shrink by puberty, so that about 40,000 remain. It is important to note that oocytes, which in the first meiotic division remain dormant for more than 35 years, may be vulnerable to damage (aging), thus contributing to the chromosomal abnormalities occurring more often in older mothers (see Chap. 28). After puberty begins, the primitive follicles repeatedly develop into mature graafian follicles. The primary oocytes also complete their first meiotic division at this point.

The primary oocyte begins to increase in size and thickness and develops a protective membrane called the *zona pellucida*. The follicle cells form a thick, fluid-filled layer around the oocyte. As soon as the follicle matures, the oocyte resumes the meiotic division to produce two cells of unequal size: the *secondary oocyte* and the *first polar body*. The secondary oocyte receives all the cytoplasm and rapidly enters the second meiotic division. At this point, ovulation occurs, and the secondary oocyte is released from the ovary. Note that the second meiotic division is completed only if the ovum is fertilized; otherwise the ovum degenerates in approximately 24 h. (See front inside cover, Plate B.)

spermatogenesis During the fifth week of embryonic life, the primitive germ cells enter the developing gonads, where they become part of the primitive sex cords. These primitive sex cords become the seminiferous tubules after birth. At puberty, the *spermatogonia,* which are the primitive male germ cells, develop into *primary spermatocytes*. The primary spermatocytes begin the first meiotic division and give rise to two *secondary spermatocytes*. These secondary spermatocytes then begin to undergo the second maturation division immediately, which gives

rise to four *spermatids*. Each spermatid contains half the number of chromosomes of the primary spermatocyte (Fig. 3-12).

When the spermatids form, they undergo a number of changes in order to develop the characteristic shape of the *spermatozoa,* the head, middle piece, and tail (see Fig. 3-13). During this process, the spermatids are embedded in the *Sertoli cells* (sustaining cells) of the seminiferous tubules, which provide the nourishment needed for spermatids to undergo changes in shape. As soon as the spermatozoa are fully formed, they enter the lumen of the seminiferous tubules and travel to the epididymis, where they attain full motility.

The mature sperm have very little independent source of nutrition when separated from the Sertoli cells. Perhaps this is why billions of spermatozoa are produced in the male reproductive life—to ensure the reproduction of the species.

fig. 3-13 Mature human sperm. (*From A. J. Vander, J. H. Sherman, and D. Luciano, Human Physiology, McGraw-Hill, New York, 1970.*)

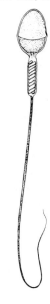

FERTILIZATION OF THE OVUM

There are many factors necessary for effective fertilization of the ovum. Coitus results in an average of 200 to 300 million sperm being deposited in the vaginal canal close to the cervical os. The sperm then have a hazardous route to travel through the uterus into the outer third of the fallopian tube where fertilization normally occurs. The distance of about 21 cm for the sperm to negotiate involves many factors which may impede their progress, e.g., incompatible vaginal or cervical fluids or a pH environment that is too acidic; possible narrowing of the cervix, uterus, or tubes; and leukocytosis in the uterus. However, by sheer numbers, many sperm (approximately 2000) reach their destination. After ejaculation, the life-span of the sperm is relatively short (24 to 72 h average) because the sources of energy and nutrition become quickly exhausted in the difficult process of moving toward the fallopian tubes.

Normally only one of the many sperm reaching the ovum will enter; the others aid the fertilizing sperm by secreting an enzyme which penetrates the zona pellucida. As fertilization occurs, a process called *syngamy* acts to protect the fertilized ovum. Syngamy is a whole set of reactions that occur at once and rapidly:

1 The ovum completes its second maturation division and extrudes a polar body (Fig. 3-14).
2 A reaction occurs in the oocyte cytoplasm, just below the cell membrane, which causes the membrane to harden and form a barrier to prevent any other sperm from entering the cell.
3 The tail of the sperm disappears, and the nucleus becomes larger, revealing its chromosomal content. At this point, it becomes known as the *male pronucleus*

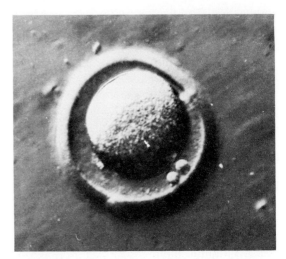

fig. 3-14 Fertilized egg with two polar bodies— 12 h. Photographed through a phase microscope 12 h after being fertilized by a human sperm. The surrounding follicle cells and extra spermatozoa have dispersed, and the two polar bodies (discarded nuclei) are seen in the perivitelline space. There is no external evidence of the very dynamic changes that are occurring within the egg for the first division into two cells. (*From R. Rugh and L. B. Shettles, From Conception to Birth: The Drama of Life's Beginnings, Harper & Row, New York, 1971.*)

(sperm nucleus before it fuses with the nucleus of the ovum.)
4 The *female pronucleus* (the nucleus of the ovum before it fuses with the nucleus of the sperm) swells.
5 The two pronuclei gravitate toward one another and fuse, thus completing the process of fertilization by restoring the full number of chromosomes to the fertilized ovum, which is now called the *zygote*. The sex of the fertilized ovum is determined by whether a sperm bearing an X or Y chromosome was successful.

cleavage

The next major step is *cleavage,* the division of the zygote which occurs 24 to 48 h after fertilization. The two daughter cells resulting from this division are half the size of the fertilized ovum; continued division results in progressively smaller cells because the zona pellucida remains intact, containing the dividing cells at the same size as the fertilized ovum. As cleavage occurs, the zygote travels down the fallopian tube toward the uterus. After several divisions the zygote begins to look like a solid ball of cells called the *morula,* resembling a mulberry (see Fig. 3-15).

implantation

At the morula stage, the dividing zygote is passed into the uterus, approximately 3 to 4 days after fertilization. The cells can now be distinguished one from another—not in their form but in their function. A group of centrally located cells become known as the *inner cell mass,* or *embryoblast* (which eventually becomes the embryo), and the surrounding layer of cells becomes the *outer cell mass,* or *trophoblast* (which eventually becomes the chorion and placenta). When the morula reaches the uterine cavity, fluid begins penetrating it, swelling the cells to form a cavity and destroying the zona pellucida (see Fig. 3-16). At this point, when the inner cell mass is separated from the outer cell mass by a fluid-filled cavity, the cells become known as a *blastula,* or *blastocyst,* and grow rapidly. This fluid-filled cavity provides nourishment for the cells as they remain free in the uterus for another 3 to 4 days (Fig. 3-17). Approximately 7 days after ovulation (or on the 21st day of a 28-day menstrual cycle) the surface cells or trophoblast layers begin to burrow their way into the lining of the uterus, which is thick and succulent (see Fig. 3-18). Implantation is accomplished by the trophoblast cells because they are able to digest or liquefy tissue by means of secreted enzymes. The blastocyst sinks deeply into the decidua

fig. 3-15 Schematic diagram of sequence of events in cleavage. *(From B. M. Patten, Human Embryology, 3d ed., McGraw-Hill, New York, 1968.)*

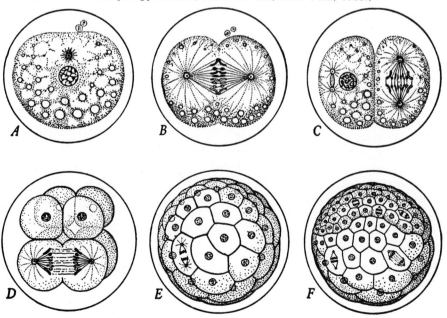

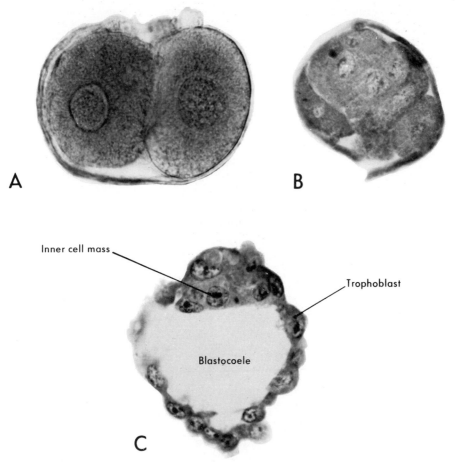

fig. 3-16 Human embryo in cleavage and blastodermic vesicle stages. (*From C. E. Corliss, Patten's Human Embryology, 4th ed., McGraw-Hill, New York, 1976.*)

(now called the *decidua basalis*). The trophoblast sends fingerlike projections into blood-filled areas that result from broken maternal blood vessels and firmly anchor the blastocyst. The trophoblastic tissue invading the decidua basalis becomes known as the *chorion*, and the fingerlike projections become known as the *chorionic villi*.

By the ninth or tenth day after fertilization, the uterine epithelium has begun to heal over the area in which the blastocyst is embedded and is now called the *decidua capsularis*.

By the end of the third month, when the growth of the embryo causes the decidua capsularis and the *decidua parietalis* (the lining of the uterus farthest from the site of implantation) to compress each other, the chorionic villi remain only in the decidua basalis (see Fig. 3-19). These chorionic villi, which are intimately associated with the decidua basalis, eventually become the placenta.

The chorion becomes one of the two fetal membranes of the placenta, the other being the *amnion*, which begins to develop by the eighth day after fertilization. The amnion starts as a small vescicle and grows into a sac which surrounds the embryo (see Fig. 3-20).

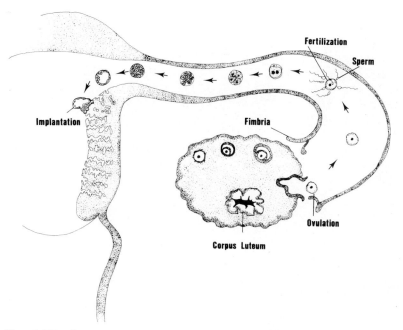

fig. 3-17 Schematic representation of events taking place during the first week of human development. (1) Oocyte immediately after ovulation. (2) Fertilization approximately 12 to 24 h after ovulation. (3) Stage of the male and female pronuclei. (4) Spindle of the first meiotic division. (5) Two-cell stage (approximately 30 h of age). (6) Morula containing 12 to 16 blastomeres. (7) Advanced morula stage reaching the uterine lumen (approximately 3 days of age). (8) Early blastocyst stage (approximately 4½ days of age). The zona pellucida has now disappeared. (9) Early phase of implantation. (Blastocyst approximately 6 days of age.) The ovary shows the stages of transformation between a primary follicle and a graafian follicle as well as a corpus luteum. The uterine endometrium is depicted in the progestational stage. (*From Jan Langman, Medical Embryology, 3d ed., Williams & Wilkins, Baltimore, 1975, p. 30; redrawn by Patricia Rodriguez-Lovink.*)

As it grows, the amnion eventually comes into contact with the chorion, and the two layers become known as the *fetal membranes.*

DEVELOPMENT OF THE EMBRYO
the germ layers

The cells of the inner cell mass begin differentiating by the eighth day after fertilization into two distinct layers: (1) *ectodermal* (the outer layer closest to the trophoblast cells) and (2) *endodermal* (adjacent to the ecto-derm). Small clefts begin appearing within the ectodermal layer and form a cavity between the ectoderm and the trophoblast layers called the *amniotic cavity*. This cavity separates the embryonic tissues from the trophoblast layer. By the tenth day, the amniotic cavity has developed a layer of cells around it called the amnion, the beginning of the membrane which will surround the fetus as it develops. The amnion cells begin now to secrete a fluid for the cavity.

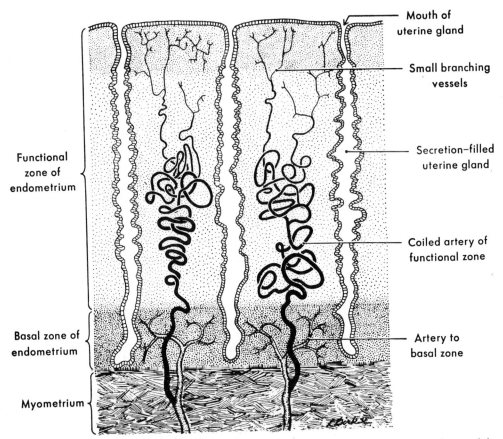

Mouth of
uterine gland

Small branching
vessels

Secretion-filled
uterine gland

Functional
zone of
endometrium

Coiled artery of
functional zone

Basal zone of
endometrium

Artery to
basal zone

Myometrium

fig. 3-18 Schematic drawing showing uterine mucosa during the secretory phase of the menstrual cycle. (*From C. E. Corliss, Patten's Human Embryology, 4th ed., McGraw-Hill, New York, 1976.*)

The cells of the endoderm begin extending in a circle beneath the ectoderm cells to enclose what becomes the *yolk sac* (see Fig. 3-20). The yolk sac functions temporarily to make blood cells for the embryo until the liver, spleen, and bone marrow can take over.

At the end of the second week of development, the two germ layers begin developing a *primitive streak,* which is a groove of cells between the ectoderm and the endoderm layers. These cells form the third germ layer, known as the *mesodermal* layer. The primitive streak establishes the long axis of the developing embryo.

The establishment of the three germ layers marks the beginning of the period of specialization, for not only are the three layers distinctly different at this point but also each layer begins its process of cell differentiation to form the varied organs and tissues of the body. Even before it can be seen under a microscope, each cell is "programmed" at a particular point in its development. The programming occurs in different ways for different tissues. For instance, some cells destined to become one type of tissue influence the cells around them to follow suit, e.g., the lens of the eye. Other cells migrate to the appropriate

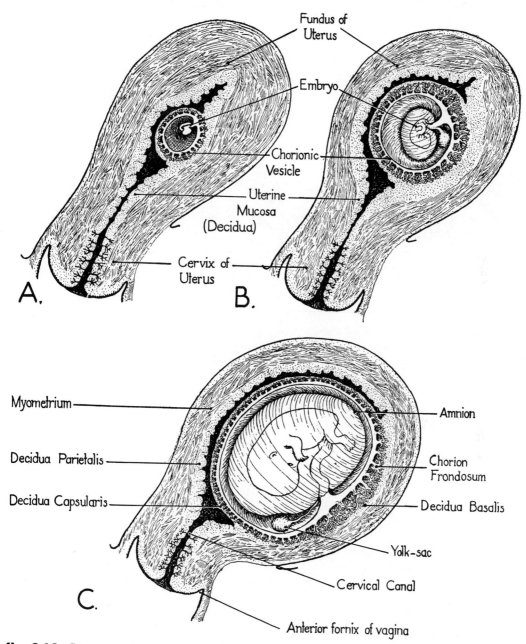

Fundus of
Uterus

Embryo

Chorionic
Vesicle

Uterine
Mucosa
(Decidua)

Cervix of
Uterus

A.

B.

Myometrium

Decidua Parietalis

Decidua Capsularis

Amnion

Chorion
Frondosum

Decidua Basalis

Yolk-sac

Cervical Canal

Anterior fornix of vagina

C.

fig. 3-19   Diagrams showing the uterus in the early weeks of pregnancy at 3, 5, and 8 weeks. (Drawn to actual size, primipara.) (*From B. M. Patten, Human Embryology, 3d ed., McGraw-Hill, New York, 1968.*)

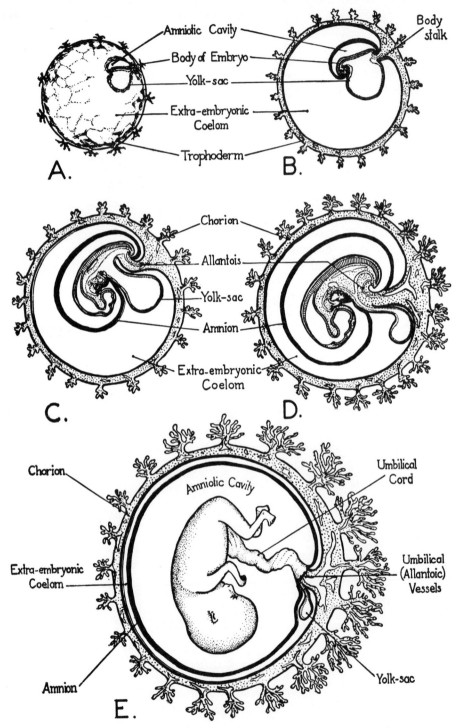

fig. 3-20 Early changes and interrelations of embryo and extraembryonic membranes. (*From C. E. Corliss, Patten's Human Embryology, 4th ed., McGraw-Hill, New York, 1976.*)

spot for development. Still others grow more rapidly than adjacent cells, causing the tissues to "fold," thus growing into the characteristic shape of the organ.

By the end of the third week, the germ layers have begun to form distinct tissues. The ectoderm layer gives rise to the central nervous system, which appears at first as a round thickening in the cephalic region of the embryo. The brain begins developing first, so that when the form of the embryo can be identified, the head appears about one-third the size of the entire body and is flexed over onto the chest (Fig. 3-21). The ectoderm also gives rise to the peripheral nervous system; the sensory epithelium of the sense organs; the epidermis of the hair, nails, and subcutaneous glands; the hypophysis; the enamel of the teeth, and the epithelial lining of many organs.

The mesodermal layer gives rise to *somites* (or segments) forming along the body of the embryo. By the end of the third week, these somites begin forming the heart, which begins to beat irregularly around the 24th day. The mesoderm also gives rise to all the connective tissue layers, the bone, muscle, blood, and lymph, the kidney and urinary tract systems, the gonads, and the spleen.

As a result of cephalocaudal folding of the embryo, much of the yolk sac (of endodermal origin) is incorporated into the body of the embryo proper. This becomes part of the abdominal cavity. Thus the endodermal layer gives rise to the gastrointestinal (GI) tract, the epithelial lining of the bladder and urethra, the thyroid, the parathyroids, the liver, and the pancreas.

THE FIRST TRIMESTER

During the fourth to the eighth week of development, the growing cells are known as the embryo. By the end of the eighth week, *organogenesis*, the period when the main

fig. 3-21   Human embryo of about 12 days' fertilization age. (*From C. E. Corliss, Patten's Human Embryology, McGraw-Hill, New York, 1976, p. 39.*)

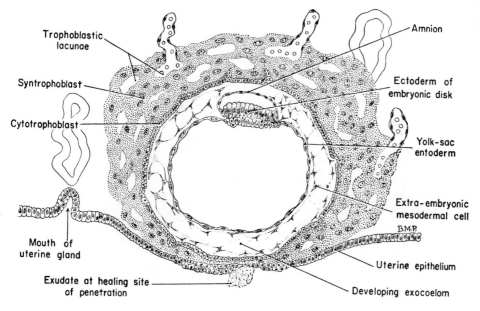

organ systems have been laid down, is completed. As a result of this organ formation, the shape of the embryo changes dramatically, so that the major features of the body form can be recognized. Thus the main systems have begun to form long before the mother becomes aware that she is pregnant.

By the end of the fourth week, the embryo is approximately 6 mm long, and the head is approximately one-third the total length. Outlines of the eyes can be seen above the primitive mouth cavity. The heart is beating asynchronously. The vertebral column is beginning to form, and the GI tract, liver, gallbladder, pancreas, and thyroid gland can be identified.

The fifth week shows greater development of the limbs, which begin as paddle-shaped buds (see Figs. 3-22 and 3-23). The face begins to look more human in form as the ear pits, jaw, nose, and eyes take shape. During this week the body stalk, which was visible at 3 weeks, begins forming a primitive umbilical cord. The body stalk forms between the trophoblast implantation in the decidua and the forming embryo. In the early stage of the body stalk, a chain of vessels provides circulation between the embryo and the chorionic villi. These vessels soon fuse into one large vein and two small arteries surrounded by connective tissue and mucus called *Wharton's jelly* which protects the blood vessels. At birth the umbilical cord will be approximately 2 cm in diameter and 50 to 60 cm long.

In the sixth week, the muscles are forming and beginning to establish nerve impulses for reflex functioning. The eyes are becoming pigmented, and the sensory retinal ends of the eye form. At this time the embryo is approximately 1 cm in length. Cartilage centers are formed in preparation for later bone development. The kidney, in rudimentary form, is beginning, and the urethra completes patent communication with the outside of the body. The penis is beginning to form, and the ovaries and testes are now distinguishable. The liver is starting to take over the job of forming red blood cells.

In the seventh week, the eyelids form, and the eyes and ears continue to develop rapidly. The palate and tongue are formed, and the neck can be seen more clearly. Bone cells are beginning to replace cartilage in the jaw, ribs, and vertebrae. Muscles are moving in a coordinated fashion—the arms and legs begin moving laterally. The ovaries and testes begin to move from their point of origin toward

fig. 3-22 Development of human hands. (a) Hand plate, 5 weeks. (b) Finger ridges, 6 weeks. (c) Definite thumb and fingers with pads, 7 weeks. (d) Regression of finger pads, 12 weeks. (*Courtesy Carnegie Institute, Washington, D. C. From R. Rugh, and L. B. Shettles, From Conception to Birth: The Drama of Life's Beginnings, Harper & Row, New York, 1971.*)

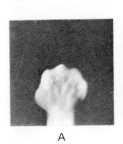 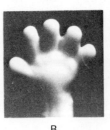 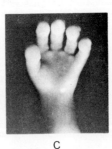 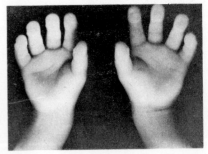

A   B   C   D

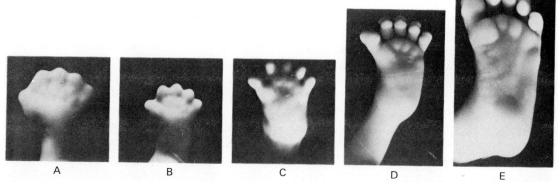

fig. 3-23 Development of human feet. (a) Foot plate, 6 weeks. (b) Toe ridges, 2 days later. (c) Heel development, 7 weeks. (d) Note walking pads, 8 weeks. (e) Regression of toe pads, 12 weeks. (*Courtesy Carnegie Institute, Washington, D. C. From R. Rugh and L. B. Shettles, From Conception to Birth: The Drama of Life's Beginnings, Harper & Row, New York, 1971.*)

their adult sites. The urogenital and rectal passages are now separate.

At 8 weeks the hands and feet are well formed. The eyes are moving toward the front of the face, and the major blood vessels are being formed. The heart is very small but has established the four chambers and is beating about 40 to 80 times a minute. The thyroid and adrenal glands are well formed, as are the taste buds. The embryo now measures 3 cm in length and weighs 2 g (see Fig. 3-24).

This embryonic period is marked by very

fig. 3-24 Human fetus, 54 days (22.5 mm or ⅞ in.) (a) Right side; (b) front; (c) left side. (*Photo by E. Ludwig. From R. Rugh, and L. B. Shettles, From Conception to Birth: The Drama of Life's Beginnings, Harper & Row, New York, 1971.*)

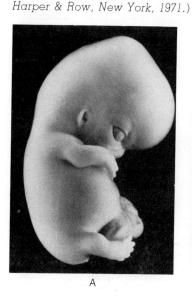

A

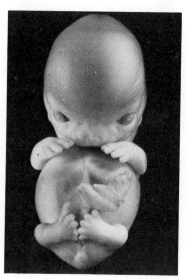

B

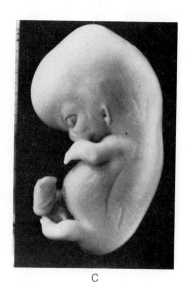

C

rapid growth and differentiation of tissue. It is characterized by extreme susceptibility to any adverse environmental influences such as radiation, infection, drugs, or smoking. The end of the embryonic period is marked by the fact that all organ systems have at least begun to form, while many are completely formed at this time (see Fig. 20-1).

The ninth week begins the third month in the first trimester of pregnancy. At this point, the embryo is called a *fetus;* the time between the beginning of the ninth week and birth is called the *fetal period* and is a time of rapid growth of the fetus. Some tissue differentiation is still occurring, of course, e.g., in the genitourinary (GU) tract, eyes, and lungs.

At 9 weeks the fetus is about 5 cm from crown to rump and weighs about 5 g. The

eyelids finish forming and seal shut for 3 months. Fingernails and toenails are forming. The heartbeat can be faintly heard with an ultrasound instrument. Finally, the genitalia of male and female are now well defined.

During the tenth week, the fetus is 6 cm from crown to rump and weighs 10 g. The head slows in its growth, and the body begins developing into proportion as a result of the rapidly growing abdominal and thoracic structures. The limbs are reaching their relative lengths. The cartilaginous skeletal system is being replaced by bone cells. Bone marrow forms and begins to function by producing blood cells. Neuromuscular interrelationships are more refined, and the fetus is actively moving. The mother may feel the first movements at this time if she is familiar with the

fig. 3-25 Human fetus at 68 days (male) (47 mm) (a) Right; (b) front; (c) left. (*Photo by E. Ludwig. From R. Rugh, and L. B. Shettles, From Conception to Birth: The Drama of Life's Beginnings, Harper & Row, New York, 1971.*)

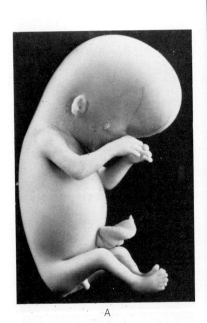 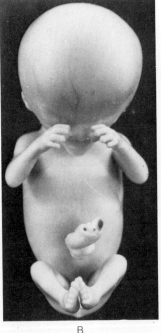 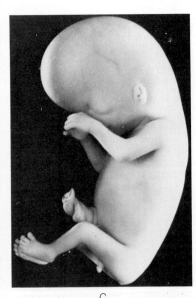

A   B   C

sensation. The movements have been described as a feeling that the fetus was blowing bubbles through a straw.

At 11 weeks, the fetus is 7 cm from crown to rump and weighs about 15 g. Tooth buds appear for all 20 temporary teeth (milk teeth). During this period, it is essential for the mother to ingest adequate amounts of calcium and minerals. Salivary glands begin to form, and the digestive tract is developing well enough so that peristalsis begins. The thyroid is complete. Insulin is forming in the pancreas and bile is being secreted by the liver. The kidneys are forming urine, which passes into the bladder and thence into the amniotic fluid.

In the last week of this trimester, the fetus is about 9 cm from crown to rump and weighs about 40 g. The thumb and forefinger develop opposition. The lungs have taken shape, and respiratory motions can be seen. The vocal cords are formed, and the swallowing reflex can be seen in response to thumb-sucking.

The end of the first trimester marks a milestone in fetal development as the fetus appears to be a miniature human being. All the organ systems have formed and continue to develop ability to function. However, the fetus is not yet viable outside the uterus because the systems cannot function properly enough for independent existence.

PLACENTAL STRUCTURE AND FUNCTION

The twelfth week marks the complete functional maturity of the placenta and membranes. These peripheral structures are crucial for the protection and nurture of the developing fetus.

amnion

The amnion appears very early in embryonic life—even before the embryo has taken form. At first, the amnion is small, but as it fills with fluid and the growth of the embryo "folds over," the amniotic cavity becomes much larger and eventually surrounds the embryo and body stalk. Later in pregnancy, the amnion expands to fill the entire space and adheres to the other membrane—the chorion.

amniotic fluid At term, the amnion contains almost a liter of fluid which forms from amniotic cells, urine, and other secretions from the lungs and skin of the fetus. This fluid is replaced about every 3 h. The secretion and reabsorption of the fluid is accomplished by the amnion cells with some assistance by the fetus through swallowing and urinating. The fluid-filled cavity serves many important functions for the fetus, namely cushioning the fetus against injury, preventing adhesions of the sticky skin, equalizing pressure, providing a medium for fetal movement, keeping the fetus at an even temperature, and providing fluid for the fetus to swallow. At term, this fluid-filled cavity provides a "wedge" to soften and dilate the cervix in labor. Amniotic fluid can also provide the physician with valuable diagnostic information in high-risk pregnancies (Chap. 27).

chorion

The chorion is derived from the trophoblast layer of the blastocyst. It is the outermost membrane and closest to the uterine lining. The chorionic villi embedded in the decidua basalis form the fetal side of the placenta. The chorionic villi enlarge by the end of the fourth and fifth months to form definable partitions which divide the placenta into segments called *cotyledons,* or little trees. Spiral arteries from the decidua basalis enter the spaces between the chorionic villi at regular intervals (see Fig. 3-18). Thus the chorionic villi become bathed with maternal blood rich in oxygen and nutrients. Exchange of fetal and maternal material takes place in many ways: osmosis, diffusion, active transport, and pinocytosis (ameboidlike action) among other more complex mechanisms (see Fig. 3-26). There is *no direct mingling* of fetal and maternal blood. However, there may be very isolated exchanges of fetal and maternal blood cells.

The so-called placental barrier is composed mainly of four layers of fetal tissue (connective tissue, fetal capillary endothelium, and two layers of trophoblast cells). This tissue becomes thinner as pregnancy progresses. Most substances can pass through this "barrier," e.g., oxygen, water, glucose, amino acids, vitamins, hormones, most viruses, many bacteria, and many drugs and chemical substances. In fact, only substances of high molecular weight or complex structure cannot pass across the placental barrier. During later months, the placenta actively exchanges antibodies which provide important protection against many infectious diseases for the newborn. Thus the placenta acts as the lungs, kidneys, endocrine and digestive systems, liver, and immune system for the fetus until these organs are mature enough to function.

placental hormones

By the end of the fourth month, the placenta produces progesterone in large enough amounts to sustain the pregnancy. In addition to progesterone, the placenta begins producing estrogenic hormones until just before the end of pregnancy. Part of the chorion produces gonadotropins which act in the same manner as the LH secreted by the anterior pituitary.

These human chorionic gonadtropins are secreted by the mother in the urine and are indicative of pregnancy. Human placental lactogen (HPL) and prolactin are also produced by the placenta to prepare the maternal body for lactation. The placenta may also be a source of a hormone called *relaxin* which is found in pregnant women.

From the twelfth week until late in the seventh month of pregnancy, the placenta continues to grow. Toward the end of pregnancy, the placental tissue begins to age, secreting hormones in decreasing amounts and becoming gradually less able to have effective exchange of nutrients, oxygen, and wastes.

THE SECOND TRIMESTER

The second trimester lasts from the beginning of the 13th week after fertilization until the end of the 26th week and is characterized by rapid growth of the fetus, particularly in height.

the fourth month (13 to 16 weeks)

The fourth month of fetal life is characterized by maturation of the musculoskeletal system. The head is less flexed on the chest. The nervous system has rudimentary control of the entire body, so that frequent arm and leg movements occur. The mother may be acutely aware of these movements by 16 to 18 weeks. The amount of movement differs. There is some evidence that fetal activity may relate to maternal emotional state; i.e., the mother's anxiety may cause an increase in maternal epinephrine which crosses to the fetus. However, it is virtually impossible to infer that the behavior or the activity of the newborn stems directly from maternal emotional states.

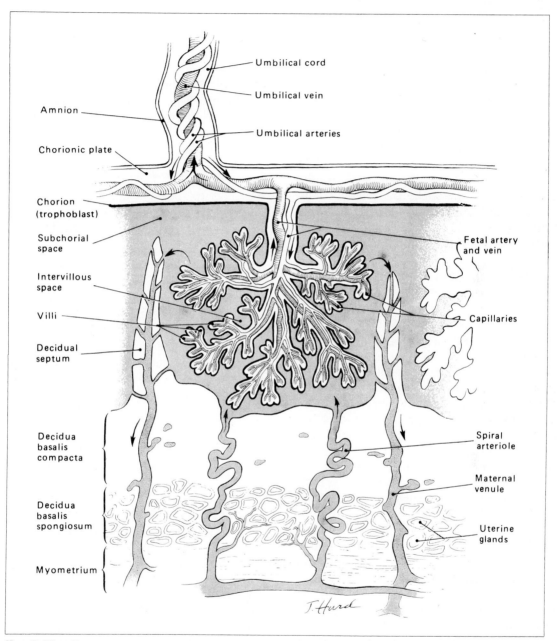

fig. 3-26 Cross section through the placenta arrows indicate the direction of maternal blood flow from arteriole back into maternal venules. Materials are exchanged across the chorionic layer lining the villi. (*From I. Telford Langley, and J. Christensen, Dynamic Anatomy and Physiology, 4th ed., McGraw-Hill, New York, 1974.*)

In the fourth month the lips are formed, and the facial contours are filling out. Fingerprints have developed, and the skin of the body is still loose, wrinkled, and pink. The brain begins forming convolutions; the cerebrum is definitely growing more rapidly and taking more space than the other parts of the brain. The heartbeat can now be heard with an amplified ultrasound fetoscope provided that the mother's abdominal wall is relatively thin.

Oocytes are forming in the fetal ovaries, and hormonal secretions begin. *Meconium,* a concentration of dead cells, mucus, bile, and other secretions, begins forming in the intestines and will later comprise the first stool of the newborn. By the sixteenth week the fetus weighs approximately 160 to 200 g and is about 14 cm in height.

fifth month (17 to 20 weeks)

During the fifth month, anabolic-catabolic exchange begins. The sweat glands and sebaceous glands secrete a fatty substance which, along with the discarded epithelial cells, form a cheeselike protective coating called *vernix caseosa.* Vernix will cover the infant until near the time of birth. Fine hair, called *lanugo,* is observable all over the body. Also eyebrows, eyelashes, and head hair appear.

The fetus now has settled into a rudimentary *circadian* (24 h) rhythm of sleeping, turning, kicking, sucking, and responding to loud noises or music. The fetus also has found its favorite position or *lie.* The mother is sometimes able to distinguish a foot or arm as it presses on her abdomen or rib cage.

Hemoglobin, which had been known as fetal hemoglobin because of its greater affinity for oxygen, now begins to form in the structure of adult hemoglobin. Respiratory movements have been identified from the eleventh week and are observed to become more regular after the eighteenth week but the alveolar structure of the lungs does not permit survival of the fetus until about the twenty-eighth week. (See Chap. 27 for evaluation of fetal breathing.)

By the beginning of the twentieth week, the fetus weighs approximately 500 g and is 19 cm in length (see Fig. 3-27).

sixth month (21 to 24 weeks)

The major occurrence during this time is the increased ossification of the skeletal structure. The bone-forming cells are very active and require a great deal of calcium for the process. The bony fetal skeleton is visible on x-ray.

The eyes are structurally complete, and the eyelids begin to open and close. The fetus is covered with a very thick vernix, and the hair on the head is getting long. Lung alveoli are becoming more mature. Certain reflexes appear, e.g., the grasp and startle reflexes, which become more refined as term approaches. Very little subcutaneous fat has been deposited; however, the skin layers are thickening on the hands and feet. The fetus now weighs about 650 to 820 g and is 23 to 24 cm in length.

the seventh month (25 to 28 weeks)

Although able to breathe, swallow, and regulate body temperature somewhat, the fetus is still dependent on maternal support. *Surfactant,* a substance essential for normal lung function, begins forming in the alveoli, preparing them to maintain expansion at birth.

Lanugo begins to slowly diminish, and the testes begin to descend into the scrotum. More reflexes become evident in the seventh month, i.e., rooting and stepping, but they are not discernible until after birth.

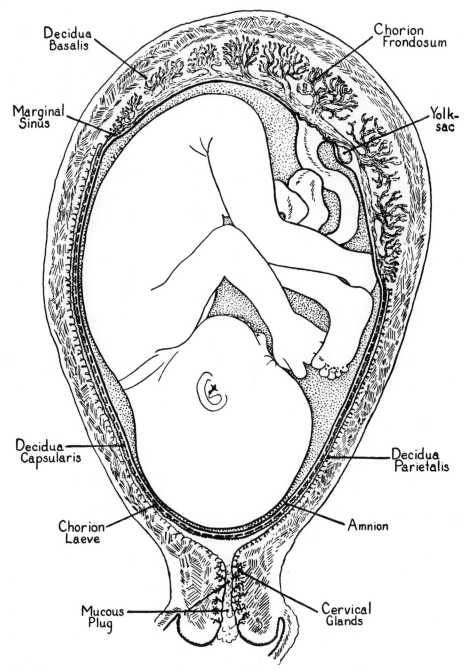

Decidua Basalis

Chorion Frondosum

Marginal Sinus

Yolk-sac

Decidua Capsularis

Decidua Parietalis

Chorion Laeve

Amnion

Mucous Plug

Cervical Glands

fig. 3-27 Diagram showing relations to the uterus of a 5-month-old fetus and its membranes. (*From C. E. Corliss, Patten's Human Embryology, 4th ed., McGraw-Hill, New York, 1976.*)

The volume of amniotic fluid will decrease to make room for the growing fetus as it occupies more space in the uterus. By the twenty-eighth week the fetus weighs approximately 1000 to 1200 g and is 28 cm long.

THE THIRD TRIMESTER

The duration of the third trimester is from the beginning of the twenty-seventh through the fortieth week after fertilization. The third trimester is characterized by the deposition of subcutaneous fat and refinement of central nervous system growth and development. The mother's diet is essential for proper growth and functioning of the brain, e.g., sufficient and appropriate protein intake. Iron is being stored in the liver for use in the newborn period, so the mother must ingest foods rich in this mineral as well as supplement her diet with iron. Again, calcium must be taken in during this trimester as the process of ossification continues.

eighth month (29 to 32 weeks)

The fetus weighs between 1300 and 2100 g and is between 32 and 36 cm long. Subcutaneous fat deposits are insulating the fetus against the impending temperature change at birth. The skin becomes less wrinkled and red. Lung alveoli are filling in, and the digestive system is maturing.

approaching full term (33 to 38 weeks)

Because of recent advances in care of the small preterm infant, the fetus can be born with excellent chance of survival at any time in this month. By 37 weeks the fetus weighs between 2500 and 3000 g and is 36 to 46 cm in length. At term, the baby will average 3000 to 3500 g and 46 to 50 cm. Activity such as turning and kicking are less frequent because the fetus is taking up virtually all the available space in the uterus. The fetus is preparing for birth by descending deeper in the maternal pelvis. Other physiological preparations for delivery include the transfer of maternal antibodies against such diseases as measles, mumps, rubella, whooping cough, and scarlet fever. These immunities will last for approximately 6 months until the infant's own immunological system is more mature. Thus, if born prematurely, the infant may be unprotected against infection.

In the ninth month the fetus has accumulated considerable meconium in the intestines which may be expelled by reflex action should the fetus encounter difficulty during labor and delivery. Otherwise, this meconium is expelled early in the newborn period.

Approximately 38 weeks or 266 days after the fusion of the sperm and ovum, a new human being is born. It is a complex and difficult adjustment for the mother as well as for the newborn because of the intimate symbiotic relationship which existed.

There often is confusion about gestational age in weeks or months. By referring to Fig. 3-28, a comparison can be made between menstrual age and fertilization age. In prenatal care, it is customary to speak of trimesters in terms of menstrual age, since the marker of the first day of the last menstrual period is identifiable by many women. However, the first phase of the menstrual cycle varies for many women, so that the *actual* fertilization age of the fetus may vary as much as 8 to 10 days from the presumed age of 14 days later than menstrual age. The use of the ultrasound biparietal diameter has aided estimation of actual age (see Chap. 27) when dates of the last menstrual period are unknown. The summary in Table 3-1 uses fertil-

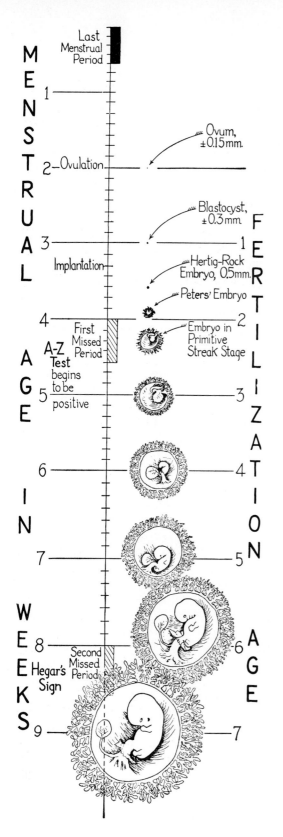

ization age, since its focus is the actual timing of fetal development.

FETAL CIRCULATION

One of the most important adjustments for the newborn is the change in circulation required for extrauterine life. Since the placenta acts as the main organ of transfer between the mother and fetus, the circulatory tree for the fetus contains special vessels that "bypass" the fetal lungs. Only a small amount of blood circulates through the fetal lungs to sustain tissue growth. The abrupt changes at birth, in both the area and the means of oxygenation (the lungs), require an immediate increase in blood volume through the lungs. The ways the fetus is suited for this change can be seen in Fig. 3-29.

Oxygenated blood enters the fetus via the umbilical *vein,* while the two umbilical arteries carry blood back to the placenta after it has circulated through the body. From the umbilical vein, part of the oxygenated blood is directed to the inferior vena cava via the first shunt, or detour, called the *ductus venosus.* Oxygenated blood from the umbilical vein also enters the portal vein to nourish the liver. After circulating through the liver, this blood enters the inferior vena cava via the hepatic vein. Therefore, blood entering the inferior vena cava from the placenta is partly oxygenated and partly unoxygenated. In addition, some blood returns from the fetal legs. This mixture of oxygenated and deoxygenated blood continues as the blood empties from the inferior vena cava into the right atrium,

fig. 3-28 Actual size of embryos in relation to mother's menstrual history (left), and fertilization age of the embryo (right). Based on a 28-day cycle. (*From C. E. Corliss, Patten's Human Embryology, 4th ed., McGraw-Hill, New York, 1976.*)

table 3-1 Development of the embryo and fetus—summary chart

time after ovulation	embryonic/fetal milestones	placental and maternal changes
fertilization age*		
3 min–48 h	Fertilization and syngamy.	
24 to 48 h	First cleavage of zygote—2-cell stage.	
3 to 4 days	Morula, 16-cell stage, enters the uterus.	
4 to 5 days	Blastocyst stage (inner cell mass and outer cell mass exists) reaches the uterus.	
6 days	Loss of the zona pellucida. Beginning of adhesion of outer cell mass (trophoblast layer) to uterine wall.	Trophoblast layer begins invading decidua basalis.
7 days	Implantation under way.	
7 to 8 days	Ectoderm and endoderm layers appear.	
8 to 10 days	Beginning of amnion and yolk sac.	
13 days	Chorion exists.	Primary chorionic villi form.
15 days	Implantation complete. Beginnings of blood vessels from yolk sac, body stalk, and chorion. Primitive streak and formation of mesoderm. Three germ layers exist.	Amenorrhea in mother. First missed menses.
18 to 21 days	Primitive nervous system folding occurs. Heart begins to twitch. Primitive eye and ear exist. Primitive red blood cells (RBC) differentiate.	Chorionic villi of placenta have circulatory core. Placenta covers approximately one-fifteenth of internal surface of uterus. Amenorrhea continues. Breast changes occur. Urinary frequency. Constipation. HCG (human chorionic gonadotropin) appears in urine.
4 weeks	Heart "folds" and begins asynchronous pulsations. Blood is pumped around the body. Yolk sac produces blood cells. Brain has differentiated into forebrain, midbrain, and hindbrain. Head large in proportion to body. Lung buds appear. GI tract and vertebral column begin. Height, 6 mm.	Placenta begins functioning in metabolic transfer. Maternal symptoms seen in third week persist. May experience "morning sickness." Chadwick's sign.
5 weeks	Limb buds appear. Rapid brain growth. Cranial and spinal nerves develop. Primitive nose, ears, and eyes form. Germ cells migrate toward gonads. Umbilical cord forming from body stalk. Heart begins forming septa.	
6 weeks	Trachea is formed. Liver produces RBCs. Simple reflexes occur. Central and autonomic nervous systems are formed. Rudimentary kidney and penis exist. Eyes begin moving to front of face. Cartilage laid down to prepare for bone formation. Lips form. Differentiation of muscles. Height, 1 cm.	

table 3-1 Development of the embryo and fetus—summary chart (*continued*)

time after ovulation	embryonic/fetal milestones	placental and maternal changes
7 weeks	Eyelids are formed. Gallbladder is formed. Liver is major site of blood cell formation. Yolk sac declines. Bone cells begin replacing cartilage. Movement of arms and legs. Height, 2 cm.	
8 weeks	Heart has four chambers and is beating rhythmically (40 to 80 beats per minute). External genitalia can be distinguished as male or female. Weight, 2 g; height, 3 cm.	Placenta covers one-third the lining of the uterus. Diagnosis of pregnancy by ultrasound by the ninth week.
12 weeks	Tooth buds appear. Bone marrow produces RBCs. Limbs have lengthened. Swallowing reflex present. Thumb and forefinger oppose. Weight, 40 g; height, 9 cm.	
16 weeks	Fingerprints develop. Frequent movements. Bladder fully formed. Weight, 160 to 200 g; height, 14 cm.	There is 200 ml of amniotic fluid present. Amniocentesis possible now (for fetal studies). Fetal heart rate can be heard with a Doptone amplified stethoscope.
20 weeks	Hair on head. Vernix caseosa and lanugo. Weight, 460 to 500 g; height, 19 cm.	Placenta covers one-half the lining of the uterus. Placenta is at its greatest size relative to the fetus and weighs 120 g. There is 400 ml of amniotic fluid present. Fetal movements may be felt earlier by a mother who has had prior pregnancies.
24 weeks	Favorite position or "lie." Eyebrows and lashes form. Ossification of bones begins. Weight, 650 to 800 g; height, 24 cm.	Placenta grows mainly in thickness rather than covering more surface area of the uterus. Mother can sense the "awake-sleep" rhythm of the fetus.
28 weeks	Lungs functional by 28 weeks. Testes begin descending. Swallowing, rooting, sucking, and stepping reflexes present. Weight, 1000 to 1200 g; height, 28 cm.	Respiratory movements in utero seen by ultrasound. Mother sometimes feels deep breaths as "hiccoughs."
32 weeks	Vernix all over. Subcutaneous fat deposits begin. Fingernails and toenails complete. Weight, 1300 to 2100 g; height, 32 to 36 cm.	Fetal movements may be so active as to prevent mother's sleeping well.
36 weeks	Maternal antibodies beginning to transfer to fetus. Weight, 2500 to 2800 g; height, 36 to 40 cm.	There is 1000 mL of amniotic fluid present, approximately.
38 weeks. Term period begins this week.	Approaches full term. Less active. Head descends into maternal pelvis. Weight, 3000 to 3500 g; height, 42 to 50 cm.	Placenta is three to four times as thick as it was at 20 weeks and weighs 500 to 650 g. There is 800 ml of amniotic fluid present. Fetal movements reduced because of limited space. Increased maternal discomforts of pressure on bladder and rectum.

table 3-1 Development of the embryo and fetus—summary chart (*continued*)

time after ovulation	embryonic/fetal milestones	placental and maternal changes
40 weeks. Considered "postterm" if born after this time.	Firm ear cartilages. Scant vernix. Weight, 3600 to 4000 g; height, 42 to 50 cm.	There is 800 mL or less of amniotic fluid.

*Refers to time after fertilization; gestational age is usually calculated from the first day of the last menstrual period, but pregnancy lasts 266 days ± 8, or 38 weeks, or 9½ months.

Source: Summary chart is compiled from many sources, but the format is based upon a chart by Florence Bright Roberts, *Perinatal Nursing*, McGraw-Hill, New York, 1977, pp. 16–18. (Used with permission of McGraw-Hill Book Co.)

and blood from the superior vena cava returns from the head, neck, and arms to the right atrium as well. Most of this blood is detoured directly into the left atrium by means of an opening fold (or flap) between the atria called the *foramen ovale.*

Blood from the lungs is emptied into the left atrium from the pulmonary veins. From the left atrium the blood flows into the left ventricle. As the ventricles contract, blood from the left ventricle enters the aorta, where 25 percent of the output supplies the head, neck, arms, and heart, while 75 percent of the output supplies the rest of the body.

The small amount of blood which enters the right ventricle without going through the foramen ovale goes to the pulmonary artery when the ventricles contract. Since the lungs only require enough blood to sustain their tissue growth, most of the blood entering the pulmonary artery is shunted through the third detour of fetal circulation, called the *ductus arteriosus,* which connects the pulmonary artery with the aorta. Finally, from the descending aorta, most of the blood flows into the internal and external iliac arteries to the umbilical arteries and back to the placenta.

The deep gasping cry that usually follows birth serves to increase the blood flow to the lung vascular bed. An immed.ate increase in pressure in the left atrium results from the increased flow through pulmonary veins, and a decrease in blood flow to the right atrium results since flow through umbilical vessels

ceases. This change in pressure causes the fold of the foramen ovale to close. At the same time, the increased flow through the aorta and the pulmonary artery causes the ductus arteriosus to constrict slowly and eventually become a ligament by 1 year of age. After the umbilical circulation ceases, the ductus venosus will also slowly collapse and become a ligament by 3 months (see Table 14-1).

Any delay in the establishment of respirations serves to defeat these changes, and in severe respiratory difficulty, the ductus arteriosus will remain open, shunting blood away from the lung bed.

The chapters that follow discuss the many ways that support can be provided for the mother and her developing fetus. The whole purpose of such health care is to ensure that a healthy infant will be born without handicaps of any kind and will then receive supportive parenting.

study questions

1 Describe the major structures of the male or female reproductive tracts. Trace a diagram and label it, checking your answers with Figs. 3-3, 3-4, and 3-5.
2 There are two major phases of the menstrual cycle. List all the symptoms for each phase and explain what each term describes. See Fig. 3-8.
3 Define the major actions of estrogen and progesterone on the female structures during the menstrual cycle.
4 Define meiosis and compare it with cell division in somatic cells.
5 Describe the major milestones from fertilization through birth:

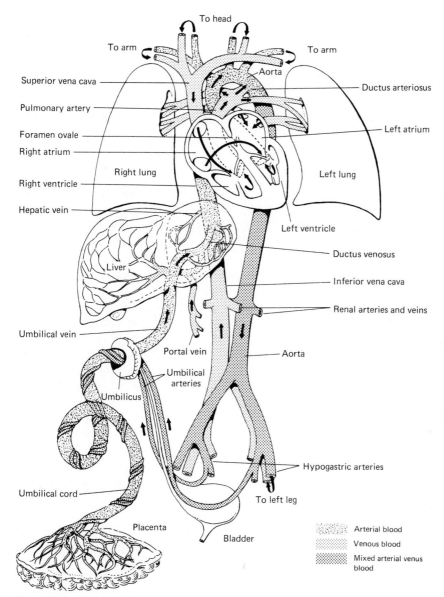

To head

To arm

To arm

Aorta

Superior vena cava

Ductus arteriosus

Pulmonary artery

Foramen ovale

Left atrium

Right atrium

Right lung

Left lung

Right ventricle

Hepatic vein

Left ventricle

Ductus venosus

Liver

Inferior vena cava

Renal arteries and veins

Umbilical vein

Portal vein

Aorta

Umbilical arteries

Umbilicus

Hypogastric arteries

Umbilical cord

To left leg

Placenta

Bladder

Arterial blood

Venous blood

Mixed arterial venus blood

fig. 3-29 Fetal circulation. (*Courtesy of Ross Laboratories, Clinical Education Aid.*)

a Define cleavage, morula, blastula, inner cell mass, trophoblast, yolk sac, amnion, chorion, placenta, embryo, and fetus.

b Describe, as if to a pregnant woman who is curious about her baby's stage of growth, what the fetus would look like at 12 weeks, 16 weeks, 20 weeks, 28 weeks, 32 weeks, and 36 weeks.

6 Identify the ways in which fetal circulation changes after respirations are established.

bibliography

Corliss, Clark Edwards: *Patten's Human Embryology, Elements of Clinical Development*, McGraw-Hill, New York, 1976.

"Fetus's Vulnerability to Foreign Chemicals," *Science News,* **109**:72, January 31, 1976.

Flanagan, Geraldine Lux: *The First Nine Months of Life,* Simon & Schuster, New York, 1962.

Hamilton, William J., J. D. Boyd, and H. W. Mossman: *Human Embryology: Prenatal Development of Form and Function,* 4th ed., Williams & Wilkins, Baltimore, 1972.

Ingelman-Sundberg, Axel and Claes Wirsen: *A Child is Born,* Delacorte, New York, 1965.

Langman, Jan: *Medical Embryology,* 3d ed., Williams & Wilkins, Baltimore, 1975.

Roberts, Florence Bright: *Perinatal Nursing,* McGraw-Hill, New York, 1977.

Rugh, Roberts and Landrum B. Shettles: *From Conception to Birth: The Drama of Life's Beginnings,* Harper & Row, New York, 1971.

4

MATERNAL CHANGES DURING PREGNANCY

MARTHA OLSEN SCHULT

Full development of the fetus takes about 266 days, or 38 weeks, after conception. When calculated from the last menstrual period (LMP), the duration is 14 days longer, i.e., 40 weeks or 280 days. Understood in calculating gestation from the first day of the LMP are the facts that women's menstrual cycles are somewhat irregular and that ovulation occurs approximately halfway through the cycle, 14 days ± 2 before the next menses (Fig. 2-1). An infant born before 37 full weeks of gestation will be incompletely developed in one or more of its body functions. A chart of the terminology related to the weeks of development is shown in Fig. 4-1. Before the end of the nineteenth week of gestation the fetus is not sufficiently matured to be able to survive out of the uterine environment. If labor begins before this time, the fetus cannot live and therefore is called *nonviable*; its birth is called an *abortion*. After the twentieth week some infants, weighing as little as 500 g, have been able to survive; therefore this period is termed the *viable*

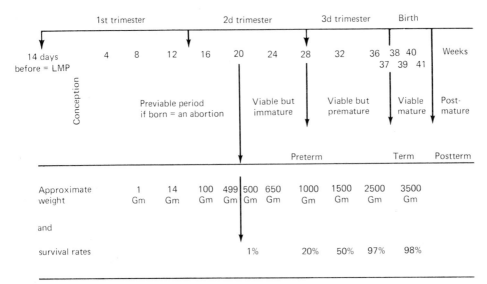

fig. 4-1 Terminology related to fetal maturity.

period. Between 20 and 28 weeks is a period of extreme fetal immaturity when the chances of survival are low. With each week after that and with each gram of weight added, the survival rates improve. *Preterm* birth is that which occurs between 20 and 37 weeks of gestation. The period of *term* birth, or *maturity,* is 38 to 42 weeks. After 42 weeks in the uterus, problems again develop, as *postmaturity* carries with it other complications.

From the very beginning of its life, the new human embryo, while traveling through the fallopian tube, is going through rapid cell division on its way to nidate in the uterine lining. It is only in the first week of its life that the embryo is virtually unaffected by outside influences such as drugs, viruses, and pollutants, except for radiation. Only during that week is it free-moving.

Between the second and twelfth weeks of life the embryo is especially susceptible to substances inhaled or ingested by the mother, substances which will travel through her circulation and may affect the fetal environment. Many of the drugs and substances that might

be taken in by the mother are harmless to the developing embryo, but others may be very harmful. Tragic experience with thalidomide and the results of rubella virus are only two examples of teratogens. Any agent toxic to cell differentiation or growth is called a *teratogen.* This includes not only agents causing structural defects but also those causing growth retardation and biochemical and behavioral effects lasting into the newborn period or even longer. Also included are agents which have been shown to be carcinogenic in later childhood, such as diethylstilbestrol.

The first 8 to 12 weeks of life of the fetus are the weeks of *organogenesis,* when the organs of the body are being formed and when there is the greatest chance of their malformation. Therefore it is most important that a woman seek prenatal care and guidance as soon as she suspects that she is pregnant.

Early prenatal care is one of our most potent ways to help prevent congenital anomalies, preterm birth, and maternal, neonatal, and infant mortality or morbidity.

PHYSIOLOGIC CHANGES CAUSED BY PREGNANCY

The hormones of pregnancy have a generalized effect far beyond their effects on the reproductive system. Likewise, the cardiovascular changes that occur during pregnancy also affect the entire body. Along with these changes is another category of effects of pregnancy known collectively as the *pressure symptoms of pregnancy.* Pressure symptoms occur as a result of the enlargement of the uterus as well as other physiologic changes that are taking place throughout pregnancy.

Many of the alterations that occur in the body as a result of the hormonal and cardiovascular changes provide the basis for the signs and symptoms of pregnancy and underlie many of the minor discomforts of pregnancy. With these variations, body systems are profoundly affected in ways that would be considered pathologic if the woman were not pregnant. These adjustments and alterations are *totally normal* during gestation. Knowing the reasons for such alterations in the body during pregnancy makes it possible for the nurse to explain the interrelatedness and meaning of the symptoms to the pregnant woman.

hormonal influences

progesterone After the woman conceives, the corpus luteum of the ovary begins to secrete increasing amounts of progesterone. Called the pregnancy-maintaining hormone, progesterone (for gestation) is necessary for nidation (implantation) of the fertilized ovum and for the maintenance of the enriched endometrium, now referred to as the *decidua.* The corpus luteum secretes progesterone for approximately 10 to 12 weeks; then it gradually diminishes in size as the placenta grows and takes over its function. Progesterone is

formed by precursors provided by both the maternal and fetal structures.

Progesterone produces a variety of effects in the body either alone or in conjunction with estrogen and other hormones. One of its principal actions is the relaxation of smooth muscles. It exerts a relaxing effect on the uterine muscles, inhibiting myometrial contractions and preventing the expulsion of the fetus from that hollow, muscular organ. Progesterone also acts to reduce the activity of tubal cilia, allowing the sperm to travel with less resistance through the fallopian tube to meet the ovum. When fertilized, the zygote can travel more slowly down the fallopian tube on its way to the uterus, all the while changing and developing in preparation for nidation (Fig. 4-2).

Progesterone acts on the smooth muscles in other parts of the body. The smooth muscles of the blood vessels are also affected, reducing vascular tone. This change allows for the increase in blood volume that occurs during pregnancy without a concurrent rise in blood pressure. In fact, during the first part of pregnancy the blood pressure may actually dip slightly. (See Chap. 23 for further discussion of these cardiovascular changes of pregnancy.) The fatigue that many women experience early in pregnancy has been attributed to the influence of progesterone plus relaxin.

estrogen Estrogen is secreted by the ovary, the adrenal cortex, and during pregnancy, by the placenta. Estrogens were the first hormones to be detected in the placenta. According to Hytten, at least 27 estrogens have been identified, all of them chemically similar to progesterone and testosterone.[1] The principal estrogen is estradiol, and the next most active estrogen is estrone. The main metabolite of estradial and estrone is estriol.

In order for estrogen to be produced in pregnancy, both fetus and placenta must be active. The fetal and maternal adrenals pro-

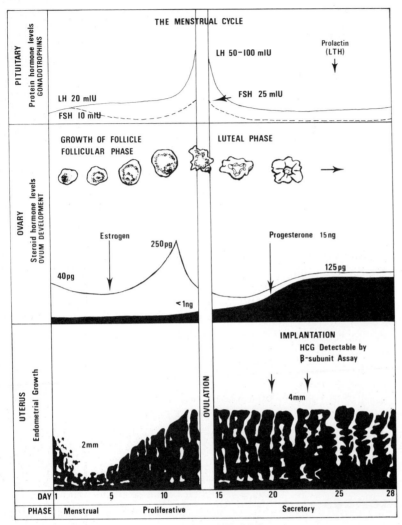

THE MENSTRUAL CYCLE

fig. 4-2 Levels of hormone during menstrual cycle and early pregnancy. (*Adapted from Hatcher, R., Contraceptive Technology, Irvington, New York, 1976–1977, Chap. 3.*)

duce precursors, and the steroid precursors are synthesized into estrogens. The metabolite, *estriol,* is excreted in the urine and is an indicator that the fetus and placenta are functioning properly. As the pregnancy progresses, the amounts of estriol should be increasing. Should there be a problem in the fetoplacental unit, the estriol levels will drop (Fig. 4-3).

The main function of estrogen during pregnancy is to control the growth and development of the uterus in conjunction with progesterone. Cervical changes are caused by the influence of progesterone and estrogen. Softening of the cervix and its spongelike consistency, the development of mucous glands, and increased vascularity are also attributed to hormonal changes. The vaginal secretions increase during pregnancy, and the walls of the vagina hypertrophy in preparation for delivery. The vascularity of the vagina, with its characteristic bluish discoloration, is also a result of the hormonal and hematologic changes of pregnancy. (See page 92 for further discussion).

The circulating progesterone and estrogens also affect the entire gastrointestinal tract. The motility of the stomach is reduced, causing a slower emptying time, and the gastric secretions are reduced by the action of estrogens and other hormones. Peristalsis throughout the entire GI tract is slowed, allowing the foodstuffs to pass more slowly, while more nutrients are extracted. Carbohydrate, protein, and fat metabolism are also affected, particularly by progesterone. It is also suggested that overall weight gain and fat depot storage can be attributed to the influence of progesterone.

Many of the breast changes that occur in pregnancy result from the influence of progesterone in conjunction with estrogens and other hormones. Estrogen influences the development of the ducts, whereas progesterone basically influences alveolar and lobule development in preparation for breast-feeding. The enlargement and mobility of the nipple and the darkening and enlargement of the areola and tubercles of Montgomery are attributed in part to the action of estrogens. The following hormones are considered to be necessary adjuncts for the development of the breasts for lactation: the pituitary hormones—prolactin, ACTH, human growth hormone, FSH, and LH; thyroid-stimulating hormone (TSH); human chorionic somatomammotropin, and other hormones secreted by the adrenals, ovary, pancreas, and placenta[2] (see Fig. 16-2).

Progesterone and estrogen in conjunction with melanocyte-stimulating hormone and the adrenal hormones cause pigmentation changes in the body. Normal body water

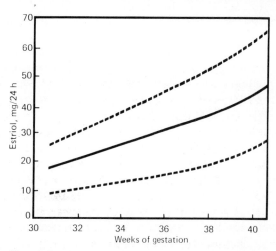

fig. 4-3 Twenty-four hour urinary estriol levels rise steadily during pregnancy. Estriol is formed by the fetoplacental unit. The fetal adrenal gland produces dehydroepiandosterone, which is metabolized by the placenta into estriol, and this is excreted by the maternal kidneys. Falling levels indicate some problem with this metabolic cycle. Serial measurements are necessary, since levels may vary during the day and from day to day.

retention during the latter part of pregnancy and increases in respiratory function are responses to estrogen and progesterone.

human placental lactogen (HPL) or human chorionic somatomammotropin (HCS) When human placental lactogen was first isolated from the placenta, it was noted that it was very similar to both human pituitary growth hormone (HGH) and prolactin. Since its effect on the mammary gland was greater than its growth-stimulating properties, it was called human placental lactogen (HPL). Later, because it possessed both somatropic and lactogenic properties, the name *human chorionic somatomammotropin* (HCS) was proposed. Both names are still in existence and refer to the same hormone.

The primary effect of HPL in pregnancy is to prepare the breast for lactation by stimulating the development of the breast and milk production. There are other possible effects attributed to this hormone, such as assisting the hormone HCG with its luteal stimulation to prolong the life and activity of the corpus luteum. Hytten and Little suggest other influences of HPL, including enhancing carbohydrate (CHO) metabolism, promoting fat storage, increasing the free circulating fatty acids, and stimulating erythropoiesis (erythrocyte production) and aldosterone secretion.[3,4]

It is also suggested that HPL could be utilized to determine the fetal state and placental functioning much the same way as estriol levels are utilized. In the maternal circulation, HPL has a short half-life of 20 to 30 min and thus could reflect recent changes in placental function. Since it is almost totally metabolized in the liver and kidneys, serum levels prove most valuable. Beginning at the fifth week of pregnancy, HPL levels rise gradually to peak at about 36 weeks. After delivery, HPL disappears within a few hours from maternal serum. Variation in levels can be rather large, depending on laboratory techniques; therefore, serial sequential readings are of more value than single tests. If there is an abnormality in the pregnancy, HPL levels tend to be lower than normal.

prolactin (PL), (PRL), (LTH) and human prolactin (HPRL)   Prolactin is secreted by both the chorionic layer of the placenta and the pituitary gland. Its major influence is indicated by its name, pro-lactin (for lactation), although the hormone has been known by many names, some of which are galactopoietic hormone, lactogenic hormone, luteotropic hormone, and mammotropin.

Little describes prolactin as having 82 groups of actions, including breast growth, osmoregulation, reproduction activity, integumentary action, synergism with steroids, and lactogenesis.[5] Drugs, exercise, and anesthesia can influence the release of prolactin.

Serum levels rise from 30 ng/mL in the first trimester to a high of 200 ng/mL at term. Amniotic fluid contains 5 to 10 times more prolactin than maternal serum. After delivery, prolactin levels diminish in 1 week if bottle feeding is chosen. If breast feeding is chosen, levels remain high during the first week and rise even higher after a feeding. Once lactation is established, however, the base level is lower, with continued peaks of release within 30 min of suckling by the infant. There is indication that prolactin plays some part in inhibiting ovulation during the period of breast-feeding (see Chap. 16).[6]

melanocyte-stimulating hormone (MSH)   During pregnancy the pituitary secretes increasing amounts of melanocyte-stimulating hormone. It is thought that this hormone, in conjunction with estrogens and adrenal hormones, contributes to the changes in pigmentation during pregnancy. The areola around the nipples enlarges and darkens. The line between the navel and the symphysis darkens and becomes known as the *linea nigra*. The faces of many pregnant women take on a characteristic appearance, known as *chloasma*, as the skin forms irregular, masklike macules on cheeks and forehead.

relaxin   Relaxin is an interesting hormone, but its activity during pregnancy is not fully understood. Secreted by the ovaries and perhaps by the placenta during pregnancy, it is thought to function in several different ways. The relaxation of the pelvic ligaments in preparation for delivery is attributed to relaxin. It is also assumed to act synergistically with estrogens and progesterone in stimulating breast growth and softening of the cervix for delivery.[7]

human chorionic gonadotrophin (HCG)   Although other gonadotrophins are formed by the pituitary gland, human chorionic gonadotrophin is exclusively produced by the cytotrophoblast of the chorion. Thus, HCG is present only during pregnancy or in a very rare chorionic growth called a *molar pregnancy* (see Chap. 22).

HCG is thought to function by controlling the secretion of FSH and LH, keeping them at a low level during pregnancy. It also stimulates the corpus luteum to continue secreting progesterone and estrogen until the placenta produces adequate levels. It is as yet uncertain whether HCG has any direct effect on the decidua in preventing menstruation from occurring or in promoting implantation.

HCG is the hormone that gives the positive results in urine-based pregnancy tests. It has been found in measurable amounts in the urine within 14 days of fertilization, the early period of very active trophoblast growth. The amount of HCG peaks at about 60 days and then drops off sharply by 100 days and remains at a low level for the remainder of the pregnancy (Fig. 4-4).

thyroid and adrenal hormones During pregnancy the thyroid gland enlarges and in many instances can be palpated in the neck. The thyroid produces increased amounts of hormone, which causes the basal metabolic rate (BMR) to rise gradually throughout pregnancy to about 20 to 25 percent above the prepregnant rate. Measurement of thyroid activity during pregnancy must take into account the increase of 25 to 50 percent of protein-bound iodine (PBI). Increased amounts of binding globulins for thyroid and for adrenal hormones accompany increased activity. There is no adverse result from these higher levels; it is a normal change needed to support fetal growth.

hematologic changes

The state of pregnancy results in normal alterations in the hematologic system. When discussing hematologic changes, it is impor-

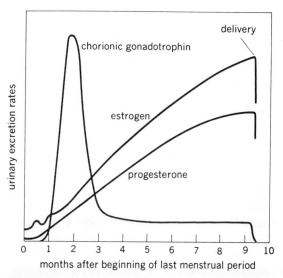

fig. 4.4 Urinary excretion of estrogen, progesterone, and chorionic gonadotropin during pregnancy. (From A. J. Vander, J. H. Sherman, and D. Luciano, Human Physiology, McGraw-Hill, New York, 1970.)

tant to remember that pregnancy is a *physiologic* state as distinct from a *pathologic* state. Some variation in the "expected normal values" is now recognized during varying stages of pregnancy.

blood volume By the tenth week of pregnancy the maternal blood volume has increased by as much as 30 to 40 percent to provide for the needs of the enlarging uterus, breasts, and placenta. Most of the blood is concentrated in the pelvic region and does not unduly change the arterial blood pressure. Blood pressure, in fact, drops slightly during the first two trimesters, returning to the normal level or slightly above during the last trimester. A combination of the vasodilating action of estrogen and the presence of an arteriovenous shunt in the placental circulation reduces pressure, much as a delta region does for a river. To accommodate the increased blood volume, however, the cardiac output increases and the pulse rises about 15 beats over the nonpregnant rate. Venous pressure in the lower extremities is affected, with an increase in femoral venous pressure from less than 10 mmHg to a level of 18 mmHg or more.[8]

hemoglobin and hematocrit   The increase in blood volume is primarily caused by an increase in plasma. The plasma volume may increase by 40 percent, while the red cell mass increases by only 15 to 25 percent. (The red cell count should remain above 3,750,000 per cubic millimeter of blood.) The result is a slight reduction in hematocrit readings but usually no significant change in hemoglobin levels. The hematocrit reading is usually 35 to 45 percent, but it may drop to as low as 30 to 33 percent. But hemoglobin levels, normally 12 to 14 g/100 mL, should fall no lower than 11 g during pregnancy. Any change below these levels is considered iron deficiency anemia, whereas a lowered hematocrit value alone is called *hemodilution of pregnancy*. The phrase *physiologic anemia of pregnancy* is still sometimes found in the literature to describe these changes, but it is misleading and is not the preferred term.

leukocytes   The leukocyte count increases during the last several months of pregnancy, and a count of 10,000 to 15,000 is not considered unusual. During and just after delivery there is a further increase in the leukocyte count, frequently to the range of 20,000 to 25,000. The count usually returns to normal within a week after delivery in the absence of other complications.

coagulation factors   Blood platelets show little change during pregnancy, with the platelet count, structure, and function typically remaining within the normal range. After delivery a transient rise in count to 500,000 to 600,000 may be observed. An increase in the levels of several of the serum-clotting factors is usual during pregnancy.

PRESSURE SYMPTOMS DURING PREGNANCY

The enlarging uterus affects a number of body functions. Symptoms caused by uterine pressure are more pronounced in the last trimester and are further aggravated if there is a multiple pregnancy. The uterus presses on the bladder during the first trimester and then again at the end of pregnancy. Uterine enlargement causes extra pressure on the arteries and veins to the extremities. Such pressure contributes toward increased femoral venous pressure, impinges on renal vessels, and precipitates hypotension as a result of compression of the vena cava in some women.

Gastrointestinal effects include constipation and hemorrhoids. Because the stomach is pushed up slightly toward the diaphragm, heartburn occurs, and some women develop a slight hiatus hernia. For others, the last few weeks include episodes of orthopnea, and lying flat in order to sleep leads to episodes of dyspnea; sleeping with two or three pillows relieves pressure on the diaphragm. Thus, like cardiovascular and hormonal changes, mechanical pressure factors affect many of the minor problems of pregnancy.

EFFECTS OF PREGNANCY CHANGES ON MAJOR BODY SYSTEMS

cardiovascular system

The increase in blood volume has several related effects that cause minor discomfort during pregnancy. The first of these is a sensation of light-headedness or fainting (syncope). The literature on this subject indicates two causes—postural hypotension and hypoglycemia. With the increase in volume of maternal blood in the pelvic region, pooling of blood can occur when the mother stands up suddenly, moving, for instance, from a horizontal position to jump up and answer the phone. A word of caution will usually prevent an episode of syncope from this cause. If the cause turns out to be hypoglycemia, the physician will advise frequent small meals during the day, with intake of quickly absorbed carbohydrate if the mother should feel faint.

Increased circulation may cause some women to have recurrent headaches as they become adjusted to the changes in volume. Emotional tension may contribute to headaches as well. Any persistent headache should be reported to the physician, as it may be a symptom of a more severe underlying problem.

varicose veins Increased blood volume contributes toward the development of varicose veins in those women so disposed and especially in those who have had preexisting varicosities. Varicose veins of the saphenous system and of the vulva and rectum (hemorrhoids) are primarily affected by the rising venous pressure in the lower extremities, induced by the enlarging uterus impinging on the venous flow. Varicosities are usually more common and pronounced in the multigravida. Besides being unsightly, they may be painful and throbbing, especially those in the vulva and rectum.

Positional change to facilitate venous return—elevation of the legs above the level of the heart or placing legs and feet on a footstool whenever sitting to avoid pressure of the chair on the lower part of the thigh—will be helpful measures. A woman with a tendency to have varicosities should wear support hose or elastic ace bandages to give support and counterpressure to the walls of the distended veins. (See Chap. 23 for further discussion of treatment.)

dependent edema Edema of the lower extremities is also related to venous return.

Standing for long periods of time and pressure of the uterus on the large veins returning from the legs tend to hinder the flow of venous return (against gravity), to the right side of the heart. Positional change to one facilitating venous return will quickly reduce this dependent, *gravity-based* edema. The side-lying position during sleep or rest is the best position for efficient kidney function. The normal woman with dependent edema should find that it has disappeared by morning after a good night's rest. Edema that persists is a warning signal to be reported to the physician.

musculoskeletal system

Many women experience low-back strain and discomfort during later pregnancy because the muscles and ligaments in the pelvic joints become somewhat relaxed, causing discomfort and pulling. It is suspected that the underlying hormone is *relaxin,* which, in conjunction with estrogen and progesterone, is preparing the body for the stretching of delivery.

posture Another factor contributing to back discomfort is the added weight and increasing abdominal girth that cause the pregnant woman to have the typical pregnant stance or walk. She leans backward to counterbalance the heavy uterus. The change in posture, unless noted and compensated for, will cause a strain on the lower back and pelvic muscles. Improper shoes may aggravate the imbalance. The mother can be taught back exercises, such as the pelvic tilt, to strengthen her lower abdominal and back muscles. A bed board under the mattress will help to align her back. Occasionally a physician advises a maternity girdle for those women whose natural abdominal "muscle girdle" is not toned well enough to support the uterus. If analgesics are needed, they should be prescribed by the physician.

leg cramps One of the most annoying problems of pregnancy is muscle cramps or spasms in the legs and feet. Some of the causes are thought to be fatigue and a decreased calcium level when there is an increased phosphorus level. Pressure on the nerves caused by the enlarging uterus may also contribute to muscle cramping.

Exercise, particularly walking, elevation of legs when sitting, and sufficient rest should help to relieve leg cramps. Standing on a cold floor and kneading the knotted muscle may relieve the cramp. Pointing the toes upward and exerting pressure downward on the kneecap helps to relieve the pain. Increasing the amount of calcium in the diet while reducing the amount of phosphorus may help to reduce cramping. To do this the physician prescribes calcium tablets and a reduced milk intake, for milk has a high content of phosphorus as well as calcium.

integumentary system

The hormones from adrenal and placental sources produce changes that are characteristic of pregnancy. The nipple and areola darken and become more prominent. A line darkens between the symphysis and the umbilicus, changing from the linea alba to what is called the linea nigra. Some pregnant women develop a pigmented area on cheeks and forehead, known as chloasma, or the "mask of pregnancy." Stretch marks, or *striae*, on the abdomen, buttocks, and breasts are not caused just by stretching (tiny tears in the lower skin layer) but are the effect of hormones from the adrenal cortex. Striae are purple-blue during pregnancy, changing to silver or brown scar tissue after pregnancy. They will never completely disappear, although they are usually scarcely noticeable between pregnancies.

The increased circulation of blood causes a variety of changes in the skin and hair. Fingernails grow faster. Many women notice *erythema,* or redness, of the palms of the hands and soles of the feet. Nosebleeds and nasal congestion are the complaint of some women. On the positive side, many who were usually uncomfortable in cold weather find themselves tolerating cold more easily during pregnancy because of the increased circulation to the extremities.

According to Hytten, instead of the usual 85 percent hair growth there is a 95 percent hair growth during pregnancy.[9] Since more follicles are active, fewer are falling out. Then with the sudden change in circulation and hormonal levels after birth, it appears that hair is coming out "in handfuls," probably because fewer follicles are active.

Sebaceous glands and sweat glands may be more active because of increased circulation. Oily skin, sometimes acne, may recur in the woman who struggled with this problem during puberty.

gastrointestinal system

The circulating estrogens and progesterone exert a relaxing effect on the smooth muscles of the entire gastrointestinal tract. The primary purpose appears to be to increase the absorption of nutrients from the intestinal tract. The motility of the stomach is slowed, gastric secretions are reduced, and stomach emptying takes place more slowly.

morning sickness Nausea is one of the most common complaints of the first trimester. For some women even the sight and smell of food bring on nausea or vomiting. Although psychologic factors, such as ambivalence toward the pregnancy, may be involved, there is a physiologic basis for nausea in the marked gastrointestinal changes. Fortunately, by the thirteenth week most women are free of morning sickness.

Women often are advised to eat a few dry

crackers before arising from bed in the morning. Dry, easily digestible carbohydrate food in the stomach may prevent symptoms. Dry, low-fat meals ensure a smaller volume of food in the stomach. Since fat slows down peristalsis, low-fat meals would not aggravate the already slowed motility that underlies these symptoms. Liquid should be consumed between meals in order to prevent dehydration. If vomiting is severe or persists at other times of day, the patient should be advised to consult the physician for treatment. Medication to stop nausea must be by prescription, not an "over-the-counter" purchase (see Chap. 20 for a discussion of antiemetics).

heartburn The cardiac sphincter between the stomach and the esophagus becomes slightly relaxed and may be opened by the pressure of the enlarging uterus, resulting in slight regurgitation of acids from the stomach. These acids irritate the mucosa, causing a burning sensation. Adding to the problems of heartburn, the increased movement of the diaphragm and the flaring of the rib cage may create a temporary, minor hiatus hernia, or an enlargement of the opening in the diaphragm where the esophagus enters the stomach.

Surgical intervention is not necessary, as the problem will disappear after the baby's birth. Remedies may include drinking milk between meals and taking small, frequent meals. Any antacid should be prescribed by the physician. Early in pregnancy, when gastric acidity is already reduced, an antacid would not be advisable. Later in pregnancy the prescription may be given for an aluminum hydroxide gel. Patients should be especially advised not to take medications containing sodium bicarbonate to relieve heartburn. (See Chap. 20.)

constipation With the slowing of peristalsis, the body is able to extract more vitamins, minerals, and other nutrients from the food that is eaten, but in the process, the body also extracts more water from the food bulk as it passes through the large intestine. Slower motility and a drier stool contribute to constipation. If the symptoms persist, hemorrhoids soon develop (see Chap. 23 for treatment). Adequate exercise, increased fluid intake, and ingestion of foods containing roughage usually will alleviate constipation. Foods with roughage are raw fruits, vegetables, and whole grain cereals with bran. If these foods are not a part of a person's usual food habit, they should be introduced gradually into the diet. These foods should be chewed well. If eaten hurriedly, flatulence and distention may be a problem. Mineral oil is not to be taken because it interferes with the absorption of fat-soluble nutrients in the small intestine. Again, any cathartic should be advised by the physician, who often prescribes a stool softener, instead of a laxative. For a summary of gastrointestinal changes, see Fig. 4-5.

renal system

With the 30 percent increase in the amount of circulating blood, there is a corresponding increase in the amount that circulates through the kidneys. However, because of increased reabsorption by the tubules of sodium and electrolytes and hence of water, there is no appreciable increase in the volume of urine produced for excretion. Toward the end of pregnancy there is even a slight reduction of urine formation, as the woman retains more body water.[10]

The renal threshold for glucose may drop slightly. A small amount of glucose may be found in the urine without being considered indicative of a problem. Later in pregnancy, *lactose,* part of the content of *colostrum* being produced by the breasts, may be found in urine. (Diagnosis of diabetic changes in pregnancy is discussed in Chap. 24.)

The ureters and bladder are composed of

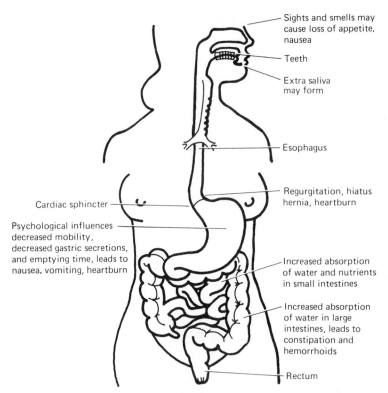

Sights and smells may cause loss of appetite, nausea

Teeth

Extra saliva may form

Esophagus

Regurgitation, hiatus hernia, heartburn

Cardiac sphincter

Psychological influences decreased mobility, decreased gastric secretions, and emptying time, leads to nausea, vomiting, heartburn

Increased absorption of water and nutrients in small intestines

Increased absorption of water in large intestines, leads to constipation and hemorrhoids

Rectum

fig. 4-5   Gastrointestinal tract showing minor discomforts during pregnancy.

smooth muscle and are therefore affected by progesterone and estrogen. The ureters dilate and relax, leading to some *stasis,* or pooling of urine. The bladder may not completely empty for the same reason; therefore infection, or *bacteriuria,* is more common during pregnancy (see Chap. 25).

nocturia   Nocturia is a common complaint among pregnant women. The basis for this problem is that fluid, affected by gravity, tends to accumulate in the lower extremities during the day. The horizontal position at night favors kidney function, and this extracellular, interstitial fluid is excreted.

Positional changes affect kidney function because of the enlarging uterus. In the supine position the uterus presses upon the renal veins and arteries, reducing effective flow to the kidneys. Therefore, it is important for the pregnant woman, especially in the advanced stages, to lie on her side whenever resting.

frequency   Urinary frequency is caused by the enlarging uterus rising out of the pelvic canal. The uterus compresses the bladder against the pelvic bones and reduces its capacity. The woman feels an urgent sensation to void even though there may be only a small amount of urine. Then, in the last weeks before delivery, after *lightening,* or tilting forward of the uterus, has occurred, the uterus again compresses the bladder to cause the same effect.

respiratory system

During pregnancy the volume of tidal air increases with the increased movement of the diaphragm and the expansion of the lower ribs laterally to allow for a larger intake of air. An increased volume of CO_2 is expelled with expiration, allowing the CO_2 from the fetus to be transferred more easily to the maternal circulation because of the decreased PCO_2 of her blood. Likewise more O_2 is inspired.

Late in pregnancy, with the increase in the size of the uterus, many women, in spite of the flaring of the ribs, experience *dyspnea.* The uterus presses against the diaphragm, and the woman may become *orthopneic.* Once she experiences *lightening,* some of the pressure of the uterus is shifted away from the diaphragm, and she can breathe more deeply and easily again.

The increased circulation may cause swelling of the vocal cords and larynx, bringing about hoarseness or deepening of the voice.

reproductive system

In pregnancy, many of the earliest and most obvious changes in a woman's body occur in her reproductive organs. The ovary ceases to produce mature ovum and instead centers its activity on releasing progesterone in order to maintain the environment necessary to nourish and provide for the fertilized ovum. The follicular-stimulating hormone and luteinizing hormone remain at a low level during pregnancy, since they are not needed to stimulate graafian follicle development or release.

In response to the increase of hormones and blood volume, the vagina and the cervix take on a bluish hue, and the cervix becomes increasingly soft and movable while the glands and mucosa secrete more mucus.

uterus The uterus no longer sheds its endometrium, since it is needed to nourish and sustain the growing embryo-fetus. The once pear-shaped, 8 cm × 5 cm × 2.5 cm uterus is growing from a 60-g weight to upwards of 1000 g. The increase in size of the uterus is dependent to a degree on the size of the fetus and placenta and the volume of the amniotic fluid. The uterus grows asymmetrically, depending on the position of the fetus in utero, and as it rises out of the pelvic cavity into the abdominal cavity it rotates slightly to the right, probably owing to the presence of the descending colon on the left side. The smooth muscles of the uterus enlarge and elongate to at least eight times their prepregnant size, allowing for this great expansion. (During the second half of pregnancy the uterine walls become very thin, allowing for better auscultation of the fetal heart and determining of the fetal position using Leopold's maneuvers).

breasts The breasts also change during pregnancy in preparation for breast-feeding. The hormones discussed earlier cause the breasts to grow and develop for the task ahead. The changes in the breasts are the result of the hormones, as well as the increased amount of circulating blood, and include changes in the areola, nipple, and tubercles of Montgomery. As the pregnancy progresses, the increased size and weight of the breasts may cause discomfort. Therefore the pregnant woman should be encouraged to wear a good supportive bra into the post-delivery period. This will prevent stretching of the ligaments and muscles which support the breasts.

Since the breasts are producing colostrum, the precursor of milk, from the fourteenth week of pregnancy, and it may leak from the breasts, the woman must be taught to keep her breasts clean and dry to prevent excoriation of the skin and nipples. Often women must wear shields or insert a clean handkerchief in each bra cup to catch the leaking fluid. If the breasts become irritated, the woman may wish to expose them to the air for brief periods each day to promote healing.

SIGNS AND SYMPTOMS OF PREGNANCY

It may be several weeks after conception before a woman suspects that she is pregnant. As changes are occurring within her body, she begins to notice symptoms, one of the first of which is *amenorrhea,* or the absence of her menstrual flow. Her breasts may become tender and feel full. She may experience morning nausea. Fatigue is another early symptom. Many women, when asked how they knew conception had taken place, stated that they "just knew something was different."

After noticing that something is different about her body and putting the symptoms together, the woman may decide to go to a clinic or private physician for confirmation of the pregnancy. (How early she goes depends a great deal on her understanding of what will take place there and how she will be received.)

The woman has experienced one or more early subjective *symptoms.* The physician will then look for *signs,* objective verification to confirm or disprove the beginning of a pregnancy. The signs and symptoms of pregnancy can be divided into two main groups: possible and positive.

Possible	*Positive*
Amenorrhea	Auscultation of the fetal heart
Breast changes	Fetal electrocardiogram
Morning sickness	
Frequency of urination	Palpation of fetal parts by examiner
Fatigue	Visualization of the fetus by means of
Abdominal enlargement	

Uterocervical changes
Vaginal changes
Positive pregnancy tests
Quickening
Ballottement

x-ray
Ultrasound visualization of the fetus

possible signs of pregnancy

Possible signs of pregnancy are those which indicate a growing embryo but at the same time could occur with another condition of medical or psychologic origin. In the past, the term *presumptive signs* has referred to those most likely to indicate pregnancy. However, such distinctions are no longer necessary. Three or more of the possible signs taken together are a fairly good indication of the presence of a growing embryo. *Positive* signs are those which establish without doubt the presence of a fetus in the uterus; they usually may be confirmed after 16 to 20 weeks.

amenorrhea Amenorrhea may be one of the earliest clues to pregnancy. In considering it as one of the signs, the physician and nurse must be aware of the possibility that other factors, such as low hormone levels, stress, anemia, and illness, can alter the menstrual cycle. The patient may suspect that she is pregnant, may worry about it, only to discover that her period is delayed for other reasons. On the other hand, some women have a diminished flow at the regular period interval for 1 or 2 months after conception and for that reason do not recognize pregnancy or seek care.

breast changes The breasts become sensitive, full, and tender because of the increased blood supply and hormone effect. The nipple and areola darken. The tubercles of Montgomery become more prominent. For many women, increased sensitivity and a tingling sensation in the breasts provide one of their first clues to the possibility of pregnancy. By 14 weeks, *colostrum,* the precursor of milk, is being produced.

morning sickness Because it occurs on an empty stomach in the morning, the nausea of pregnancy is particularly easy to identify. Psychic factors plus hormone changes contribute to morning sickness. About 50 percent of pregnant women experience this bothersome nausea and vomiting. If the vomiting becomes excessive, so that it endangers the baby or the mother, the condition is referred to as *hyperemesis gravidarum* (see Chap. 24).

frequency of urination Frequency is caused by the pressure of the enlarging uterus as it rises out of the pelvic area. The bladder, compressed by the uterus, sends a message of urgency to void even though it may contain only ¼ to ½ cup of urine. Frequency is also present when there is a bladder infection, but the frequency of early pregnancy does not have the other symptoms of infection—burning and pain on urination.

fatigue All the metabolic changes that are under way seem to cause an unusual amount of fatigue and sleepiness for a woman in early pregnancy. During later pregnancy, fatigue comes from the changes in body posture and the extra weight that must be carried everywhere.

abdominal enlargement Most primigravidas do not notice marked changes in abdominal size until the second trimester. By the sixteenth week the woman usually finds that she can no longer button her skirt or slacks. However, some multigravidas notice

tightening of their clothes almost immediately after one missed menstrual period.

The rising of the uterus into the abdominal cavity is gradual and has completely occurred at about the twelfth week. From that time, the height of the fundus above the symphysis is a guide to the duration of the pregnancy because the uterus rises about 1 cm a week (Fig. 4-6). MacDonald's rule for calculating the duration of pregnancy is as follows: *measurement of height of fundus above symphysis (in cm) × 8/7 = duration of pregnancy (in weeks).* A second rule for calculation is to divide the height of the fundus by 3.5 to determine the duration in lunar months (Fig. 4-7). The measurement is thrown off by obesity, multiple pregnancy, and an abnormally small or large amount of amniotic fluid.

Abdominal enlargement may occur in cases of *pseudocyesis* (pseudopregnancy), when the woman, believing that she is pregnant, goes through many of the preliminary signs. The physiologic basis for such a pseudocyesis has been documented by Brown and Barglow, who showed that the corpus luteum

fig. 4-6 Height of the fundus by weeks of gestation.

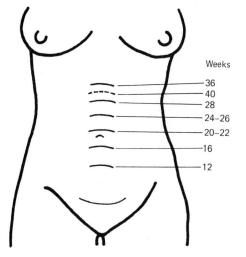

Weeks

36
40
28
24–26
20–22
16
12

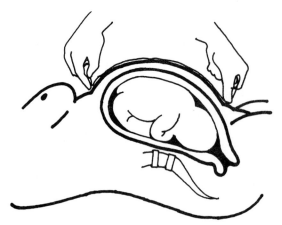

fig. 4-7 Measurement of fundal height.

can remain active under influence of stress-induced hormones, even though conception has not occurred.[11]

uterocervical changes With increased circulation and hormonal activity the uterus and the cervix become increasingly soft. The softness is noted first as a spot on the anterior side of the uterus just above the uterocervical junction. This softening is known as *Ladin's* sign and may occur as early as the fifth week of pregnancy. The softening of the cervix itself is called *Goodell's* sign. In addition to these two signs, the lower uterine segment becomes very compressible. On bimanual examination of the junction, the fingers of the examiner seem to touch, apparently compressing the area to paper thinness. This is *Hegar's* sign and can be demonstrated as early as the sixth week. Before the use of isoimmunologic tests for pregnancy, Hegar's sign was a very valuable indication of pregnancy.

The tight, long, smooth cervix that guards the entry to the uterus changes by softening and by forming a large number of mucus-secreting glands near the external *os* (opening). These glands secrete a thick, tenacious mucus which plugs the cervical canal effec-tively, closing off the os during pregnancy and thereby forming a barrier to help protect the uterine contents from vaginal organisms. When labor begins and the cervix begins to open, these glands are shed in the form of a *plug* of mucus.

vaginal changes Because of the increased blood supply to the pelvic region the vaginal mucosa and the cervix take on a bluish-purple coloration known as *Chadwick's* sign, or *Jacquimeier's* sign, demonstrable by the eighth week of pregnancy.

There is an increased supply of glucose to the cells of the vagina, as well as a general hypertrophy of the vaginal folds. The cervical secretions increase throughout pregnancy and may constitute a hygiene problem for the woman. *Leukorrhea,* or the increased secretion of cervical mucus, is thin, watery, milky white and may be profuse enough to necessitate the wearing of a vaginal pad in later pregnancy. The secretions should not cause itching or irritation to the tissues unless there is an infection present. For hygienic reasons the pregnant woman is advised to cleanse the entire perineal area and keep it dry to prevent chafing. A mild vinegar and water solution is an effective external cleansing agent, but douches should not be used unless prescribed by the physician.

If the discharge becomes yellowish or thick and white, causes pruritus, or has an odor, it is probably caused by one of the normally present organisms in the vaginal tract. The most common of these are *Trichomonas vaginalis* and *Candida albicans* (see Chap. 25). Medications are prescribed in the form of vaginal suppositories, gels, or solutions applied to the mucosa. The husband or sexual partner should also be treated, because of the possibility of reinfection. In order to prevent reinfection, the use of condoms is advised until both partners have completed the course of treatment.

positive pregnancy tests   There are two basic types of laboratory tests for pregnancy: biologic and isoimmunologic. Both types are based on the presence or absence of HCG in the urine (see Fig. 4-4).

In biologic tests, the urine of the possibly pregnant woman is injected into an animal; resultant changes in its gonads are caused by HCG. In the *Friedman* test, the urine is injected into a rabbit; in the *Aschheim-Zondek* (A-Z) test, a mouse is used; and in the *Hogben* test, a frog or toad is used. If the woman is pregnant, the HCG will stimulate ovulation or the development of spermatozoa in the animal within a few days. These tests are all approximately 97 percent accurate. Urine can yield positive results 4 weeks after conception has occurred. Unfortunately, these tests require the breeding and sacrifice of test animals and thus are expensive.

The second method of testing for pregnancy, the *isoimmunologic* test, has virtually eliminated the cumbersome, time-consuming biologic tests because urine testing can be done in the clinic and takes from 2 min to 2 h, with a 95 percent accuracy rate.

One of the commonly used agents is the Pregnosticon test.* Instructions for use require that the patient void to give a fresh specimen; only a few drops of urine are necessary. The test is based on an antigen-antibody reaction; HCG is the antigen, and the serum from rabbits immunized against HCG is the antiserum. If no clumping of the HCG-coated latex particles occurs when mixed with the urine and antiserum, the test is considered positive for pregnancy. If clumping or agglutination occurs, the test is negative. A positive test can be found 12 days after the first missed menstrual period, or about 26 days after conception.

A new home pregnancy test has been released to the general public and is sold in drugstores. The cost is under ten dollars. The kit can be used only once, so the woman must wait until at least 9 days *after* the day she expected her period to begin to allow for an adequate level of HCG. The test is claimed to be 95 percent accurate and takes 2 h to complete.†

quickening   By the sixteenth to eighteenth week a primigravida will begin to feel the baby move within her uterus. Known as *quickening* or "feeling life," it is for many women a most significant point in their pregnancy. Even the woman who is anxiously waiting for the sign may mistake it for flatulence, for the flutter of fetal movement is so slight. A multigravida, being more experienced, may feel movements by the fourteenth to sixteenth week.[12]

ballottement   While doing a vaginal examination, the examiner may tap the cervix in order to feel for the rise and then the fall of the fetus within the amniotic fluid. This movement of the fetus in response to such a stimulus is known as *ballottement*.

It is usually done after the sixteenth week of gestation.

positive signs of pregnancy

There are *three types* of positive indication of a growing fetus: hearing or recording the fetal heart, feeling the fetal parts or movements, and visualizing the outline of the fetus by x-ray or ultrasound.

auscultation   Auscultation of the fetal heart rate (FHR) is possible at about the

---

*Pregnosticon Dri-Dot, trademark, Diagnostic Products, Organon, Inc., West Orange, N.J. 07052.

†e.p.t., Trademark for in-home early pregnancy test, marketed by Warner/Chilcott, Morris Plains, N.J. 07950.

twentieth week after the LMP with a fetal stethoscope. An electronically amplified sound can sometimes be heard by the twelfth to sixteenth week. The fetal heart rate is most clearly audible through the back of the fetus. Therefore, the stethoscope is placed over that site after the abdomen has been palpated (Fig. 4-8). It is important that the examiner differentiate between the mother's pulse and the fetal heart sound. The usual fetal heart rate varies from 120 to 160 beats per minute, approximately twice that of the maternal pulse (70 to 90). Both heart rates should have a regular rhythm. When listening to the heart the nurse may hear a slurring or blowing sound known as a *souffle*. The sound of the blood as it surges through the umbilical cord is called the *funicular souffle;* as it passes through the uterine vessels on the maternal side, it is called the *uterine souffle.* The funicular souffle is at the same rate as the fetal heart, since the baby's heart propels the blood through the umbilical cord. The uterine souffle sounds at the same rate as the mother's heart rate.

fetal electrocardiogram   A fetal electrocardiogram may, on rare occasions, be included as a positive sign of pregnancy, for electrodes applied to the mother's abdomen by 14 to 16 weeks can pick up the almost doubled rate of the fetal heart. This method is useful in diagnosing the presence of a multiple pregnancy or in confirming fetal death, but it is used less often today because the ultrasound method is available.

palpation of fetal parts   Palpation of the fetal shape or body movement by the examiner is the second type of positive indication of pregnancy. By the twentieth week the examiner can usually differentiate between fetal kicking and what the mother may have described. By the twenty-sixth week the baby can be felt through the abdominal wall, and various parts identified. However, this

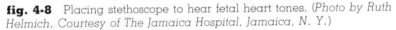

fig. 4-8   Placing stethoscope to hear fetal heart tones. (*Photo by Ruth Helmich. Courtesy of The Jamaica Hospital, Jamaica, N. Y.*)

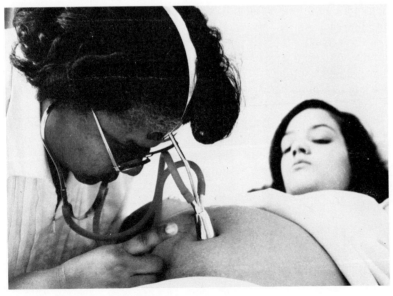

sign can never be used as a sole indication of pregnancy, for some women have muscle tumors (myomas) in the uterine wall that could be misleading.

visualization of the fetus   Visualization of the fetal outline or skeleton is possible by means of x-ray and ultrasound. Calcification of the bones takes place after the first trimester, so that the fetal skeleton shows more clearly after this time. However, x-ray merely to identify pregnancy is never done during the early part of pregnancy.

ultrasound   On the other hand, ultrasound has not been proved to be harmful and can pick up very early the fetal heart beat and the outlines of the fetal head in the enlarged uterus (see *Chap. 27* for further discussion). Ultrasound is not available everywhere but is becoming an increasingly useful tool in obstetrics (Fig. 4-9).

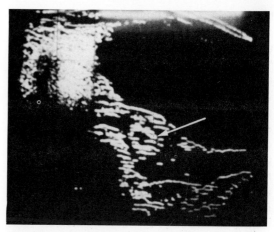

fig. 4-9   Ultrasonography indicating an embryo of 6 weeks' gestation. Gestational sac at 6 weeks. (Fetal heart tones can be confirmed by Doppler effect after the ninth week.) (*Photo courtesy of Horace E. Thompson, M.D., University of Colorado Medical Center, Denver, Col.*)

DETERMINING OBSTETRIC STATUS

gravidity and parity

The terms in Table 4-1 are special to obstetrics and are used as a shorthand way of referring to a woman's obstetric situation. As you learn more about pregnancy these terms will take on meaning. For example, if a patient has a *gravida IV, para 0* listing, it implies that she has been pregnant four times, but has never been able to carry an infant to term. Thus, she may have some underlying medical problem and may be tremendously anxious about the current pregnancy when she is seen in the clinic.

Gravidity and parity are described in two different ways. The first system explains only the number of times the woman has conceived

(gravidity) and the numbers of times she has delivered an infant of more than 20 weeks' gestation (parity).

A woman's gravidity refers to her state of having conceived a baby or of being pregnant

table 4-1   Gravida and para terminology

Gravid = pregnant, the state of being pregnant
Gravida = a pregnant woman
Gravidity = the number of times a woman has been pregnant
Primigravida = a woman who is pregnant for the first time
Multigravida = a woman who has been pregnant more than once (usually used for one who has delivered more than once, also)
Para = a woman who has delivered a *viable* infant (over the age of 20 weeks), whether alive or stillborn
Parity = the *number* of *times* a woman has delivered a viable infant*
Nullipara = one who *never* has borne a viable child (para 0)
Primipara = a woman who has had *one delivery* of a viable infant or infants (para I)
Multipara = a woman who has had *two or more* deliveries of viable infants (para II, III, IV, etc.)

*The birth of twins, triplets, etc., counts as one delivery.

regardless of the length of time she is or was pregnant. The term makes reference only to the number of pregnancies, not to the number of babies which may or may not result.

In the first system, parity refers to a woman's deliveries after 20 weeks of gestation (age of viability). If the woman has miscarried or aborted before her twentieth week, it is recorded as part of her gravidity, but not in her parity. Parity does not refer to babies—only to *deliveries* of viable babies. Whether or not the baby was born alive or dead is not taken into account when referring to parity; only deliveries are counted.

The second system describes only her parity, but in more detail. The parity is listed in four categories: term deliveries (T), preterm deliveries (P), abortions (A), and offspring now living (L). Shortened, these terms equal *T-P-A-L*. To determine gravidity from parity, add T, P, and A. (Always remember to include the current undelivered pregnancy, should the woman be coming into the clinic or the labor room.) Whether the viable (age in weeks) infant survived or not does not alter the parity. Remember the number of children resulting from her deliveries are counted only in column (L), living. Multiple births count only as one para but show in the column of living children (if they survived). Some institutions add a fifth category, multiple births (M), to make parity more accurately reflect what happens. Parity, like gravidity, is a shorthand reference system.

Transfer between the systems can be made as in the following examples (see Tables 4-1 and 4-2).

duration of pregnancy

The usual length of time from conception to birth is 266 days, but some races have a shorter gestation period. For instance, in some areas, black women have a period of pregnancy of about 8 days less than Caucasian women. (This difference may merely reflect socioeconomic factors such as poverty, nutrition, etc.) Some women, particularly primigravidas, go beyond the average period by 1 or 2 weeks without difficulty.

estimating duration Several terms are used to designate the date the full-term preg-

table 4-2 Comparison of gravidity and parity

Case A	This woman is pregnant; she has had one delivery at term and has one child living.
Case B	This woman is not presently pregnant; she has had one delivery at term, one abortion (spontaneous or induced), and has one living child.
Case C	This woman is pregnant; she has had three deliveries at term, one preterm delivery, and two abortions. She has four living children.
Case D	This woman is not presently pregnant; she has had one preterm delivery (at 33 weeks) and has two living children.

	System 1			System 2			
	gravida	para		term	preterm	abortion	living
Case A	II	I	Case A	1	0	0	1
Case B	II	I	Case B	1	0	1	1
Case C	VII	IV	Case C	3	1	2	4
Case D	I	I	Case D	0	1	0	2 (twins)

nancy is expected to end. The most commonly used terminology to designate this approximate date are estimated date of confinement (EDC), estimated date of delivery (EDD), and "due date."

Since the exact day of conception is rarely known, calculation is done from the first day of the last menstrual period. If the length of pregnancy is estimated from the first day of the last menstrual period, the duration becomes 14 days longer, or 272 to 280 days. (All calculations are based on a 28-day cycle in which ovulation occurs 14 days ±2 after the period starts, even though 50 percent of all women have a shorter or longer interval between menses.) Using Nägele's rule, the estimated time for delivery is figured as follows:

LMP + 7 days − 3 months + 1 year = EDD

This can be reduced to a formula set as follows:

	Day	Month	Year
LMP =	15	11	1979
	+7	−3	+1
EDD =	22	8	1980
	(day)	(month)	(year)

It should be kept in mind that only a very small percentage of women (4 percent) actually deliver on their EDD. It is merely an estimation. An actual delivery date 2 weeks either way is not unusual.

In the event that the woman cannot remember her LMP or when her menstrual cycle is so irregular as to make the date of conception unknown, other means can be used to determine when the infant will be born. The height of the fundus can be measured and MacDonald's rule used. If the mother is sure of her quickening date, Rawlings and Moore suggest a method of calculation:[13]

Date of quickening + 20 weeks and 2 days
= EDD for a primigravida

Date of quickening + 21 weeks and 4 days
= EDD for a multigravida

This method is more exact and requires the use of a calendar for accuracy. For example:

Primigravida's date of quickening =
Mar. 20, 1979
+ 20 weeks and 2 days

= Aug. 9, 1979

Multigravida's date of quickening =
Nov. 26, 1980
+ 21 weeks and 4 days

= Apr. 27, 1981

A combined calculation using both methods probably would give a more accurate EDD than either one used alone.

Perhaps the most dominant theme during pregnancy is that of growth and development. The experience of pregnancy is unique for every woman because the process is experienced differently in every case. And yet the experience is universal, in that the same basic physiologic processes are occurring in every pregnant woman. Chapter 5 will discuss the care given to the pregnant woman based on these changes occurring in pregnancy.

study questions

1 Trace the hormones of the menstrual cycle and identify which are continued in higher levels during pregnancy. Which are inhibited?
2 Describe at least five effects of the increase in blood volume.
3 Why does blood pressure fall slightly during the first trimester? What happens to the pulse?
4 List the possible and positive signs of pregnancy. Which minor discomforts result from the signs of pregnancy?
5 Identify the pressure effects of the enlarging uterus on the surrounding organs and vessels of the body. What are interventions which can be suggested to the pregnant woman who is in the third trimester?
6 Make your own list of minor discomforts of pregnancy and the instruction that can be given to a pregnant woman about methods of alleviation without medication.

7 Practice listing the parity and gravidity of different women you observe in the clinic. Does the birth of twins count as one or two deliveries?

references

1 Frank E. Hytten and Isabella Leitch, *The Physiology of Human Pregnancy,* 2d ed., Blackwell, Oxford, 1972, p. 193.
2 B. Little and R. B. Billiar, "Endocrine Disorders," in S. L. Romney (ed.), *Gynecology and Obstetrics: The Health Care of Women,* McGraw-Hill, New York, 1975, Chap. 26, p. 401.
3 Hytten and Leitch, op. cit., pp. 212–214.
4 Little et al., op. cit., pp. 395–398.
5 Ibid., p. 401.
6. B. H. Yuen, W. R. Keye, Jr., and R. B. Jaffee, "Human Prolactin: Secretion, Regulation, and Pathophysiology," *Obstetrical and Gynecological Survey,* **28**(8): 527, 1973.
7 Hytten and Leitch, op. cit., pp. 203–204, 214–215.
8 Ibid., p. 84.
9 Ibid., pp. 104–105.
10 Ibid., p. 153.
11 E. Brown and P. Barglow, "Pseudocyesis: A Paradigm for Psychophysiological Interaction," *Archives of General Psychiatry,* **24**:221, 1971.
12 R. C. Benson, *Handbook of Obstetrics and Gynecology,* 4th ed., Lange, Los Altos, Calif., 1971, p. 38.
13 E. E. Rawlings and B. A. Moore, "The Accuracy of Methods of Calculating the Expected Date of Delivery for Use in the Diagnosis of Postmaturity," *American Journal of Obstetrics and Gynecology,* March 1, 1970, pp. 676–679.

bibliography

Hellman, L. M., and J. A. Pritchard: *Williams' Obstetrics,* 14th ed., Appleton-Century-Crofts, New York, 1971.

Homburg, R. G. Potashnik, B. Lunefeld, and V. Insler: "The Hypothalamus as a Regulator of Reproductive Function," *Obstetrical and Gynecological Survey,* **31**(6): 455, 1976.

Hytten, F. E., and I. Leitch: *The Physiology of Human Pregnancy,* 2d ed., Blackwell, Oxford, 1972.

Romney, S. L. et al.: *Gynecology and Obstetrics: The Health Care of Women,* McGraw-Hill, New York, 1975.

Rugh, R. and L. B. Shettles: *From Conception to Birth: The Drama of Life's Beginnings,* Harper & Row, New York, 1971.

5

PRENATAL CARE

CHRISTINE D. SOUTHALL

INTRODUCTION

Prenatal care can best be termed preventive, protective care of the mother and the growing fetus during its development. Everything done for the mother is based on the physiologic and psychologic changes that take place in these most important 9 months.

Some women experience pregnancy as an exhilarating, exciting, welcomed occurrence, whether planned or "accidental." It may be their raison d'etre, the way to verify their feminine role. But for others, when pregnancy is unplanned, unexpected, or definitely unwanted, it may be a frightening time, a nuisance, or at least an interruption in their career plans. For all women, it is definitely a fact of life. Once conception has occurred, no amount of emotional acceptance or rejection will cause the growth process to stop.

Approximately 95 percent of all pregnancies are normal in every respect; the others are called high-risk, complicated pregnancies. Prenatal care is directed toward preventing complications, modifying those that occur, and supporting the mother during this period in order to allow her to carry the fetus to the full term of growth. The prenatal phase of the perinatal cycle is the most crucial period for the development of the baby and for its healthy outcome. Nursing care during this phase is totally concerned with the education and supportive care of the parents.

While private care during pregnancy offers perhaps the most personal care, most women in our society currently receive their prenatal care through some type of clinic. It is because of this that the clinic has been used to generalize nursing and patient care. Principles of care during the prenatal stage of the cycle do not differ.

SEQUENCE DURING PRENATAL VISITS

A nurse usually has the first contact with a patient following the registration procedure. Ideally, every clinic patient should be briefed by a nurse on what she can expect during the rest of her visit. (To do this effectively in large clinics, some nurses have made introductory films or videotapes.)

The patient should be assured of the confidentiality of her record and of the importance of having a complete history for background information that will be useful in assessing the current pregnancy. This background information and family history are usually taken by the nurse, after which the patient's weight, height, and urine specimen results are noted on the chart. The physical examination, including a vaginal examination for signs of pregnancy and possible infection, is performed by the physician or midwife during either the first or the second visit. Following this, blood tests are performed for screening.

If a pregnancy test is needed, it is done at this time, and the result is made available before the woman leaves the office.

The interval for subsequent visits may vary; the usual pattern is one visit per month until the thirty-second week, after which the visits may be scheduled every 2 to 3 weeks because signs of beginning complications are more likely to occur as the patient nears term.

The patient needs to know that on subsequent visits, the brevity of the examination does not mean poor care. The blood pressure, urine, and weight can be explained as important indices to the physician of a healthy progression of her pregnancy.

medical history

A complete medical history is taken at an early visit, with the interview often conducted by the nurse. The physician should know of previous operations and illnesses which might have an influence on the course of the pregnancy. For example, it would influence the mother's care markedly if she were a diabetic or had a heart condition from a childhood bout with rheumatic fever. The following diseases are important in a medical history:

Past Illnesses
syphilis, gonorrhea
heart disease
diabetes
tuberculosis
measles
rickets
hypertension
anemia
sickle-cell disease
kidney infection

Past Surgery
abdominal
pelvic
perineal
spinal
lower-back

Family History of Illness
any genetic diseases
hypertension
diabetes
heart disease
cancer
tuberculosis

Included in the history would be the family history, for any disease that might be genetically carried would alert the examiner to possible disorders that could influence the health of the mother or fetus.

social history

A brief questionnaire, such as the one shown in Table 1-2, may elicit social and family factors which may complicate the pregnancy outcome. Discretion is important, and pertinent facts are recorded on the chart. Social habits, such as customary amount of drinking or smoking, may be included in this part of the record. (The patient should be assured of the privacy of her record.)

obstetric history

Information about onset, regularity, and duration of menses, as well as any problems associated with it, should be included in the history. Gravidity and parity will be determined. Any problems occurring during these pregnancies and deliveries, as well as any physical or mental problems in these infants, any neonatal complications or stillbirths, must be noted. Previous attempts at conception and any problems of infertility, plus experience with success or failure of contraceptive methods, are included. Once the history is obtained, the EDD is established and any present complaints are noted.

All these facts may be gathered by interview with several staff members in the clinic, but the purpose is the same—to assist in determining the direction of care for the individual patient. The physician needs to "know" the patient's idiosyncrasies in order to individualize care, and the nurse must always counsel and teach each patient according to her peculiar life circumstances, without generalizing information.

physical examination

At the first visit, a complete physical examination will be made. For many healthy women, this may be the first time they have ever been examined; certainly it will be the first time for several of the tests they will have. Therefore, explanations of each procedure will greatly ease anxiety.

general examination *Ears, eyes, nose, and throat* (EENT) are examined to determine any infections, abnormalities, dental caries, or gum problems. The condition of blood vessels can be seen when the fundus of the eye is examined with a fundoscope.

Skin and hair often give clues to the overall health of the woman. A skilled examiner can gain a general impression fairly rapidly by observing the color, turgor, and condition of the skin.

Neck and chest yield information about the thyroid gland, the lymph nodes of the axillary area, and the breasts. *Breasts* are examined for asymmetry, dimpling and retraction of the nipple or skin surface. With the patient supine, the breast is palpated for masses. Every woman can and should be taught about breast self-examination during her pregnancy examinations.

Heart and lungs are auscultated for irregularities in function. The findings, coupled with a medical history, may permit diagnosis of a borderline cardiac condition during this first examination.

Extremities are examined for varicose veins and edema. The physician notes any signs of infection or restriction of movement.

Abdominal examination is done to determine the presence of any tenderness or mass. The size and shape of the uterus and the fundus usually are measured at each visit, to permit recording of the rate of fetal growth (Fig. 4-7). Patients often are very tense about abdominal palpation and need help in relaxing enough to allow the examiner to complete the task.

pelvic examination The external genitalia are examined for any lesions, scars or infections. Then, a vaginal speculum is inserted to provide a clear view of the cervix (Fig. 5-1). The color, condition, and amount of leukorrhea from the cervix are observed. At this time most physicians take a Papanicolaou test to screen for cervical cancer cells and take a specimen of cervical mucus for detec-

tion of gonorrhea. The speculum is removed, and a bimanual examination is performed to determine pelvic size and uterine consistency (Hegar's sign). A few pelvic measurements are made at this time: the *biischial diameter* is the distance between the ischial tuberosites (normally 8 cm or more), and the *diagonal conjugate* is the distance between the lower margin of the pubic bone to the promontory of the sacrum (normally 11.5 cm or more) (Fig. 5-2). (Measurements are discussed in detail in Chap. 10.)

fig. 5-1 (a) Insertion of the speculum. (b) Inspection of the cervix. To avoid discomfort, the speculum is inserted at an angle which will decrease its transverse diameter at the introitus; it is then rotated to the midline. The cervix is exposed by opening the blades with thumb pressure. The cervix is inspected, and specimens are obtained for cytologic examination. (*From S. L. Romney et al (eds.), Gynecology and Obstetrics: Health Care of Women, McGraw-Hill, New York, 1975.*)

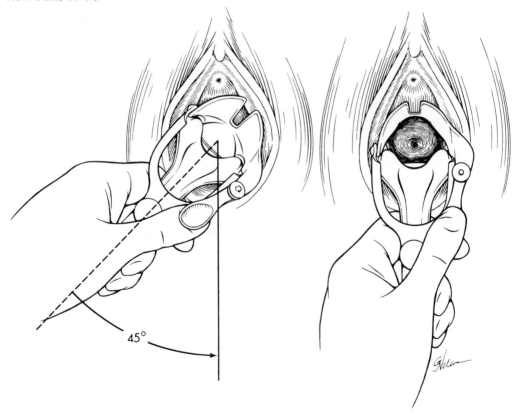

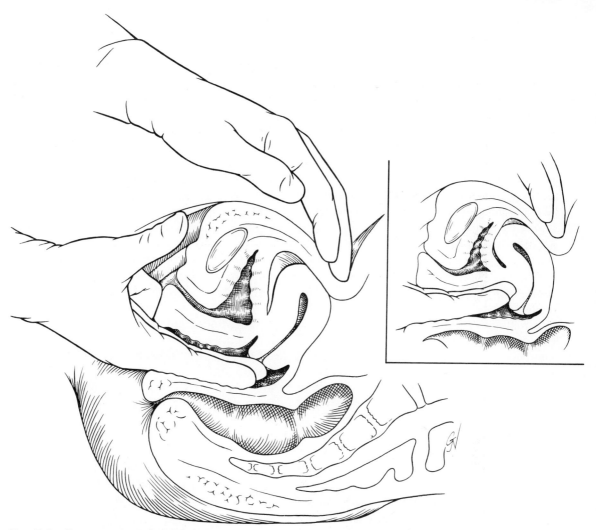

fig. 5-2 Bimanual examination. Palpation (a) of the cervix to determine size, shape, and consistency and its relation to the axis of the vagina, and (b) of the uterus for size, shape, consistency, mobility, and tenderness. Its anterior position is best determined when the corpus can be "grasped" between the fingers of the two hands. (From S. L. Romney et al. (eds.), Gynecology and Obstetrics: Health Care of Women, McGraw-Hill, New York, 1975.)

vital signs At every visit the vital signs will be taken and recorded. Of these signs, the blood pressure is the most significant and diagnostic indication of potential problems. An early base-line reading is important to have for comparison with later changes. A slight drop in pressure is expected in the first 24 weeks, with a return to normal or slightly above base line in the last trimester. Any elevation over base line of 30 points systolic and 15 points diastolic may be an indication of hypertension or preeclampsia (see Chap. 23). Older women often have preexisting high blood pressure. Early documentation during the prenatal clinic visits helps to diagnose and treat this type of hypertension.

laboratory tests

Urine tests can detect hormonal, cellular, and chemical products in the urine. The first visit includes the most thorough testing for glucose, protein, and cells. If glucose is indicated, a blood sample will be drawn and screening for diabetes carried out (see Chap. 24). At every later visit a dipstick test is made for glucose and protein levels. The nurse directs the patient to obtain the urine specimen collected free of vaginal secretions which, being protein, would falsely affect the results of the albumin test. Most clinics ask for a clean voided midstream urine sample: easily used kits are available or can be constructed with cotton balls and warm water. If an antiseptic is included, the woman must rinse well. If a culture and sensitivity test of urine are ordered, a clean voided specimen is preferable over a catheterized one. Culture of urine is usually done in the second trimester, since bacteruria is a common condition during pregnancy (see Chap. 25).

Blood tests are done as part of the initial examination of the pregnant woman's status. Complete blood count, hemoglobin, and hematocrit will indicate the normality of her hematologic system. Hematocrit will be repeated at 32 weeks. Blood is typed as to group—A, B, AB, or O—and for the presence or absence of the Rh factor. In the event that the mother is Rh-negative, the father should be typed. A test for *antibody titer* is done for all women who potentially could have an antibody buildup in their own blood against the fetal Rh-positive erythrocytes inherited from an Rh-positive father (see Chap. 29).

Screening for some genetically carried diseases is possible, and specific screening for thalassemia and sickle-cell trait will be done on women of Mediterranean or African ancestry. (The effect of these problems is discussed in detail in Chap. 22.)

By state law, every pregnant woman in the United States must be screened for syphilis. The serology test usually is done at the first visit and, depending upon the clinic policy, may be repeated before labor begins.

Many clinics are now screening for the presence of the rubella antibody. Any woman with a low antibody titer (under 1:20) is a candidate for rubella immunization immediately after delivery (see Chap. 25).

Many clinics require that the woman have a routine chest x-ray. This early x-ray shows heart size and can be used as a base-line view if later cardiac symptoms develop. X-rays are also done to screen high-risk populations for tuberculosis. Tuberculosis incidence varies, depending on risk factors of poverty, poor nutrition, and numbers of recent immigrants in an area (see Chap. 25).

Most private obstetricians do not order chest x-rays for their patients, considering them to be less exposed and thus less likely to have contracted tuberculosis. In any case, when a pregnant woman has a chest x-ray, her abdomen should be shielded by a lead apron to prevent scatter. Although the amount of radiation for a chest film (and dental films) is very small, precautions of this sort should never be ignored.

referrals

Before the end of the first visit, the woman will receive a referral to the dentist; this is done for three reasons: (1) since patients sometimes neglect their teeth when they are not pregnant, this practice provides dental screening for a large group of women; (2) if sufficient calcium is not ingested, decay may occur; (3) an assessment of the state of the patient's dental health from the beginning of pregnancy contributes toward the total health picture.

Other referrals in the clinic setting may include one to the nutritionist for evident nutritional problems or one to the social worker. For example, routine referral to social service would be made for a very young mother, an emancipated minor, a woman who is involved with drugs, or one who has family problems needing social service assistance.

The clinic patient should be provided with information regarding the availability of help, if and when she needs it between visits. In contrast to a private physician, the clinic is not available after hours. In order to provide assistance, many hospitals have set up a telephone system, usually in the admitting labor area. This allows a patient to reach professional counsel when trouble arises. Such reassurance is important to patients who perhaps in the past have found clinics to be somewhat inaccessible and impersonal.

subsequent visits

At each subsequent visit, the uterus is evaluated for growth consistent with estimated gestational age. In the last trimester, Leopold's maneuvers are carried out to determine the position of the fetus (see Fig. 5-3). The mother is questioned about fetal movements, and the fetal heart tones are obtained, at 12 to 16 weeks, using an ultrasonic stethoscope (Fig. 5-4) or by 20 to 24 weeks with a conventional stethoscope.

Urine tests are evaluated. If protein is present, other screening tests must be done for kidney function or for developing preeclampsia. If glucose is present, a glucose tolerance test is recommended. In the later part of pregnancy, lactose may disturb glucose tests, and screening should be done with test materials which differentiate between lactose (from colostrum reabsorbtion) and glucose. Testing with Clinistix or Tes-Tape will do so.

At each visit the mother will be asked to report any unusual symptoms, while a brief examination will rule out edema of the extremities, excessive weight gain, and rising blood pressure. Without causing her alarm, the warning signals of problems should be taught so that she can identify symptoms which should be reported.

PRENATAL EDUCATION

Nurses counsel prenatal patients, both in clinics and in private offices. The nurse may be deluged with questions on each visit if she is perceived by the pregnant woman as a person who will listen and answer questions. (Nurses can choose to take the role of educator or can avoid this role by spending all their time with technical tasks.)

In the clinic sequence, the woman, when seen by the teaching nurse, is likely to be tired and hungry. It is therefore best to keep the initial nursing conference short and to the point; an offer of milk or juice may be most welcome. The nurse elicits questions from the woman on any point not understood in the process she has just been through.

Emphasis should be placed on giving the client a sense of the availability of supportive services throughout the pregnancy, as well as the feeling that there is concern for her well-being. Since explanation of the examiner's findings (shown on the patient's chart) is reassuring, the nurse goes over the chart and the recommendations with the client and plans with her for the next visit.

Conferences are personal and sensitive for both the woman and the nurse. The setting should be chosen to ensure privacy, relaxation, comfort, and freedom from as many distractions as possible. Knowledge of interviewing techniques is helpful. Sensitivity to the length of the conference, the nature of information sought and the response given is important. Women who do not ask questions

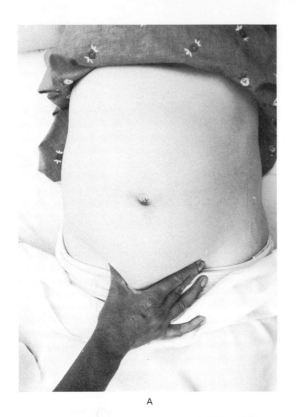

A

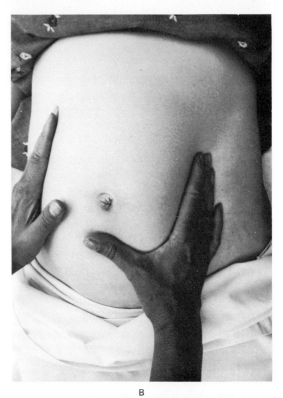

B

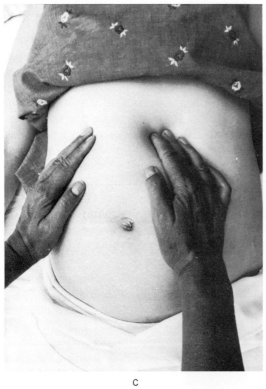

C

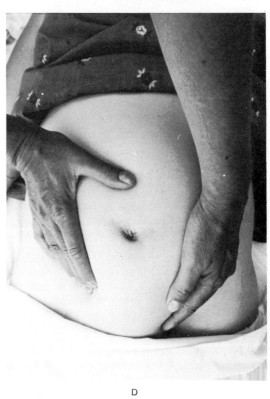

D

may be very inquisitive. Some who ask many questions may be anxious; others may simply need to socialize.

A woman's attitude toward pregnancy is largely dependent upon whether or not she has chosen to have a baby. Because so many women have the options of practicing family planning or of having an abortion, feelings are usually positive.

Observers who studied the needs expressed by pregnant women found that basic psychologic needs did not vary in relation to economic status or class but that parity of the mother and her educational level significantly influenced the frequency of her questions and the anxieties that she expressed. "Frequency of concerns related to childbirth, family, subsequent pregnancies and finances increased as education level decreased."[1]

Tanner has identified the basic developmental phases through which most women pass during pregnancy. During each trimester, questions and interests reflect the phase with which the woman is involved. As Tanner states:

Pregnancy is a period of disequilibrium involving profound endocrine and general somatic as well as psychologic changes. This constitutes a significant turning point in the life of the individual, the resolution of which will affect future adjustments.[2]

first trimester

First-trimester needs vary according to whether the pregnancy is a first or subsequent

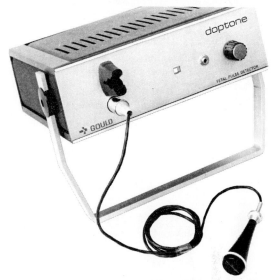

fig. 5-4 Doptone for auscultation of fetal heartbeat. Amplified heart sounds can be heard early in the second trimester. (*Courtesy of Gould, Inc.*)

one. A first pregnancy is like any other "first" experience. Curiosity and concern are felt about the unknown that lies ahead. Even the most carefully planned educational program will not fully relieve the accompanying anxiety generated from anticipation.

Although the woman may choose to become pregnant in the beginning there will always be an ambivalence until the idea of being pregnant becomes a reality and an acceptance of the growing fetus, or *integration*, takes place.[3]

Most pregnant women are concerned during the first trimester with the changes in their own bodies and how these changes will affect

fig. 5-3 Leopold's maneuvers. (*a*) With thumb and forefingers, press into the lower abdomen just above the symphysis. If the part is hard, round and freely movable, it is the head and is not engaged. If it is firmly fixed, the head is probably engaged. (*b*) Press gently with the palms on each side of the abdomen. The general examination will reveal if the oval shape of the fetus is parallel with the long axis of the mother. Press deeply to feel the smooth curve of the back as contrasted to the uneven feel of the extremities. (*c*) Palpate the fundus with the fingers. The breech feels soft and irregular, and the head feels hard, round, and freely movable. (*d*) Using the first three fingers of each hand, press deeply into the pelvis, moving toward the inlet. The head can usually be felt higher on the side opposite the fetal spine because the head is flexed. (*Photos by Ruth Helmich.*)

their lives. Some of their expressed concerns have to do with:

1 Normality of symptoms of pregnancy ("Should I worry?" "Am I normal?" "What shall I do?")
2 Changes in life-style that will result from the pregnancy ("I wonder how pregnancy will make me different?")
3 Changes in relationship with the woman's partner ("How will he accept this pregnancy?" "How will it change sexual responses?")
4 Medical care—the sequences and reasons for visits ("How can I get help between visits?")

The woman may appear to be very self-concerned and will reflect the ambivalence of the phase through which she is going. Because she probably will not be able to focus on instructions concerning future events such as labor, delivery, child care, or contraception, such topics are best discussed in later visits.

Signs of difficulty with first-trimester tasks Signs of difficulty with achievement of the first-trimester tasks may be demonstrated as exaggerated discomforts, such as severe nausea, sleeplessness, and fatigue. The woman may demonstrate that she cannot yet accept the pregnancy by seeking reassurance from several sources; she may make appointments with different medical offices to corroborate the diagnosis. In addition, she may have unresolved anger, feel depressed, and be hostile toward her sexual partner. Interventions may assist her to resolve these conflicts. Certainly, she will need support while she works through these feelings. Chapter 7 discusses the normal ambivalence of the first trimester and the support which can be offered.

nutrition and drugs During the first trimester, emphasis on nutrition should begin.

Adequate intake is of such importance that the whole of prenatal teaching should include nutrition as a priority. Chapter 6 identifies normal weight gain during pregnancy and the ways in which diet must be adjusted to achieve a healthy pregnancy.

Drugs used by the woman must be identified as early as possible during the first trimester because the early stages of embryonic development are the most susceptible to injury by chemicals. Chapter 20 discusses drugs which are injurious to the growing fetus.

second trimester

By the end of the first trimester, discomforts from physiologic changes have usually disappeared. The expectant mother is well on her way to settling down to exactly what she needs to do for herself and the growing baby. Her concerns begin to shift from her own bodily changes during the first trimester to the growing baby. It is during the second trimester that the baby takes on its own identity as a separate being. The psychologic task of perceiving the fetus as a growing baby, separate from herself,[4] is normally completed by the end of the second trimester.

If the nurse wants to test the mother's perception of the baby's individual identity, she can ask how the mother responded to the feeling of quickening. Mothers who have successfully accepted the baby's presence usually respond in positive ways. In general, the mother is interested in protecting the health of the infant, and her concerns will now reflect her awareness of the infant's needs. The more general concerns are as follows:

1 Nutritional intake ("Am I gaining too much?" "Too little?")
2 Amount of exercise, travel ("What restrictions are necessary?")
3 Progression of fetal growth ("How big is the baby this month?")
4 Warning signs of problems

5 Changing body image (how reflected in clothes, hygiene, hair, skin)

6 Changes in sexual desires (concern about restrictions and misconceptions)

signs of difficulty with second-trimester tasks Signs of difficulty with second-trimester tasks may include continuing anger and depression because of lack of acceptance. Numerous physical complaints and a focus on her own concerns, rather than turning in this trimester to the thought of the developing fetus, may indicate problems. It often becomes evident in this trimester that a person is not yet able to plan or look forward to being a parent. Clues to difficulty in parenting may become evident in this self-involvement or in childish behavior.

If the woman visited the clinic initially after missing two periods, by the second trimester she is returning for her second or third visit. The process she will be going through does not frighten her. She relaxes and socializes with other women.

Individual conferences are continued, as suggested earlier. By this time, however, most women have begun to participate in group discussions or the teaching program that the particular clinic may have set up. Most of the woman's waiting time in the clinic should include giving, sharing, and receiving information. Various approaches are used in clinics toward this end. One useful way is to schedule the group conference into the sequence of the visit, in 30-min segments, staggering the appointments, so that no one has to wait too long. The specific topic for discussion may be posted for sessions in a given morning or afternoon. Thus, if an expectant mother missed a session, she can elect to sit in on the discussion of the current topic (Fig. 5-5).

Several nurses may be assigned to conduct "bench conferences" on a selective basis with women who, by appearance (bodily attitude) or other nonverbal signs, indicate a need for private discussion. Closed-circuit TV, videocassettes, and a variety of cartridge films may be utilized in small groups for information purposes. By whatever means the staff may choose to disseminate information, the goal is usually to utilize the available time for client-based concerns.

With each recommendation for health maintenance, the nurse should give a reasonable explanation based on the physiology of pregnancy. There are few hard-and-fast rules today; recommendations are tailored to each woman's life-style, the aim being to bring her to an acceptable level of health, and to maintain her at that level, while preventing problems.

exercise, rest, relaxation Exercise and rest should be discussed in terms of relieving minor discomforts of pregnancy during the second and third trimesters. For most women, especially if they are working, the activities of the home provide enough activity and exercise. Physicians often recommend long walks as the best form of exercise when the woman is not employed outside the home. Rest intervals with feet elevated will help prevent edema and will improve lower-extremity circulation.

Muscle-toning exercises are taught as early as the need is indicated; e.g., if a patient lives in a walk-up apartment, discussion of the best way to climb stairs without strain may be helpful. Ways of stooping, bending, and lifting are often taught earlier than exercises for labor and delivery.

Relaxation is sought in individual ways and discussed whenever there are problems. (See Chap. 9 for preparatory exercises for labor and delivery.)

sexual intercourse Questions regarding intercourse usually come from women who are pregnant for the first time and are anxious to follow instructions to the letter. In the ab-

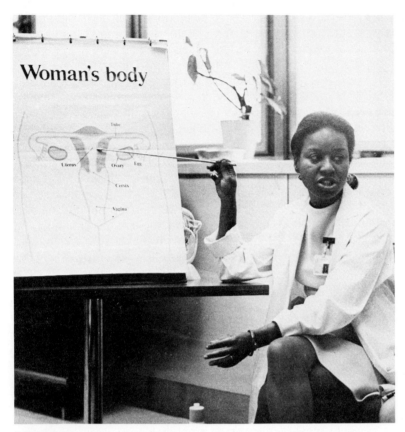

fig. 5-5 Teaching in the clinic. (*Photo by Nancy Goodman.*)

sence of complications, however, there is no advice peculiar to pregnancy. Couples may continue their sexual relationship as usual. Some men have reported that there is a difference in the feeling of the vagina. This, of course, results from the physiologic changes which have taken place.

In the past, intercourse was restricted at intervals during the first 3 months, and again 6 weeks before delivery, because of fear of complications. Now, physicians merely advise the couple to use common sense about position and pressures.[5] Chapter 7 discusses some of the sexual fears and fantasies women may experience.

employment Socioeconomic factors, cultural considerations, safety aspects, and the therapeutic value of work all help in determining whether to continue one's employment. A consultation with the physician or midwife gives direction to the expectant mother. Frequent periods of rest may be needed in the third trimester, and sitting or standing for long periods should be avoided.

smoking Excessive smoking is detrimental to the growing fetus. The weight difference is directly proportional to the number of cigarettes smoked.[6]

There is a strong inverse relationship between maternal smoking and mean birthweight of offspring. The mean birthweight decreases over 400 grams in Whites and over 250 grams in Negroes and the low birthweight rate more than doubles between babies of nonsmokers and those smoking over 30 cigarettes a day.[7]

In another large survey, data from the Ontario Perinatal Mortality Study (50,000 births) found that birth weight had the strongest correlation with smoking. Women who smoked more than one pack a day had twice as many infants weighing under 2500 g, abnormalities of the placenta were more common, and these factors led to a higher perinatal mortality.[8] Finally, real-time ultrasound scanning has demonstrated that smoking depresses fetal breathing movements, in utero for up to 30 min. The long-term effects on the fetus are not known.[9]

alcohol The fetal alcohol syndrome is a specific pattern of malformations and includes prenatal and postnatal growth retardation, mental retardation, and small head size. Minor abnormalities of the eye, face, heart, joints, and external genitalia may also occur when the mother has been a severe chronic alcoholic for several years. The infants were affected directly in proportion to the amount of alcohol ingested.[10] Therefore, until further studies can clarify its effects on the fetus, it seems wise at this time to counsel a very low alcohol intake or none at all during pregnancy.

travel After midpregnancy, trips of over 2 to 3 h by car, train, or plane are unwise, because of the prolonged sitting time. If a trip has to be made, the woman should change positions frequently and, if driving, stop to walk around at least every 2 h.

Prolonged sitting or standing is associated with a marked increase in sodium retention, a change caused by the postural effect on the dynamics of blood flow through the kidneys. Sodium retention leads to water retention (see Chap. 23) and consequently to edema, first in the lower extremities and then, when severe, throughout the body.[11]

SEAT BELTS According to the 1967 American Medical Association Committee on Medical Aspects of Auto Safety, seat belts continue to be an important safety factor for pregnant women. Lap and shoulder belts provide the best protection, with the lap belt fastened, of course, below the bulge of the uterus.

hygiene during pregnancy Most women practice good daily hygiene. Sensitivity can be exercised in the case of a mother who has special needs. A reminder can be given to women about safety during bathing, the most important point to make, since baths, both tub and shower, can be taken right up until the time of delivery.

Increased vaginal secretions may be bothersome during pregnancy. Discussion will help women to recognize leukorrhea as normal (Chap. 4); they should be taught to report to the physician if it becomes excessive enough to necessitate the wearing of a pad, if it is odorous or discolored, or if it causes itching. Douching is not advised, and tampons, feminine hygiene suppositories, creams, and jellies are usually prohibited unless ordered by the physician. Perineal care several times a day should relieve any discomfort that might occur.

preparation for breast feeding The prenatal period is the ideal time to discuss breast feeding with the mother. The advantages of this method of feeding can be presented in prenatal classes, with each mother being given an opportunity to express her feelings and to ask questions. There are many myths in our society about breast feeding:

that it spoils the figure; that a woman with small breasts cannot produce enough milk; the breast milk is too thin for the baby; that breast feeding is too complicated; etc. Some women are embarrassed by the idea of breast feeding; others find it repugnant. Much depends on the woman's feeling of comfort with her own body. Often a woman will find resistance on her husband's part. Open discussion at home or in the childbirth education class may reduce his concerns. If he remains adamant, she probably should not breast-feed because tension over this issue can reduce her ability to produce milk. La Leche League, an organization dedicated to the promotion of breast feeding, has excellent literature available and in most parts of the country has members ready to help new mothers in preparing for breast feeding and to give assistance and support after the baby is born.

NIPPLE AND BREAST CARE Opinions differ widely on the importance of prenatal nipple care and whether or not it has any effect on successful breast feeding. It is certain, however, that positive thinking and looking forward to the experience help. If the mother is given routine, practical instructions on how to care for her breasts and nipples during her pregnancy, this may stimulate her interest in breast feeding and give her a positive attitude toward it. Once the breasts enlarge, support is needed. Breast tissue will stretch if not supported during pregnancy and the lactation period. A variety of supportive brassieres is available; nursing brassieres can be used during pregnancy (Fig. 16-9).

Daily washing of the breasts and nipples is the only care that is necessary during most of the prenatal period. Soap should be used sparingly, if at all. Beginning in the eighth month, a small amount of colostrum should be hand-expressed from the breasts daily. The mother learns now how to express fluid

from the ducts and can later help prevent painful engorgement when lactation begins.

Daily gentle "pulling out" of the nipple during the last few months of pregnancy is also recommended. A treatment for flattened nipples, it also helps to toughen the nipple and prevent soreness from developing during nursing. Conditioning the nipples for nursing can also be done by rubbing them with a rough terry towel after bathing. Inverted nipples are relatively uncommon; unless they are noticed and treated during pregnancy the mother may have difficulty with feeding the infant. The inverted nipple retracts when pressure is applied to it between the thumb and forefinger, and folds back into itself. A hand breast pump will draw out the nipple and, if used several times a day during pregnancy, will help correct inversion. Often inversion corrects itself spontaneously once the baby is put to the breast.

the warning signals Sometime during the early prenatal visits, each woman should be instructed about when to notify the physician of problems. Warning signals of problems other than the normal minor discomforts should be clearly taught. Unknowingly, a woman may endure a pathologic change in her condition, assuming that it is "just one of those things that happen." Every pregnant woman should be taught to report any of the following signals *immediately* should they occur anytime during pregnancy. Warning signals can be divided into groups as below:

Bleeding. Any bleeding during pregnancy is abnormal. It may warn of impending abortion, a poorly implanted placenta, or a sudden separation of the placenta. And a few women have vaginal bleeding from cervical erosion due to chronic infection.
Infection. Signs of infection in any part of the body are warning signals, but during

pregnancy, those conditions that might affect the fetal condition are especially serious. Fever, chills, and signs of kidney, bladder, or vaginal infection are all reportable.

Pain. Pain during the course of pregnancy is usually abnormal. The abdominal aching and perineal pressure of prelabor or the "catching," brief pain in the side due to a pulling sensation of the round ligament as it supports the uterus are exceptions. Occasionally, pain radiates through the groin or down the line of the sciatic nerve as a result of pressure on the nerves in the pelvic region.

Preeclampsia. A group of signs and symptoms related to developing preeclampsia may demonstrate as (1) severe continuous headache, (2) edema in face, hands, or legs upon arising in the morning, (3) scanty, concentrated urine, (4) visual disturbances. Any of these must be reported at once, as the preeclampsia syndrome can develop very rapidly.

third trimester

No matter what the background of the mother, her needs in the third trimester will be expressed in approximately the same ways. She focuses on the outcome of the baby, the process of labor, her own changing physical condition and emotions, and her figure during this last trimester. Even multiparas have questions about the differences in labor and delivery with each baby. If a program has been designed for education in childbirth for the last trimester, it usually begins about the thirtieth week of gestation. By this time the mother has been working through her emotional task of separation from the fetus in preparation for its delivery. She is getting ready to take up the care of the infant.[12] Concerns expressed in this trimester tend to be about:

1   The baby's well-being (questions on birth defects, signs of fetal well-being, how birth affects the infant, effect of medication and anesthesia)
2   The costs of having a baby (fees, having to stop work, expenses for equipment)
3   The process of labor and delivery (pain, fears, misconceptions, when to come to the hospital)
4   Family (how other children will accept the infant, how to plan for them during hospitalization, how father will respond to the infant)

The changing contours of the woman's body become more prominent; backaches, leg aches, lower abdominal pressure, ligament pain, fatigue, extra weight, concern about normal dependent edema, and anxiety over the warning signals of preeclampsia all cause her to be impatient for labor to begin.

Thus the woman is eager to learn any methods and techniques to relieve discomforts and those which will be of assistance to her during the later part of pregnancy and during the labor process. She will use exercises and practice breathing in these weeks when she would not have done so before. If this is a first pregnancy, she will need instruction to reduce the fear of the unknown in labor. If it is a second or third pregnancy, a review is usually welcome. The approach to childbirth education will vary according to the method used in each hospital. The one commonality is to reduce the fear-tension-pain cycle by information and discussion of sources of anxiety (see Chap. 9). Usually, after discussion, an informational brochure is given to each woman to reinforce the material.

Counseling continues on an individual basis and may now include preparation for the baby. Many women still cannot focus on baby care. The outcome of the pregnancy is as yet unreal. Therefore, postdelivery classes should be held on the unit for those who become aware that they do not really know what to do for the new infant.

Many women are superstitious about buying anything for the infant before its birth; to do so might risk death or injury to the child, they have been told. The nurse may acknowledge that this is a belief that some do hold and can skillfully turn the conversation to a discussion of the equipment that will be needed by the new baby, even though layette purchasing can begin any time the mother wishes. The father or grandparents may have this task during her hospitalization, but the mother will want to know how to plan. The only important fact to emphasize is that planning should be in advance of taking the infant home. Mothers who have limited apartment space and/or income will usually welcome suggestions on how to economize.

signs of difficulty with third-trimester tasks Signs of difficulty with third-trimester tasks include a continuing high level of anxiety about self, the process of labor, or the discomforts of pregnancy. If the woman neglects health practices or cannot prepare for or focus on needs of the coming infant during this phase, it may be that she cannot adjust to what is happening in her body.

When Light and Fenster questioned women after delivery, they found that concerns took a different order of priority than before delivery.[13] High on the list at that time was the concern about how to prevent subsequent pregnancies; indications are that the woman after delivery is highly motivated to learn about contraception. Therefore, future plans are not usually explored until after the baby's birth.

Of course, not every woman follows the "average pattern." Nurses can become skilled in individualizing the teaching and support of patients during prenatal care. Table 5-1 correlates the developmental concerns of pregnancy with signs and symptoms and nursing interventions.

study questions

1 For each trimester, list at least five needs any woman would have, regardless of ethnicity or educational level.

2 Read Table 5-1 carefully. Correlate pregnancy concerns with teaching points for each trimester.

3 Why is a syphilis screening test mandatory? Check Chap. 25 to assist your answer. Should a screening test for gonorrhea also be done on most patients?

4 Why might rubella screening be important to do early in pregnancy? How can it be shown that a woman subsequently had a light case of measles? Check Chap. 25, before you answer.

5 Practice Leopold's maneuvers on a patient in the last trimester. Identify where the fetal heart is best heard.

6. Identify the ways a nurse can assist in the prenatal examination. What points may need interpretation later, during the counseling session?

7 If a young primigravida is frightened at the thought of a pelvic examination, how would you intervene?

8 How would you interpret warning signals to a woman who is 20 weeks pregnant? Which symptoms occur more commonly after 20 weeks?

9 Plan how you would teach a woman regarding the effects on her baby if she smokes two packs of cigarettes a day.

references

1 H. K. Light and C. Fenster, "Maternal Concerns during Pregnancy," *American Journal of Obstetrics and Gynecology,* **118**(1):47, 1974.

2 L. M. Tanner, "Developmental Tasks of Pregnancy," in B. S. Bergersen, et al., *Current Concepts in Clinical Nursing,* Mosby, St. Louis, 1969, Chap. 28, p. 293.

3 Ibid., p. 292.

4 Tanner, op. cit., p. 293.

5 Barbara Quirk and Ruth Hassanein, "The Nurse's Role in Advising Patients on Coitus during Pregnancy," *Nursing Clinics of North America,* **8**(3):501, 1973.

6 M. B. Meyer, B. S. Jonas, and J. A. Ronascia, "Perinatal Events Associated with Maternal Smoking During Pregnancy," *American Journal of Epidemiology,* **103**:464, 1976.

7 K. R. Niswander and M. Gordon (eds.), *The Women and Their Pregnancies, The Collaborative Perinatal*

table 5-1 A correlation of the process of pregnancy with nursing interventions

developmental tasks and concerns	signs and symptoms	nursing interventions
First trimester (1 through 14 weeks post-LMP or 1 to 12 weeks postconception) *Tasks* Acknowledgment of the pregnancy. Acceptance of the fetus within her. Must work through conflicts with her own mother to begin to take up her own future mothering role. *Frequent concerns* Normality of symptoms, future changes in lifestyle. Changes in relationship with partner. Cost of care and now to manage. Normality of ambivalence to being pregnant. *Signs of difficulty with first-trimester tasks* a. Exaggerated discomforts such as nausea, sleeplessness. b. Excessive need for reassurance that she is pregnant. c. Anger and rejection of idea of pregnancy. d. Depression, crying, extreme mood swings. e. Distance from sexual partner.	**1 to 4 weeks postconception** *Subjective* Amenorrhea, but some women may have spotting at the time of the expected period. Fatigue, thought to be caused by the ovarian hormone relaxin. Nausea, may be caused by decreased maternal blood sugar, decreased gastric motility. Peak period from 60 to 100 days postconception parallels. HCG elevated levels. Soreness, tingling of the breasts. *Objective* Elevated basal body temperature owing to the presence of the corpus luteum. **5 to 8 weeks** *Subjective* Enlarging uterus causes pressure on bladder, frequency of urination. Desire for sexual relations may decrease. *Objective* Breasts enlarge, areola darken. Enlarged Montgomery's follicles. Mucous plug formation in the cervical canal. These signs present by 5 to 7 weeks: Ladin's—softening on the anterior side of the uterus above the uterocervical junction. Goodell's—softening of the cervix.	**First prenatal visit** Instruct on the importance of seeking early prenatal care and avoiding any drugs during weeks 1 to 12 unless prescribed by physician. Teach the importance of adequate sleep, rest periods, sitting with legs elevated, exercise, using good body mechanics. Suggest intake of dry carbohydrate foods before arising, eating small, frequent carbohydrate foods, and eliminating greasy, spicy foods. Teach about avoiding over-the-counter medications for nausea. Isoimmunologic test can be positive 26 days postconception. An early symptom of pregnancy. Advise wearing supportive bra. Client using BBT can see sustained temperature elevation on graph. Become aware of clients' concerns and begin teaching at those points. Other instruction must wait until anxiety has been diminished. In the absence of pain, burning on urination, or hematuria, reassure the client that these are caused by the pressure of the growing uterus. Omit fluids after 6 P.M. to prevent nocturia. Explain that sexual desires vary during pregnancy for both physical and psychological reasons. Advocate the use of a supporting bra, with adjustable cups, wide adjustable straps, and a smooth interior to prevent irritation. First visit lab work includes: blood type, Rh, CBC, hemoglobin, hematocrit, urinalysis, and often serology. High-risk population are screened for tuberculosis, sickle-cell disease. Vaginal or cervical smears taken for gonorrhea and other infections, and a PAP test may be done. Instruct client to bring first-voided specimen for biologic tests, but obtain fresh-voided specimen for isoimmunologic test.

table 5-1 A correlation of the process of pregnancy with nursing interventions (continued)

developmental tasks and concerns	signs and symptoms	nursing interventions
	Hegar's—softening of the lower uterine segment. Positive pregnancy test for HCG using biologic methods.	
	9 to 12 weeks	
	Subjective	
	Nausea subsides by 12 weeks. Frequency subsides by 12 weeks.	
	Objective	
	Gingivitis, hypertrophy of the gums.	Check on intake of foods rich in vitamin C. Advise dental checkup. Caution use of lead apron if need dental x-rays.
	Weight gain of 0 to 3 pounds. Some may lose weight.	Dietary teaching: Weight gain should average 1 lb a month in the first trimester, and 11 lb in each of the second and third trimesters (0.8 lb/week).
	Chadwick's sign—now present at 8 weeks, bluish discoloration of the vagina.	
	Height of the fundus is at the symphysis, rises about 1 cm per week thereafter. 12 weeks—fetal pulse detected by ultrasonic techniques.	Teach to report these warning signals of problems: in first and second trimester, vaginal bleeding, fever, chills, pain, persistent vomiting, leaking of fluid from the vagina.
Second trimester (15 to 28 weeks post-LMP or 13 to 26 weeks postconception)	**13 to 16 weeks postconception** *Objective* Colostrum is present.	Advise the use of cream to soften crusts formed by colostrum. Remove the crusts as part of bathing. Avoid soap on the nipple.
Tasks Conceptualizes the fetus as a separate being.	Profuse, thin, white vaginal discharge, leukorrhea. Report if pruritis, or foul odor: *Candida albicans*, trichomonal infections common	Suggest the use of a solution of vinegar and water externally; use of loose, cotton undergarments; vulval pads can be used, change frequently; tampons are contraindicated.
Manages the shifts in dependency from the role of daughter to the role of wife. Completes the working through of conflicts with her own mother.	Abdominal appearance of pregnancy. Height of the fundus is halfway between symphysis and the umbilicus.	Advise against tight, constricting clothing or wearing shoes with a heel higher than 1 ½ in. Reinforce good body mechanics, introduce the pelvic rock exercise and body toning exercises.
	17 to 20 weeks *Subjective*	
Mimicry, role playing to help assume the role of mother.	Quickening—maternal perception of first fetal movements.	Instruct client to report any cessation of fetal movement lasting longer than 24 h.
	Often, increased sexual desire.	Reinforce concept that variations in sexual interest do occur and that her partner may not understand these variations.

table 5-1 A correlation of the process of pregnancy with nursing interventions (*continued*)

developmental tasks and concerns	signs and symptoms	nursing interventions
	Objective Increase in total blood volume which contributes to light-headedness or fainting; occurs by 10 to 14 weeks, peaks at 8 ½ months (34 to 36 weeks).	Good communication is essential. Advise her to move slowly when moving from a horizontal position.
Frequent concerns: Nutritional intake. Changing body image. Changing life-style and sexual needs. Progression of fetal growth. Warning signs of problems.	The formation of varicosities of the saphenous system, vulva, and rectum. Headaches.	Avoid constricting bands around legs and long periods of sitting and standing. Use of support hose and elevation of legs at a 90° angle at least twice a day may be indicated. Report severe headaches—do not take aspirin in large doses. Report visual disturbances; edema of the face, hands, or legs in the morning; scanty, concentrated urine.
Signs of difficulty with second-trimester tasks a. Lack of acceptance of pregnancy. b. Depression, anger, anxiety continues. c. Numerous physical complaints and focus on own concerns. d. Indications of no family support. e. Indication of inability to plan ahead. *Preparation for the new family member:* Includes siblings Prepares to deal with sibling rivalry Buys equipment, baby clothes (unless cultural, socio-economic restrictions)	Hemodilution of pregnancy is result of increased plasma (40%) and small RBC increase. Hemoglobin of 11.0 to 12 g, and hemotocrit may be 30 to 33%. Fundus is slightly below the umbilicus. **21 to 24 weeks** *Subjective* Pelvic joints are relaxing as a result of the hormone relaxin. *Objective* Skin changes in pigmentation—chloasma of the face, linea nigra of the abdomen, striae gravidarum. Increased perspiration. Dilation of the right ureter owing to pressure from the dextro-rotated uterus **25 to 28 weeks** *Subjective* Leg cramps owing to decreased calcium when there is an increased phosphorus level; fatigue. *Objective* Fetal parts are palpable. Fundus is above umbilicus. Bal-	Include iron-bearing foods in diet. Fetal heart tones are audible with stethoscope. Reinforce good body mechanics; use of squatting position, tailor sitting. Reassure patient that while these cannot be prevented, the pigmentation will fade after delivery. Teach hygiene if necessary. Since urinary stasis and resultant pylonephritis may result, reinforce the need to report any signs of infection. Side-lying position facilitates kidney efficiency from now on. Advise exercise, particularly walking, elevation of legs; as a substitute for milk, calcium tablets may be ordered to achieve calcium-phosphorus balance.

table 5-1 A correlation of the process of pregnancy with nursing interventions (*continued*)

developmental tasks and concerns	signs and symptoms	nursing interventions
	lottement—the rebound of fetal parts.	
	Braxton Hicks contractions—painless, intermittent contractions.	Explain that these occur throughout pregnancy and are not labor contractions.
	Hemorrhoids	Replace hemorrhoids if possible, if external. Advise using ice on the area; using knee chest position for up to 15 min. Teach diet to avoid constipation.
Third trimester (29 through 42 weeks post-LMP or 27 through 40 weeks postconception)	**29 to 32 weeks** *Subjective* Fatigue recurs.	Anticipatory guidance about availability of classes in preparation for childbirth; inform of the signs of labor, be aware of unrealistic attitudes toward labor; employment will be terminated usually by the seventh month; travel involving trips of over 2 to 3 h are unwise; if necessary, the woman should be instructed to change position frequently and to stop car and walk around.
Tasks Acceptance of pregnancy. Continues to view fetus as a separate individual. Acceptance of physical and psychological changes.	May feel faint in the supine position owing to the pressure on the inferior vena cava, which prevents the return of blood from the lower extremities.	Advise the use of a side-lying position such as a modified Sims' position.
Frequent concerns: Baby's well-being and factors affecting this. Anxiety over fantasies of deformed baby. Expenses. Process of labor and delivery. Acceptance of baby by other children. Present discomforts.	Sexual desire again decreases because of physical discomfort. Constipation owing to slowed peristalsis, pressure of uterus on lower colon, rectum, hemorrhoids. Heartburn resulting from pressure of uterus on stomach causes mild hiatus hernia, regurgitation of stomach acid into esophagus.	Counseling about variations in desires, alternative sexual practices, and reassurance that this experience is normal. Avoidance of constipation by a regular elimination routine, liberal fluid and roughage intake, and exercise is best. Home remedies, over-the-counter preparations, and enemas are to be avoided. Antacids may be ordered by the doctor. Advise small meals and sitting up after eating. Advise against over-the-counter preparations.
Signs of difficulty with third-trimester tasks a. High level of anxiety about self, process of labor. b. Continued nonacceptance. c. Behavior which neglects health practices.	*Objective* Blood pressure returns to the prepregnancy level after a slight drop owing to vasodilation. Pulse rate has risen to 15 beats per minute over normal because of increase in cardiac work. Fundus is midway between	Monitor blood pressure for changes. A bp of 140/90 or an increase of 30 mmHg in systolic or 15 mmHg in diastolic pressure is considered a symptom of preeclampsia. Reinforce instructions to notify physician of preeclampsia symptoms. Prenatal visits will be every 2 weeks until

table 5-1 A correlation of the process of pregnancy with nursing interventions (*continued*)

developmental tasks and concerns	signs and symptoms	nursing interventions
d. Lack of support from family or spouse. e. Lack of preparation for or focus on needs of new baby. Preparation for labor and delivery. Becomes impatient for ending of pregnancy; mood swings occur again as ambivalence about future is demonstrated.	the umbilicus and the xiphoid. **33 to 36 weeks** *Subjective* Backache. Changes in gait. Shortness of breath and other pressure symptoms increase (heartburn, feeling of fullness after eating, constipation, varicose veins, dependent edema in extremeties, hemorrhoids). **37 to 40 weeks** *Subjective* Lightening—descent of the presenting part into the true pelvis. Aching in lower abdomen. *Objective* Fundus just below the diaphragm until lightening, then appears to tip forward.	the ninth month, when they will be weekly. If patient plans to breast-feed, teach her to express colostrum. For flat or inverted nipples, teach rolling motion to assist in making them more prominent. Reinforce use of good body mechanics, supportive shoes, sometimes girdle; use of heat, analgesics, and rest as ordered by physician. Remind patient to limit her activities to avoid dyspnea; pillows may be needed at night. Symptoms will disappear when lightening occurs. Relaxation and breathing techniques; support husband as coach. Teach signs of effective labor: Contractions increasing in intensity and frequency. Do not stop with walking. Mucous plug, "bloody show," expelled. Membranes may rupture anytime and should be reported to physician.

Source: Adapted from A. Tully, "Pregnancy," in *Blakiston Handbook of Clinical Nursing*, McGraw-Hill, New York, Chap. 9, 1979.

Study of the National Institute of Neurological Diseases and Stroke, Saunders, Philadelphia, 1972, p. 72.

8 D. Rush and E. H. Kassim, "Maternal Smoking: A Reassessment of the Relationship with Perinatal Mortality," *American Journal of Epidemiology*, **96**: 183, 1972.

9 F. A. Manning, "Fetal Breathing Movements as a Reflection of Fetal Status," *Postgraduate Medicine*, **61**:116, 1977.

10 J. J. Mulvehill and A. M. Yeager, "Fetal Alcohol Syndrome," *Teratology*, **13**:345, 1976.

11 J. Atkinson, "Salt, Water, and Rest as a Preventative for Toxemia of Pregnancy," *Journal of Reproductive Medicine*, **9**(5):224, 1972.

12 Tanner, op. cit., p. 293.

13 Light and Fenster, op. cit., p. 50.

bibliography

Bruser, M.: "Sporting Activities During Pregnancy," *Obstetrics and Gynecology*, **32**:721, 1968.

Combs, A. W., D. L. Avila, and W. W. Purkery: *Helping Relationships: Basic Concepts for the Helping Professions*, Allyn and Bacon, Boston, 1971.

David, M. C.: "The First Trimester of Pregnancy," *American Journal of Nursing*, **76**(12):1945, December 1976.

McBride, A. B.: *The Growth and Development of Mothers*, Harper & Row, New York, 1973.

Pirani, B. B. K.: "Smoking During Pregnancy," *Obstetrical and Gynecological Survey*, **33**(1):1, 1978.

Richardson, S. A. and A. F. Guttmacher (eds.): *Childbearing—It's Social and Psychological Aspects, Williams & Wilkins*, Baltimore, 1967.

Slatin, M.: "Why Mothers Bypass Prenatal Care," *American Journal of Nursing*, **71**:1388, 1971.

Steinberg, J.: "Radiation and Pregnancy," *Canadian Medical Association Journal*, **109**:51, 1973.

Wells, G. M.: "Reducing the Threat of a First Pelvic Examination," *American Journal of Maternal Child Health*, **2**(5):304, September/October 1977.

Williams, B.: "Sleep Needs During the Maternity Cycle," *Nursing Outlook*, February 1967, p. 292.

6

NUTRITION DURING PREGNANCY

BEATRICE LAU KEE

NUTRITIONAL NEEDS DURING PREGNANCY

preparation for pregnancy

Nutritional preparation for pregnancy does not begin just prior to conception. Nor does it begin in adolescence. It should be a lifetime process for the mother-to-be. It is known that the nutritional health of the newborn depends upon the nutritional status of the mother at the time of conception as well as upon her nutritional practices during pregnancy. It is important for her to have adequate stores of nutrients in her body tissues to provide for all the nutrient needs of the fetus. The adequacy of nutrient stores is a result of a lifetime of good eating practices rather than a quick transformation from poor to good nutrition when pregnancy occurs.

Infants and young children, still under parental influence, usually are well fed. They usually continue good eating habits in their school years until they reach adolescence. Adolescent boys usually have ravenous appetites that go along with their linear growth and activity. By eating large quantities of food to meet the demands of their appetites, their nutrient needs usually are met. Girls do not fare as well.

Adolescent girls usually are not as active as boys, nor do they grow as tall; therefore their caloric needs are not as great. Usually concerned about maintaining slim figures, they may cut down their caloric intake or omit meals and follow bizarre weight-losing schemes at the expense of good nutrition.

Dietary studies have shown that the most prevalent nutritional problem among adolescent girls today is iron deficiency anemia, shown by low hemoglobin and hematocrit levels and by diets with low iron levels. The problem may be magnified among adolescent girls from lower socioeconomic backgrounds.

In order to be in good nutritional health, the daily food plan shown in Table 6-1 is suggested for the adolescent girl and adult woman prior to pregnancy.

table 6-1 Daily food guide—basic four food groups

food group	important nutrients	recommended daily amounts

Milk	Calcium
	Protein
	Riboflavin
		Adolescents: 4 cups
		Adults: 2 cups
		Equivalents:
		  8 oz fluid milk or
		  1 oz cheddar cheese = 1 cup milk
		  ½ cup cottage cheese = ½ cup milk
		  ½ cup ice cream = ¼ cup milk

Meat	Protein
	Iron
	B vitamins
		Two servings.
		One serving is equivalent to:
		  2 oz lean, cooked meat, poultry, or fish
		  2 eggs
		  1 cup cooked dry peas, beans, or lentils
		  4 tablespoons peanut butter

Fruit/
vegetable
	B vitamins
	Iron
	
	Vitamin C
	
	Vitamin A
		Four or more servings.
		One serving is equivalent to:
		  ½ cup vegetable
		  ½ cup fruit
		One serving of citrus fruit or other fruit or vegetable rich in vitamin C daily; and
		One serving of a dark green or deep yellow vegetable or fruit *every other* day

Breads/
cereals
(whole
grain or
enriched)
	B vitamins
	iron
		Five servings; four, if one is a breakfast cereal
		One serving is equivalent to:
		  1 oz dry ready-to-eat cereal or
		  ½ cup cooked cereal, rice, spaghetti, macaroni, or noodles

This plan represents approximately 1500 and 1800 kcal for the adult and adolescent, respectively. If skim milk is used instead of whole milk, the caloric content is reduced by approximately 80 kcal for each cup of milk. Additional calories are obtained from accompanying free-choice foods. The Recommended Dietary Allowances for adolescent and adult women can be seen in Table 6-2.

adaptation of diet during pregnancy

According to an old Chinese tradition, a baby is a year old when it is born. Actually, at birth the newborn is nutritionally 9 months old. The mother's nutrient reserves at the time of conception and her nutritional intake during pregnancy are essential factors in the nutritional health of the infant. If a woman begins in poor nutritional health, it is absolutely essential for her to have first-rate food intake during her pregnancy.

It is known that during the first part of pregnancy, gastrointestinal motility is slowed to enable the nutrients to be absorbed more efficiently in the small intestines. Better absorption of nutrients helps meet the nutrient demands of the first trimester before the woman realizes that she is pregnant. When

table 6-2 Recommended dietary allowances (revised, 1973)

age, yr	females, 11–14	females, 15–18	females, 19–22	females, 23–50	pregnant females	lactating females
Weight, kg, lb	44, 97	54, 119	58, 128	58, 128		
Height, cm, in	155, 62	162, 65	162, 65	162, 65		
Energy, kcal*	2400	2100	2100	2000	+300	+500
Protein, g	44	48	46	46	+ 30	+ 20
Fat-soluble vitamins:						
Vitamin A activity, RE+	800	800	800	800	1000	1200
IU	4000	4000	4000	4000	5000	6000
Vitamin D, IU	400	400	400		400	400
Vitamin E activity, IU	10	11	12	12	15	15
Water-soluble vitamins:						
Ascorbic acid, mg	45	45	45	45	60	60
Folacin, μg	400	400	400	400	800	600
Niacin, mg	16	14	14	13	+2	+4
Riboflavin, mg	1.3	1.4	1.4	1.2	+0.3	+0.5
Thiamine, mg	1.2	1.1	1.1	1.0	+0.3	+0.3
Vitamin B_6, mg	1.6	2.0	2.0	2.0	2.5	2.5
Vitamin B_{12}, μg	3.0	3.0	3.0	3.0	4.0	4.0
Minerals:						
Calcium, mg	1200	1200	800	800	1200	1200
Phosphorus, mg	1200	1200	800	800	1200	1200
Iodine, μg	115	115	100	100	125	150
Iron, mg	18	18	18	18	18+‡	18
Magnesium, mg	300	300	300	300	450	450
Zinc, mg	15	15	15	15	20	25

*kcal = kilocalories.
+RE = retinol equivalents.
‡This increased requirement cannot be met by ordinary diets; therefore, the use of supplemental iron is recommended.
Source: *Recommended Dietary Allowances*, revised, 1973, Food and Nutrition Board, National Academy of Sciences–National Research Council.

she does recognize the pregnancy, she should evaluate her dietary pattern (often with nursing or nutritionist help) to make sure that she is receiving all the foods necessary to provide the balance needed by the fetus.

maternal needs during pregnancy   If during each day of the entire gestation the mother adds 300 kcal over and above her base-line, nonpregnant daily intake, she will supply the caloric needs for the estimated average 12.5-kg (27.5-lb) weight gain. The figures are calculated by taking into account the reduced energy expenditure during the last trimester.

Realistically speaking, it is neither practical nor desirable for anyone to count a daily caloric intake. Therefore, the best way to evaluate intake during pregnancy is for the mother to record and observe her *rate* of weight gain. If she is gaining too rapidly or not gaining enough, her diet can be further evaluated.

weight gain   The "energy cost" of making a baby is about 80,000 kcal for the normally active homemaker in the United States. Of course, the working mother, or one more active than usual, may need to take in proportionately more calories. Barring excessive fluid retention, her caloric intake, then, can be measured by periodic weighing. Many sets of figures are given for normal sequence of weight gain, all of which are averages. The growth and development sequence of the infant would indicate that the least weight is gained in the first trimester and the most toward the end of pregnancy.

The first trimester may include a loss of weight, or a gain of up to about 3 lb, or 1.5 kg. Each week after the twelfth, about 0.8 to 1 lb, or 400 to 500 g, should be gained in a normal pattern. Hytten gives the following rates of weight gain:[1]

By 10 weeks 650 g (about 1.5 lb)
By 20 weeks 4000 g (about 9 lb)
By 30 weeks 8500 g (about 19 lb)
By 40 weeks 12,500 g (27.5 lb)

Overweight women are usually advised to gain approximately 20 lb, whereas women of normal weight should gain at least 25 lb. Each woman is individual in her response to her pregnancy, and dietary counseling must be flexible. A large increase (2 lb/week or more) or a decrease in weight should be evaluated as to its cause. For this reason, the woman is weighed during every prenatal visit, with the weight recorded on the chart and compared with the previous weight.

In the past, many physicians advised their patients to limit their weight gain during pregnancy to avoid a difficult and prolonged labor and delivery. Women were anxious to follow this advice so that they would return more quickly to their normal size after delivery.

It is important to recognize that if adequate calories are not available to provide for maternal and fetal growth, proteins will be utilized for calories. This negates the use of proteins for fetal tissue synthesis, which is essential for normal development. Therefore, inadequate food intake sometimes has resulted in undernourished, low-birth-weight infants and some birth defects—thus the new recommendations of the Committee on Maternal Nutrition of the National Research Council that the healthy woman should gain *at least* 25 lb. Nurses can interpret these facts to the mother who is anxious about regaining her figure and who may be skimping on her food intake.

Careful study of the components of weight gain in a normal pregnancy has detailed the elements of the average 12.5-kg increase.

	No. of grams
Fetus	3300
Placenta	650
Amniotic fluid	800
Uterus	900
Breasts	450
Maternal blood	1250
Maternal fat stores	5200
	12,500 (12.5 kg, 27.5 lb)

The maternal stores once thought to be protein were found to be fat. The increase of fatty tissue is gained in proportion to the total weight gain and cannot be considered as excessive weight, for this fat probably is stored in preparation for lactation.

If weight gain is excessive and there appears to be no abnormal retention of fluid, a moderate calorie restriction may be advised to slow down the rate of weight gain. The mother is instructed to limit intake of sugar, butter, margarine, oil, fried foods, gravies, and rich desserts. Skim milk may be substituted for whole milk. The nurse should never advise her patients to omit bread and potato from the diet. These foods provide valuable nutrients and are necessary for her health. Any reduction from the recommended diet should be by prescription from the obstetrician and be under his supervision.

changes in nutrients

protein needs To meet the nutrient needs for the growth and health of the fetus, and for the growth of the maternal accessory tissues, an additional *daily intake* of 30 g protein is recommended. The base-line recommendation for women of childbearing age is 46 g daily; thus, 76 g daily is recommended during pregnancy.

Protein is needed for the growth of the fetus, uterus, mammary glands, and placenta, and for formation of amniotic fluid and plasma. These additional needs are over and above the normal anabolic needs of the woman.

Foods providing high-value, complete proteins are meat, fish, poultry, eggs, and milk. Plant sources are useful but are usually incomplete proteins. Vegetables, cereals, nuts, dried peas, beans, and lentils are sources of about one-third of the protein in North American diets. In some cultural groups the proportion of protein from plant sources increases (Table 6-3).

calcium needs Even though calcium absorption is more efficient during pregnancy, additional intake of calcium is needed, especially during the period of bone formation and growth of the fetus. The recommended daily amount during pregnancy is 1200 mg (see Table 6-4).

Calcium is unevenly distributed in foods. The highest amount is found in milk and milk products. A small quantity is found in dark green leafy vegetables. An intake of approximately 4 cups of milk daily will meet the calcium needs during pregnancy.

iron Before pregnancy the average woman absorbs about 10 percent of the iron in her diet. The additional needs for the increased maternal blood volume and fetal stores are partially compensated for by the lack of men-

table 6-3 Protein content of major foods

Food	Amount	Approximate protein content, g
Lean meat, fish or poultry (cooked)	1 oz	7
Egg	one	7
Milk	8 oz	8
Pasta	½ cup	3
Peas, split	½ cup	7
Beans, dry cooked, drained	½ cup	7

table 6-4 Calcium in milk food group

food	amount	calcium content, mg
Whole milk	8 oz	288
Skim milk	8 oz	296
Modified skim	8 oz	352
Cheddar cheese	1 oz	213
Cottage cheese	½ cup	115
Yogurt	8 oz	271

struation and by the increased iron absorption by the body. During the third trimester, almost three times the usual amount of iron can be absorbed by the body. At the same time, the fetus is demanding iron from the mother to form red cells and to accumulate stores that should last from 3 to 6 months after birth.

If iron intake is inadequate, the fetus will not develop these iron stores, and the mother will become anemic. Therefore, a daily intake of 18 mg is *essential* during pregnancy. Since it is very difficult to get the needed 18 mg iron daily in the diet, many physicians recommend an iron supplement (see Table 6-5).

Iron deficiency anemia is common in those women who have diets deficient in proteins, leafy green vegetables, dried peas, beans, and enriched breads and cereals. Teenagers most commonly have iron-deficient diets and may need extensive counseling to correct their nutritional habits. Where a clinic population has a history of poor diet, iron (taken orally) is usually prescribed (see Table 6-6).

vitamins The additional intake of B vitamins is obtained with the foods added for the calorie and protein intake. *Folacin* (folic acid) is found in proteins and leafy green vegetables. Many doctors now advise supplementation of 200 to 400 μg folic acid.

VITAMIN C   Additional intake of 15 mg vitamin C is recommended during pregnancy. Since the North American diet is likely to be low in

vitamin C, special emphasis should be given to foods which provide this nutrient. Ascorbic acid is unevenly distributed in foods, but certain foods stand out as high vitamin C sources. To provide the Recommended Dietary Allowance of 60 mg vitamin C, the woman should take one of the following foods daily:

Fruits

Orange juice	½ cup
Orange	1
Grapefruit	½
Grapefruit juice	½ cup
Tangerine juice	½ cup
Papaya	⅔ cup
Strawberries	¾ cup

Vegetables

Broccoli, cooked	½ cup
Cauliflower, cooked	1 cup
Greens, cooked (kale, collards, mustard, turnip)	1 cup
Green pepper	1

VITAMINS A, D, E, K   The recommended intake of vitamin D, 400 IU, is supplied by 1 qt fortified milk. Cheese, which often is used as a milk substitute, is a good source of calcium but is not fortified with vitamin D.

Vitamins A, D, E, and K are fat-soluble and are stored in some measure in the body. Therefore, excess intake is not recommended and may be harmful to the developing fetus. Counseling about self-medication with vitamins is important, since in this culture many women are accustomed to taking large doses of vitamins during dieting periods or because a neighbor has recommended vitamin ingestion for a variety of ills. Water-soluble vitamins are excreted by the body and overdose is not harmful, but fat-soluble vitamins are dangerous in high doses. Most obstetricians prescribe a low-dose multivitamin during pregnancy. Instructions to the mother will include cautioning her to take just what is prescribed.

table 6-5 Iron content of foods

food	amount	iron, mg
meats group		
Pork liver, fried	3 oz	24.9
Calf liver, fried	3 oz	12.2
Beef liver, fried	3 oz	7.5
Heart, beef, braised	3 oz	5.0
Beef, lean, broiled	3 oz	3.0
Pork, roast	3 oz	2.7
Egg, cooked	1 large	1.1
Haddock, breaded and fried	3 oz	1.0
Tuna, canned	2 oz	1.0
Frankfurter	1, 2 oz	0.8
vegetable-fruit group		
Baked beans in tomato sauce	½ cup	2.6
Red kidney beans, canned	½ cup	2.3
Prune juice	½ cup	0.9
Spinach, cooked, drained	½ cup	2.4
Raisins	½ cup	1.6
Peas, cooked	½ cup	1.5
Beet greens, cooked, drained	½ cup	1.4
Prunes, dried, uncooked	4	1.3
Broccoli, cooked, drained	1 cup	1.2
Apple juice	½ cup	0.3
Potato, baked	1 medium	0.7
Beets, cooked, drained	½ cup	0.5
bread-cereal group		
Bran flakes, 40%	1 cup	12.4
White bread, enriched	1 slice	0.6
Whole wheat bread	1 slice	0.6
Corn flakes	½ cup	0.2
Farina, enriched, cooked	½ cup	5.0
Macaroni, enriched, cooked	½ cup	0.7
Noodles, enriched, cooked	½ cup	0.7
Rice, enriched, cooked	½ cup	0.7
milk group		
Milk, whole	1 cup	0.1
Cheddar cheese	1 oz	0.3
Cottage cheese	½ cup	0.3

Source: From C. F. Adams, "Nutritive Value of American Foods in Common Units. Handbook No. 456" U.S. Dept. of Agriculture, 1975.

nursing intervention

One of the most important aspects of prenatal care is that of nutritional counseling for the mother. The nurse has many opportunities to advise and teach patients concerning maternal and infant nutrition. She can teach pregnant women informally in a prenatal clinic or physician's office. Formal teaching can be done in mothers' or parents' classes. Opportunities

table 6-6 Daily diet plan in pregnancy

food	base-line diet	diet during pregnancy
Milk	Adult: 2 cups	4 cups
	Teen-ager: 4 cups	4 cups
Meat, fish, poultry, eggs, nuts, dried peas or beans	2 servings (2 oz each)	2 servings (3 oz each)
Vegetable/fruit: Include:	4 servings	4 servings
High-vitamin C fruit or vegetable	1 serving daily	1 serving daily
Dark green or deep yellow vegetable	1 serving every other day	1 serving daily
Bread/cereal, enriched or whole grain	5 servings	5 servings
	(4, if one serving is a breakfast cereal)	

to teach about infant feeding also occur at the bedside of the postpartum unit and in a postpartum follow-up visit to a new mother.

When the pregnant woman understands that what she eats has an influence on her unborn baby, she will usually try to cooperate with a diet plan. One way of stating this simply is found in a pamphlet from The National Foundation—March of Dimes, "Nutrition and Birth Defects Prevention".[2] "Malnutrition comes from not eating enough of the right foods. Malnutrition is different from hunger: you can eat just about anything and hunger will go away. But you have to eat the right kinds of food for malnutrition to go away."

The nurse may have to work closely with the pregnant woman to determine her dietary habits, because different sources of essential nutrients are "favorite foods" in different cultural groups. The nurse who works in a prenatal-care setting should become informed of the cultural patterns of her area.

Every woman seeks the highest level of health for her growing baby and can respond positively to diet counseling that begins "where she is," i.e., that takes into consideration her life style and the foods to which she is accustomed.

study questions

1 At which period of gestation is good nutritional status most important for the development of a nutritionally healthy infant?
2 How much weight should a healthy woman gain during pregnancy? At what rate should this weight gain take place? How many calories are needed daily to provide for this weight gain? Why is positive calorie balance essential for the development of the fetus?
3 Why is calcium important during pregnancy? How much milk is recommended? What milk substitute is a good source of calcium but a poor source of vitamin D?
4 The Recommended Dietary Allowances for iron are not increased for pregnancy. Why? When are fetal iron stores accumulated? What foods are good sources of iron? What are the consequences of an inadequate iron intake during pregnancy? Why are iron supplements recommended?
5 What are the basic foods which are needed to provide adequate nutrition prior to pregnancy? What foods should be added during pregnancy?

references

1 Frank E. Hytten, and Isabella Leitch, *The Physiology of Human Pregnancy*, 2d ed., Blackwell, Oxford, 1972, p. 285.
2 "Nutrition and Birth Defects Prevention," The National Foundation—March of Dimes, White Plains, N.Y. 10602.

bibliography

Adams, Catherine F.: "Nutritive Value of American Foods in Common Units: Agriculture Handbook No. 456," USDA, Washington, 1975.

Bradfield, Robert B., and Thierry Brun: "Nutritional Status of Mexican-American," *American Journal of Clinical Nutrition,* **23**(6):798, 1970.

Committee on Maternal Nutrition/Food and Nutrition Board, *Maternal Nutrition and the Course of Pregnancy,* National Research Council, National Academy of Sciences, Washington, 1970.

Fernandez, Nelson A.: "Nutritional Status of the Puerto Rican Population: Master Sample Survey," *American Journal of Clinical Nutrition,* **24**(8):952, 1971.

Holey, Elizabeth S.: "Promoting Adequate Weight Gain in Pregnant Women," *American Journal of Maternal Child Nursing,* **2**(2):86, 1977.

Jacobson, Howard N.: "Nutrition and Pregnancy," *Journal of the American Dietic Association,* **60**(1):26, 1972.

"Nutrition in Pregnancy and Lactation, Report of a WHO Expert Committee," *World Health Organization Technical Report Series No. 302,* 1965.

Recommended Dietary Allowances, Eighth Revised Edition, 1973, National Research Council, National Academy of Sciences, Washington, 1974.

Rosso, Pedro: "Nutrition and Abnormal Fetal Growth," *Contemporary OB/GYN,* **2**(3):53, 1973.

Shanklin, D. R., et al.: "Nutrition and Pregnancy: An Invitational Symposium," *Journal of Reproductive Medicine,* **7**:199–219, 1971; and **8**:1–12, 1972.

Weigley, Emma S.: "The Pregnant Adolescent," *Journal of the American Dietetic Association,* **66**(6):588, 1975.

7

THE PREGNANCY EXPERIENCE

NANCY T. BLOCK

PREGNANCY, A DEVELOPMENTAL CRISIS

Life is not a static state but a dynamic process. Every form of life is characterized by a fairly predictable series of crises—changes or events which expose the individual to stress and even danger but which when successfully struggled through and mastered lead to new stages of growth and further development of the individual's creative potential. Failure to master such crises, on the other hand, results in stagnation, maldevelopment, and illness.

Human life has many interrelated facets—genetic, anatomic, physiologic, psychologic, and social, to name a few—all of which are involved in this process, affecting each other at every developmental stage. Pregnancy, particularly a first pregnancy climaxing in the birth of a child to a previously childless couple, is experienced by them as a major developmental crisis, leading to the new stage of parenthood. As such, it is both a hazardous and a potentially creative event for mother, father, and infant simultaneously, tapping into all the interrelated aspects of life and personality.

One of the basic psychologic requirements for healthy, organized human growth and development is a sense of meaning and purpose. This serves as a framework within which individuals can integrate and act upon their experiences with their own feelings, the outside world, and other beings to whom they relate. In all times and cultures, humans have attributed a special significance to the reproductive process, perceiving it as a means of participating in the ongoing creative processes at work in the universe. Religious ceremonies and social practices connected with puberty, conception, pregnancy, delivery, and early infancy are ways of giving expression to this essential dimension of human experience, which tends to be disregarded by our modern technique-oriented health care system.

In the midst of crowded waiting rooms, noisy labor rooms, and harried delivery rooms, it is all too easy to lose sight of the unique significance of each delivery, together with the preceding months of preparation, for the particular human beings involved. However, certain progressive medical centers are now acknowledging the importance of helping couples experience the bringing of a new life into the world as an emotionally meaningful as well as medically safe event. Although no one knows exactly what babies experience at the time, parents' reactions have been studied and described in detail.

the importance of emotional factors

This chapter is intended to sharpen the nurse's awareness of feelings and attitudes and their tremendous importance in achieving good health both during and after pregnancy. Emotional and physical well-being are intimately linked together. This means that a maternity nurse tunes in to the mother's state of mind as attentively as to the baby's heartbeat and evaluates the position of the mother within her family as carefully as the position of the fetus within its mother.

Furthermore, medical personnel must understand that people are exquisitely sensitive to the attitudes of those on whom they must depend. In this case the prospective parents, looking to the obstetric team for assistance and support, may be greatly affected in the way they experience and deal with pregnancy, delivery, and parenthood by the team's response. Therefore, it is important that nurses and doctors do not simply observe the progress of the pregnancy in a clinical way, noting problems as they arise. They must also provide understanding and encouragement to the patient and her family.

Is this asking too much of the busy professional? Actually, doctors and nurses who make the effort to know and relate to their patients' feelings usually find their work easier, more enjoyable, and far more effective.

An obstetric team, then, should know the answers to the following questions:

1 How is a healthy woman likely to feel and think throughout her pregnancy and delivery?
2 How can her husband and older children be expected to react?
3 Where may things go wrong emotionally?
4 What should be the roles of the medical people involved, and how are they likely to feel?

Let us consider these questions in order.

parents' reactions

As women's personalities and backgrounds differ, so each woman's reaction to pregnancy is somewhat unique. Furthermore, no two pregnancies are identical for the same woman. After all, each time she is pregnant, she carries a different child, under different circumstances. Fathers' reactions, of course, vary in a similar way from individual to individual and from pregnancy to pregnancy. However, investigators who have studied and worked closely with large numbers of "pregnant parents" find that certain patterns of feelings and behavior are fairly predictable at different stages of pregnancy for both parents.

Prospective parents tend to be frustrated, bemused, troubled, or ecstatic by turns, and bursting to talk to someone. They are usually anxious to be reassured that their changing moods constitute a normal human experience rather than a sign of mental imbalance. It is helpful for the obstetric team, from the beginning of pregnancy, to encourage them to express these feelings, both to the medical personnel and to other prospective parents. Pregnant women tend to restrict private discussions with the obstetrician to physical symptoms and concerns. Therefore, additional prenatal classes which provide both information and support are a valuable complement to the medical team's services.

We begin, then, by considering the changing feelings of the average pregnant woman, remembering that her reactions are closely tied to those of family, friends, and medical helpers.

THE FIRST TRIMESTER: ACCEPTING PREGNANCY

In studies of the pregnancy experience, it has been noted that the trimesters of pregnancy demarcate fairly clearly a series of developmental tasks which must be achieved if parenthood is to begin well. If there is difficulty in progressing from acceptance of the preg-

nancy to the second task, that task will not be completely incorporated and movement into parenthood will be hindered. It seems important, then, to understand the progress that parents must make as the months of pregnancy go by and to assist them whenever possible in achieving these steps in development.

Life's earliest and most urgent needs are for food, sleep, warmth, and close affectionate human interaction. Their fulfillment provides life's first experience of love, which develops trust and provides a basis for future relationships and learning. The physical and psychologic stresses of pregnancy reawaken these needs. Sleeping, eating, and affection become major issues again in early pregnancy, just as they were in early childhood. It is often said—and not always sympathetically—that pregnant women want to be "babied." This is quite literally true, and for good reason.

The shifts in her body hormones cause the pregnant woman to feel strange and often disturbing sensations. Her appetite is changed—she may actually be quite nauseated or experience unusual cravings. She feels tired and sleepy much of the time. Her emotions are difficult to control; she may feel like laughing or crying without much explanation. Her activities may be restricted. All of this interferes with her routines, focuses her attention inward on herself, and forces on her a change of pace. She becomes aware of a process taking over her body and mind, her present and her future, over which she has little control.

The symptoms which are thrust on a woman in early pregnancy seem to be nature's way of ensuring that she gets the extra rest and attention she needs for the tremendous new task she has undertaken. She is also forced to confront and deal with the resulting changes affecting her life.

Pregnancy is a time of increased emotional activity and openness in the family. Husbands and children are drawn into the excitements and uncertainties. Indeed, prospective parents are surprised at the richness and unpredictability of their own feelings, scarcely recognizing themselves as the "commonsensical" beings which they were formerly and which they will become again once the pregnancy is over.

ambivalence

Pregnancy is an unmistakable sign of femininity; it is also proof of sexual activity. Most women who accept and take pride in their sexual identity, and who are in a favorable position to bear and raise a child, welcome the discovery that they are pregnant.

Many women, however, are somehow embarrassed by or dissatisfied with their sexual role. Some reject femininity in obvious outward ways, claiming that pregnancy and motherhood are unfair burdens thrust upon the female sex. Such a woman might feel resentment or humiliation at becoming pregnant. She might, of course, seek an abortion—or she might refuse to face the fact of her pregnancy. She may suffer from fears of pregnancy relating to her mother's experience. If her mother died at her own or a sibling's birth, she may feel frightened, or even guilty. If her mother had difficulty in becoming pregnant or in carrying a pregnancy to term, or if she is past the menopause and therefore infertile, the pregnant daughter may feel that she is competing with and thereby denigrating her mother.

For some women, becoming pregnant may satisfy a need to compete with men, as it is something no man can do. Other women who envy males their physical characteristics may imagine that the fetus is a male organ. Pregnancy may be reassuring for the time being, but the woman's illusion concerning the new "appendage" is bound to be shattered before long, leaving her more dissatisfied and depressed than ever.

Psychoanalysis has shown that, in many cases, a girl has a strong unconscious wish for a baby as evidence of the love of her own father—a little girl's first romantic attachment. Since she has learned very early that he actually belongs to another female, her mother, she shifts her hopes to a baby, as though it were a gift from her father which will be her very own and love her unconditionally in his place. The fantasy is strengthened if her mother's love and support have been inadequate in which case the baby may be viewed as an emotional substitute for both parents. Many unmarried teenage girls, especially lonely ones who lack parental guidance and affection, allow themselves to become pregnant for this reason.

Of course, they are bound to become disillusioned and to make poor mothers, because the baby, it soon turns out, demands far more love and attention than it can immediately repay, from the very girl who desperately wishes to be loved and protected herself. Such an immature, emotionally deprived mother may neglect or abuse her child after birth, or care for it mechanically and capriciously as if it were a doll. As the shocking occurrence of serious mistreatment of children in our country rises, it is the increasing responsibility of the medical and allied professions to be alert to such potentially abusive mothers very early in pregnancy. Psychiatric help, or possibly even abortion, might be offered to them, though resistance to suggestions may be great.

In some unusual cases, a woman who desperately wants a child develops *pseudocyesis,* or false pregnancy. Remarkably convincing physical changes may occur, as the woman herself steadfastly believes she is pregnant. Psychiatric help is obviously needed in persistent pseudocyesis.

fantasies

There are a number of fantasies which a woman may experience in early pregnancy.

She may feel and imagine that she and the baby are one and interchangeable. This is not hard to understand. The tiny embryo is deep down and hidden inside her, like one of her own organs. It has given no sign yet of having a life of its own. The mother has felt no separate movement, heard no separate heartbeat. Her own body shape, especially in a primipara, remains deceptively normal for some time. Yet she knows there is a baby within. Sometimes she fancies that she is the baby.

A similar fantasy, one which is common to young children and may recur in pregnancy, connects conception with eating, as though the baby, like food in the mother's digestive tract, may be eliminated.

These fantasies make it easy to deny the real facts and implications of pregnancy, which many women, particularly unwed adolescents, tend to do at first. Some neglect for several months to seek confirmation of their pregnancy and prenatal care, greatly jeopardizing a successful delivery. One might say this is a sign of regression, this *ambivalence*—failing to accept her new responsibility to herself and her anticipated child, and, instead, playing the child herself, depending upon others to bring her to the doctor or clinic for necessary medical attention.

THE SECOND TRIMESTER: DEVELOPING A NEW IDENTITY

By the end of the first trimester, the bulge of the growing uterus and the passage of time have helped convince nearly every pregnant woman that, beyond any doubt, she is to become a mother. Soon, the baby's movements will be proof positive. This brings her abruptly upon one of the most absorbing and important psychologic tasks of her life—pondering what

it means to be a mother, and even more basically, a woman.

To be sure, she has done some thinking about this long before her pregnancy, and she will probably continue to consider and reconsider her role from time to time throughout the rest of her life. But there is a certain urgency—a deadline when she will suddenly *be* a mother—imposed by pregnancy.

child vs. mother

Some consider pregnancy a woman's greatest time of personal scrutiny. It is like a long mirror, a 9-month "moment of truth," in which she faces herself as a woman and takes inventory. She can neither avoid the confrontation nor hasten it, and during the wait she has time to explore her inner world, where the questions are written large, "Who am I?" and "Who am I to become?"

Deep within her, she recognizes that a transformation is about to take place. When pregnancy is terminated in delivery, she will have become, once and for all, a parent. At the same time, childhood is symbolically left behind, though many "child" longings remain within every adult. With mixed feelings, she prepares to step over the one-way threshold into parenthood.

Every woman has received some kind of preparation for parenting, whether positive or negative. Even if she is still in her teens, she has years of infancy, childhood, and adolescence behind her. Bit by bit, during that time her personality was taking shape, her hopes and expectations were being formed, and her ideas of womanliness were developing. She considered many models, tried out some, adopted a few. The whole process was gradual; changes were almost unnoticed as they occurred. Now, pregnancy opens up a window to review her past. She relives childhood feelings, experiences, and relationships, trying to bring them into focus from her new perspective.

As she looks backward and inward, sensing herself a child again, the chief person she confronts is her own mother. She may become quite obsessed with thoughts of their relationship. She may reexperience a confusing mixture of feelings—tender affection, frustrated anger, admiration and scorn, rebellion and dependency—which were present in years past. She must soon step out on stage as a full-fledged mother herself and usually wants very much to be a good one.

conflicts about motherhood

Understandably, some women will experience considerable difficulty in assuming this new role. An extreme case may be a woman who grew up without a mother figure and is bewildered for lack of any kind of model in her own experience. If she did have a mother, whom she perceived as a very bad example, it may still be difficult for her to construct a different pattern for her own motherhood. She will find it almost impossible to give to her child what she has not received herself. If she is fortunate, other "mothering" people in her life—relatives or friends—have filled this need. Even supportive doctors, nurses, and other professionals can be of some help to her, for they not only care for *her,* but they can demonstrate to her some practical child-care techniques that will make her more competent and confident in actually handling her infant.

A pregnant woman, especially a primipara, who does not appear to be experiencing some struggles is a cause for concern. She may be mentally blocking out her pregnancy because of fear or resentment. On the other hand, she may have the fantasy that her own mother is the baby's mother and will therefore take care of it, while she herself is only an intermediary, or even a rival. If she lives with her mother, who does take over child care following delivery, she may fail to develop as a parent in her own right.

The teenage girl is still in the throes of the adolescent struggle for autonomy versus lingering dependency needs. If she becomes pregnant in competition with or in defiance of her mother, she may have great difficulty in resolving her feelings. If her mother offers a poor role model, or if the girl rejects what her mother can indeed offer, she may be looking fruitlessly to transient boyfriends, siblings, or even her baby to fulfill her emotional needs.

dependence on the father

Normally toward the end of the second trimester, the expectant father becomes more involved in the pregnancy. Practical and financial concerns require his attention. But beyond that, his wife may begin quite actively to draw him into the experience. She insists that he must feel the baby move, putting his hand on her enlarging abdomen. She may begin classes to prepare for childbirth, urging him to participate with her. Her desire for intercourse is likely to decrease during pregnancy, but she may wish to be held and caressed.

Does she require this attention of her husband simply because he is most available? Is he supposed to substitute for her own mother as comforter and protector? Perhaps. At any rate, the pregnant woman shifts her preoccupation from her mother to her husband, and begins to work out her mixed feelings toward him, much as she has already done toward her mother.

She feels in turn dependent or competitive, insecure or confident, tender or resentful, toward him. These feelings are frequently expressed as fears for his safety or as fluctuating moods. Needless to say, the husband, unless he is a flexible and confident man, may become confused and overwhelmed. He may withdraw from his wife emotionally, or actually desert her, unless he is helped to cope with her changeable behavior.

THE THIRD TRIMESTER: PREPARATION FOR DELIVERY

By the third trimester, the pregnant woman has usually accepted her pregnancy and coming motherhood. Arrayed in maternity clothes, she is the center of attention wherever she goes, proud of her obvious accomplishment. Folklore has it that a woman is most radiantly beautiful when she is "great with child"—the "madonna mystique," one might call it. In exalted, dreamy moments, she feels special, instrumental in the rite of creation, destined to bring forth a new life. She is eager for the event.

common concerns

Yet the pregnant woman must recognize what will be required of her. Her developmental task is to become ready for delivery and then to take up the role of parent to the new infant.

To relieve anxiety, she becomes absorbed in various matters—the medical details of the coming delivery; clothing; equipment; a name for the baby; household preparations for her absence at the hospital; her own increasing awkwardness; and minor but annoying physical symptoms. Her legs and back may ache, her breath comes short, her bladder won't wait, and she can't reach down to put on shoes and stockings. Still, if she has a job outside the home, she may prefer to keep working until the last minute if allowed to, even though nature is giving her the message to slow down. A mother who already has one or more young children may not be able to slow down anyway. Indeed, older children, sensing that a new competitor is arriving

soon, may become more demanding of her attention than usual.

Naturally, there are particular anxieties about whether something will go wrong with the delivery, and whether the baby will emerge normal and healthy. Such concerns frequently appear in dreams at this stage.

sexual intercourse

Sexual relations become very awkward toward the end of pregnancy. Both husband and wife require some ingenuity, as well as mutual understanding, tenderness, and a sense of humor to work out their sexual adjustments. The pregnant belly is a real obstacle which comes between them. In addition, the wife's changing sexual feelings and physical shape may repel her husband, while she herself tends to be uncomfortable and self-conscious. Usually, in the course of a normal pregnancy, an obstetrician will impose few restrictions on sexual activity, unless there are such medical indications as bleeding or a history of prenatal complications. Frequently the couple themselves will limit intercourse unnecessarily, out of fear or ignorance, at this time when intimacy and mutual support are especially vital to their relationship.

Because many couples are reluctant to discuss intercourse, some member of the medical team should routinely and explicitly deal with the issue early, and perhaps raise it again in the third trimester, to elicit questions, doubts, and fears. If coitus must be restricted for medical reasons, alternative avenues of reciprocal sexual gratification may be suggested, such as mutual masturbation by manual or oral means.

anxiety about labor

If false labor occurs, it may be frustrating and bewildering to the pregnant woman, especially if she is ignorant or misinformed about what to expect. She will be offered all kinds of advice by relatives, friends, and neighbors who consider her pregnancy a community affair.

Finally, she is indeed in labor. The average woman then presents herself at some hospital. She may be accompanied by her husband, another relative, or a friend, or she may come alone. Ideally, she will have become familiar with the hospital during her pregnancy, in preparation for this event, though frequently it is totally strange to her. As she progresses through labor and delivery, she may be reassured by the familiar faces and voices of nurses and doctors whom she knows and has come to trust. On the other hand, if she is a clinic patient in a busy city hospital, she is more likely to find herself unable to recognize a single familiar person.

REACTIONS OF THE FATHER

Let us now consider how the expectant father has been faring for 9 months. He has his own predictable assortment of feelings. Some of them are due purely to his maleness or his own personality. Others are reactions to the particular way his wife rides out her pregnancy "trip."

traditional attitudes

Expectant fathers in this country have traditionally been pushed into the background. They are said to feel like "fifth wheels" throughout the pregnancies and deliveries of their wives. The increasingly frequent man who asserts himself often finds himself in a kind of "lion's den" of jealous female relatives and sphinxlike doctors and nurses, all making him feel most unwelcome and uncomfortable.

However, he is beginning, fortunately, to gain more appropriate recognition as father of the child.

The news that his wife is pregnant is almost always a source of tremendous pride to a man, for he takes it as evidence of his masculinity and his power to create life. He may also anticipate a child, particularly a son, as a symbolic extension of himself, adding potentially to his life-span and accomplishments. It is unfortunate when, as so often happens, a man feels that his responsibility ends here (except, perhaps, to provide financial support to his family). Playing the part of emotional father to the expected baby, and husband to its mother, is a much more demanding role than that of becoming a biologic father through one act of intercourse.

tasks, fantasies, and conflicts

Probably, every pregnant woman seems like a strange and unfamiliar creature to her husband at times, and he must adjust to her in some way. He frequently needs reassurance that he is not the cause of her emotional fluctuations. He also needs someone to whom to vent his own feelings (in case his wife is not in the mood to listen).

Furthermore, he has his own psychologic tasks to perform which parallel those of his wife. He, too, must recognize and accept the fact of the new child who will soon intrude upon *his* life, making him a parent also.

Our society renders this task especially perplexing for men because of the curiously irrational notion that men are not supposed to be tender, caring, patient human beings. A "real man" is portrayed in movies, comic books, and folklore as tough, domineering, and unemotional. Who is to set the matter straight for the expectant father?

In addition, a number of inner fears and

conflicts may crop up during pregnancy to plague the expectant father and handicap him in developing his new role.

Some men, harboring deep neurotic conflicts over their own sexual identity, with unconscious fears of being feminine or homosexual, cannot allow themselves to be "soft" in any way. Instead they are impelled to be hard, brusque, and defensive, and tend to make poor husbands and fathers unless they receive psychiatric help.

One of the natural feelings which a man often has to confront when his wife becomes pregnant is that of envy. As a little boy, he may have learned his mother was having a baby, and wished that he could perform an equally marvelous feat. If he said so, he was probably laughed at and told, "Only girls can have babies!" As he now watches his wife's abdomen enlarge and feels the movements of the fetus with his own hands, he is again reminded that *he* cannot bear a child. If he is otherwise insecure about his own abilities and worth, and his relationship with his wife is strained, he may at this time stay away from her as much as possible, keeping busy with his work, other hobbies, or associations which build up his sense of identity and achievement. He may seek out a girl friend at this time, for reassurance. He thus resorts to rejecting or competing with his wife, instead of supporting her in what is actually their joint production, the pregnancy.

Occasionally an expectant father will actually identify or compete with his pregnant wife strongly enough to experience the "couvade syndrome." This term is derived from a French word meaning "to sit on" or "hatch," and refers to a psychosomatic condition mimicking pregnancy—the male version of pseudocyesis. This may include a variety of symptoms such as nausea, weight gain, abdominal distension, or pain, and is occasionally severe enough to require psychiatric intervention.

The immature man who married in order to acquire the permanent, undivided attention of a "mother" for himself will, of course, begin to feel uneasiness and jealousy over the approach of a serious rival for his wife's attention. These feelings only tend to increase after the birth of the child unless he can discuss them and discover creative ways of handling them. The more confidently he can begin assuming supportive and caring roles as husband and father, the more readily he can give up competing with his own child. Parental preparation courses during the pregnancy, which include some practical instruction in child care for both parents, can be extremely useful to such fathers.

Besides competing with his own wife and child, the American husband very frequently feels that he has to compete with the obstetrician in importance to his wife and to the whole production. If he feels totally overshadowed and displaced, he may withdraw his interest and support altogether. It is an alarming fact that many fathers, especially of the lower socioeconomic classes in our urban areas, tend to desert their families, or at least fail to take on appropriate responsibilities in child support and upbringing. Yet they can hardly be blamed, it seems, when they are so frequently given the message by the experts that babies are none of their business!

support of the father

It is the opinion of this writer that one of the most urgent tasks of the obstetric team ought to be the proper care of the fathers of the babies who are being born daily in our nation's hospitals, both private and public. Alert and sympathetic professionals who support the father's self-esteem may help keep him in the picture at this crucial time, to the enormous benefit of the family and society. Like his wife, he needs to be educated and encouraged to play his role well. His presence ought perhaps to be required, as a matter of course, at certain prenatal office visits, instructional activities, labor room, and delivery area, with the option of attending the delivery itself to signify his full participation in producing children.

Although attitudes are changing, hospital personnel, for various reasons, have often opposed the father's active involvement. Some of these reasons reflect practical concerns, which can usually be resolved if there is a willingness to do so. Other reasons are rooted in unconscious attitudes of the staff, which will be discussed toward the end of this chapter.

THE DELIVERY EXPERIENCE

Having weathered the 9 months of pregnancy, the couple come—hopefully, together—to the final act of labor and delivery, the culmination of the whole experience. Some couples with a strong determination to share this experience firsthand, avoid going to a hospital altogether for fear of being separated, and arrange for home delivery, whatever the medical risks.

Some hospitals allow the husband in the labor and delivery rooms if he is properly prepared and motivated. Actually, many couples still prefer to leave the delivery itself in the hands of the medical team, with minimal participation themselves—she well sedated and he waiting somewhere outside; but all expectant parents ought to feel that they have the right to some choice in the matter.

The well-prepared couple will have discussed matters with the doctor and made certain decisions in advance, such as the place and expected method of delivery. They should know, as far as possible, what to anticipate and how to assist in the physiologic process of birth, by proper breathing and relaxation.

Nevertheless, there are the inevitable pain, anxiety, and uncertainties which tax both the medical and psychologic expertise of the support personnel. When proper preparation is lacking, or the hospital regulations are cumbersome and its personnel insensitive, the laboring mother's anxiety can easily escalate into panic—especially if she finds herself alone among strangers. Her inability to relax and cooperate may in turn cause unnecessary complications in the delivery.

Some women panic even under ideal conditions, and need sedation. Medical complications may call for further analgesia or anesthesia. In view of this, it is imperative to prepare every expectant mother, especially the "natural childbirth" enthusiast, for the possibility that a need for medication might develop after all. She should be relieved of the fear, in advance, that she would be a "failure" in any way because of that.

Among the foremost questions in a laboring mother's mind are, "Can I do it?" and "Can I trust those who have to help me in this inescapable ordeal?" Being forced to depend on others, if her relationship with them is not good, may cause her feelings of anger and helplessness. Frank discussions with the medical team before the stresses of delivery arise will vastly increase rapport.

role of the professional staff

If all goes well, the completion of the delivery, with the first sight and feel of the new baby, is for the parents an experience of incomparable fulfillment, and for the attending staff a moment of deep satisfaction. All share the elated feeling of having successfully completed an ambitious but rewarding family project.

The doctors and nurses have a legitimate place emotionally as "parent figures" to the new parents. The actual relative ages of the participants is unimportant. Medical personnel, who are in the dominant position with their expertise and authority, can be either "bad parents"—judgmental, belittling, and domineering—or "good parents"—supportive and encouraging the couple to feel that *they themselves* have actually done a good job. The parturient mother has never worked harder in her life, and the father, perhaps, never agonized so much. They are entitled to enjoy a sense of accomplishment. Furthermore, they will be needing all the confidence and self-assurance they can muster for the difficult early period after they bring the new baby home from the hospital (Fig. 7-1).

impact of hospital policies

The hospital delivery and postnatal routines are significant in confirming the parents' central importance to their child. The mother needs to be reasonably well awake during and immediately after the delivery, though as free of pain as possible, to appreciate what she has done. Studies of parental attitudes toward their children suggest that both parents should be allowed to see and hold their infant at the earliest practical moment in order to establish a strong emotional bond between them. Such bonding, or the lack of it, may profoundly affect their future relationship. True, there may be no father in the picture at delivery. Or the mother herself may have strong negative feelings about her baby, in which case it should not be thrust at her. Nevertheless, the message she receives from the medical team ought to be, "This is *your* baby—your accomplishment, and your responsibility."

The opposite message may be conveyed by certain hospital practices whereby technically underweight babies are overzealously

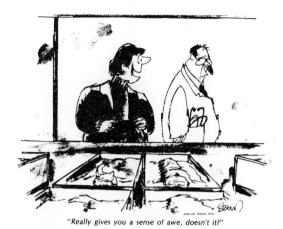

"Really gives you a sense of awe, doesn't it?"

fig. 7-1 *(From American Medical News, January 19, 1976, by permission.)*

guarded from contact with their parents because of convenience to the nursing staff and fear of infection. The luckless parents may scarcely be allowed a glimpse of their child, who is kept "safely" at the back of the nursery. Hour by hour, their anxieties mount while their confidence wanes, until the moment of discharge from the hospital when they are abruptly handed a mysterious, fragile bundle to deal with. Small wonder if they feel frightened and inadequate! (See Fig. 7-2.)

siblings' needs

Where there are older children in a family, their needs must be considered in addition to those of the parents and the newborn. They tend to feel left out of the pregnancy and birth, and therefore become more demanding or babyish themselves. Their unhappy behavior, in turn, increases difficulties for both parents. Older children's competitive needs to feel important can be turned to very good use at this time by involving them in discussions of what is happening and enlisting their willing participation. Assignment of small but significant tasks within the household (elevating their status to competent helpers), along with

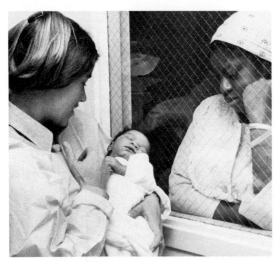

fig. 7-2 The nurse enjoys the baby while the mother is guarded against touching by a reinforced window! (*Photo courtesy of St. Luke's Hospital, New York.*)

some extra attention in their own right, can transform a very threatening experience into a happy and creative one for the newborn's siblings. Some obstetric centers, recognizing this concern, allow older children to visit their mother and the new baby in a special area.

POSTDELIVERY PITFALLS

A few words must be said here about postpartum emotional disturbances, which are relatively common and seem to stem from a number of causes, some of which may be preventable. These disturbances may occur days, weeks, or months following delivery.

The grieving of a mother who has given up a baby for adoption, or whose baby was born dead or deformed, is normal. She must be allowed to undergo the mourning process, and may benefit from some help in working through the burdens of self-blame, guilt, and anger which she will experience (Fig. 7-3).

A woman who is subject to psychotic breakdowns of one sort or another is likely to suffer a relapse in the postpartum period. She should be carefully followed for at least 2 months after delivery, and given prompt psychiatric attention if any signs of psychosis develop.

In addition, many apparently healthy women, following normal deliveries, experience a prolongation or exaggeration of the common, brief, "after-baby blues," which seem to be hormonally related. Such depressions can also reach psychotic proportions, endangering the well-being and even the lives of the mother, the baby, and other family members through violence or neglect. Again, psychiatric attention is urgent.

In some cases, alertness of the medical staff to psychologic problems during pregnancy may forestall a postpartum crisis. A pregnant woman who seems to have an unrealistic concept of the demands and dependency of a newborn baby on its mother, or who appears unduly immature herself, depending heavily on the obstetrician, nurses, and relatives for constant attention, is a prime target for trouble. She can be helped somewhat by the obstetric staff even during her brief prenatal contacts. She should be seen regularly by the same doctor, nurse, or counselor, who would recognize and acknowledge her feelings but give her positive support, so that "growing up" internally to her new role is not so difficult.

Many women never truly accept their babies' separateness, even after birth. Feeling somehow incomplete or unfulfilled without the child—as though it were indeed a vital organ or appendage—they tend to keep at least one of their children bound to themselves emotionally throughout life, to satisfy their own unconscious need. They may suffer depressions, not only postpartum but whenever the child leaves the home in later years. Such women generally require extended psychotherapy for improvement.

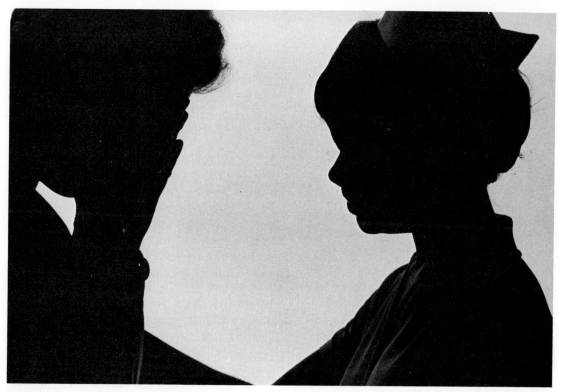

fig. 7-3 Nursing intervention as depression begins may avert more complex problems. (*Photo by Larry Mulvehill.*)

Men have been found to experience their share of difficulties as well, apparently rooted in feelings of rivalry for the mother and more likely to occur after the birth of a son. Relatively little attention has been paid by clinicians and researchers to postpartum problems of fathers—a further indication, perhaps, of society's tendency to underplay their role (Fig. 7-4).

PSYCHOLOGIC PROBLEMS OF THE PROFESSIONAL STAFF

Most of this chapter, up to this point, has been aimed at helping obstetric teams to understand their patients. In order to be truly effective in helping their patients, however, medical professionals require a special degree of self-understanding. Being human, just as their patients are, they are subject to needs and attitudes of their own which may interfere seriously with their competence. Recognizing and dealing with these personal feelings may be the most difficult professional task which they need to face.

the need to control

A major psychologic issue for health care professionals is that of *control*. People, as a rule, try to control things they are afraid of. A doctor's or nurse's determination to control

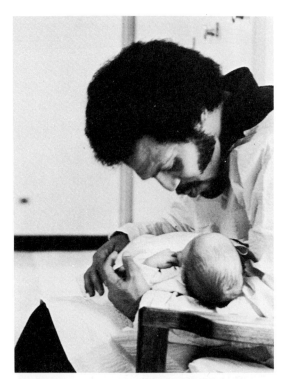

fig. 7-4 A father needs time with his new baby. (*Photo by Andrew McGowan.*)

disease and eliminate untimely death is commendable, but it is bound to fail at times. Death, disease, and unforeseen complications continue to occur in spite of the greatest human skill and dedication. If a person is frightened and angered by these forces, feeling helpless or guilty because he cannot forestall them, he may take out his feelings on his fellow workers, or even on the patient who is already the victim of circumstances.

Obstetricians may exercise their needs to control upon their women patients in inappropriate ways, such as failing to allow them to express their feelings or to participate in decisions. An authoritarian attitude may extend beyond medical to personal matters, such as how many babies to have and when, or what birth control methods to use when several safe options are available. Or it may dictate the conditions of delivery, without consideration for the patient's feelings and convenience. Nurses have their own ways of overcontrolling patients, particularly through setting up inflexible or insensitive hospital routines.

feelings of envy

A somewhat different problem tends to apply mostly to male obstetricians but may be of concern also to female professionals; that is, some sort of *envy* of the pregnant woman's accomplishment in bearing children. A young nurse or female doctor who has never been pregnant herself, especially if she is having difficulty conceiving, may feel that she is being outdone, and thus may unconsciously resent the patients committed to her care. An older single or postmenopausal female may have similar feelings toward expectant mothers. If she happens to work in the newborn nursery, she may tend to become openly possessive toward the babies and punitive toward their mothers, depriving them of contact with their infants or belittling their competence. When the time comes for mother and child to leave the hospital, such a nurse has been heard to exclaim reproachfully, "Are you taking *my* baby home?"

The obstetrician has available a different, though no better, avenue of expressing envious feelings without directly competing for possession of the baby. He or she may express a need to take credit for the whole birth process by patronizing the expectant mother, dismissing her role with such words as, "Don't worry, little mother, I'll have this baby for you!"

As noted earlier, some "mothering" is needed by the pregnant patient. She may appropriately look to her doctors and nurses, as well as to her own parents and husband, for support and concern. Too often, however, medical people tend to exclude the patient's family from involvement, thereby keeping her emotionally dependent on themselves. In causing expectant fathers and other relatives to feel less than welcome and important to the successful outcome of pregnancy, the medical staff may reveal their need to compete for the patient's affection and gratitude.

aids to the staff

It is to be hoped that medical people will have the wisdom and courage to confront and correct their own unhelpful attitudes, for the benefit of their patients as well as themselves. It has proven useful for an entire obstetric service to initiate frank discussions of cases or situations which have aroused emotional problems for the staff. Regular airings of tensions, anxieties, and feelings of guilt or anger among the professional staff, if properly conducted, can be both instructional and therapeutic. Also helpful are informal reading seminars based on such pertinent writings as Arthur and Libby Colman's book, *Pregnancy, The Psychological Experience,* Klaus's studies on maternal needs, and Brian Bird's book, *Talking with Patients.* Individuals with persistent psychologic problems might do well to seek personal psychotherapy.

Finally, a special word. Although the modern approach to patient care is via the *medical team,* and although the nurse is the key person on the team with regard to regular, direct contact with the patient, he or she may hesitate to contribute openly some valuable observations, insights, and skills. As the team approach to medicine grows in acceptance, so the special role of the nurse should increase in recognition and respect. Timidity and false modesty generate only discomfort and distrust. Team members, to be truly effective, must feel free to share and contribute as equals, though their particular responsibilities differ, in their common effort to serve people who seek their help.

study questions

1 Why must psychologic factors be considered in the management of pregnancy?
2 Especially during a first pregnancy, what developmental task faces the parents during the first trimester? The second? The third?
3 Identify some clues that would indicate problems in completing these tasks.
4 What particular feelings and concerns does a pregnant woman typically experience during each trimester of pregnancy?
5 Describe some common feelings and attitudes of expectant fathers.
6 What interventions can be used to promote good emotional health in a family during pregnancy, delivery, and the immediate postdelivery period?
7 What psychologic problems should be referred for psychiatric treatment?
8 Identify psychologic needs and attitudes on the part of the obstetric team which may prove detrimental to the families with whom they work. How may these be corrected?

bibliography

Abernathy, V.: "Identification of the Women at Risk for Unwanted Pregnancy," *American Journal of Psychiatry,* **132**(10):1027, 1975.

Barclay, R. L. and M. L. Barclay: "Aspects of the Normal Psychology of Pregnancy: The Midtrimester," *American Journal of Obstetrics and Gynecology,* **125**(2):207, May 1976.

Benedek, Therese: "The Psychobiologic Approach to Parenthood," in E. J. Anthony and T. Benedek (eds.), part II *Parenthood, Its Psychology and Psychopathology,* Little, Brown, Boston, 1970, pp. 109–206.

Bibring, G. L.: "Psychological Aspects of Pregnancy," *Clinical Obstetrics and Gynecology,* **19**(2):357–371, June 1976.

Bird, Brian: *Talking with Patients,* Lippincott, Philadelphia, 1955.

Chappel, John N., and Robert S. Daniels: "Puerperal Psychosis," *Hospital Medicine,* June 1969, pp. 115–122.

Colman, Arthur D., and Libby Lee: *Pregnancy: The Psychological Experience,* Herder and Herder, New York, 1971.

Deutsch, Helene: *The Psychology of Women,* vols. I and II, Bantam Books, New York, 1973 (paperback ed.).

Erikson, Erik H.: "Eight Ages of Man," in *Childhood and Society,* Norton, New York, Chap. 7, 1963.

Hott, J. R.: "The Crisis of Expectant Fatherhood," *American Journal of Nursing,* **76**(9):1436, September 1976.

Howells, John G.: "Childbirth Is a Family Experience," in J. G. Howells (ed.), *Modern Perspectives in Psycho-obstetrics,* Brunner-Mazel, New York, 1972, Chap. 7, pp. 127–149.

Jessner, Lucie, et al.: "The Development of Parental Attitudes during Pregnancy," in E. J. Anthony and T. Benedek (eds.), *Parenthood, Its Psychology and Psychopathology,* Little, Brown, Boston, 1970, Chap. 9, pp. 209–244.

Klaus, M. H. and J. H. Kennell: *Maternal-Infant Bonding,* Mosby, St. Louis, 1976.

MacFarlane, A.: *The Psychology of Childbirth,* Harvard, Cambridge, Mass., 1977.

Masters, W. H., and V. E. Johnson: *Human Sexual Response,* Little, Brown, Boston, 1966.

"Men Also Can Suffer from a Postpartum Reaction," *Frontiers of Psychiatry: Roche Report,* December 1, 1977.

Nadelson, C.: " 'Normal' and 'Special' Aspects of Pregnancy," *Obstetrics and Gynecology,* **41**(4):611–620, 1973.

Obrzut, L. A. J.: "Expectant Fathers' Perception of Fathering," *American Journal of Nursing,* **76**(9):1440, September 1976.

Richardson, A. C., and L. D. Webber: "The Noetic Dimension of Human Reproduction," *American Journal of Obstetrics and Gynecology,* July 15, 1971, pp. 808–822.

Sherefsky, P. M. and L. J. Yarrow, *Psychological Aspects of a First Pregnancy,* Raven, New York, 1973.

Shields, D.: "Psychology of Childbirth," *The Canadian Nurse,* November 1974, pp. 24–26.

Wagner, N. N. and D. A. Solberg: "Pregnancy and Sexuality," *Medical Aspects of Human Sexuality,* March 1974, pp. 44–66.

Wessel, M. A.: "Expectant Fathers Can Also Suffer Pangs of Pregnancy," *Medical Opinion,* September 1976, pp. 48–53.

8

MODERN MIDWIFERY

DOROTHEA M. LANG

A phone rings in the midwifery office, and a concerned voice asks for the midwife. What might be her concern? It is a young pregnant mother asking a seemingly simple question about a "little ache" in her side. For the next 18 min the midwife's friendly yet detailed questions regarding other possibly related symptoms which might, or might not, point to the simplest muscle strain or to the warning signs of a developing complication of pregnancy finally result in a reassuring answer. This young mother was at the end of her eighth month of pregnancy. This midwife and her colleagues have managed the patient's care since the day of her positive pregnancy test. Last Wednesday she had her prenatal checkup, and the midwife will see her again the day after tomorrow, when she arrives at the hospital in early labor, and throughout the delivery, and then with the baby at feeding time and for her first month's postpartum visit, and for interim counseling.

This is a modern midwife, a *certified nurse-*

midwife (C.N.M.), who functions as a part of the professional obstetric team.[1] She might be employed by a hospital, by a medical center, by an affiliated community-based maternal and child health service, or by an obstetrician-midwife group practice.[2,3] She manages the complete maternity care for mothers with an essentially normal course of pregnancy. She always functions with readily available medical consultation should any sudden medical complications arise. Today's modern midwife is prepared to function in all areas of woman's health maintenance concerned with reproductive processes, including family planning and childbirth. Perinatal care and newborn health management are integral parts of midwifery practice.

Midwifery management of labor and birth in most countries takes place in the patient's home, and over 80 percent of the world's babies are delivered by nonphysicians. Most of these infants are delivered at home. The American midwife, the C.N.M., usually performs the delivery functions in a hospital setting, where the majority of the mothers in the United States currently deliver. Being aware that familiar homelike surroundings and close family support can have a relaxing influence on the laboring mother, the midwife attempts to integrate these family-centered supportive measures into today's hospital setting, where, in case of sudden complications, the mother or baby can benefit from the most modern emergency facilities.[4]

Midwifery practice endorses the philosophy that each woman has the right to personalized health care and the right to acquire family health education which will help her to understand her own psychophysiologic functions as a woman, wife, and mother. Therefore, a midwife is committed to provide each woman with quality health care. This means that along with quality physical care, there must be educational opportunities provided which will guide the family members to the security they desire through personalized family planning; this individualized education will enable them to have quality in the childbirth experience itself and have satisfaction in the nurturing of the newborn, as well as help them to acquire the ability to form rewarding family relationships within the cultural setting of their choosing.

Although a professional midwife's functions may vary slightly from setting to setting, she will function in any or all of the described typical patient-care activities.

TYPICAL ACTIVITIES IN THE CARE OF PATIENTS

Traditionally the obstetrician follows his or her patients from office to hospital; similarly, today's professional midwife, the certified nurse-midwife, is the consistent and continuing link between the community-based ambulatory care center, office, or clinic and the inpatient services of the affiliating hospital. She acts as a liaison between the community hospital health care teams and serves as a "patient advocate" throughout all units of the hospital.[2]

In the ambulatory care center the midwife may care for approximately eight to ten prenatal revisit patients and one or two new prenatal patients during a 2-h prenatal session. The same number of patients can usually be cared for in the postpartum or family planning session.

At all times, whether in the hospital or in the community, in areas pertaining to obstetric management, the C.N.M. works with the readily available consultation and supervision of a physician.

A typical day for a nurse-midwife may start in a prenatal care center in the community. After a new maternity patient has been admitted to the center, attended a public health nurses's "new-patient orientation conference," and had her laboratory work completed, the mother is introduced to the midwife.

The midwife evaluates the laboratory findings and, through a friendly interchange of feelings and concerns, obtains a complete medical and obstetric history, adding any other pertinent information to the family history which may have been previously taken by the nurse. The patient then is ushered onto the examining table, and the midwife performs the total physical examination, including breast examination, auscultation of heart and lungs, abdominal palpation, complete pelvic examination and evaluation, and the taking of a Papanicolaou smear (Fig. 8-1).

Throughout her clinical work-up, the midwife encourages questions from the patient, thus providing information on maternity care, family planning, and general health maintenance. This on-the-spot discussion of problems related to the mother's discomforts or facts regarding growth and development of the fetus is most reassuring to the mother.

After the patient's total physical and emotional findings have been evaluated, the appropriate midwifery management is implemented; this includes the initiation of appropriate referrals and the prescribing of approved medications, vitamins, and treatments. Should findings reveal early signs of complications or obstetric problems, the physician is contacted, and consultation is provided to the midwife as necessary. If the patient is found to have a medically complicated condition, she is referred to the obstetrician for management.

During a revisit appointment, the prenatal patient is individually counseled by the midwife regarding her interim history. Each mother is encouraged to select the degree to which she (and her husband and family) wishes to participate in the birth process. Classes in preparation for childbirth and responsible parenthood, while optional, are offered and

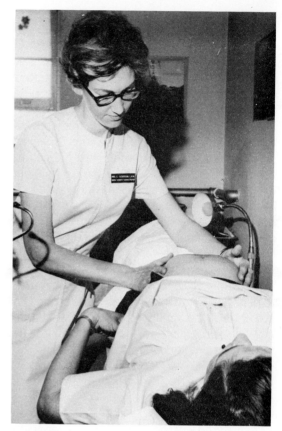

fig. 8-1 Nurse-midwife examines mother to determine fetal position. (*Photo by Ruth Helmich.*)

encouraged.[5] Personalized information and support are provided by the midwife throughout the maternity cycle. Newborn health care is emphasized, and family planning counseling is offered.

In the hospital, the professional midwife (C.N.M.) manages the complete obstetric course of mothers with a normal or near-normal labor. Mothers with minor complications are comanaged with the resident and the attending medical staff. The physician manages the medical problems, and the midwife manages the course of labor and performs the spontaneous delivery.

It has been adequately demonstrated that C.N.M.s can successfully manage the obstetric course of mothers who have no medical complications. A 5-year report of one of New York City's midwifery services demonstrated that certified nurse-midwives, as part of a medically directed obstetric-perinatal team, can also successfully manage the care of mothers with certain complications, such as mild preeclampsia, hypertension, premature ruptured membranes, prematurity, persistent posterior position, shoulder dystocia, anemia, severe varicosities, and drug addiction, and maintain a low perinatal mortality.[6]

When a patient-client arrives at the hospital in labor the midwife will perform the admission physical examination, evaluate the status of labor, secure appropriate comfort measures, and provide reassurance as needed by the patient and her family members. The attending obstetrician or the resident in charge of the unit is notified of the admission and the physical findings. Depending upon the policies of the unit, a physician will evaluate the status of the patient's heart and lungs to determine if general anesthetics could be administered in the event that emergency surgery or a cesarean delivery is required.

Throughout labor, the midwifery management includes supportive care and continuity in implementing those childbirth concepts that the client believes in and has learned during her preparation for labor sessions. This type of continuity of personalized care is of utmost importance in attempting to eliminate or minimize the need for medication during labor and birth.[7]

During the course of labor, the physician and obstetric nurse in charge of the unit are kept informed of the course of labor, and the midwife consults with the obstetrician or the maternal-fetal perinatologist whenever she or the supporting nursing team notices any deviation from normal. Any necessary treatments, infusions, and medications, such as sedatives and analgesia, are prescribed by the midwife in accordance with the Approved Certified Nurse-Midwife Orders, as described in each hospital's *Midwifery Policy Manual*.

Throughout labor and delivery, every possible comfort measure and relaxation technique is employed by the obstetric team. As long as the course of labor and delivery is normal, the midwife will perform the delivery (Fig. 8-2). If required, the midwife provides local anesthesia or gives a pudendal block prior to performing an episiotomy. She manages the third stage of labor and prescribes oxytocics as needed. She repairs the episiotomy or any lacerations if indicated and manages the fourth stage of labor.

The midwife provides immediate care of the newborn and, if necessary, performs simple resuscitation. She confirms the official

fig. 8-2 Nurse-midwife shows newly delivered infant to its mother. (*Photo by Ruth Helmich.*)

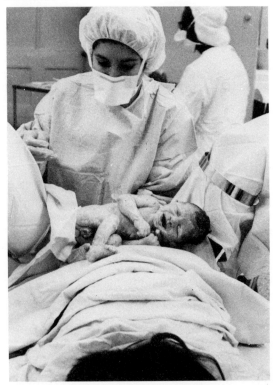

Apgar score and signs the birth certificate. Early mother-newborn interaction is also encouraged by the midwife, as nonmedicated or minimally medicated mothers should be given the opportunity to hold (and breast-feed) their newborn before they leave the delivery room. The father should be given the opportunity to hold his newborn, and as soon as possible, family members or other significant persons are encouraged to share those early moments of joy.[8]

At all times, the nurse-midwife works in close cooperation with the maternity nursing team. Management of the patient depends to a great degree also on the nurses' findings and their observations of the patient. The midwife regularly reviews and compares the medical, midwifery, and nursing notations on the records and participates actively in the team conferences on care of the patient. Whenever the midwife provides maternity nursing care, she follows the nursing policies of the unit. Frequently she will provide consultation to nursing students and the members of the maternity nursing team. She participates in the development of new policies for care of patients and new tools for their education. The midwife is an expert in the management of normal labor and childbirth. As such, at many medical centers she is also involved with the education, demonstration, and supervision of midwifery and medical students during their course experiences in normal labor and delivery.

Postdelivery care includes individual visits by a midwife to each of her patients in the postpartum unit. As part of the perinatal team, the midwife checks each newborn during the daily newborn nursery visits and makes every effort to visit mother and baby in the postpartum unit at feeding time, offering counseling as indicated.

To follow through with the education which every patient-client received during the prenatal period, the midwife continues to instruct the mother, emphasizing postpartum self-care, newborn care, and family adjustment. Instructions are also given regarding postpartum and pediatric health care appointments.

As desired by the patient, the midwife may prescribe contraceptives. Family planning counseling is an integral part of patient education.

The continuity of care which such arrangements can provide is self-evident. According to feelings that have been expressed by mothers, it is most satisfying and comforting for them to see a familiar person in the hospital, one whom they have learned to trust during their prenatal period, and to know that they will see her again in the community clinic or office for the postpartum, family planning, and interconceptional care.

THE UNIQUENESS OF THE MODERN PROFESSIONAL MIDWIFE

In every society the consumers and the providers of health care develop a common understanding of the functions and responsibilities of each member of the health care team. Within the past decade the American public, through its public media, has voiced a strong demand for the "return of the midwife" to function on the health team. Today's public is searching for the midwife who will provide "complete" maternal and women's health maintenance care for the "healthy" woman.

the independent and dependent role of the midwife

The midwife's functions are well known to most of the families of the world. In the United States the education of the professional midwife or certified nurse-midwife is based on a careful balance between the *preventive* and *curative* aspects of health care. The balance is carefully adjusted according to the *interdependent* role of the midwife as she functions as a professional member of a health team in a specified facility or a geographic region.

The prime emphasis of midwifery education is on the *preventive* components of health care, because, as part of the team, the midwife is expected to function as an independent expert in the management of perinatal care of the "healthy." The second most important emphasis is on the *curative* aspects of health care, because whenever a patient-client encounters obstetrical or medical problems, the midwife must be able to detect and diagnose the earliest signs of a complication and refer for appropriate medical consultation. The physician then functions in the prime management role, and the midwife assumes more of the dependent management role as she provides continuity of supportive patient care services. In this instance, she assists the patient in her adjustment to the transitions from the preventive health team to the curative health team and, hopefully, back to the preventive health team.

the midwife in community-based and hospital-based care

Because of the intensive educational preparation, the certified nurse-midwife is prepared to provide comprehensive family-centered services in "well-being" health care *and* in "acute sickness" health care.

The midwife's ability to function in the community *and* in the hospital is of utmost importance to the family, because the midwife is the continuous link between the two areas of health care. No matter where the care is being provided, a healthy mother's prenatal care or labor and delivery care will require a ready access to an acutely responsive perinatal team that will be able to manage the high-risk complications if and when such emergencies arise. During such an emergency the midwife can accompany the mother and provide continuity of care throughout the physician's management of the complicated medical problems. When the acute emergency is over, the midwife will again continue the care in the community as long as the client's health status remains in the low-risk category.

the midwife as a client advocate

Those who take an advocate role must know their clients as individuals and as members of the families from which they came and to which they and their babies will return. The midwife *knows* the maternity patient thoroughly because of her repeated prenatal contacts with the mother and her family, over a period of months—sometimes years—not just by a single interview from across the table.

An advocate must know the patient-client in at least five ways: within the realm and context of the physical, psychological, educational, economic, and spiritual-religious frame of the client's existence.

Perinatal care advocacy must also relate to the newborn baby. The midwife considers the parent *and* the baby as the "complete patient package" before and after birth. As the midwife has a good awareness of the medical diagnosis of pregnancy, she simultaneously attempts to make a diagnosis of the patient's factual and emotional understanding of the pregnancy and the meaning it has for the mother, father, and family. During each prenatal visit or home visit the midwife becomes more familiar with the deep-rooted needs and strengths of a mother's existence as an individual, as a family member, and as part of the cultural environment to which the mother/baby belong.

the midwife as an educator of the patient-public

As the midwife provides personalized *physical* care, she also provides opportunities for *family life education* which will guide the woman and her family toward "self-preservation of health."[9] People learn best when they *need* to know and at a time when they want to know. Midwives come in contact with the patient-public at the most educable points of life.

preadolescent/teenager The body and emotional changes of the preadolescent/teenager trigger a natural curiosity and a search for answers to difficult questions regarding the organs of reproduction, emotions, hygiene, sex, and contraception. Individualized attention from a midwife appears less threatening to this age group.

pregnant woman A missed menstrual period causes a woman to seek professional assistance to check out her suspicions of pregnancy through a pregnancy test or physical examination. This is an obvious opportunity for the midwife to offer preventive medicine and health education and "health-preservation" counseling, all of which the midwife is trained to provide.[10]

care of mother during pregnancy and delivery Comprehensive prenatal care is a vital base for comprehensive perinatal care. As the midwife provides direct prenatal management, she also encourages emotional and physical preparation for childbirth to help the mother prepare herself for a satisfying perinatal experience. The midwife provides educational sessions at the patient's request. The midwife's knowledge of the special needs of each mother/family is integrated into the midwife's individual management of each healthy mother's labor and delivery. A midwife also provides important continuity of supportive care for those mothers at perinatal risk who will be managed by the obstetrician-perinatologist.

care of the infant While learning to nurture the infant, a mother usually seeks guidance for successful breast-feeding and other mothering techniques.[11] The midwife provides this guidance and also utilizes this opportunity to integrate other infant "health-preservation" education.

interconceptional family planning patient Immediately after delivery and shortly thereafter, a mother is usually concerned with her body's adjustment to the nonpregnant state. Simultaneously, she is usually motivated toward seeking family planning measures. Mothers initially request these services from the familiar midwife who also delivered her baby.[12,13]

guidance in parenting for couples New parents or individuals who are anticipating a rapidly approaching new adult role as parent frequently seek out a professional who can help them with educational sessions on "parenting." The importance of good parenting is well documented to assure optimal growth and development of a newborn, the infant, the child.[14]

the midwife as an educator of professional team members

All perinatal team members must know the important aspects of management of mothers with an essentially healthy, uncomplicated course of pregnancy and childbirth. The midwife, as the acknowledged expert in the management of the healthy mother, is the choice educator and clinical instructor for midwifery, medical, and nursing students. Many leading medical centers around the world have employed professional midwives as professors for the education of "perinatal care of the healthy."

MIDWIFERY IN THE UNITED STATES

Midwifery as currently practiced in the United States must be understood through the richness of its heritage, which comprises the work of tireless pioneers in the midwifery profession and the sustaining support of friends outside the profession. This fine heritage enables the modern midwife to function as a coequal with other professionals in today's health teams and health care programs.

Historically, the profession of midwifery precedes almost every other profession. The earliest biblical writings mention midwifery as a personalized service that women offered to women.[15] Since that time, the profession has been perpetuated mostly by the apprentice-tutorial pattern of education, the traditional form of education throughout early civilizations until the twentieth century.

Compared with the other women of their time, midwives were usually the most educated, and they rightfully earned respect from the families in the communities which they served. These midwives were the only professionals who officially assisted at birth, cared for the newborns, and provided supportive services to the mother and family.

In American history, the earliest colonial records tell us that the midwife was a very important person in the newly settled territories. The services of a midwife were guaranteed by several charter companies as an inducement to women to travel to the new lands. In 1641, the General Court of Massachusetts showed its respect and esteem for midwives by ordering that they, along with "physicians and chirurgeons," should have transportation first on all ferry boats in the colony.[16]

In the early nineteenth century, a new vogue of employing physicians to assist in childbirth was brought from other countries. Soon the use of forceps was introduced, and the hospital was encouraged as the place for delivery and for the education of physicians in midwifery/obstetrics.[17]

As the immigrants continued to flock to the New World, they brought with them their midwives, who often neither spoke English nor were familiar with the American customs and practices of hygiene. Vast misunderstandings between the medical hierarchies and the midwives developed and inevitably were magnified by the complex health problems that prevailed during these decades. Midwives were not invited to practice in hospitals, and because of the lack of opportunities for formal and progressive midwifery education, they had little chance to keep pace with new approaches to health care and could not become part of the American obstetric scene.[16,17]

At the turn of the century (1900), worsening social and health conditions in the urban areas contributed to infant and maternal mortality. The low status of women at that time furthered the atmosphere in which all midwives were blamed for the deaths of infants born at home during those preantibiotic times. As a result the midwives were gradually discouraged from practicing in most urban areas.

In 1905, New York City became concerned about the fact that over 3000 practicing midwives were delivering 40 percent of all babies in the city. Many tried to condemn the midwives; others suggested that the work of the midwife could and should be raised to higher planes by proper education and state licensure. Two years later the Board of Health started to license midwives.[18,19]

One early attempt to bring the midwife into the mainstream of health care was initiated by the New York City Health Department when, in 1911, it opened the Bellevue School of Midwifery, the first American school of midwifery. In this educational program, midwives and obstetricians worked as a team in providing maternity care. The school's midwifery students included women from New York City and surrounding states, some immigrant midwives, local lay-midwives, birth attendants, and some nurses. However, the school closed in 1936, when less than 10 percent of New York City's births were attended by midwives.[18,20]

In 1925, the late Mary Breckinridge founded the Frontier Nursing Service (FNS) to provide primary health care for people in the mountain counties of Kentucky. Realizing the special maternity care needs of the area, Mrs. Breckinridge went to England to study midwifery and to recruit professional midwives for the Kentucky program. Because some of these professional midwives were also professional nurses, this service is recognized as the first nurse-midwifery service in America.[21] The first recognized school of nurse-midwifery in the United States is the Maternity Center Association School of Nurse-Midwifery.[22] It was organized in association with the Lobenstein Midwifery School and Clinic and accepted its first student group in 1932. Thereafter, most schools required nursing education and experience as a prerequisite to American midwifery education.

Acceptance of the full scope of the nurse-midwife's services by American hospitals seemed painfully slow. As a result, many of the nurse-midwifery graduates became educators of maternal and child health in schools of nursing or actively encouraged the family-centered approach to childbirth by demonstration, graduate nurse education, and parent education.[22,23] Many midwifery graduates also chose challenging consultation assignments in maternal and child health programs with the U.S. Children's Bureau or state health departments which enouraged educational preparation in midwifery. Some graduates went overseas to travel and work under government auspices or to serve as missionaries, providing leaderhip in international health.[20,22]

Pioneering endeavors of the Maternity Center School of Nurse-Midwifery and the Frontier School of Midwifery stimulated several demonstration programs in the 1940s and 1950s. One education program was established at the Tuskegee Institute in Alabama, which between 1941 to 1946, was mainly supported by funds from the United States government. Other nurse-midwifery education programs developed at Yale, Johns Hopkins, Columbia, and the Catholic University-Catholic Maternity Institute.[24] Hospital-based formal midwifery education was initiated in 1958 by Dr. Louis Hellman when he invited the transfer of the Maternity Center School of Nurse-Midwifery into the hospital-medical center setting, at the Kings County Hospital in affiliation with the Downstate University of New York in Brooklyn, New York. Gradually over the next 20 years additional educational programs were developed at the universities of Utah, Mississippi, Illinois, South Carolina, Kentucky, Minnesota, California, Georgetown, St. Louis, Loma Linda, and Emory and at the Meharry Medical College, the New Jersey College of Medicine, and by the United States Air Force.[28]

In 1964, the Roosevelt Hospital in Manhattan became the first voluntary hospital to employ midwives to function as part of the obstetric team to provide comprehensive maternity and family planning care.[26,27] New York City's Maternal and Infant Care Project (MIC) pioneered in the regional approach of integrating midwives into the hospital-based and community-based obstetrical-perinatal care teams of a citywide maternity care program.

Acceptance of midwives by the consumers of care was overwhelmingly positive.[28]

As obstetric nurses, midwives, obstetric residents, and obstetrician-gynecologists worked together in an increasing number of hospitals, mutual respect, trust, and colleague-team relationships developed. The team approach was exemplified in the "Joint Statement on Maternity Care," which was published in January 1971 by the American College of Obstetricians and Gynecologists (ACOG), their Nurses Association (NAACOG), and the American College of Nurse-Midwives (ACNM). With this statement, midwifery entered the mainstream of American health care, as it specifically provided that, as part of a medically directed health team, "qualified nurse-midwives may assume responsibility for the complete care and management of uncomplicated maternity patients."[29] In his Health Message of 1971, the president of the United States mentioned the allocation of funds for the education of nurse-midwives, and federal guidelines for the Maternal and Infant Care Projects across the country included recommendations that certified nurse-midwives be employed on the health care teams.[30]

Public media started to carry information on the return of the "midwife in modern style."[31,32] Large numbers of nurses applying for entrance into the nurse-midwifery educational programs encouraged new programs to develop. An up-to-date listing of these educational programs may be obtained by writing to the American College of Nurse-Midwives, 1012 Fourteenth Street, N.W., Suite 801, Washington, D.C. 20005.

The media has also created a public awareness of the growing importance of the midwifery profession.[33] Suddenly, the desire to become a professional midwife is being voiced by an increasing number of women who have no educational background in nursing. Many of these women have a science-related college education, are certified child-birth educators, are birth attendants, or function in a health-related profession. These women are searching for a midwifery education program that is geared to the "post-health science" candidate, thereby creating two routes into professional midwifery: the postnurse route and the post-health science route.[34,35] Proponents of this idea insist that graduates from both routes should attain the same high standard of education and experience for practice and that all graduates should sit the same national certification examination.

In May 1971, the American College of Nurse-Midwives initiated the National Certification Examination to standardize the basic competency level of the professional midwife practitioner.

International recognition was given the American midwife as early as 1956, when the American College of Nurse-Midwives (ACNM) became a member of the International Confederation of Midwives (ICM). The ICM selected the United States as the site for its Golden Anniversary International Congress. In 1972, the triennial congress was held in Washington, D.C. The ACNM had the honor of hosting over 2000 midwives from over 100 countries.[36,37]

Thus in the United States, professional midwifery has taken its rightful place among the health professions in today's modern health care system.

DEFINITIONS IN MIDWIFERY

midwifery

Midwifery is the art and practice of combining the scientific, philosophic, and human approach to the provision of health maintenance of women in their normal reproductive processes, including childbirth, with involvement of the family and/or significant others. Midwives practice within a health team and a framework of an organized regional or local health service with qualified medical consultation.

certified nurse-midwife

A certified nurse-midwife (C.N.M.) is a professional midwife who possesses evidence of being certified according to the requirements of the National Certifying Board of the American College of Nurse-Midwifes. Such a person is entitled to use the initials C.N.M. after her name. She is educated in two disciplines: nursing and midwifery. A nurse-midwife may be further qualified by having a baccalaureate, master's, or doctoral degree in public health administration, nursing, or a health-related science.

international definition of midwife

A midwife is a person who, having been regularly admitted to a midwifery educational program fully recognized in the country in which it is located, has successfully completed the prescribed course of studies in midwifery and has acquired the requisite qualifications to be registered and/or legally licensed to practice midwifery.

the sphere of practice The midwife must be able to give the necessary supervision, care, and advice to women during pregnancy, labor, and the postpartum period; to conduct deliveries on her own responsibility; and to care for the newborn and the infant. This care includes preventive measures, the detection of abnormal condition in mother and child, the procurement of medical as-

sistance, and the execution of emergency measures in the absence of medical help.

The midwife has an important task in counseling and education—not only for patients but also within the family and community. The work should involve antenatal education and preparation for parenthood and extends to certain areas of gynecology, family planning, and child care.

She may practice in hospitals, clinics, health units, domiciliary conditions, or any other service.*

birth attendant

The birth attendant is internationally recognized as a health worker who fulfills a useful role in areas where health services are not sufficiently developed. In most countries, only on-the-job orientation and working experience enable the birth attendant to assist women during childbirth and in the immediate postpartum period, including newborn home care.[38]

american college of nurse-midwives

The ACNM is the professional organization for certified nurse-midwives in the United States. It establishes the standards for the practice of midwifery, provides a national certification mechanism for the professional midwife, and offers guidelines and accreditation for midwifery educational programs in the United States. The ACNM collaborates with all other professional groups who share its primary concern for quality maternal-infant health care for all women and babies. The early roots of the organization were formed in

*This international definition was accepted by the ICM Membership in 1972, as well as by the Joint Study Group on Maternity Care, FIGO, WHO.[37,38]

1929, and the ACNM was incorporated in 1955.

international confederation of midwives

The International Confederation of Midwives (ICM) is an international organization whose membership consists of national groups of midwives. It was established with the belief that the profession of midwifery will be advanced by greater international cooperation and that this will promote the health and well-being of the family throughout the world. This international organization was founded in 1922.[39]

study questions

1 From the section, "Typical Activities in Care of Patients," identify the functions and responsibilities of the C.N.M and compare them with nursing and physician functions and responsibilities. Where is there an overlap? How are the roles complementary?
2 What is meant by interdependent/independent/dependent roles?
3 In the early 1900s, what factors led to the decline of midwifery practice?
4 Identify four factors that have led to an increased acceptance of professional midwifery practice today.
5 Identify a new trend in the practice of midwifery by persons who are not nurses.
6 How does the definition of a certified nurse midwife in the United States differ from the international definition of a midwife?

references

1 *Qualifications, Standards and Functions,* The American College of Nurse-Midwives, Washington, D.C., 1975.
2 D. M. Lang, "Providing Maternity Care Through a Nurse-Midwifery Service Program," *Nursing Clinics of North America,* **4**(3), 1969.
3 S. T. Gatewood and R. B. Stewart, "Obstetricians and Nurse Midwives: The Team Approach in Private Practice," *American Journal of Obstetrics and Gynecology,* [123](1):35, September 1975.
4 B. Carrington, "A Sample Pattern for Family Centered Maternity Care," *Journal of Nurse-Midwifery,* **12**(1), spring 1977.
5 V. H. Elinds, *The Rights of the Pregnant Parent,* Waxwing Productions/New York, Two Continents, Ottawa, 1976.
6 M. A. Schmidt, *Midwifery Service Progress Report: Maternity, Infant Care and Family Planning Projects,* Department of Health, New York, 1972.
7 D. B. Haire, *The Cultural Warping of Childbirth,* International Childbirth Association—Special Report, International Childbirth Association, Hillside, N.J., 1972.
8 M. H. Klaus and J. H. Kennell, *Maternal and Infant Bonding,* Mosby, St. Louis, 1976.
9 D. M. Lang, "The Professional Midwife on the Perinatal Team," *Journal of Nurse-Midwifery,* **12**(1), spring 1977. 1977.
10 G. S. Brewer and T. Brewer, *What Every Pregnant Woman Should Know,* Random House, New York, 1977.
11 K. Pryor, *Nursing Your Baby,* Harper & Row, New York, 1963.
12 B. Seaman and G. Seaman, *Women and the Crisis in Sex Hormones,* Rawson, New York, 1976.
13 M. Nofziger, *A Cooperative Method of Natural Birth Control,* Book Publishers, Nashville, Tenn., 1976.
14 T. W. Thevenin, *The Family Bed: An Age-Old Concept in Childrearing,* P.O. Box 16004 Minneapolis, MN 55416, 1975.
15 The Holy Bible, Exodus 1:16.
16 C. G. Fox, "Toward a Sound Historical Basis for Nurse-Midwifery," *Bulletin, American College of Nurse-Midwives,* **14**(3), 1969.
17 R. W. Wertz and D. C. Wertz, *Lying In: A History of Childbirth in America,* Free Press, New York, 1977.
18 D. Harris, "The Development of Nurse-Midwifery in New York City," *Bulletin, American College of Nurse-Midwives,* **14**(1), 1969.
19 D. Harris, E. F. Daily, and D. M. Lang, "Nurse-Midwifery in New York City," *American Journal of Public Health,* **61**(1), 1971.
20 M. T. Shoemaker, *History of Nurse-Midwifery in the United States,* Catholic, Washington, D.C., 1947 (ACNM Archives).
21 M. Breckinridge, *Wide Neighborhoods, A Story of the Frontier Nursing Service,* Harper & Row, New York, 1952.
22 *Twenty Years of Nurse-Midwifery, 1933–1953,* Maternity Center Association, New York.
23 H. Corbin, H. "Historical Development of Nurse-Midwifery in this Country and Present Trends," *Bulletin, American College of Nurse-Midwives,* **4**(1), 1959.

24 *Education for Nurse-Midwifery,* American College of Nurse-Midwives, Washington, D.C., 1958.

25 *What Is a Nurse-Midwife?,* American College of Nurse-Midwives, Washington, D.C., 1975.

26 J. Borsellega, The Role of the Nurse-Midwife in a Voluntary Hospital, *Bulletin, American College of Nurse-Midwives,* **7**(4), 1967.

27 B. Brennan, J. R. Heilman, *The Complete Book of Midwifery,* Dutton, New York, 1976.

28 A. Simon, "A Satisfied Patient Views Nurse-Midwifery," *Bulletin, American College of Nurse-Midwives,* **17**(2), 1972.

29 American College of Obstetricians and Gynecologists (ACOG), the Nurse Association of the American College of Obstetrics and Gynecologists (NAACOG), and the American College of Nurse-Midwives (ACNM), "Joint Statement on Maternity Care (and Supplement)." *ACOG Newsletter,* February 1971.

30 *Health Message from the President of the United States, Relative to Building a National Heatlh Strategy,* 92d Cong., 1st Sess. H.R. Doc. 92-49, Feb. 18, 1971, p. 9.

31 J. Klemensrud, "Midwives Carry New Image into the Hospital Delivery Room," *The New York Times,* Sept. 20, 1972.

32 D. Lang, "The Midwife Returns Modern Style," *Parents Magazine,* October 1972.

33 D. Lang, "What is the Future of the C.N.M., in *21 Century Obstetrics Now,* NAPSAC, National Association of Parents and Professionals for Safe Alternatives in Childbirth, Marble Hill, Mo., 1977, vol. I.

34 The National Midwives Association, *N.M.A. Newsletter,* **1**(1), 1977.

35 I. M. Gaskin, *Spiritual Midwifery,* Book Publishing, Tenn., 1978.

36 *New Horizons in Midwifery,* International Confederation of Midwives, London, 1973, p. 220.

37 Internation Federation of Gynecology and Obstetrics and The International Confederation of Midwives, *Maternity Care in the World,* 2d ed., C. M. Printing Services, Hampshire, England, 1976.

38 "The Midwife in Maternity Care," *Report of a WHO Expert Committee,* WHO Technical Report Series, no. 331, 1966.

39 M. F. Myles, *Textbook for Midwives,* London, Churchill Livingstone, 1975.

9
EDUCATION FOR CHILDBIRTH

CONSTANCE R. CASTOR

Girls and boys are informally educated for the childbirth experience from their own birth. Depending on their culture, this education varies in its positive and negative qualities. The availability of formal programs of prenatal education is a rather modern phenomenon. The change to the nuclear family in our society reduced the natural education source of mothers, aunts, and cousins in the extended family. Now, with the general movement toward self-awareness and responsibility for becoming pregnant, parents in unprecedented numbers are seeking to prepare themselves for the childbirth experience.

In preparation classes, through organized learning programs, parents can acquire information and specialized skills which will permit the woman to remain relatively comfortable and in control of herself during labor and delivery. She can participate actively in the process with no sacrifice of safety to either herself or the fetus.

METHODS OF PREPARATION

There are currently two major approaches to preparation for childbirth in the United States: psychophysical methods and psychoprophylactic methods.

psychophysical method

The psychophysical method evolved out of the natural childbirth movement of the forties and fifties, which was founded on the writings and work of Dick-Read, Thomas, and Goodrich. The program of education and exercise is directed toward breaking the fear-tension-pain cycle. Fathers are welcomed to class and are prepared for labor as well. The psychophysical method is the oldest approach to prepared childbirth in this country. Such courses frequently incorporate general prenatal education with specific labor techniques which the woman can apply as she chooses.

maternity center association   The *Maternity Center Association* has long been in the forefront of a family-centered approach to preparation for childbirth. Initially, the education and techniques it advocated were based on Read's work. As time passed, its approach encompassed the philosophies of others, such as Goodrich and Thomas. It remains the prime example of the psychophysical approach. The Maternity Center encourages a program of physical and mental preparation for birth; the inclusion of the husband; the creation of a warm, supportive environment during labor; and specific activities, such as abdominal and chest breathing, for the management of labor.

Bradley method of husband-coached childbirth   *The Bradley method of husband-coached childbirth* is another example of a psychophysical method. Dr. Robert Brad-

ley has based his method on his observations of animal behavior during birth. Most of the techniques for labor are derived from this "imitation of nature." Bradley describes these techniques as meeting the laboring mother's need for:

1   Darkness and solitude
2   Quiet
3   Physical comfort
4   Physical relaxation
5   Controlled breathing
6   Closed eyes and the appearance of sleep

Bradley pioneered the rejection of a typically passive role for the husband. Instead, he created a central role for the husband as overseer and director of his wife's labor preparation and conduct. The manner of emphasis on the husband may be interpreted by some contemporary women as paternalistic and overbearing. The transference of the dominant male authority figure from physician to husband neglects in part the woman's need to take responsibility for her own behavior.

Kitzinger method   A careful reading of the writings of Sheila Kitzinger, clearly demonstrates the blurring of distinction between psychophysical and psychoprophylactic methods. Kitzinger adamantly believes in the conscious participation of the mother. Her program is structured to achieve a rhythmic coordination and harmony in the body and in labor. This results in emotional preparedness for birth.

Kitzinger's approach advocates an elaborate system for relaxation which includes the husband as a helper. The system was developed from the "Method School" of acting. Nonetheless, it includes thorough training in active relaxation. Although it does not claim to be part of a conditioning process, it certainly creates a new type of adaptive behavior for the mother.

Kitzinger's second approach to "harmony in labor" utilizes breathing techniques, starting with slow breathing and progressing to shallow, rapid breathing for the final moments of the first stage of labor. Finally, Kitzinger integrates physical exercises, relaxation, and breathing in extensive preparation for the second stage of labor.

With the changes in contemporary society and with the continued refinement in the education of parents, the differences between psychophysical and psychoprophylactic methods are rapidly disappearing.

psychoprophylactic method

The psychoprophylactic method of childbirth preparation was introduced in the early sixties through the efforts of Marjorie Karmel and her book, *Thank You, Dr. Lamaze.* The method evolved out of the application by the Russians of Pavlovian classical conditioning to childbirth. Popularly known as the *Lamaze Method,* psychoprophylaxis was originally characterized by a rigid and somewhat dogmatic approach. This can be attributed to the climate of the times in which it was introduced.

Today, although differences in technique can be observed as it is practiced throughout the world, the central thrust of psychoprophylaxis remains a highly structured system based on conditioning, discipline, and concentration. On the surface, many of its techniques are similar to those of the psychophysical approach. Indeed, it can be said that the methods have mutually influenced one another. A closer evaluation of the actual teachings reveals a greater intensity in psychoprophylaxis, with a central emphasis on the role of conditioning. It is believed that the woman must undergo a period of highly disciplined training which teaches her to substitute new responses to the stimulus of labor contractions. The necessity for sound prenatal education and reduction of psychic tension is recognized as well. The support of a knowledgeable labor coach is inherent to the technique. In most Western countries, including the United States, the coach is the father. Within this and subsequent chapters, the word "husband" may be used interchangeably with the person who will assist, coach, and encourage the woman—perhaps a parent, boyfriend, close friend, or other close relative.

The psychoprophylactic method is sometimes referred to as a nonpharmacologic analgesia, but it recognizes that the various obstetric modalities can be added to the prepared woman's efforts as circumstances warrant.

hypnosis

Hypnosis is an effective approach to the alleviation of pain in childbirth, but it is impractical as it depends on a sufficient supply of trained physicians. Through hypnosis, the woman learns to enter a trancelike state, focusing intently on the hypnotist or on prearranged self-hypnotic suggestions, which significantly reduce attention to outside stimuli. Some observers feel that there may be elements of self-hypnosis in the other methods discussed, but this has not been adequately demonstrated.

general classes

Many physicians teach childbirth classes in their offices. General information is given on the pregnancy and labor process. Most physicians who take the time to educate their patients find a reduction in numbers of questions and a heightened sense of cooperation on the part of the couple.

leboyer delivery

Wide exposure to both the film and the book by Dr. Leboyer, *Birth Without Violence,* has resulted in large numbers of couples seeking the kind of childbirth experience he describes.

Although Leboyer's approach is not specifically a method for childbirth, he has championed the creation of a warm, human, and gentle environment for birth. This approach can be integrated with any of the popular childbirth methods, since it is directed to the satisfaction of the physiological and emotional needs of the mother and child and not to methodology.

Leboyer seeks to minimize what he considers to be the trauma of birth, and he appeals to the physician to take responsibility for this by (1) eliminating unnecessary stimuli and (2) encouraging the maternal-infant bond.

The Leboyer philosophy includes patience, emotional support, good communication, and education as integral parts of obstetrical management. He emphasizes a gentle, controlled delivery, specifically avoiding stress on the craniosacral axis. He postulates that such stress interferes with the baby's well-being, particularly initiation of breathing, irritability, and other central nervous system symptoms. He feels that a gentle waterbath at birth restores lost body heat, relaxes the craniosacral axis, and puts the infant in harmony with its environment.

Leboyer is also concerned with unnecessary stimulation of the newborn at birth. It should be stressed that the key word here is *unnecessary.* In no instance does Leboyer sacrifice safety and health of baby or mother for any aspect of his approach to birth. Leboyer can be said to have a humanistic philosophy which implicitly fosters the mother-infant bond.

summary

It should be understood that preparation for childbirth provides the modern couple with the means to cope effectively with the stress of pregnancy, birth, and the early postpartum period. The psychophysical and psychoprophylactic methods are similarly based on (1) accurate information to reduce anxieties and fears which are recognized to accentuate pain; (2) the acquisition of specific techniques of relaxation, muscular control, and respiratory activity to reduce or eliminate the pain of labor; and (3) the creation and maintenance of a calm, supportive environment. A comparison of these methods is given in Table 9-1.

MECHANISM OF PAIN CONTROL

In the past, much of the effectiveness of preparation for childbirth was attributed by some to good education, dedication, courage, distraction, and luck. Grantly Dick-Read believed reeducation and antepartal and intrapartal support were essential in helping a woman achieve control during labor. Concentration and distraction played a part as well, as the woman practiced mental disassociation and performed relaxation and breathing activities. Lamaze and other proponents of psychoprophylactic preparation for childbirth believed that classical Pavlovian conditioning was the element responsible for the management of labor. This explanation was based on the principle of cortical excitation-inhibition. Women were deconditioned from harmful attitudes by an educational process and conditioned to perform various motor and neuromuscular skills during labor. These conditioned responses were thought to take precedence in the stimulus-response cycle

table 9-1 Comparison of methods of preparation for childbirth

	Read	Bradley	Kitzinger	psychoprophylactic methods	
				adapted Lamaze (US)	classic Lamaze
Rationale	Women negatively influenced by cultural conditioning Need to break fear-tension-pain cycle	Attempts to imitate other mammal's instinctive conduct in labor through intelligent reasoning	Mental and physical harmony produce a creative childbirth experience	Behavioral conditioning of mother produces reliable and constructive responses to demands of labor	Pavlovian conditioning raises threshold of pain by creating a zone of inhibition in cortex
Provision of support for mother	Medical labor attendants	Role of husband and physician central	Husband or significant other	Husband or significant other Medical labor attendant	Medical labor attendants, including a "monitrice" or specialized labor attendant
Prenatal physical exercise	Strenuous physical exercise thought inherent to preparing the body for labor	Rigorous exercise based on rationale of athletic qualities of labor	None specifically prescribed	Nonstrenuous program of physical fitness to increase comfort in pregnancy	"Body-building" exercise to prepare for "athletic event" of labor
Labor techniques	Create positive mental attitude Use of abdominal breathing for most of labor Use of panting Passive relaxation exercise Pushing technique	Imitation of sleep through position and use of abdominal breathing Deep mental relaxation Pushing technique	Rhythmic breathing: slow to shallow as labor progresses Refined relaxation technique Detailed pushing technique and exercise stressed	Rhythmic breathing: slow to shallow but *not* panting nor rapid Refined active relaxation and body awareness Detailed pushing technique	Diaphragmatic breathing: slow and rapid; use of panting and vigorous blowing Neuromuscular disassociation exercises Pushing technique
Comments	Mystical overtones Diluted in practice by others from Read's original premise	Absolutes in methodology Domineering role of husband Role of techniques secondary	Adaptive approach to teach women to approach labor with confidence	Flexible but structured program to integrate physical, emotional, and mental responses during labor	Often practical with rigid and dogmatic qualities

and were registered in the cortex as an area of excitation which subsequently inhibited or interfered with the registering of painful stimuli in the brain.

More recent investigations on pain by Melzack suggest a fuller explanation for the effectiveness of psychoprophylactic childbirth preparation. According to this theory, referred to as the *gate-control* theory, the central nervous system is capable of effectively blocking or reducing pain under certain conditions. It is suggested that local physical stimulation, such as the stroking activity done in labor, can balance the pain stimuli by closing down a gate type of mechanism thought to exist in the cord. Activity within the cord itself, such as is created when the woman performs various neuromuscular and motor skills, further modifies the transmission of pain. Finally, selective and directed cortical activity, such as the various cognitive activities related to analyzing and directing one's behavior and concentrating on breathing and relaxation skills, is proposed to activate and close the gating mechanism as well.

This theory points out the need for the creation and maintenance of a supportive environment and the development of trusting relationships as essential to the structuring of an atmosphere in which the various higher mental activities can be successfully implemented.

Perhaps other elements of behavior and learning, such as behavioral modification, also operate to create this highly structured system of preparation. Further exploration of these related areas is necessary before definitive explanations can be made.

THE VALUE OF PREPARATION FOR CHILDBIRTH

Although family-centered maternity care was an academically accepted concept for dec-

ades, it was not applied consistently. Husbands were included in prenatal classes but were permitted limited or no actual participation during labor. Their involvement was generally confined to the hours of waiting, at home or in the waiting room. If the husband was admitted to the labor room, it was under closely regulated conditions. Some institutions promoted rooming-in and flexible visiting hours, but the focus still remained on the needs of the staff for control, rather than on the needs of the family for support and time to be together.

More recently, this situation has dramatically changed. Informed couples sought to share this experience; prepared husbands began to be included as part of the supporting group throughout labor and delivery. Only then did family-centered maternity care become a practical experience as well as an academic idea.

need for a coach

The practitioners of the psychoprophylactic method of prepared childbirth, in particular, have strongly advocated the active participation of the husband or of a labor coach. It has been recognized that not only does the laboring woman desperately want to help herself (which preparation provides) but also the presence of a caring person, knowledgeable in what should be done for support, has a discernibly calming effect during this time of physical and emotional stress. Although proponents of various methods of childbirth preparation suggest that the husband may be best suited for this role, room must be made for the many situations where the father is not part of the woman's current environment.

In studies of husband-coached childbirth, the couple's relationship, both as husband and wife and as parents, was found to be affected. Each spoke of the other in new appreciation; the bond seemed to be strengthened; couples had new perspectives on their marital and parental roles. These subjective findings are now gaining the attention of behavioral scientists, who are verifying in objective studies the validity of such observations.

effects of preparation

The effects of preparation for childbirth are seen during the prenatal period as both men and women acquire information, gain appreciation for each other's role, and evaluate and develop realistic goals. The anxieties of pregnancy are not limited to the woman but extend to her husband or mate, creating the *pregnant couple.* Parent education in preparation for childbirth must deal with these anxieties as well. Such preparation seeks not only to present the husband with the same factual information as his wife but also to give him a sense of importance and relevance during the birth experience. He gains an appreciation of the physical effort of birth as well as the assurance that he, too, will be prepared to function in specific and definite ways as part of the childbirth preparation team.

In the psychoprophylactic method of prepared childbirth, the woman learns how to integrate the physical, emotional, and intellectual aspects of her personality so that she can work as a harmonious and focused unit throughout the complex demands of labor. This response is in contrast to that of the unprepared woman who remains out of focus as labor approaches and who finds the physical and emotional responses in labor dominating and opposing rational thought processes.

Through disciplined learning and through the concentrated application of technique and information during labor, the prepared woman is better able to cope with the strenuous demands of labor. She controls her body and checks the inclination of "flight"; she works cooperatively *with* the process of labor, enhancing the work effort during all stages. She has learned to minimize fatigue by reducing unnecessary and distracting activity, both during contractions and in the contraction intervals. By sophisticated and conscious control of her body, she effects a significant reduction of psychic tension and its components of anxiety, fearful anticipation, and heightened perception of pain. (The need for analgesics, anesthetics, and obstetric intervention is dramatically reduced, with benefit to both mother and baby.)

During birth, the prepared woman works more efficiently and is able to cooperate. Because she has been intellectually prepared to understand the mechanism of the second stage, she can use her body more effectively, again with benefit to herself and the baby (Fig. 9-1).

Immediately after birth, the woman will be characteristically excited and pleased with her efforts. With the absence of analgesics or anesthetics, or a reduction in their use, potential aftereffects, such as alterations in vital signs, mental confusion, anxiety regarding the baby, headaches, are eliminated.

The cooperative efforts of the mother to enhance the work of labor and reduce or eliminate the use of medication and anesthetics produce important benefits to the newborn. Apgar scores are consistently good in normal infants; in low-birth-weight and defective babies, such lack of depression and improvement of oxygenation may have an important impact on their survival.

summary The total result of preparation for childbirth extends beyond the specific performance of technique during labor into an improved physical and emotional readiness for parenthood for both husband and wife and discernible benefits to the newborn.

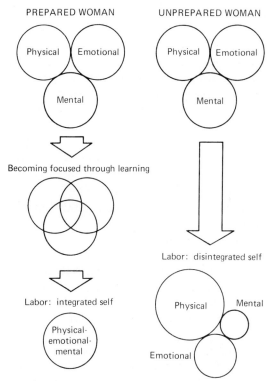

PREPARED WOMAN   UNPREPARED WOMAN

Physical Emotional   Physical Emotional

Mental   Mental

Becoming focused through learning

Labor: disintegrated self

Labor: integrated self

Physical   Mental

Physical-emotional-mental   Emotional

fig. 9-1 Results of childbirth preparation. Through preparation for childbirth, the woman learns to integrate herself physically, emotionally, and intellectually so that she remains focused and in control throughout labor. The conditioning process allows her to meet each contraction with an appropriate technique; she substitutes new, learned responses to the stimuli (contractions), which significantly reduces or eliminates pain. By contrast, the unprepared woman remains out of focus, so that her reactions disintegrate under the stress of labor. Anticipatory anxiety and the contraction itself signal "pain"; she responds with diverse and inappropriate reactions, breath holding, muscular tension, psychic tension, unnecessary activity, crying out, and loss of control. (*From Castor, "Participating in Childbirth: A Parents' Guide," 2d ed., Council of Childbirth Education Specialists, New York, 1973. By permission of the author.*)

selection of physician, clinic, and hospital

Parents-to-be should select their doctor, clinic, and hospital on the basis of their decision to be a prepared couple in the birth experience. Couples will be concerned with hospital facilities and policies. Most prepared women desire the atmosphere and milieu of a family-centered maternity care unit as a continuation of their prenatal education and labor participation. The medical community is finally responding with significant changes directly related to consumer demands.

Until recently the outlook for the clinic patient was bleak. The impersonal nature of many clinics, the staffing procedures, and other clinic policies made it difficult for the woman to be assured of a supportive situation or a sympathetic acceptance of the idea of prepared childbirth. As effective teaching practices are being perfected for the clinic situation, as clinic personnel are being educated regarding the benefits of preparation for childbirth, and as cultural differences are receiving more respect, effective classes are being formed in many clinic settings. It remains with the woman or couple to seek that clinic which provides the opportunity for sharing this experience. Word-of-mouth communication and public relations efforts will acquaint the community with the availability of these programs.

Participation in programs of preparation should not be limited to parent-initiated requests. As physicians, nurses, and hospitals become more familiar with its concepts and more comfortable with its practical implementation, all pregnant women when first entering prenatal care should be introduced to the availability of preparation and education for birth.

The couple needs to understand that many physicians and health care facilities still may not be enthusiastic proponents of husband-coached childbirth but rather will reflect a more modest acceptance and willingness to help the woman help herself within the bounds of good obstetric practice.

sources of classes for preparation

The growing interest in prepared childbirth and the concurrent trend in obstetrics toward minimal use of pharmacologic agents have created an ever-increasing demand for classes in prepared childbirth. This need is being met by expanded parent education programs of hospitals, health agencies, specialized interest groups, and private practitioners.

Parent education courses offered by health agencies and institutions have commonly been general in approach and content. The classes vary in length from three to eight sessions and may be taken at any point in pregnancy. Informal group discussions led by a resource person focus on various aspects of pregnancy (hygiene, nutrition, exercise) and a general introduction to labor, delivery, postnatal recovery, and the newborn (care, feeding). The aim has been to help parents gain an understanding of the pregnancy-birth continuum, and to understand and cope with anxiety, rather than to teach specific techniques of prepared childbirth. More of these institutional programs are now incorporating techniques for labor, often in addition to the general prenatal series. The curriculum is then expanded to include some or all of the content discussed below. Many agencies prefer to continue the general courses, which they feel meet the total community's needs, and to refer interested parents to the childbirth educator in private or group practice.

The Red Cross offers free prenatal classes and baby care classes. Taught by a registered nurse, these classes usually are attended by women during the day. Visiting nurse services may offer classes to groups of pregnant women, especially to young teenagers in community agencies. In fact, the interest level is high enough so that classes could be started in many noninstitutional sites.

Concern for quality has emerged with the sudden upsurge of interest. Several groups now prepare childbirth education specialists. (Information about further preparation can be obtained from the Maternity Center Association and Council of Childbirth Education Specialists.)

the childbirth educator

One of the most important sources for classes in specific techniques of prepared childbirth is the nurse engaged in private or group practice as a childbirth educator. As a private practitioner, the childbirth educator provides a program which incorporates current trends in technique and philosophy, whereas institutions must be responsive to more general community needs and more fixed hospital policies.

The course is more structured in format and extends for five or six weekly sessions near the end of pregnancy. The focus is on specifically preparing a couple for the work of giving birth. The program includes a presentation of the philosophy and goals of prepared childbirth, emotional and physical changes of pregnancy, detailed analysis of the stages of labor, and expectations for the immediate postpartum period. Central to the program is the learning of specific techniques and physical conditioning exercises. Parents are usually referred for baby care classes and hospital tours.

It is hoped that in future developments, complete childbirth preparation will be provided within the context of the woman's total prenatal and postnatal care, as an integral part of her physician's, hospital's, or clinic's program.

BARRIERS TO PREPARATION FOR CHILDBIRTH

When seeking the barriers to preparation for childbirth, the woman's culture, education, attitude, family, and economic status must be considered. In certain cultural groups, the lack of interest by the woman's husband or family, or their overt opposition to and degrading of her interest, is a sufficiently strong factor to deter her consideration of childbirth preparation programs *unless* such preparation is an integral part of her prenatal care, as suggested earlier. If she views her husband's active participation as essential, even though he might not oppose her interest, she is likely not to choose the course.

Other cultural, social, temperamental, or maturational factors influence the woman and her involvement. Such preparation for childbirth may violate sexual taboos, cultural expectations, or family structure. If the woman has unresolved conflicts about her sexuality, this pregnancy, and/or motherhood, the probability of her participation will be reduced.

Lack of participation may logically arise out of lack of information or misinterpretation. Although somewhat interested in the idea of learning to help herself, the woman may be unaware of the availability of classes in her community and, lacking strong motivation, fail to seek out such information.

She may be uninformed as to the basic concepts of childbirth preparation, especially if she is a member of a lower socioeconomic or a culturally deprived group. With a smattering of information, she may misinterpret the purpose and goals of these programs. These particular deterrents can be significantly modified by the accurate presentation of the purpose and availability of classes to the whole community.

Fatigue and other physical factors may seriously affect her attitude toward and her motivation in seeking out and attending classes. Intrinsic to her attitude is her self-image and her concept of the uniqueness of her role in the childbirth experience. If she lacks positive feelings about herself as a worthwhile person, as a mature individual able to cope with her life situation, she is apt not to consider this preparation. In addition, whether or not she and her husband see preparation for childbirth as a worthwhile expenditure of effort and money will influence consideration and choice of prenatal education.

During the final trimester, women typically become introspective and preoccupied with the outcome of the pregnancy. Such questions as "Will I be all right?" and "Will my baby be healthy?" typify the mother's emotional reactions. She should be considering the implications of the birth of the baby, and yet these very implications are a source of anxiety. A healthy response is to seek out sources of information, including classes in childbirth preparation.

If a woman's anxiety level is extremely high, however, she may avoid the very thing that would help her to cope—counseling and education. Nurses who are in touch with women during the third trimester need to bear in mind the dominant psychological needs of this period and take the initiative in suggesting sources of education as well as in creating a climate conducive to honest questions and counseling.

Other factors are influential in excluding participation. Classes must be made available at convenient times and locations for the couple, and the cost must be reasonable for all socieconomic groups. Childbirth educators in private or group practice must make known their willingness to accept reduced fees if low-cost programs are not otherwise available.

The attitude of the various authority figures responsible for her prenatal care cannot be overlooked. Unless a woman is highly motivated, rejection of the concepts of childbirth preparation and participation by doctor or nurse will block her from participating in a program.

In many instances, several factors are present simultaneously which effectively block preparation.

summary

We can say that classes in preparation for childbirth are becoming more widely available throughout the country. Programs are being broadened to include women and couples from low economic groups as well as the middle class.

Couples interested in active participation in the birth experience can be expected to investigate and select prenatal care and hospital on the basis of interest in and support of family-centered preparation for labor and postpartum care.

At the present time, many women and couples do not enter prenatal preparation or are excluded from participation despite its acknowledged benefits; for example, the teenager, the unmarried, those from minority groups, the immature, and the very frightened are seldom seen in class unless a special attempt is made to include them. Accurate information and an inclusion of preparation as an intrinsic part of prenatal care may serve to eliminate many of these barriers.

NURSING APPROACH IN CHILDBIRTH EDUCATION

The goals of parent education will determine the content of classes. The central goal should be the reduction of anxiety and fear through the dissemination of accurate information. The direction and depth of this information will be determined by the needs and interests of the participants. Keeping in mind the need to reduce anxiety, reinforce the normalcy of childbirth, and enhance each couple's self-esteem, the childbirth educator evaluates class objectives, content, and approach.

In presenting factual information pertaining to pregnancy, labor, and the postpartum period, the teacher directs the discussion to the needs, awareness, and intellectual capacities of the group. The content must be appropriate, relevant, and readily understood. There must be sufficient detail to give the couple an accurate and realistic picture of labor, presented in a positive manner which will enhance self-esteem and not heighten preexisting anxieties. Effective learning can then take place. Since the classes take place in the third trimester, there must be an awareness of how the concerns and anxieties of the couple are focused. Concerns about the baby's normalcy, the woman's ability to give birth safely, and the ambivalence regarding parenthood are the major focus during this period.

Childbirth educators work to create a pleasant, relaxed atmosphere, establishing themselves as concerned and knowledgeable resource persons, so that the couples can verbalize questions and underlying anxieties without fear of rejection. Thoughtful and appropriate answers must be given, which reflect awareness of the meaning of the question. Does a husband simply want a piece of information, or is he expressing a particular anxiety? In asking about medication, is the woman reflecting on her goals or her fears for herself or for her baby?

As an atmosphere of acceptance, knowledgeability, and self-awareness is established, the couple will begin to see themselves as unique and yet within the normal context of childbearing. The group experience itself assists in developing this attitude. The couple's reactions and feelings are no longer mysterious or capricious but become more manageable and understandable. Independent and self-sufficient women in particular are helped to accept their new dependency needs and vacillating energy states.

As the couple perfects various neuromuscular and respiratory skills related to childbirth, effective childbirth educators see to it that important communication skills are also established. They provide opportunities for the exploration of feelings, continually involving the husbands in nonthreatening ways. As the classes progress, the nurse-teachers underscore the validity of the man's role both in class and during the childbirth. They direct comments and questions to the husbands, asking them to solve specific labor problems. Basic to all this is the introduction of the husband's role as chief supporter—or coach—from the very first session. His role is continually built as the important caring person needed by his wife during labor. In a more general way, childbirth educators encourage a mutual respect for the specific roles of both husband and wife during the childbirth experience. They foster the concept of birth as a family experience and of the couple as an informed and cooperating team.

Through this learning experience the couple becomes independent, knowledgeable, and cooperative, and learns that it can manage a stress situation. The skills and confidence thus developed will, it is hoped, encourage the growth of the couple as a family unit, able to deal with the ongoing stresses of family life.

basic goals of childbirth education

1 Minimize anxieties, correct misconceptions, and reduce fear by providing factual information on pregnancy, labor, and the postpartum period in detail and terms suitable for pregnant couples.

2 Teach neuromuscular, motor, and respiratory skills. Proficiency in these skills will enhance the woman's response to labor and her ability to deal with it intelligently and cooperatively.

3 Provide an accurate framework of reference for the pregnant couple in which they will see their responses, concerns, anxieties, and fears appropriately.

4 Create a setting in which cooperative, independent, and knowledgeable parents can effectively utilize both verbal and nonverbal communication skills.

5 Develop a relaxed and open atmosphere conducive to learning and growing in self-awareness.

content of classes

introductory class The introductory class sets the tone of acceptance and credibility. The learning process by which the couple increases in self-awareness and ability to master the skills essential to control in labor begins. The childbirth educator excites the couple with the potential for control and comfort during labor when utilizing the techniques to be taught. The presentation is such that each couple determines its own needs and goals within the context of preparation for childbirth and begins to learn how these needs and goals will be met during the classes. It is in this session that the couple can be helped to see themselves as a pregnant couple for which certain physical and emotional reactions are entirely normal.

The teacher facilitates group interaction by making introductions using first and last names. (Couples should feel that they are all together as people about to become parents who share a mutual desire to learn how to help themselves.) Introductions should be limited to simple information: name, parity, due date, community, and hospital. Describing occupations might unnecessarily divide the group along socioeconomic lines.

General comments as to the purpose of the course are made. Realistic goals are presented and some basic concepts introduced. Parents need to understand that they will establish their own goals as the class evolves. Although couples are easily overwhelmed by a too-complex explanation of theory and methodology, a discussion of the basic principles upon which the techniques operate is important.

Since the class is still a collection of persons and not as yet a group, couples respond more readily to concrete and factual details as opposed to theoretic concepts. Using visual aids, such as the Maternity Center's *Birth Atlas* (Fig. 9-2), the childbirth educator pre-

fig. 9-2   Using visual aids, the childbirth educator discusses the birth process with the parents.

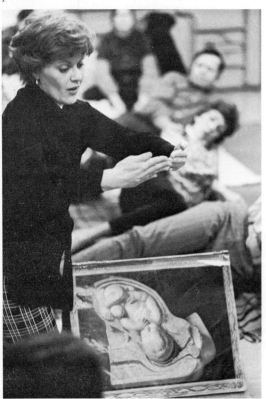

sents pertinent information on conception and the trimesters of pregnancy. By discussing this in a parallel outline of fetal development and maternal changes, the childbirth educator reinforces the reality of the baby and the understanding of self. Using words like, "Now your baby's heart can be heard," helps the couple to identify *their* baby, particularly if it is their first. Comments such as, "Many women feel very tired at this point," or, "You may have become very nervous about being home alone," not only establish the nurse's insight into pregnancy but again enhance self-awareness.

Physical conditioning exercises are appropriate to this first class (Fig. 9-3). Couples are anxious to *do* something. These exercises (described in Figs. 9-4 to 9-9) basically serve to increase the woman's sense of well-being and physical comfort during pregnancy. They are directed, not toward the development of muscular strength, but toward improvement of circulation, ventilation, body awareness, and posture.

The couple also begins the mastery of neuromuscular control and the development of teamwork. Controlled relaxation is the foundation upon which all other techniques are applied. The woman begins to develop her body awareness. She learns how to be comfortable, to detect tension in her body, and to facilitate relaxation. Her husband begins to learn to detect tension in his wife by touch and observation. Together they concentrate on achieving the active (vs. passive) relaxation necessary for control during labor. The husband is encouraged to touch and stroke his wife in ways to enhance relaxation and rest. Stroking always accompanies the verbal cue, "Relax," so that stroking itself soon becomes a signal for relaxation.

intermediate classes   Building on the information and rapport of the introductory class, the childbirth educator expands sub-

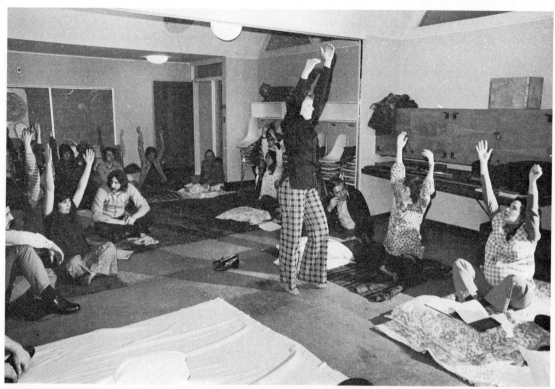

fig. 9-3 The childbirth educator starts the class with a warm-up exercise, which also helps to improve ventilation and increase the woman's sense of well-being.

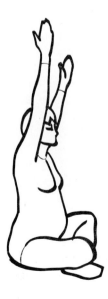

fig. 9-4 Tailor reach exercise: The woman alternately reaches (in a rhythmic pattern) with arms stretched toward the ceiling. This exercise tones both upper chest and upper back muscles, and promotes good ventilation. (*From Castor, "Participating in Childbirth: A Parents' Guide," 2d ed. Council of Childbirth Education Specialists, New York, 1973. By permission of the author.*)

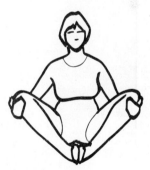

fig. 9-5 Tailor Press exercise: The woman learns to use thigh muscles to press knees toward floor, using slight resistance with hands. This exercise helps to relieve hip tension and low backache. (*From Castor, "Participating in Childbirth: A Parents' Guide," 2d ed., Council of Childbirth Education Specialists, New York, 1973. By permission of the author.*)

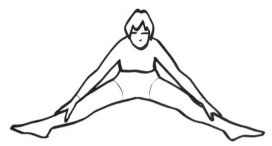

fig. 9-6 Tailor stretch exercise: Sitting up on the floor and bending from the hips, the woman stretches forward, sliding her hands toward her ankles. This exercise also relieves hip tension and low back distress. (*From Castor, "Participating in Childbirth: A Parents' Guide," 2d ed., Council of Childbirth Education Specialists, New York, 1973. By permission of the author.*)

sequent classes with a logical progression. Content is carefully structured to parallel the interest and awareness of the couple, their understanding of the mechanism of labor, and their emotional responses during labor, as well as the development of labor itself. Couples need a clear understanding of what happens, how the mother will feel and react, how she can cope with each particular phase, and how her husband can support and direct her efforts.

In teaching the second stage, for instance, the childbirth educator needs to be alert to the anxiety about and fear of giving birth. Attitudes of sexuality, fear of safety, misconceptions relating to the second stage, and

fig. 9-7 Childbirth educator demonstrates the back roll exercise, which is used as a passive pelvic tilt for pregnancy and as a preparation for the expulsive technique to be learned later on.

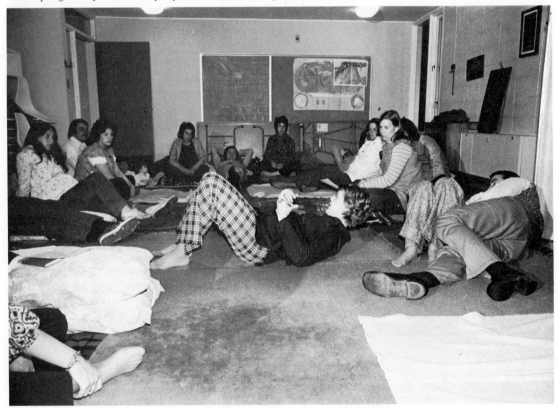

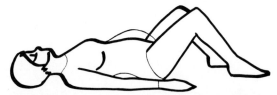

fig. 9-8 Pelvic tilt exercise: Using abdominal and buttock muscles, the woman rotates the pelvis up, pressing small of back against the floor. Knees are bent to stabilize the pelvis. This exercise relieves low backache and hip tension, as well as toning the abdominal muscles. (*From Castor, "Participating in Childbirth: A Parents' Guide," 2d ed., Council of Childbirth Education Specialists, New York, 1973. By permission of the author.*)

inaccurate information contribute to these fears of pain and injury held by both husband and wife. It is essential that the couple gain an accurate and positive understanding of the mechanism of birth and a realistic expecta-

tion about their ability to work with the birth process.

concluding class The couple's proficiency in technique and knowledge of labor must be reviewed and evaluated. One effective technique is the use of role playing in a variety of real-life situations. Their responses can be evaluated by the group to determine the most effective and appropriate approach.

The nurse can introduce material pertinent to the postpartum period. Couples need a basic awareness of the physical changes and emotional and social adjustments of the recovery period.

They also need to be prepared for the rather "unfinished" qualities of their newborn, as well as his demands and needs. The impact of the firstborn, both in terms of the mother's physical recovery and the parents' adjust-

fig. 9-9 Bent leg lift exercise: The pelvis is stabilized by bending the knees and tilting the pelvis up. The woman alternately bends each knee over the abdomen, extends the leg toward the ceiling, lowers it, and slides it along the floor to the starting position. This exercise relieves low backache and hip tension and tones the leg muscles. (*From Castor, "Participating in Childbirth: A Parents' Guide," 2d ed., Council of Childbirth Education Specialists, New York, 1973. By permission of the author.*)

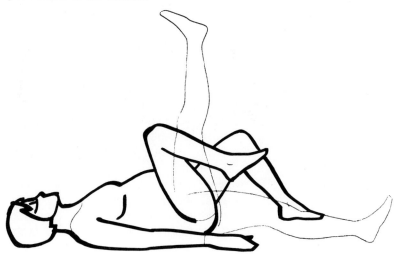

ments to being parents, must not be minimized.

First-time mothers need to be made aware that they will not suddenly be transformed into the romanticized image of motherhood but will grow into an ability to mother.

Many primigravidas are unprepared for the various aspects of physical recovery, such as lochial flow, involution, breast engorgement, fatigue, and emotional lability. A brief discussion of what to expect aids understanding of the physiology of the recovery period, as well as providing a few practical suggestions for dealing with this recuperative and restorative period.

sample class outline: psychoprophylaxis

I. Introductory class
   A. Introduce self and fellow class participants.
   B. Discuss basic purpose and goals of the course.
   C. Present information pertaining to the basic concepts of psychoprophylaxis.
   D. Discuss highlights of conception, fetal development, maternal reactions, and physical changes, using visual aids.
   E. Teach physical conditioning exercises, discussing rationale and using demonstration and group participation.
      1. Tailor press
      2. Tailor stretch
      3. Tailor reach
      4. Pelvic tilt
      5. Bent-leg lift
      6. Perineal control (Kegel exercise)
   F. Teach basics of controlled relaxation, using demonstration and group participation: (Figs. 9-10 and 9-11)
      1. Achieving comfort
      2. Facilitating relaxation

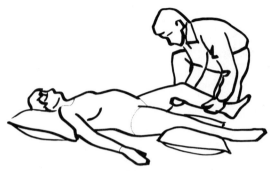

fig. 9-10 Controlled relaxation: In this neuromuscular technique, the woman learns to consciously facilitate relaxation while her husband learns how to enhance their teamwork through new verbal and nonverbal communication skills. (From Castor, "Participating in Childbirth: A Parents' Guide," 2d ed., Council of Childbirth Education Specialists, New York, 1973. By permission of the author.)

      3. Self-detection of tension and relaxation
      4. Husband/coach's detection of tension and relaxation
      5. Role of touching and stroking to enhance relaxation
      6. Use of precise verbal cues
      7. Development of gross muscular control
II. Intermediate classes (three of four)
   A. Perfect controlled relaxation technique
   B. Introduce and develop the mechanism of labor, using visual aids.
   C. Discuss related maternal reactions and emotional responses to the mechanism of labor.
   D. Teach various labor techniques in which the couple needs to become proficient, using demonstration, visual aids, and group participation:
      1. Integration of controlled relaxation
      2. Rationale for respiratory techniques (Fig. 9-12)

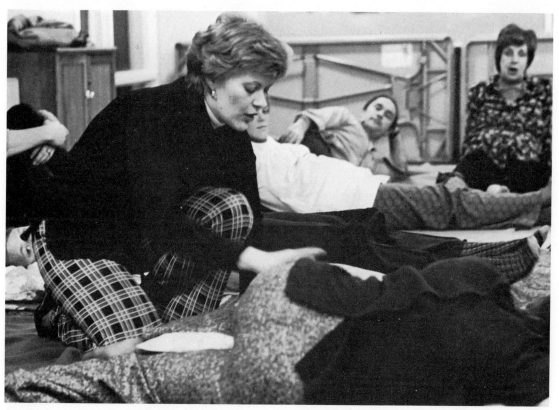

fig. 9-11 The nurse demonstrates how to encourage and facilitate relaxation.

3. Rhythmic chest breathing
   a. Slow rate
   b. Modified rate
4. Shallow chest breathing
   a. Combined with rhythmic chest breathing (modified rate)
   b. Rhythmic pattern of shallow breathing and short blows
5. Recognizing, preventing, and dealing with hyperventilation
6. Expulsion techniques
   a. Overcoming fear of pushing
   b. Integrating controlled relaxation (especially perineal)
   c. Effective use of abdominal muscles in directing pushing effort
   d. Correct position to enhance the work effort (Fig. 9-13)
   e. Respiratory patterns to enhance work effort
   f. Effective coaching in expulsion
   g. Control of pushing effort
7. Managing back labor
E. Develop the couple's confidence and self-awareness, through discussion.
F. Introduce couples to various community resources, e.g., baby care classes, visiting nurse services, family planning services.
G. Review class content through role playing, nonthreatening question periods, and class participation.
H. Acquaint couples with local hospital facilities and policies, using tours, visual aids, and discussion.

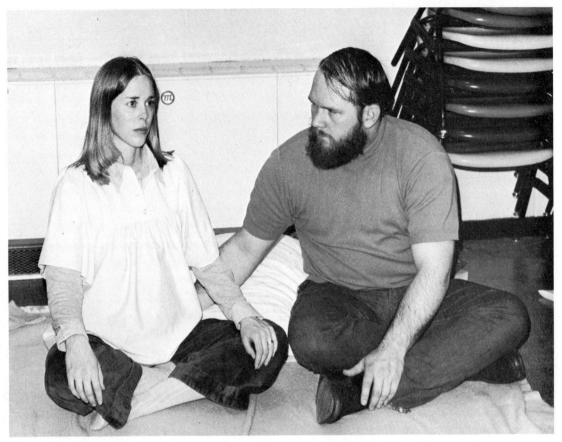

fig. 9-12 Practicing breathing technique for labor. The woman's coach is learning how to evaluate her breathing patterns and how to enhance relaxation under stress.

III. Goals and content of concluding class
   A. Complete review of mechanism of labor, maternal reactions, labor techniques, and husband's role, through discussion, role playing, and visual aids.
   B. Discuss immediate postpartum period, using group discussion:
      1. Physical recuperation
      2. Emotional responses
      3. Emotional needs
      4. Hospital facilities: recovery area, postpartum unit, nursery
   C. Discuss newborn, using group discussion.
      1. Appearance at birth
      2. Care of infant in delivery room
      3. Characteristics of newborn during first few days
      4. Need for mother's physical contact
      5. Feeding, if pertinent to class needs
   D. Discuss postpartum period at home, using group discussion:
      1. Physical changes
      2. Emotional needs and responses
      3. Simple exercises to improve muscle tone and sense of well-being
      4. Husband's needs and role

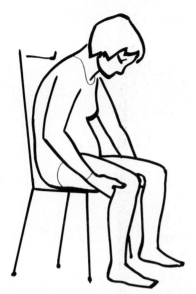

fig. 9-13 Explusive technique: The woman must learn to master her body for effective and efficient work during the second stage of labor. She learns how her position, respiratory rhythm, and voluntary muscular activity enhance the pushing effort. Her coach learns cue words to remind her of the correct technique.

By first learning the expulsion techniques when sitting in a hard chair, the woman becomes aware of how her body works while in a more comfortable position for advanced pregnancy. Once she has perfected this, she learns how to do these same actions in the more common labor position (Fig. 9-11). (*From Castor, "Participating in Childbirth: A Parents' Guide," 2d ed., Council of Childbirth Education Specialists, New York, 1973. By permission of the author.*)

study questions

1 Select three of the prenatal exercises illustrated and demonstrate them to your classmates. Integrate what you know about proper body alignment during pregnancy and the rationale for each exercise.
2 Observe a complete series of childbirth preparation classes. Compare the basic goals of childbirth education with your observations of the classes.
3 Observe a complete series of childbirth preparation classes. After each class, describe the nurse's interactions with the couples. Note the ways, both verbal and nonverbal, the teacher makes individuals com-

fortable, facilitates communication, and creates a positive learning environment.
4 Review the section, "Barriers to Preparation for Childbirth." Discuss at least three women or couples from your experience who illustrate one or more of these situations. Describe how this person was affected.

bibliography

Bing, Elisabeth: *Six Practical Lessons for an Easier Childbirth*, Bantam, New York, 1969.

Bradley, Robert A.: *Husband Coached Childbirth*, Harper & Row, New York, 1974.

Chabon, Irwin: *Awake and Aware*, Dell, New York, 1969.

Chertok, L.: *Motherhood and Personality*, Lippincott, Philadelphia, 1969.

Goodrich, F. W. Jr.: *Preparing for Childbirth*, Prentice-Hall, Englewood Cliffs, N.J., 1966.

Kitzinger, Sheila: *The Experience of Childbirth*, Penguin, Baltimore, 1972.

Lamaze, Ferdinand: *Painless Childbirth*, Simon & Schuster, New York, 1972.

Leboyer, Frederick: *Birth Without Violence*, Alfred Knopf, New York, 1975.

Melzack, R. and K. Casey: "Neutral Mechanisms of Pain: A Conceptual Model," in *New Concepts of Pain and Its Management*, Davis, Philadelphia, 1967.

Richardson, S. and A. Guttmacher: *Childbearing—Its Social and Psychological Aspects*, Williams & Wilkins, Baltimore, 1967.

Siegele, D.: "The Gate Control Theory," *American Journal of Nursing,* **74**(4):498, 1974.

Sumner, P. E., J. P. Wheeler, and S. G. Smith: "The Labor-Delivery Bed—Simplified Obstetrics," *Journal of Reproductive Medicine*, **13**(4):, 158, October, 1974.

Tanzer, D.: *Why Natural Childbirth?* Doubleday, Garden City, N.Y., 1972.

resources

TEACHER PREPARATION COURSES:
Council of Childbirth Education Specialists, 168 West 86th St., New York, N.Y. 10024 (psychoprophylaxis).
Maternity Center Association, 48 East 92 St., New York, N.Y. 10028 (psychophysical).

PARENT-LAY GROUPS:
National Association of Parents and Professionals for Safe Alternatives in Childbirth (NAPSAC) P.O. Box 1307, Chapel Hill, N.C. 27514
International Childbirth Education Association (ICEA) P.O. Box 5852 Milwaukee, Wis., 53220
American Society for Psychoprophylaxis in Obstetrics (ASPO) 1523 L St. N.W., Washington, D.C. 20005

10

THE PROCESS OF LABOR AND DELIVERY

SUSAN E. ANDERSON*

Labor is the process by which the uterus expels or attempts to expel the fetus, placenta, and amniotic sac. Labor is accomplished by the rhythmic contractions of the uterus. Pressure against the cervix created by the fetus and amniotic sac results in effacement and dilation of the cervix, which allows for passage of the fetus from the uterus, through the cervix and birth canal, and into the extrauterine environment. In order to accomplish this process, there must be an intricate interrelationship among the "powers," the "passage," and the "passenger." The powers are the uterine contractions. The passage is the bony pelvis, the cervix, the vagina, and the introitus. The passenger is the fetus and amniotic sac. Normal labor requires that the powers be sufficient to expel the fetus, that the passage be of adequate size to allow descent and expulsion of the fetus, and that the passenger

*Recognition is given to Jean C. Metzger, who was the original author of the chapter The Process of Labor in the first edition of this text.

be of average size and in a position to allow negotiation of the passage via the mechanism of labor. Each of these factors is discussed in this chapter in regard to the normal labor process.

THE POWERS

The uterus is a hollow, pear-shaped, muscular organ located in the pelvic cavity between the bladder and the rectum. The uterus is divided into two unequal parts: the *corpus,* the upper, triangular portion, and the *cervix,* the lower, cylindrical portion. The corpus is divided into the *fundus,* the convex part of the uterus above the insertion of the fallopian tubes; the *body,* the portion between the fundus and the isthmus; and the *isthmus,* the segment located just above the internal os of the cervix (Fig. 10-1).

The musculature of the uterus consists of bundles of smooth muscle united by connective tissue. During pregnancy the uterus enlarges 500 to 1000 times in capacity. Uterine enlargement during pregnancy involves both stretching and hypertrophy of muscle cells and is most marked in the fundus.

The uterus is supported by the broad ligaments, the round ligaments, and the uterosacral ligaments. The broad ligaments extend from the lateral margins of the uterus to the pelvic walls. The round ligaments are situated between the folds of the broad ligaments and extend forward and upward over the external iliac vessels, through the external abdominal ring, and along the inguinal canal to terminate in the labium majus. The uterosacral ligaments extend from the posterior and upper portion of the cervix to the sacrum.

Blood is supplied to the uterus by two main routes. Uterine arteries connect to the hypogastric arteries from the internal iliac arteries. Ovarian arteries are direct branches of the aorta. There is a progressive augmentation of blood flow to the uterus during pregnancy.

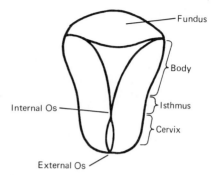

fig. 10-1 Anatomical landmarks of the uterus.

The nerve supply to the uterus is chiefly from the sympathetic nervous system, but the parasympathetic nervous system is also involved. The sympathetic fibers cause contraction and lead to vasodilation. The sympathetic fibers maintain tone, while the parasympathetic fibers effect the intermittent contractions. The nerve supply of the uterus is more regulatory than primary, allowing labor to occur even if all nerves to the uterus are severed. The eleventh and twelfth thoracic nerve roots carry sensory fibers from the uterus, transmitting the pain of uterine contractions to the central nervous system. Sensory nerves from the cervix and upper portion of the birth canal pass to the second, third, and fourth sacral nerve roots, while sensory nerves from the lower birth canal pass through the ilioinguinal and pudendal nerves. The pain of labor is caused by stretching of the cervix, contraction of the uterus, stretching of the lower uterine segment, stretching and distention of the birth canal and perineum, and tension and torsion on the ligaments supporting the uterus.

The motor fibers to the uterus originate at the seventh and eighth thoracic vertebrae. This separation of sensory and motor levels permits the use of caudal, epidural, and spinal anesthesia. See Chap. 20 for more detail on analgesia and anesthesia.

uterine contractions

Normally the uterus begins contracting effectively after 280 days of gestation (post-LMP). However, irregularities in the menstrual cycle make precise calculation of gestational age difficult, and 14 days in either direction has generally been accepted as within normal limits. The contractility of the uterus varies as pregnancy progresses (Fig. 10-2). Contractions occur infrequently throughout pregnancy. These contractions are called *Braxton-Hicks* and are usually sporadic and non-rhythmic. During the last month of gestation these Braxton-Hicks contractions increase in frequency and may occur every 10 to 20 min. They can be palpated by an observer and may be experienced as discomfort by the mother. If measured electronically they rarely exceed 20 mmHg. (See Chap. 27 for more detail on electronic monitoring.) These contraction patterns account for most cases of false labor.

The contractions of true labor provide the powers with which to efface and dilate the cervix, to expel the fetus, and to accomplish placental separation and expulsion. Uterine contractions originate in the fundus, where there is the highest concentration of muscle cells. The contraction then spreads downward

fig. 10-2   Contractions throughout pregnancy: frequency (F), duration (D), and intensity of uterine contractions in relation to uterine activity, as observed in different phases of gestation, labor, and postpartum. During gestation, uterine activity is low, less than 25 Montevideo units. (Montevideo unit = product of frequency and intensity of uterine contractions in each 10-min period.) Prelabor begins a rapid increase in myometrial contractility. The highest pressures are during the second and third stages. Within 24 h the myometrial activity declines rapidly. The initially high pressures after delivery are required for uterine hemostasis (*Redrawn from Helmuth Vorherr, in N. Assali and C. R. Brinkman (eds.), "Pathophysiology of Gestation: Maternal Disorders," Academic Press, New York, 1972, vol. 1, chap. 3.*)

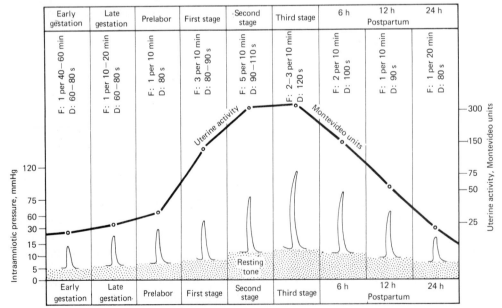

into the lower segment. As the muscle fibers shorten and thicken with each contraction the cervix is slowly and progressively drawn into the lower segment. This process is called *effacement.* The force of the contractions, along with the pressure of the presenting part and amniotic sac, causes the cervix to open or *dilate.* See Fig. 10-3*a* and *b.* Contractions can also loosen the amniotic sac from the uterus and cause spontaneous rupture of the membranes.

Each contraction is characterized by a rhythmic pattern. This pattern consists of an *increment,* increasing intensity; an *acme,* the peak; and a *decrement,* decreasing intensity (see Fig. 10-4). Between each contraction is a rest or relaxation period. This allows the fetus and uterine muscles to recover from the stress of the contraction. Contraction patterns that do not have an interval of relaxation between contractions are pathological and require immediate medical intervention. Contractions can be monitored by palpation of the fundus by the observer, by electronic monitoring, and by visually observing the

change in uterine contour as contractions occur (see Fig. 10-5).

initiation of labor

Initiation of contractions at the time of fetal maturity is a topic of much discussion and research. Several theories have been proposed regarding the initiation of labor. These theories generally have two foci. One focus is on the stretching of the uterus and is the basis for early onset of labor in multiple gestations and polyhydramnios. The other, more popular focus is on hormonal stimulation of the uterine muscle. This has been the basis of theories proposing that the onset of labor is caused by increasing estrogen, decreasing progesterone, or increased levels of prostaglandins.

The latest research by Liggins supports a theory favoring a local mechanism involving the fetal membranes and deciduum that controls prostaglandin release. This theory proposes that the onset of labor is mainly the

fig. 10-3 Degrees of effacement and dilation. (*a*) Primigravida. (*b*) Multigravida. (*Courtesy of Ross Laboratories, from "Phenomena of Normal Labor."*)

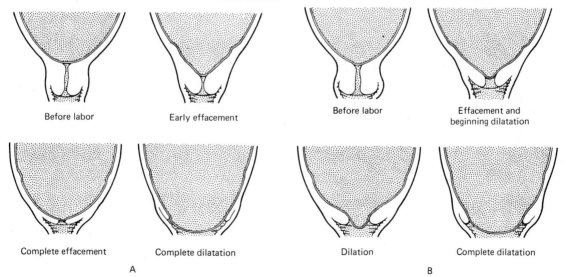

| Before labor | Early effacement | | Before labor | Effacement and beginning dilatation |

| Complete effacement | Complete dilatation | | Dilation | Complete dilatation |

A   B

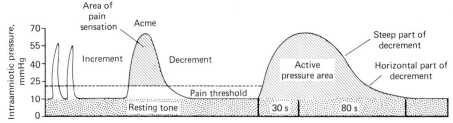

fig. 10-4 Intensity, shape, duration, active pressure area, and area of pain sensation of uterine contractions. The contraction is a bell-shaped curve, with a steeper slope during increment. The relaxation phase (decrement) lasts for two-thirds of a contraction. The resting tone (lowest intraamniotic pressure between contractions) amounts to 10 mmHg and is considered as the active pressure area. The pain threshold is the intrauterine pressure above which a contraction is painful—about 10 to 15 mmHg over resting tone. (*Redrawn from Helmuth Vorherr, in N. Assali and C. R. Brinkman. (eds.), "Pathophysiology of Gestation: Maternal Disorders," Academic Press, New York, 1972, vol. 1, chap. 3.*)

outcome of a genetically determined maturational event in the amnion and/or chorion. Fetal and maternal hormones may modulate, but rarely control the time of birth.[1]

THE PASSAGE

The pelvis is the bony ring through which the body weight is distributed to the lower extremities. It consists of four bones: the sacrum, the coccyx, and the two innominate bones. These bones are joined together by four joints: the sacrococcygeal, which joins the sacrum and coccyx; and the symphysis pubis, which joins the two innominate bones (see Fig. 10-

6). During pregnancy these joints are relaxed by a hormone called relaxin.

The pelvis is divided into the true and false pelvis at the linea terminalis (see Fig. 10-7). The false pelvis is of no obstetric significance and varies considerably in different women. The true pelvis provides the bony passageway. For a normal delivery this passage must be of adequate size and shape to allow delivery of an average-size fetus. Pelves are classified according to the shape of the inlet (see Fig. 10-8). The typical female pelvis is gynecoid. The inlet is almost round, with the transverse diameter being slightly greater than the anterior posterior diameter (see Fig. 10-9).

fig. 10-5 Change in abdominal contour as contraction occurs. Dotted line indicates contraction.

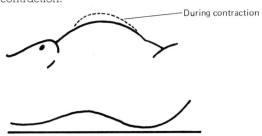

fig. 10-6 Anatomical structures of the bony pelvis.

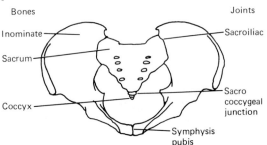

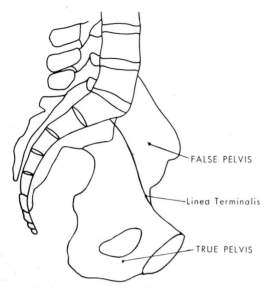

fig. 10-7 True pelvis and "false pelvis," divided by the linea terminalis. (*Courtesy of Ross Laboratories. Clinical Education Aid No. 18.*)

The pelvis is theoretically divided into four planes: the pelvic plane of inlet, the pelvic plane of outlet, the plane of greatest pelvic dimension, and the midpelvic plane.

1 The pelvic inlet is assessed by three measurements: the diagonal conjugate, the obstetric conjugate, and the conjugate vera (see Fig. 10-10). The diagonal conjugate is the most significant pelvic measurement. It measures the distance from the lower margin of the symphysis pubis to the sacral promontory. This can be measured on the vaginal exam by placing the tip of the middle finger on the sacral promontory and then marking where the symphysis pubis touches the index finger. If the measurement is 11.5 cm or greater, the pelvic inlet is of adequate size. The conjugate vera and obstetrical conjugate

fig. 10-8 Types of pelves. (*a*) Platypelloid. (*b*) Android. (*c*) Gynecoid. (*d*) Anthropoid. (*Redrawn from Ullery and Castallo, "Obstetric Mechanisms and Their Management," Davis, Philadelphia, 1957, p. 39.*)

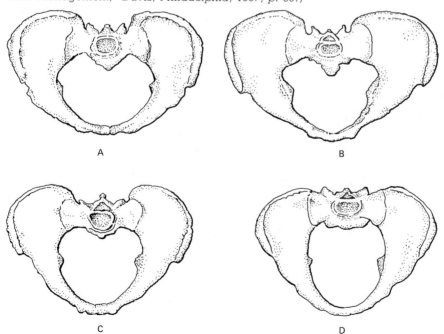

A

B

C

D

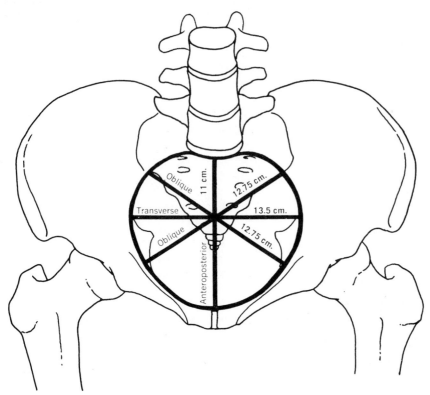

Oblique 11 cm.

12.75 cm.

Transverse 13.5 cm.

Oblique 12.75 cm.

Anteroposterior

fig. 10-9 The pelvic inlet, bounded by the linea terminalis. (*Courtesy of Ross Laboratories, Clinical Education Aid No. 18.*)

can be approximated by subtracting 1.5 to 2 cm from the diagonal conjugate.[2]

2 The pelvic outlet is assessed by measurement of the transverse diameter, which is the distance between the ischial tuberosities; a measurement of 8 cm or greater is considered adequate.[3] This diameter can be assessed using a Thom's pelvimeter or a closed fist.

3 The plane of greatest pelvic dimensions extends from the middle of the posterior surface of the symphysis pubis to the junction of the second and third sacral vertebrae (see Fig. 10-10). This plane is of no obstetrical significance.

4 The midpelvic plane can be assessed only by roentgenograms. Inadequacies in this plane may be suspected if the ischial spines are prominent, if the pelvic side walls are convergent, or if the concavity of the sacrum is shallow.

The pelvis should also be assessed for the following characteristics. The pubic arch must allow passage of the fetal head as it extends during the birth process. The angle of the arch should be 90° or greater.

The ischial spines are evaluated for prominence. The sacrum and coccyx can be palpated by the examining fingers. The coccyx should be freely movable. The anterior surface of the sacrum is assessed for its curvature. The length of sacrospinous ligaments can be estimated by placing one finger on the ischial spine and the other on the sacrococcygeal platform.[4]

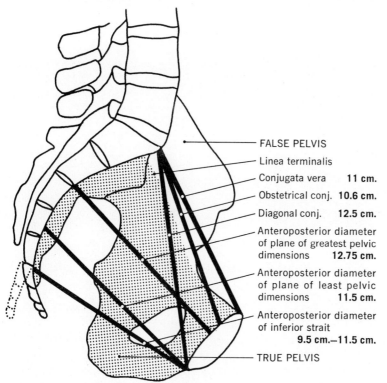

FALSE PELVIS
Linea terminalis
Conjugata vera   **11 cm.**
Obstetrical conj. **10.6 cm.**
Diagonal conj.   **12.5 cm.**
Anteroposterior diameter
of plane of greatest pelvic
dimensions   **12.75 cm.**
Anteroposterior diameter
of plane of least pelvic
dimensions   **11.5 cm.**
Anteroposterior diameter
of inferior strait
9.5 cm.—11.5 cm.
TRUE PELVIS

fig. 10-10 Diameters of the pelvic planes. (*Courtesy of Ross Laboratories, Clinical Education Aid No. 18.*)

X-ray pelvimetry can be useful in determining the size and shape of the bony pelvis, but several other factors must be taken into consideration when assessing the adequacy of the pelvis. These factors are the progress of labor, force of contractions, moldability of the fetal head, presentation, position, and size of the fetal head.[5] With the growing concern regarding radiation exposure, however, ultrasound is being used more often as a means of assessing fetal size and position.

THE PASSENGER

In order to negotiate the maternal passageway, the fetus must fit through the bony pelvis.

The methods by which the fetus is able to accommodate are termed the feto-pelvic relationship. The fetal head is the largest, least compressible, and most common presentation. The fetal head consists of seven bony plates separated by suture lines (see Fig. 10-11). Since these bony plates are poorly ossified, they can be readily compressed, resulting in an overlapping of the bony plates, called *molding*. Molding allows the fetal head to adapt to the shape of the bony pelvis. The head assumes its normal shape 2 to 3 days after delivery (see Plate D. and Fig. 14.8).

The presenting diameter of the fetal head will vary greatly depending on the degree of flexion or extension. Ideally, the head should be flexed so that the smallest diameter, the suboccipitobregmatic, is presenting.

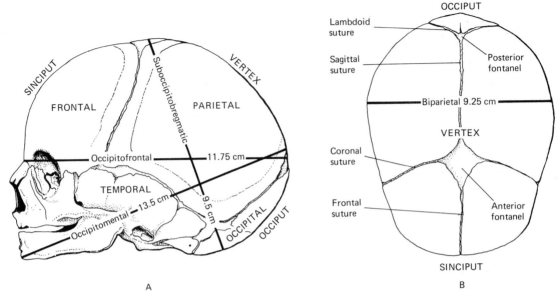

fig. 10-11 (a) side view of the fetal skull. (b) Vertex view of the skull. (*Courtesy of Ross Laboratories, from "Phenomena of Normal Labor."*)

lie

Lie refers to the relationship of the long axis of the fetus to the long axis of the mother. Well into the third trimester the fetus has ample room and may still be found in a variety of positions in the course of a week. During the last few weeks of gestation as the fetus approaches maximum size and the amount of amniotic fluid decreases, the lie becomes relatively stabilized. In 99 percent of pregnancies at term the fetus exhibits a longitudinal lie. A transverse lie is abnormal and is usually cause for operative delivery.

attitude

Attitude refers to the position of the parts of the body of the fetus in relation to itself. Most commonly the fetus assumes what has come to be called "fetal position," with back curved, head flexed, and knees flexed, with thighs resting on abdomen and lower legs across the abdomen. Arms are at sides or are flexed and crossing over the chest.

presentation

Presentation refers to that portion of the fetus presenting in the pelvic inlet. There are three major presentations: cephalic, breech, and shoulder. The incidence of these presentations is 95 percent cephalic, 3.5 percent breech, and 0.5 percent shoulder. The presentation determines the *presenting part,* which is that part of the fetus closest to the cervix and is the part that can be felt by the examining finger in the vagina.

position

Position refers to the relationship between a point of reference on the presenting part and the four quadrants of the maternal pelvis. The point of reference in a cephalic presentation is the occiput; in a face presentation, the chin

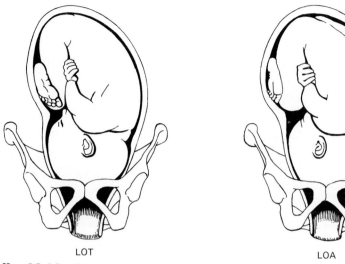

fig. 10-12 Positions assumed during internal rotation. (*Courtesy of Ross Laboratories, Clinical Education Aid No. 18.*)

(mentum); and in a breech presentation, the sacrum. Most commonly at engagement the fetus is in the LOT position (left occiput transverse) and changes to LOA (left occiput anterior) as it descends. This means that the occiput of the fetus is directed toward the left abdominal surface as the fetus descends through the birth canal (Fig. 10-12 and 10-13).

Fetal position and presentation can be assessed by abdominal palpation, vaginal examination, roentgenography, and ultrasound. Abdominal palpation is performed by using Leopold's maneuver. Upon vaginal examination the fontanels and suture lines can be palpated to determine the position of the fetus. (Fig. 10-14). If vaginal examination and abdominal palpation are inconclusive, x-ray or ultrasound may be used to give precise fetal position and presentation.

station

Station refers to the level of the presenting part in the pelvic midplane (Fig. 10-15). When the presenting part is at the level of the ischial spines it is said to be at a zero station. Levels above the spines are designated by negative values, −1, −2, −3. Levels below the spines are designated by positive values, +1, +2, +3, +4, down to the pelvic floor.

THE MECHANISM OF LABOR

In order to negotiate the bony pelvis the fetus must go through certain maneuvers. These

fig. 10-13 Position of suture lines and fontanels in LOA position.

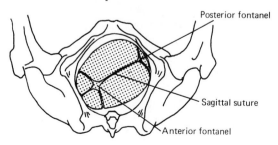

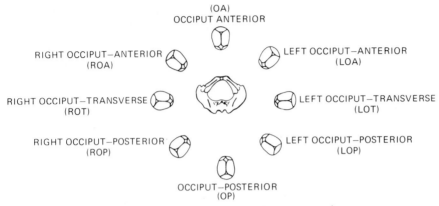

fig. 10-14 Positions of the fetal head. *(From Romney et al., Gynecology and Obstetrics: the Health Care of Women, McGraw-Hill, New York, 1975.)*

maneuvers are referred to as the mechanism of labor or the cardinal movements. The mechanism of labor for an LOA position is described in Fig. 10-16.

A   Head at entrance to the true pelvis, partially engaged.

B   The presenting part is *engaged* and *descending* into the midpelvis transversely to accommodate the largest diameter of the pelvis. As the head descends, it *flexes*, probably as a result of the resistance encountered.

C and D   *Internal rotation* occurs when the

fig. 10-15 Station in relation to descent of the fetal head. *(Courtesy of Ross Laboratories, from "Phenomena of Normal Labor.")*

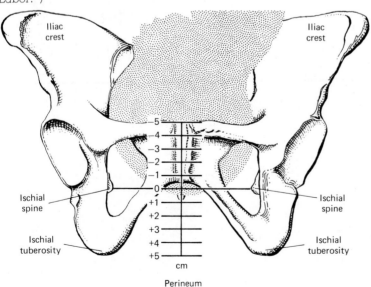

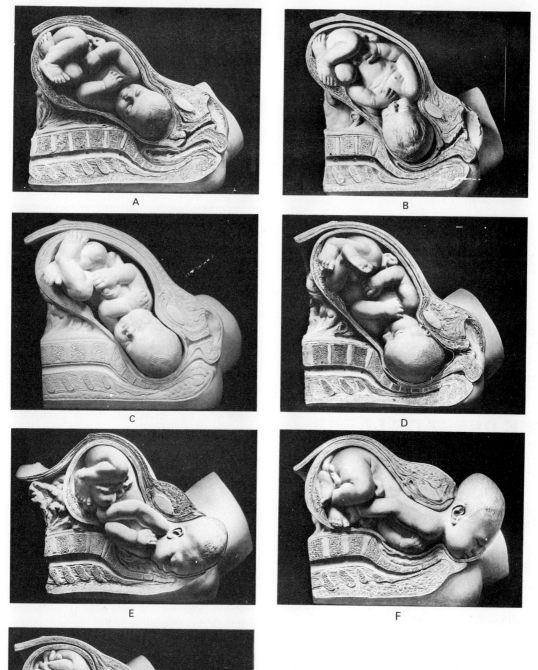

fig. 10-16 Mechanisms of labor in the vertex position (LOA). (*a*) Head at the entrance to the true pelvis. (*b*) Engagement and flexion completed. (*c* and *d*) Internal rotation in progress. (*e*) Crowning. (*f*) Extension completed. (*g*) External rotation and beginning delivery of shoulders. (*Reproduced with permission from "A Baby is Born," Maternity Center Association, New York, 1964.*)

head reaches the pelvic floor. The fetal head must rotate to accommodate the larger anteroposterior diameter of the pelvic outlet.

E   The head crowns as it presents at the introitus.

F   *Extension* allows the head to negotiate the pelvic arch. Completion of extension results in delivery of the head.

G   *External rotation* involves two movements. After the head is born, it turns to realign itself with the shoulders, which are in the transverse diameter of the pelvic inlet. The second movement involves the rotation of the shoulders to the anterior posterior diameter of the pelvic outlet.

Expulsion or birth of the baby occurs as the anterior shoulder slips under the symphysis. The posterior shoulder and remainder of the body follow easily.

THE ONSET OF LABOR

The onset of labor is usually equated with onset of regular contractions as experienced by the mother. Evaluations in the last weeks show that some effacement and dilation of the cervix have taken place before labor. In fact, some patients, unaware of contractions, may report for a routine appointment and be found to have an almost fully effaced and partly dilated cervix.

One study showed the average dilation of nulliparas to be 1.8 cm and of multiparas 2.2 cm when they were examined within 3 days of delivery. Nulliparas came into labor with an average effacement of 70 percent, multiparas with 61 percent. Very few patients come into labor without some dilation. Those who have not dilated adequately are considered to have a potential labor problem.

Readiness for labor is the key factor in how long the body will take to accomplish the work of the first stage. Some of the work of getting ready for labor evidences itself with characteristic signs.

signs of approaching labor

1   Strong *Braxton-Hicks contractions* may persist for several hours at a time with a fair degree of regularity. The contractions may sometimes be recognized in that they tend to be low in the pelvis or groin rather than in the back or over the fundus, and they may be relieved, rather than aggravated, by walking.

2   *Lightening* usually occurs in the nullipara approximately 10 to 14 days before onset of active labor. This settling of the fetus into the pelvic cavity is characterized by relief from pressure in the upper part of the abdomen and by renewed pressure on the pelvic organs, with increased urinary frequency as one symptom. This descent usually does not occur in the multipara until after the onset of active labor.

3   The *mucous plug* (cervical secretions), which has acted as a safeguard against ascending infection during pregnancy, is usually expelled shortly before or at the time of labor. This is called *show* when it becomes mixed with the blood from small breaks in cervical capillaries as a result of dilating activity.

4   Although the earliest indication of labor for a primigravida may be lightening, other women experience increasing pressure sensations throughout the pelvic area. Multiparas particularly complain of perineal or groin pressure. Loss of weight and varying energy levels are particularly apparent just prior to labor.

stages of labor

Classically, labor has been divided into three (or four) stages.

First stage—from onset of labor to full effacement and dilatation of the cervix

Second stage—from full dilatation through descent and birth of the baby

Third stage—from birth of the baby through delivery of the placenta

A fourth stage is sometimes defined as the period of recovery—1 to 2 h following delivery of the placenta.

first stage The first stage is divided into latent and active phases. The latent phase technically extends from the beginning of effacement (long before labor becomes evident) to approximately 4-cm dilatation of the cervix. Various terms are used to describe divisions of the latent phase—*prodromal* and *early* are used in this text. The *active phase* describes active dilation of the cervix from 4 to 10 cm. This phase is divided into the accelerated period and the transition period by one method, or the acceleration phase and phase of maximum slope by another method.

In addition, Friedman has redefined the phases of labor by functional divisions to describe the dilatational phase and the pelvic phase[6] (Fig. 10-17).

Preparatory phase
    = latent and accelerated phases
Dilatational phase
        = phase of maximum slope
Pelvic phase
    = rim of cervix (9 cm) through birth

ASSESSMENT OF PROGRESS   Progress of effacement, dilation, and descent can be determined only by internal vaginal examination. (Rectal examinations can be done but are less accurate and are more likely to cause infection.) These determinations should be made as often as needed to keep aware of progress, but not *more* often than needed. It is most important to maintain strict asepsis to avoid introduction of bacteria into the birth

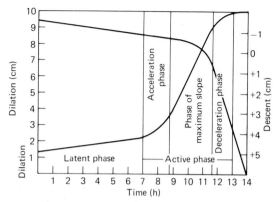

fig. 10-17   Normal labor curve, with functional divisions. (*From Friedman, "Normal Labor Curve," Clinical Obstretrics and Gynecology, 16(1) 176, 1973.)*

canal. Sterile gloves are used, and pouring antiseptic solution, such as Zephiran Chloride, over the glove for lubrication is routine procedure. With the patient in the dorsal recumbent position in the labor bed, the examiner separates the labia widely before introducing the first two fingers, in order to avoid contaminating the gloves. Some labor room policies require the wearing of a mask by the examiner, and cleansing of the whole perineum prior to examination.

In assessing the progress of dilation, use of *centimeters per hour,* rather than total number of hours, makes possible early recognition of a labor problem. Friedman gives the time for the latent phase (prodromal and early) for the nullipara as an average of 8.6 h, but not more than 20, and for the multipara an average of 5.3 h, but not more than 14. During active dilation the pattern for the nullipara averages 3 cm/h and at least 1.2 cm, while that for the multipara averages 5.7 cm/h, rarely less than 1.5 cm.

When the cervix is almost completely dilated, the patient may experience an increase in pain and frustration. There may be an increase in bloody show, caused by small fissures in the cervical rim as it completes dilation and the final stretching around the presenting part. Shortly, the characteristic grunt is heard as the pressure of the presenting part on the pelvic muscles and rectum stimulates a reflex expulsive response. Strong abdominal and diaphragmatic muscles are brought involuntarily into action to move the fetus through the remainder of the birth canal.

The contractions are now expelling the fetus from the uterus, which gradually decreases in length, becoming thicker in the fundus. As the uterus contracts, the supporting round and uterosacral ligaments pull the fundus forward and the cervix back, so that the fetus is directed behind the pubis and into the sacral curve.

It is important to remember that descent does not *begin* at this time—the fetus has been descending slowly and progressively since it became engaged.

rupture of membranes Membranes will usually rupture toward the end of the first stage if they have not done so previously. If the break is high, there may be only a trickle of fluid, and this only during a contraction. If there is a question as to whether or not membranes have ruptured prior to or after admission, *nitrazine paper* will give a neutral or alkaline reaction in the presence of amniotic fluid in a usually acid vagina. A microscopic test can be performed by making a smear of fluid and observing for ferning.

Whenever the membranes rupture, it is important to check the fetal heart beat. If the rupture is accompanied by a gush of fluid, the umbilical cord may be washed downward, and be compressed between the presenting part and the cervix. If membranes are ruptured artifically (ARM) by the physician, the FHT (fetal heart tone) should be checked before and after the procedure.

fetal response to labor The fetus is passive in the birth process and is wholly dependent on its environment for survival.

The stresses of the labor and delivery, in themselves, may leave the infant poorly equipped for the major adjustments which must be made in the first few minutes following birth. If the labor process is overlong, if the contractions are long and intense, and particularly if intervals between contractions do not allow for full circulatory recovery, problems may be expected.[7]

Prolonged bradycardia is associated with acidosis, which decreases responsiveness to resuscitative measures. Infants who are depressed from analgesic or anesthetic drugs which have crossed the placental barrier tend to have lower cord blood oxygen levels, to be more acidotic, and to respond more slowly, either independently or with resuscitation.[8] Choice of drugs, as well as timing and dosage of these agents, is therefore of extreme importance.

It has been possible to observe the fetal response to the labor process both electronically and by auscultation, the former process being more accurate and reliable. Such observation is usually coordinated with the measurement of contractions previously discussed, so that the relationship can be readily seen (see Chap. 27 for details).

If electronic recording equipment is not available, auscultation of the fetal heart must be carried out to evaluate the status of the fetus. The frequency for taking the FHT is determined by the findings, but should not be less than every 10 to 15 min in the active phase of the first stage nor less than every 5 min in the second stage. The monitor recording should be checked at the same intervals.

Indications in the mother for immediate readings and close follow-up would include:

1 Rupture of membranes
2 Anything which might reduce maternal blood pressure and therefore diminish blood supply to the fetus via placental circulation. The latter might include a drug reaction, reaction to conduction anes-

thesia, hypertonic contractions, supine hypotension, or hemorrhage.

While the specific underlying problem is being remedied, oxygen administered to the mother as a supportive measure will help to prevent oxygen deprivation to the fetus (see Acute Fetal Distress, Chap. 27).

The fetal heart is best heard through the upper part of the back of the fetus. Thus, if the fetus is in the LOA position, the FHT will be heard best to the left and slightly below the level of the umbilicus early in the first stage, and correspondingly lower as the baby descends.

Auscultation can be done with an ordinary stethoscope but it is easier to hear the rhythm with equipment which amplifies the heart sounds. Gentle pressure must be put on the area, sufficient to overcome the distance created by adipose and other intervening maternal tissue. The fetoscope adds bone conduction vibrations to those heard. The Doptone and other similar devices magnify and broadcast the sounds (Fig. 10-18).

It is difficult to hear the FHT during a strong contraction, but it is important to get a 30-s reading during the decrement, and another 1 min later for comparison, when electronic monitoring is not available.

Patterns are more meaningful than an isolated reading. Using graph paper to record would help in seeing both patterns and their relationship to contractions.

When describing the FHT, the base-line level of the heart rate should be termed as follows:[8]

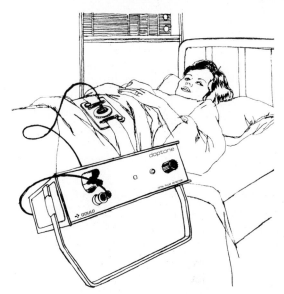

fig. 10-18 Doptone for fetal heart monitoring. *(Courtesy of Gould, Inc.)*

	Beats per minute
Marked tachycardia	Above 180
Moderate tachycardia	161–180
Normal range	120–160
Moderate bradycardia	100–119
Marked bradycardia	100 and below

Many normal labors are not being monitored routinely at the present time; however, the trend is toward increasing use of monitoring equipment. It is considered advantageous for evaluation purposes, especially during active dilation and descent.

second stage The major function of the second stage of labor is *descent*. To accomplish this, the resistance of the vaginal canal, the muscles and fascia of the pelvic floor, plus the superficial muscles, fascia, and connective tissue of the vulva and perineum, must be overcome. The patient must add her voluntary expulsive efforts during contractions to achieve the pressure needed for this process.

With these forces functioning adequately, the descent of the fetus should be constant and continuous, the rate of progress dependent upon the resistance met. Friedman has defined normal limits of descent as a guide to aid in recognizing problems early. The guide is for normal presentations, uncomplicated by any malposition or other known problems. For the nullipara whose birth canal has not been previously distended, the fetus can be expected to descend at least 1.5 cm/

h, descending in most cases at 3 cm/h. In the multipara the fetus can be expected to progress faster than 2.1 cm/h, most often at about 5 cm.[9]

The pelvic floor, made up chiefly of the levator ani muscles and their fasciae, must be displaced downward and outward by the fetal head. The resistance is variable and can be evaluated on internal manual examination.

The folds of the vagina stretch to form a lining membrane for the canal. The fascial layers are thinned as they stretch, making them and the vagina susceptible to tears.

During contractions the perineum will be seen to bulge progressively. Fecal particles may be passed because of pressure on the rectum. The anus opens, and hemorrhoids, if present, swell. Gradually the labia separate, the slit becoming progressively larger until the fetal scalp is seen. Between contractions the head is forced back by the elasticity of the muscles of the pelvic floor. After a few contractions the labia have flattened with distension, and the head maintains the perineal opening during the relaxation phase. This is called *crowning* (Fig. 10-16e).*

The skin over the perineum glistens as it is stretched to its limit. If there is adequate elasticity, the occiput will progress, with the head in flexion, until the largest area is encircled. The occiput emerges and then the face and chin slip out over the perineum by extension of the head.

The delivery of the head should not be hurried. If progress seems too fast, either for adequate stretching of the perineum, or to avoid rapid decompression of the head, the mother can be coached to pant rather than push during the contractions. The doctor may then ask her to exert some pressure *between* contractions so as to ease the head out under better control. *Forcible* pressure must never

*Another definition of *crowning* will also be found—that of the largest circumference of the presenting part being encircled by the vulva.

be put on the head to restrain its progress. If there is question that the perineum may tear, or if the pressure and time required for adequate perineal stretching are causing fetal distress, the physician will perform an *episiotomy*. Following this, the head slips out easily.

As soon as the head is born, the nose and mouth are cleared of mucus and amniotic fluid to prevent their aspiration when the infant first breathes. The physician feels for the cord. If it is wrapped around the neck, he attempts to slip it over the head. If the length is inadequate, the cord is clamped and cut. Usually the anterior shoulder advances to the pubic arch, which acts as a pivot. The posterior shoulder moves forward over the perineum, allowing the anterior shoulder to be carefully delivered first. Then, while watching the perineum carefully and applying steadying pressure, the posterior shoulder is delivered. The rest of the body slips out easily.

There are differences of opinion regarding whether the cord should be cut before or after draining the residual volume of placental blood to the fetus. The prevailing opinion is that this extra blood increases the likelihood of *hyperbilirubinemia* in the neonatal period.

third stage Immediately after the birth of the infant, there may be a slight flow of blood until the uterus contracts firmly around the placenta. Close observation is maintained to see that it remains well contracted. With the contraction, the site of placental attachment becomes smaller than the placenta itself. In most instances, by 1 to 5 min several indications that the placenta has separated and moved into the lower segment and vagina will be noted:

1 The uterus becomes smaller and spherical.
2 There is a slight gush of blood from the vagina.
3 The umbilical cord lengthens by several inches.

4 The uterus may rise in the abdomen because the separated placenta displaces it upward.

If the patient is awake, the physician will probably ask her to bear down to deliver the placenta (Fig. 10-19). If she is anesthetized, fundal pressure may be exerted after ascertaining firm uterine contraction, but this must be done with great care. The placenta must be inspected to be certain that it is complete, i.e., that no parts have been left in the mother.

In some instances, separation may take somewhat longer. At no time may traction be put on the cord or membranes when still attached, as they may tear, leaving fragments attached to the uterus, or worse, traction could cause inversion of the uterus.

If there is delay in separation of the entire placenta, resulting in considerable bleeding, or if the placenta is found to be incomplete, the placenta or what is left of it must be removed manually. Many physicians are doing this procedure routinely to shorten the third stage and therefore minimize bleeding. Obviously this must be done with care and with meticulous asepsis. The patient *must be* anesthetized; then the cervix and vagina must be carefully inspected so that they can be repaired if necessary and blood loss prevented.

The first hour following delivery is a critical

fig. 10-19   Birth of the placenta. (*Reproduced with permission from "A Baby is Born," Maternity Center Association, New York, 1964.*)

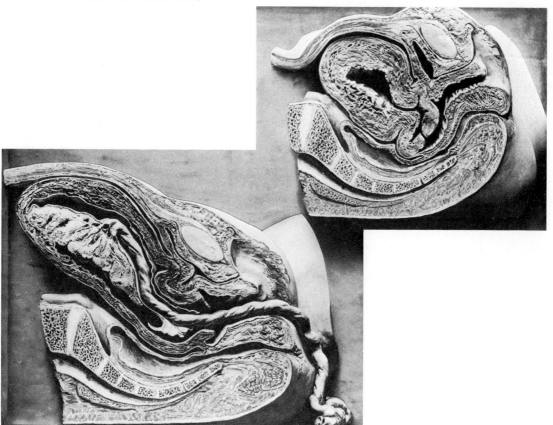

period for the mother. The blood vessels and myometrium are intertwined in such a way that natural ligatures are created when the uterus is contracted. Careful and frequent observations must be made to see that firm contraction is maintained until clotting can take place.

Nursing care of the laboring mother is discussed in Chap. 11. Complications of labor and delivery are discussed in Chap. 26.

study questions

1 By abdominal palpation you find that the fetus is in LOA position. Describe your findings as you perform Leopolds maneuver.
2 Amy has been admitted to the labor room but is not sure she is really in labor. How would you differentiate between true and false labor?
3 List three signs indicating the onset of labor.
4 In order to negotiate the bony pelvis, the fetus must perform the seven cardinal movements that make up the mechanism of labor. Describe each of the movements, the pelvic plane involved, and the critical pelvic diameter.
5 Describe the first stage of labor according to the following criteria: divisions of first stage, expected dilation, and time parameters.

references

1 G. C. Liggins, C. S. Forster, S. Grieves, and A. L. Schwartz, "Control of Parturition," *Biology of Reproduction*, **16**(1): 39, February 1977.
2 Louis Hellman, Jack Pritchard, and Ralph Wynn, *William's Obstetrics*, 14th ed., Appleton-Century-Crofts, New York, 1971, p. 301.
3 Ibid., p. 305.
4 C. M. Steer, *Moloy's Evaluation of the Pelvis in Obstetrics*, 2nd ed., Saunders, Philadelphia, 1959, p. 54.
5 M. S. Cooperstein, "The Use of Pelvicephalography of the Unengaged Head in the Nullipara with Cephalic Presentation at Term: Prepartum vs. Intra-partum Studies," *Journal of the American Osteopath Association*, **76**: 683, May 1977.
6 Emanuel Friedman and Marlene Sachtleben, "Station of the Fetal Presenting Part. IV: Slope of Descent," *American Journal of Obstetrics and Gynecology*, **107**(15): 1032, 1970.
7 Mario Zilanti, Carlos Segura, et al., "Studies in Fetal Bradycardia During the Birth Process, II," *Obstetrics and Gynecology*, **42**:842, 1973.
8 Edward H. Hon, *An Introduction to Fetal Heart Monitoring*, Corometrics Medical Systems, Wallingford, Conn., 1973, p. 52.
9 Friedman, op. cit., p. 1034.

bibliography

Anderson, S. F.: "Childbirth as a Pathological Process: An American Perspective," *American Journal of Maternal Child Nursing*, **2**(4):240, July 1977.

Friedman, E.: *Labor: Clinical Evaluation and Management*, Appleton-Century-Crofts, New York, 1967.

———: "The Functional Divisions of Labor," *American Journal of Obstetrics and Gynecology*, **109**:274, 1971.

"Intrapartum Evaluation of the Fetus," *Journal of Obstetric, Gynecologic, and Neonatal Nursing*, vol. 5, no. 5, Suppl., September-October 1976.

Oxhorne, H. and W. R. Foote: *Human Labor and Birth*, Appleton-Century-Crofts, New York, 1968.

Smith, B. A., R. M. Priore, and M. K. Stern: "The Transition Phase of Labor," *American Journal of Nursing*, **73**:488, 1973.

11

NURSING DURING LABOR AND DELIVERY

CONSTANCE R. CASTOR

Labor is work and progress. It is the work of regular uterine contractions which results in progressive cervical changes and culminates in the birth of a baby and the expulsion of placenta and membranes. This work requires the integration of both physical and mental effort and total concentration if the woman desires to be an active participant during labor. The following discussion is oriented to the psychoprophylactic method of childbirth preparation but includes comments about adaptation of care for the nonprepared woman.

SIGNS OF LABOR

The preparation for this work is an ongoing process throughout pregnancy which accelerates during the final weeks. The uterus has accommodated the growing fetus by the elongation and hypertrophy of its muscle fibers as well as the formation of a few new fibers.

There is simultaneous development of a network of *fibroelastic tissue,* permitting a significant increase in strength and elasticity, imperative to the accomplishment of labor.

cervical changes

The softening of cervical consistency noted earlier in pregnancy becomes more pronounced in the last few weeks of pregnancy, in response to hormonal influence. The cervix is said to *ripen.* The degree and timing of this softening may vary for each woman, but the cervix will be "ripe" within the week of delivery.

During the entire pregnancy the vagina has been prepared for the stretching process by forming extra blood vessels, increasing secretory action, and developing increased elasticity. There is a generalized relaxation of the tissue, and a deepening of the vaginal folds.

metabolic changes

Metabolic changes characteristic of the latter part of pregnancy may produce varying energy states which alternately result in a sense of increased work capacity (energy spurt) and increased fatigue. The woman's metabolism increases to facilitate the work of labor and may result in weight loss of several pounds in the two final weeks.

During antepartal education, women learn to recognize this possibility and pace their activities, trying not to deplete energy stores and resting as the body demands. It is not unusual for women to undertake ambitious projects, only to be frustrated by quickly fading energy. They might also experience a *nesting* impulse to get things in order for the baby. The urgency of this impulse is not always understood by husbands and families.

Although the first indication of labor for a primigravida may be *lightening,* other women may experience increasing pressure sensations throughout the pelvic area. Multiparas especially complain of perineal or groin pressure (Fig. 11-1).

The *mucous plug* (cervical secretions), which has acted as a safeguard against ascending infection during pregnancy, is usually expelled shortly before or at the time of labor. Referred to as the *show,* this is often the first indication of the beginning of labor. Although the show most frequently occurs within the 24 h immediately prior to labor, it may be observed several days before.

The amniotic membranes most often rupture during the active phase of labor. A few women experience a *premature rupture of membranes,* before the onset of labor. The amniotic fluid usually leaks in small amounts, as there are no contractions to exert force.

Although a tear is present, and the fluid is leaking, the body continues to manufacture amniotic fluid; therefore, a *dry birth* is impos-

fig. 11-1 Lightening—a release of pressure on the diaphragm as the fetal head descends into the true pelvis to engage.

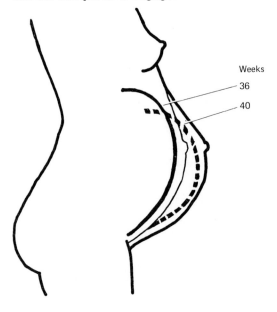

sible. The physician should be notified when the membrane ruptures, since another protective barrier has been removed and infection may follow if labor does not begin within 12 h. At this time, the baby's position, presenting part, and condition should be checked by the physician.

Some women experience episodes of diarrhea, intermittent backache, or generalized abdominal cramping immediately before labor begins.

The mother may experience very early irregular contractions and be convinced that she is in labor. These misleading signs indicate prelabor, often called *false labor*. The contractions prove ineffective, irregular, and poorly defined (i.e., without much increment or decrement). The abdomen remains relatively soft and can be indented with gentle finger pressure. Activity—showering, walking, busyness—generally causes the contractions to cease. On examination, no marked cervical dilatation is noted, and the presenting part has not begun to descend.

The woman experiencing false labor is often embarrassed, discouraged, and susceptible to fatigue. A skillful nurse can be a source of encouragment and renewed self-esteem in emphasizing the vague nature of early labor, even to the trained observer. Ready access to the physician or other attendant for labor evaluation in the office or clinic examining room also helps to diminish the woman's feelings of frustration. With antepartal education, women become more sophisticated in judging the quality of contractions, as false labor seldom requires special techniques.

summary

Prelabor is characterized by:

1 Contractions at irregular intervals, constant or irregular duration, and constant or irregular intensity

2 Lack of progressive cervical effacement or dilatation
3 Failure of presenting part to descend
4 Absence of a show
5 Walking produces relief

Advancing labor is characterized by:

1 Contractions of increasing frequency, increasing duration, and increasing intensity
2 Cervical effacement and dilatation progresses
3 Descent of presenting part
4 Intensification with walking
5 Presence of a show

Imprecise, sketchy, or unintelligible information to the pregnant woman regarding contractions and labor, both in clinics and in private practice, is a major factor in the repeated trips or phone calls to physician, clinic, or hospital which result from anxiety. The nurse can be a calming influence in this period of heightened stress by planning and implementing a realistic plan for the dissemination of accurate and appropriate information, in terms understood by the woman.

PHASES OF LABOR

The medical terminology used to describe labor has become highly technical with the advent of sophisticated monitoring equipment and devices. The obstetrical nurse, while knowledgeable of this terminology, is required to use descriptions and terms which communicate to parents and other nursing personnel as well as to physicians.

For the purpose of determining appropriate nursing action, we will describe the first stage of labor as having *latent* and *active* phases.

the latent phase: prodromal period

The latent phase includes both a *prodromal* or "warming-up" phase and a building up of contractions typical of *early* labor. There is frequently no clear-cut distinction between these periods.

The prodromal phase is characterized by irregularity and variability, but differs from false labor in that significant cervical changes occur, the baby may begin to descend, and there is a progression in contractions, however erratic. The prodromal phase should be seen as an essential period of intermittent contractions which are irregular in frequency, mild in intensity, and poorly defined.

This phase can be confusing to the woman until progress becomes evident. During antepartal instruction, the preparatory aspect of the prodromal phase is emphasized. This knowledge reduces the incidence of early hospitalizations during this period.

contractions   Contractions (1) are characteristically short (Fig. 11-2)—30 to 40 s in duration; (2) come at irregular intervals, from 20 to 5 min: and (3) may be interpreted as intestinal cramping or intermittent backaches. Diarrhea may occur.

duration   In the primigravida, the duration of this phase is highly variable—from zero to many hours. If a multipara experiences this phase, its duration is usually under 6 h. Confident and well-prepared women frequently are unaware of this phase until the contractions are better defined.

work   As part of the continuum of labor, cervical changes occur in response to contractions. The descent of the presenting part and the effacement process continue slowly. Although the membranes are usually intact at this time, should they rupture, the clear, odorless fluid generally escapes in small spurts with each contraction.

woman's mood   Just as the physical characteristics of the prodromal phase are variable, so are the woman's reactions. She is comfortable; her mood may be described as excited, ambivalent, and/or anxious. With antepartal preparation, her most frequent reac-

fig. 11-2   Contraction: prodromal phase. Contraction duration: 30 to 40 s (A–B); intervals: 2 to 5 min (A–C); strength: mild and irregular. (*From Castor, "Participating in Childbirth: A Parents' Guide," 2d ed., Council of Childbirth Education Specialists, New York, 1973.*)

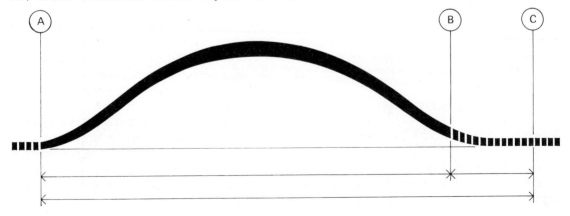

tions are a sense of excitement ("This may be it!") tempered by ambivalence ("Am I ready? Can I handle it?"), until a predictable pattern is established and she begins to use appropriate techniques. Her mood parallels the ambivalence of the first trimester.

comfort measures and techniques
The woman should be encouraged to keep occupied with activities which divert her attention but do not tire her. She should be encouraged to rest periodically when this phase occurs during the day.

She should urinate often to prevent bladder distention and interference with labor. Her diet is usually restricted to easily digested foods and liquids which will sustain her for the long work of labor but which will neither be a safety hazard if an anesthetic becomes necessary nor result in distracting nausea and vomiting. Many physicians now encourage the prepared woman to consume *small* amounts of sweetened tea, water, gelatin desserts, or toast with jelly.

If she awakens with mild contractions,the woman is encouraged to get up, take a warm shower and cup of tea, and then try to sleep. When she understands that the more pronounced contractions of active labor *will* awaken her, rest becomes possible.

If a woman is unduly apprehensive at this time, she may utilize the technique of *controlled relaxation.*

the coach Circumstances may indicate that someone other than the father act as coach: friend, relative, or nurse. The role of the coach remains essentially the same. The mother primarily needs the coach to be available during the prodromal phase to indicate love and concern for her. Although it is not necessary for the father to return home at this point, if he is already there (e.g., during a weekend or evening) he should be alert to signs of tension in the mother. He then can coach her in relaxation techniques. He reminds her to empty her bladder and maintain fluid intake as permitted. The record of labor duing this phase should simply include hourly comments on duration, interval, and strength of contractions.

nursing approach If the childbirth educator can be available for consultation during the earlier phases of labor, suggestions on technique, aid in maintaining the self-confidence of the couple, and validation of their appraisal of labor are very supportive.

The office or clinic nurse, who may be in contact with the couple during this phase, can give encouragment and interpret instructions from the physician in a manner which is positive and supportive. The nurse needs to be oriented to the emotional susceptibility of the laboring woman, realizing that positive remarks are understood by her as important, meaningful encouragement.

If they have come to the hospital or clinic too early, the couple should not be sent home with an abrupt dismissal. Here is a good opportunity for important reinforcement of learning, in which the nurse can underscore the need for rest and the maintenance of fluid balance and energy reserves and remind them of the nature of the labor process. The couple at this point see themselves as amateurs and appreciate a few moments of specific directions relevant to their needs.

If a unique situation occurs in which the woman is hospitalized, the nurse's focus should be on the maintenance of a restful and relaxed environment. In cases where the woman has elected to use a method of childbirth preparation and will have her husband remain with her, the husband also should be encouraged to rest. If he returns home to rest, both he and his wife need to be assured that he will be summoned promptly when labor becomes active. The nurse must take responsibility for carrying out this promise.

If the husband remains in the labor room with his wife, he should be encouraged to keep his wife occupied with diversional activity as he would do at home, and he can assume most of the responsibility for her comfort.

The nurse will monitor both the woman's and baby's conditions by observing vital signs, fetal heart tones, and contractions. Despite the fact that the woman is not yet in active labor, the nurse should make frequent visits to the woman so that she does not feel abandoned.

summary of nursing intervention during the prodromal period   If the nurse is in contact with the woman at this time, the nurse will:

1   Assess the phase of labor and condition of the mother
2   Assess the condition of the fetus
3   Take appropriate nursing action:
    a   Complete prescribed admission procedures
    b   Establish a relaxed and supportive environment
    c   Ascertain if the mother has had any preparation for childbirth and reinforce this teaching
    d   Encourage restful and diversional activities
4   Evaluate nursing intervention and make any necessary modifications

the latent phase: early period

Progressive labor patterns become established during the early phase. The pace of labor is more consistent, with better-defined contractions at more predictable intervals. This is the longest, but easiest, phase of labor. The woman will be comfortable during most

of the phase without any specific labor technique.

contractions

1   Most of the contractions have a duration of 30 to 45 s and are of moderate strength.
2   Increment, acme, and decrement of the contractions are better defined and more apparent.
3   Contraction intervals become more regular, from 10 to 5 min apart. Earlier in the phase they are closer to 10 min apart; as the phase concludes, intervals shorten to 5 min.

During classes, parents are reminded that some degree of irregularity will be present throughout labor, but that within a given period of time, most contractions will conform to a specific pattern.

duration   Friedman includes the early period as part of the preparatory (latent) phase. In his timetable, both the prodromal and early periods combined will *average* 9+ h for primigravidas and 6+ h for multiparas.

work   Cervical changes become more evident during this phase, as the contractions work to almost complete effacement and bring dilation to 4 cm. Usually the presenting part gradually moves deeper into the pelvis. The rupture of membranes does not profoundly influence labor in the early phase.

mood   During the earlier part of this phase, the woman is comfortable and in control. Her mood is confident. If she has not experienced the prodromal phase, she may feel the flush of excitement and anticipatory anxiety characteristic of the beginning of regular contractions.

As the phase progresses, she finds herself increasingly drawn into the experience of labor, in contrast to the peripheral attentiveness of the beginning of labor. The woman's confidence in herself, and in her coach, is reinforced as she begins to apply techniques appropriately.

The unprepared woman, on the other hand, may experience divergent reactions. Her perception of her comfort level may be drastically altered by anxiety. Relaxation and self-directed activities may be difficult as concern for her own and her baby's well-being increases. Accurate perception of contractions may also be affected.

comfort measures and techniques

The prepared couple should be encouraged during classes to view the woman's work in labor as a close parallel to that of a long-distance runner or swimmer. Warm-up completed, the race is begun. Runners pace themselves with controlled effort, coordinated muscular effort, and rhythmic breathing patterns. They resist the impulse to panic into premature speed in response to the efforts of other competitors. In this same way, the prepared couple relies upon the effectiveness of their training program and upon their ability to interpret labor correctly, to make appropriate responses.

At the beginning of the early phase, the woman continues diversional activity, interspersed with rest periods.

The woman is confronted with a sense of urgency to deal with the progressively stronger contractions as the phase continues. She finds she can no longer walk or talk through a contraction; she pauses as it begins, perhaps takes a little gasp of air, or may perceptively tense. These are indications that she should begin the active use of learned techniques.

She utilizes the skill of *controlled relaxation,* by taking a deep breath as the contraction begins, relaxing her body completely as she exhales, letting it concentrate on the contrac-

tion. She may breathe normally as she permits the contraction to work. This ability to let the body work without interference by concentrating on the controlled relaxation skills may be sufficient to deal with tension. If not, she can begin controlled breathing activities.

BREATHING TECHNIQUES The couple has learned a series of precise respiratory techniques so that in labor the woman may effectively pace the intensity of her labor pattern with the appropriate respiratory pattern. The woman has learned the necessity of rhythmic respirations, and her coach has learned the importance of monitoring her efficiency and technique.

The couple learns that certain aspects of the techniques remain constant and are in fact basic to all respiratory effort.

1   *Chest breathing,* which is said to diminish diaphragmatic interference on the uterine fundus, is employed throughout. The woman feels as though she is breathing higher and higher in the chest as she progresses with the techniques, using more of the intercostal muscles and an increasing shallowness of respiratory depth.

2   A *deep breath* initiates and concludes each contraction. This is an important signal for both the woman and her coach. The woman has learned to relax consciously as she exhales this breath, in preparation for the work of the contraction. The coach reminds her of this by stroking or saying "Relax." These beginning and ending breaths make each contraction into a single entity that terminates, as opposed to the sense of relentless contractions. The demarcation also facilitates the use of contraction intervals for rest.

3   A *focal point* increases the woman's concentration and diminishes distraction. It serves to direct her attention to dealing

with the contraction constructively, rather than running from it. This point of focus may change from time to time.

4 *Verbal* and *nonverbal cues* are used in practice to indicate when the woman will use a breathing technique, e.g., "Contraction begins . . . contraction ends." The conditioning to such verbal cues is readily transferred to the actual contraction. At times, these may even be used by the coach during labor, if the woman has become drowsy, tired, or uncertain as to the actual onset of each contraction. The coach may stroke and touch parts of the mother's body to facilitate relaxation and to communicate caring.

5 A *comfortable position* is important for effective relaxation and efficient respiration. It has been determined that the usual recumbent flat position not only may interfere with the progress of labor but may cause undesirable intraabdominal pressure on the large blood vessels. The woman may assume any safe position. She usually chooses a tailor-sitting, side-lying, or semi-Fowler's position.

The first respiratory pattern she will use is *rhythmic chest breathing,* at the slower rate of about eight breaths per minute. The inhalation is through the nose, and the exhalation through the mouth, stressed and slightly prolonged. In rhythm with the breathing, the woman can use a circular *stroke* over the abdominal area, using her fingertips. This type of stroking, known as *effleurage,* enhances her comfort and becomes another precise motor skill on which to concentrate. It may be done with one or both hands, or by her coach. This type of breathing is continued for as long as it is effective (Fig. 11-3).

With the advance of dilatation as the phase progresses, the woman may need to progress in breathing activity as well. If so, she modifies the rhythmic chest breathing by increasing the rate to 16 or 20 breaths per minute, continuing with the rhythmic stroking.

the coach The need for active coaching usually coincides with the woman's use of specific breathing activities. The coach assists with the controlled relaxation technique, observes breathing technique for rhythmic quality and correct performance, and makes note of progress. He reminds the woman to empty her bladder and to take sips of water if permitted. The coach helps her to determine what position is most comfortable, to initiate the use of technique, or he may suggest that she progress with techniques if the one she is using is not effective.

nursing approach The need for positive encouragement and validation of the couple's own observations remains constant throughout labor. The prepared couple is well informed in the mechanics of labor and has worked hard to develop teamwork and skills. The couple needs to be kept posted on the progress of labor. When such progress is slow, as it typically is with first babies, the nurse's wise choice of words means the difference between perseverance and discouragement; for example, contractions should be referred to as such, rather than as "pains."

The nurse should demonstrate respect for the bond which exists and grows between the members of the couple as they work together. If knowledge of technique permits, the nurse may make alternate suggestions, confirm the couple's choice of technique, or even take over while the coach has a coffee break. If the coach indicates that his suggestions on technique are different, the nurse should defer to him, understanding that the couple's confidence is based on a familiarity which has grown with weeks of practice; they are not rejecting the nurse personally.

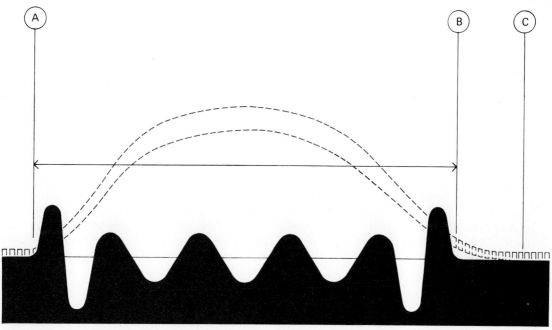

fig. 11-3 Latent phase and rhythmic chest breathing. Contraction duration: 30 to 40 s; intervals: 10 to 5 min (A–C); strength: mild to moderate, regular. Rhythmic chest breathing at rate of 8 breaths per minute. Deep breath begins and ends each contraction. (*From Castor, "Participating in Childbirth: A Parents Guide," 2d ed., Council of Childbirth Education Specialists, New York, 1973.*)

During the admitting procedure and continuing throughout the monitoring of labor, the nurse should interfere as little as possible during a contraction.

summary of nursing intervention during the latent phase During the latent phase, the nurse should:

1 Assess phase of labor and condition of mother:
   a Take baseline vital signs, blood pressure, pulse and respirations, and temperature
   b Ascertain the quality of contractions, their duration and intervals
   c Observe for show and rupture of membranes
   d Determine progress made at home by questioning the couple about contractions, appearance of show, and condition of membranes
   e Observe the mother's behavior and state of mind
2 Assess condition of fetus:
   a Listen to fetal heart tones for quality and rate
   b Palpate position, lie, and presentation
   c Attach external electronic equipment if it is to be used
3 Take appropriate nursing action during admission procedures:
   a Complete record taking, including listing allergies and last food-fluid intake
   b Give perineal shave (total or partial)
   c Give admitting enema (as ordered)
   d Obtain urine specimen (clean voided, especially if show is present)

e Make accurate identification of the mother
f Provide for care of personal belongings
g Perform a vaginal examination (depending on setting, these exams may be a nursing function)
h Draw blood for hematocrit, type, and cross-matching (as ordered)
4 Establish a comfortable, relaxed, and supportive environment by:
  a Introduction and welcome to the couple
  b Familiarizing the couple with facilities and equipment
  c Using quiet, calm voice
  d Assisting the woman into a comfortable position
  e Providing the woman with comfort aids: pillows, blanket, washcloths, emesis basis, drinking cup, ice chips, comfortable chair, supply of clean bed pads
  f Determining if the mother has taken a course in prepared childbirth and reinforce its goals
5 Evaluate nursing intervention and make any necessary modifications

active phase: accelerated period

The active phase includes a period of *accelerated,* progressive dilatation with well-defined contractions at frequent intervals and a *transition* period immediately preceding complete dilatation. Friedman refers to this as the dilatational phase, describing it as the time when contractions reach maximum slope.

At the midpoint of cervical dilation, contractions become strong and consistent in quality, with shorter rest intervals. This phase demands the total concentration of the laboring woman and the encouragement of those attending her, if she is to remain in control.

contractions

1 The duration of contractions now consistently extends from 50 to 60 s; they are of moderate to strong intensity.
2 Contractions have a well-defined curve and a distinct peak (acme) lasting from 40 to 50 percent of each contraction (Fig. 11-4).

duration The phase varies widely in length, but it averages 2 to 3½ h. It is now calculated in terms of centimeters of dilation and descent per hour. The primigravida usually progresses at 1.2 to 3 cm of dilatation per hour, and the multigravida, at 1.5 to 5.7 cm/h.

work The work of this phase includes further effacement of the cervix while rapid dilatation from 4 to 8 cm is taking place. The woman may plateau at 5 cm, as if resting for the next "climb," but the phase is short for both nulliparas and multiparas. Signs of entering transition are often clearly demonstrated as nausea and vomiting, trembling legs, and perspiration begin (see physical reactions of transition period).

mood The carefree, confident, talkative mood which often characterizes the early phase is quickly replaced by an intense, total absorption in the work of labor. As the phase continues and fatigue increases, the woman's confidence begins to waver; she requires active supportive measures.

The unprepared mother may now exhibit a disorganized pattern of behavior. Apprehension increases and sentences become fragmented. The mother may become irritable, unable to cope if left alone, and beg to be "put to sleep."

comfort measures and techniques
The woman must now direct her conscious

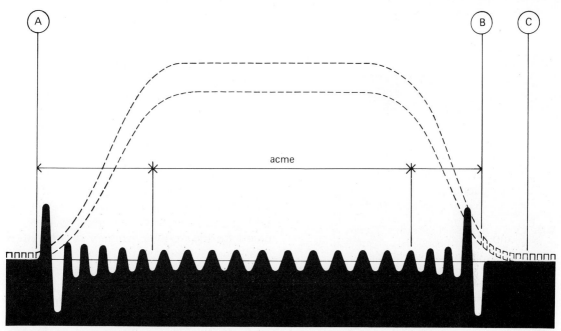

fig. 11-4 Active phase and shallow breathing. Contraction duration: 50 to 60 s (A–B); intervals: 5 to 3 min (A–C); strength: strong, well-defined peaks. Shallow breathing is coordinated to the intensity of each contraction. Rhythmic chest breathing, at the increased rate of 16 to 20 breaths per minute, is used during this increment and decrement; shallow breathing is used for the acme. (*From Castor, "Participating in Childbirth: A Parents' Guide," 2d ed., Council of Childbirth Education Specialists, New York, 1973.*)

efforts to *controlled relaxation.* She becomes aware of the critical importance of this concentration to her ability to deal with the contractions.

In order to deal with the more intense contractions of the active phase, the woman progresses to a *combined pattern* of the modified rhythmic chest breathing and shallow breathing. She matches the increment and decrement with the rhythmic chest breathing pattern; she utilizes the lighter, faster shallow breathing for the acme. The rhythmic *stroking* is continued if the woman finds it soothing. As the contractions demand, she may use the *shallow breathing* for the entire contraction, permitting greater flexibility in rate and depth. When employing this technique, the woman breathes lightly and evenly, both inhaling and

exhaling through her slightly opened mouth. The rate is just fast enough to ensure respiratory exchange (as opposed to simply moving tidal air) with minimal effort and depth of respirations (Fig. 11-5).

"BACK LABOR" Should the woman experience so-called *back labor,* because of either a posterior position of the fetus or a focus of tension, she and her attendants must organize response and action for effective control. While using appropriate breathing techniques, the woman directs her total concentration on releasing tension both generally specifically in the sacrum, perineum, buttocks, and thighs. She avoids lying on her back; her coach applies firm counterpressure to the sacral area. Some women find relief by

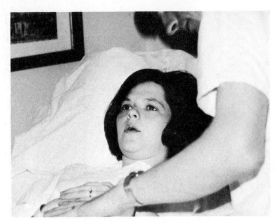

fig. 11-5 In active labor, this mother is seen concentrating on relaxing and on shallow chest breathing. Her husband is checking the contraction to help her coordinate the breathing to the contraction.

the application of cold or warm compresses or by doing the pelvic rock exercise, rounding the back and tilting the pelvis forward.

Ice chips, if allowed, and cool-water mouth rinses are refreshing (mouthwash is nauseating). Some women prefer to suck on sour lollipops between contractions. Talcum powder will make stroking of either abdomen or back easier.

HYPERVENTILATION   If, despite good teaching, adequate practice, and good coaching, a woman begins to *hyperventilate,* a respiratory imbalance of decreased CO_2 levels will develop. She must rebreathe her exhaled air from a small paper bag or her cupped hands. This usually quickly corrects the imbalance and relieves the symptoms of dizziness, light-headedness, and tingling.

the coach   The need for active coaching increases with the active phase. As the contractions heighten and occur more frequently, the woman's perspective becomes distorted. She needs to be reminded to take one con-

traction at a time. Her coach helps her accurately focus on the contractions by counting off each 15-s interval with the contraction. During the contraction, her degree of relaxation is observed; specific instructions are given to facilitate relaxation, especially during the peaks.

nursing approach   Although the couple has learned various skills, this does not mean the total abolition of discomfort or the elimination of all sensations of labor. The couple understands that medication, anesthetics, and other obstetric techniques may be indicated for the accomplishment of the stated goal.

In observing labor and the woman's reactions, the nurse relies on the woman's judgment of her comfort. She may appear to be in distress when actually she is concentrating and working hard. Comments such as, "You're working very hard," "Having a baby is hard work. You're doing a good job," or "That contraction was not easy, but you managed it," underscore the nurse's appreciation of the work of labor and the effectiveness of the woman's efforts.

Even with expert teaching, an occasional couple enters labor with unrealistic goals and exaggerated reactions. In dealing with this kind of couple, the nurse continually directs them toward realistic and attainable goals, reinforcing what is known to be stressed in prenatal preparation. "As you learned in class . . . ," is a helpful emphasis.

With the unprepared woman, the nurse needs to be skillful in relating to the mother in order to calm her and encourage her. Ideally, provision should be made for a nurse to remain with the mother. Although she may not have a complete frame of reference, this mother also needs to be informed of her progress and the baby's condition in terms she can understand. The nurse's manner needs to be direct and positive, and using simple terms, the nurse can coach some relaxation and breathing techniques.

summary of nursing intervention during active phase: accelerated period During the accelerated period, the nurse should:

1 Assess condition of the mother and phase of labor:
   a Continue to check vital signs
   b Observe contractions by palpation or monitor
   c Note show and condition of membranes
   d Observe mother's behavior and state of mind
   e Perform vaginal exams, if a nursing function in that setting
2 Assess condition of fetus:
   a Palpate position
   b Check fetal heart tones (quality and rate) by fetoscope or monitor
   c Observe activity
   d Observe amniotic fluid for color
3 Take appropriate nursing action during admission procedures as described earlier. (Multiparous women come to the hospital during this phase.)
4 Maintain a relaxed, comfortable, and supportive environment:
   a Use a courteous attitude when entering and leaving the room
   b Introduce new personnel
   c Interpret appropriate information in a positive manner
   d Enhance physical comfort of both mother and father
   e Be aware of techniques being used by the couple
   f Support efforts of the couple
5 Take appropriate nursing action in assisting the physician and performing tasks as directed by him. These might include:
   a Preparing for artificial rupturing of membranes. In explaining this, emphasis should be placed on the painlessness of the procedure, the need for sterility, and the effect it will have on the progress in labor. Following this procedure, the nurse is expected to closely monitor contractions, the mother's condition, and the condition of the fetus.
   b Administering sedatives and analgesics, if required. Dosages usually will be significantly reduced for the prepared mother. The coach should be reminded that responses are dulled and that the mother requires active coaching.
   c Assisting with the administration of regional anesthetics as necessary
6 Evaluate nursing intervention and make necessary modifications

active phase: transition period

As cervical dilation nears completion, the woman enters the most intensive and demanding part of the first stage. Fatigue, the inconsistency and discomfort of the contractions, and the intensity of labor make control difficult.

Friedman places most of this period in the pelvic phase, as the fetus begins its descent through the pelvis in preparation for entry into the birth canal.

contractions The pattern of contractions intensifies as the uterine muscles work to complete dilation.

1 The duration of these contractions can be palpated at 60 to 90 s.
2 Intervals shorten to 3 to 2 min.
3 Contractions build rapidly into very strong peaks, which last about two-thirds of the contraction. The contraction also subsides

quickly, but the woman often feels as though it never totally disappears as the uterine tonus rises (Fig. 11-6). Some multiparas experience multiple peaks.

duration   In a woman having her first baby, this final phase usually lasts up to 1 h; the advanced phase is completed in 20 to 45 min for multiparas. This phase may also be calculated in terms of fetal descent (see Fig. 10-17).

work   The cervix now dilates fully, from about 8 to 10 cm, with the baby pushed deep into the pelvis and against the cervix. This produces a heavy show as more cervical capillaries rupture. The presenting part may cause strong sensations of pressure in the rectum, back, groin, or perineum. Many women feel as if they must have a bowel movement and will call for a bedpan.

mood and physical reactions   The woman becomes agitated and intense during the transition period. The physiologic changes of labor and fatigue make her irritable, restless, and discouraged. She finds it difficult to cope with contractions; relaxation during the brief rest intervals is almost impossible. She may sweat profusely, become chilled, or alternate between these reactions. Her legs may tremble and cramp. She may complain of nausea or a backache. She may feel overwhelmed and discouraged; she wants to give up. Her perspective is severely distorted.

The use of appropriate labor techniques and the presence of a coach enable most

fig. 11-6   Transition phase contraction. Contraction duration: 60 to 90 s (A–B); intervals: 3 to 2 min (A–C); strength: intense. Contraction may have multiple peaks. The increment and decrement are brief; to the woman the contraction does not seem to entirely subside, since the tonus has risen. (*From Castor, "Participating in Childbirth: A Parents' Guide," 2d ed., Council of Childbirth Education Specialists, New York, 1973.*)

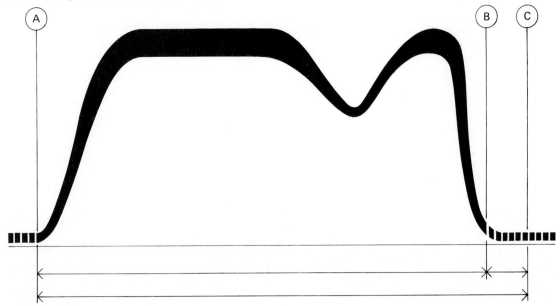

prepared mothers to cope with the intensity of this period. The nurse will observe most of this behavior nonetheless.

comfort measures and techniques To handle this tough period, the woman must deal with each contraction with a rhythmic pattern of *shallow breathing and short puffs.* The sequence is usually three or four shallow breaths and one puff, which can be altered to meet the contraction's intensity. A sequence of one shallow breath and one puff is particularly effective for strong peaks or sensations of pressure. If she experiences the urge to push before dilation is complete, she uses a repeated blow-blow-blow until given permission to bear down (Fig. 11-7).

To assist in her efforts to relax between contractions, restore respiratory balance, and foster a sense of well-being, the woman uses the *rhythmic chest breathing* at its slowest rate, eight breaths per minute during the brief intervals.

Stroking (effleurage) is irritating and distracting during the advanced phase, but the woman may find relief in supporting the lower abdominal area with her hands.

the coach Coaching must be specific and direct. The woman's reactions frequently require active and continual direction. The coach must insist that she take one contraction at a time, because she anticipates them all and panics. She must be reminded to use the *rhythmic chest breathing* between contractions. The coach may have to touch the abdominal area lightly to help her discern the absence of a contraction. Communication,

fig. 11-7 A rhythmic pattern of shallow breathing and short puffs is used to control the intense contractions of the transition phase. Rhythmic chest breathing is used between contractions to aid relaxation and restore respiratory balance. (*From Castor, "Participating in Childbirth: A Parents' Guide," 2d ed., Council of Childbirth Education Specialists, New York, 1973.*)

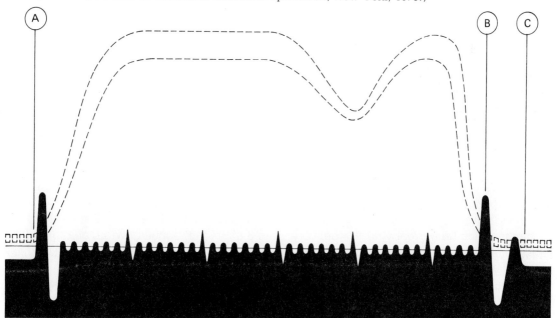

both verbal and nonverbal, is very important to her ability to remain in control. The coach cannot allow her to waste the rest periods, no matter how brief, in purposeless activity or tenseness.

nursing approach The woman's need for the reassurance of the nurse intensifies. The nurse's continued interpretation of the physician's findings and her support and encouragement of the couple's efforts increase their tolerance and enhance their effectiveness. A woman at this point in progress must not be left alone. The nurse, therefore, plans the various preparatory activities—seeing to the coach's gowning, checking on delivery-room setup and required equipment, arranging for one person to remain with her at all times. During this phase, the nurse is expected to monitor the fetal condition more frequently. This needs to be done skillfully, so as not to interrupt the woman's activities. The nurse is alert to any sudden changes in the position of the fetal head, particularly with multiparas, in whom dilation may dramatically progress from 8 to 10 cm in a few minutes, with concurrent descent of the baby into the birth canal.

summary of nursing intervention during active phase: transition period Intervention remains focused on points previously discussed:

1 Assess condition of the mother and phase of labor
2 Assess condition of the fetus
3 Take appropriate nursing action in assisting the physician and performing tasks as directed, including readying the delivery room and transfer of the mother
4 Maintain a relaxed, comfortable, and supportive environment
5 Evaluate nursing intervention

second stage

With full dilatation, the forces of labor focus on descent. The baby must pass through the dilated cervix, maneuver down through the pelvis, then distend the vagina, pass through the perineal muscles, and emerge. Controlled and efficient voluntary bearing down by the woman contributes to an effective and safe delivery. Bearing-down efforts add about 40 lb of pressure to the uterine contraction work. Fortunately, the expulsive action of the uterus, the woman's sense of renewal, and prior instruction will enable her to be an effective and active assistant.

contractions The tumultuous quality of the transition period subsides. Once again the contractions become regular and predictable.

1 Duration of contractions is 90 to 100 s.
2 Intervals change to 4 to 2 min, with a well-defined rest period.
3 Increment, acme, and decrement are well defined and consistent. Contractions are strong. The uterus can be seen rising up within the abdomen during each contraction; the fundus perceptibly lowers (Fig. 11-8).

duration With the cooperative efforts of the prepared woman, it takes 20 to 90 min to accomplish the second stage for a primigravida, with an average duration of 40 to 60 min (and 20 pushes). Lack of muscle resistance in a multipara usually reduces the second stage to 10 to 40 min (and 10 pushes). In the primigravida, fetal descent is at a rate of 1.5 to 3 cm/h. In the multigravida, at a rate of 2.1 to 5 cm/h.

work The mechanical work of labor involves the *flexion, descent,* and *rotation* of the

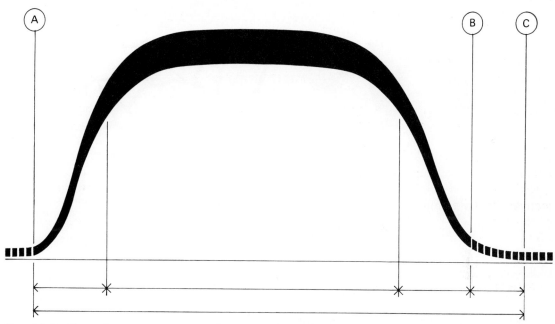

fig. 11-8 Second-stage contraction. Contraction duration: 90 to 100 s; intervals: 4 to 2 min; strength: intense but defined. Increment and decrement lengthen, helping to make contractions more manageable. (*From Castor, "Participating in Childbirth: A Parents' Guide," 2d ed., Council of Childbirth Education Specialists, New York, 1973.*)

baby's head through the pelvis and vaginal canal. Indeed, birth is impossible without these maneuvers (see Fig. 10-16).

mood The irritability, discouragement, and agitation which marked the final hour of the first stage rapidly disappear at full dilatation and the beginning of the woman's cooperative efforts. As she senses active progression with each push, and as the contractions resume a more manageable pattern, the woman gets the feeling of a second wind, a renewal of energy and stamina. Modesty is replaced by a greater work sense; position and bodily covering are unimportant to her.

The father's encouragement to sustain the immense pushing effort is very important to her, and she focuses intently on him. Although she becomes oblivious to peripheral activity, she is susceptible to confusion if conflicting directions are given or several people attempt to direct her. The woman's pushing effort may be timid and inefficient at first. As she senses that the harder she pushes the better it feels, and as she is specifically directed by her coach, her efforts become rhythmic and efficient (Fig. 11-9).

The unprepared woman may completely lose control. The great force of labor may make her feel as though her body is rushing on without her. She may utter loud screams at the peak of the contraction. She frequently is unable to follow directions unless they are simple and repeated. She thinks she *is* bearing down, but everyone keeps telling her to "push!"

It is important that the woman be prepared for the sensations which accompany expul-

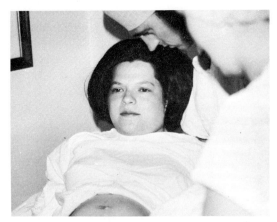

fig. 11-9 The mother is in the pushing position. Her husband gives her the necessary cues as she bears down with the contraction. It is obvious that she is concentrating and working hard.

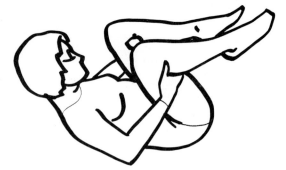

fig. 11-10 The woman concentrates on pushing at the peak of each contraction. To do this, she takes a series of deep breaths during the increment and then holds her breath, bearing down with the abdominal muscles while consciously relaxing the perineum to enhance pushing efficiency; she quickly exhales, inhales, and holds her breath several times during each peak. During the decrement, she takes several deep breaths. (*From Castor, "Participating in Childbirth: A Parents' Guide," 2d ed., Council of Childbirth Education Specialists, New York, 1973.*)

sion so that they can be put in proper perspective: the distention of the vaginal tissue: the increasing pressure on the perineum; rectal pressure; the absence of perception of the contraction itself with the pushing effort. As the baby exerts greater and greater pressure on the perineal musculature, her pushing effort may temporarily diminish. She may also feel the full weight of the responsibility of getting this baby out, which can be overwhelming to her unless her efforts are continually encouraged and unless her progress is continually noted. Some women require detailed direction; others need only occasional reminders (Fig. 11-10).

A tremendous sense of relief accompanies the birth of the head. Though some women report that it feels good to push, most women will be absorbed in a great work effort and the overriding urge to get that baby out.

comfort measures and techniques
Technique focuses on controlled relaxation, correct positioning to influence favorably the axis of the birth canal, effective use of the abdominal muscles and diaphragm, and the

direction of pushing effort toward the vagina. The woman learns to push during the peak of each contraction, permitting the contraction to build by taking a series of deep breaths. She learns to push several times during the peak, which, for many women, seems to maintain pushing efficiency better than one sustained push. She restores respiratory balance by taking several deep breaths as the contraction declines. Pushing effort must come from the abdominal muscles, and not consist simply of straining in the throat. Between contractions she must rest, utilizing controlled relaxation once again. She learns to cooperate with the physician's instructions during the delivery of the head, controlling her pushing effort by utilizing the shallow breath and blow sequence to control the strong urges to expel the baby at once (Fig. 11-11).

The woman is also prepared for the *episiotomy* and understands its place in normal delivery. Since this is often feared out of ig-

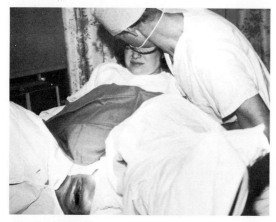

fig. 11-11 As the mother bears down with the contraction, the baby's head comes down onto the perineum, causing it to bulge. *Caput* is seen.

norance and misinformation, the episiotomy is carefully explained as being a painless procedure, even without local anesthesia, when done at the peak of a contraction, as pressure from the baby's head causes a natural anesthesia to the perineum. As the physician enlarges the vaginal outlet with surgical scissors, the woman experiences a sensation not unlike being unzipped. She now pushes the baby out with decreased resistance. (Local anesthesia is, of course, used in most instances.) (Figs. 11-12 and 11-13.)

the coach The implications of the coach's continued involvement through delivery are now being more completely understood. The former banishment of the father at this time, after hours of active involvement, caused an acutely felt emotional wrenching. He felt left out, and his wife felt isolated.

In contrast, the father's presence at the birth of their child can be a profound experience for the new parents and orients them in a beautiful way to parenthood as a mutually shared effort.

The father remains at the mother's side, speaking directly into her ear, if need be. He also has learned the correct pushing technique so that he can encourage her efforts. Both in practice and in delivery he uses cue words:

(Breathe) *In, out; in, out; hold* (your breath)
Relax key areas (jaw, mouth, perineum)
Push out (use the abdominal muscles; push out through the vagina)
Release air

He repeats the sequence several times for each contraction and slowly counts to help her sustain pushing for each 20- to 30-s block.

He reminds her to maintain a correct position with her sacral area flat, so that the

fig. 11-12 Birth of head in OA position (left); rotating to ROA (right).

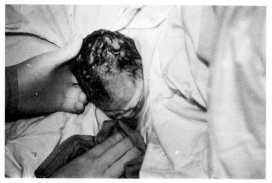

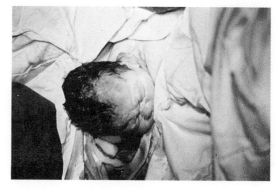

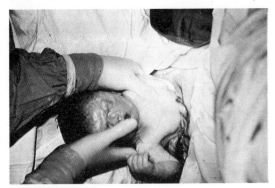

fig. 11-13 Birth of body.

pelvis is in a slight tilt upward and knees are flexed.

Between contractions, he encourages her to relax by speaking in soothing tones, stroking, or using a cool cloth.

nursing approach The nurse plays a dual role during the second stage, as she or he assists the physician in assuring the safe delivery of a healthy baby and undergirds the efforts of the couple.

Recognizing that a woman most often relates best to a single source of direction, the nurse defers to the father or the physician, except for general encouragement. However, if the woman's efforts falter, the nurse should recognize that she needs specific directions, not general statements such as "Push!" General directions are frustrating, because the woman feels she *is* pushing. The nurse can help the husband give specific, detailed help.

When the hospital prohibits the father's presence during the second stage, the nurse assumes the coaching role.

The unprepared mother is in desperate need of encouragement and reassurance. She needs someone to hang on to—both physically and emotionally.

summary of nursing intervention during second stage During the second stage, the nurse should:

1 Assess the phase of labor and the condition of the mother
2 Assess condition of fetus
3 Maintain a supportive and safe environment
4 Take appropriate nursing action in assisting the physician and performing tasks as directed. These may include:
  a Efficient transfer of mother to delivery table *between contractions*
  b Adjusting the lighting
  c Explaining activities: perineal scrub, draping, fetal monitoring, administration of intravenous solutions or medications
  d Preparing equipment necessary for delivery and immediate care of the newborn
5 Assess condition of the newborn (discussed in detail in Chap. 14):
  a Take Apgar score
  b Monitor physical condition and vital signs
6 Take appropriate nursing action in care of newborn:
  a Clear air passages
  b Take care of cord
  c Provide prophylactic eye care, *after* parents have held baby
  d Make identification of infant
  e Provide warmth
  f Provide necessary physical contact between mother and baby
7 Evaluate nursing intervention

third stage

The placenta, having completed its intricate life-sustaining function, now separates from the wall of the uterus as it once again contracts. The uterus, now considerably smaller, rises up and assumes a globular shape. The placenta is painlessly expelled as the mother pushes for the last time.

contractions and duration Mild contractions of approximately 1-min duration occur 5 to 30 min after the birth of the baby and then continue at longer intervals through the recovery period. The uterine contractions exert pressure which causes the placenta to move into the lower uterine segment or upper part of the vagina, from which the woman can then push it out (Fig. 11-14).

mood Following the birth of the baby, the mother usually is exhilarated and talkative, irrespective of the length or intensity of labor and/or delivery. She feels very close to the father; she reaches out physically and emotionally for her baby. Her prevailing reaction is one of elation, tempered with a sense of new responsibility: parenthood. The transition into parenthood can be facilitated by the continued support of the professional maternity care specialist, the provisions for contact with the infant, and the physical care of the new mother (Fig. 11-15).

The mother may express annoyance at having to exert herself to push out the placenta or at the repair of the episiotomy. Also, she is highly perceptive at this time and will pick up any signals of anxiety or concern. If any variance from the norm occurs, she needs accurate information and positive reassurance.

comfort measures and techniques The mother appreciates anything which increases her comfort, such as wiping her face, giving her ice chips, or adjusting the delivery table.

the coach This is a sharing time, as the couple waits for the completion of delivery.

fig. 11-14 (a) Expulsion of placenta, a and b (*Photo by Ruth Helmich.*)

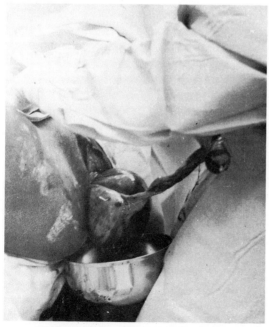
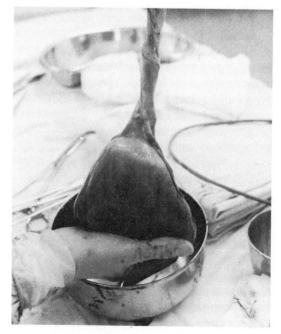

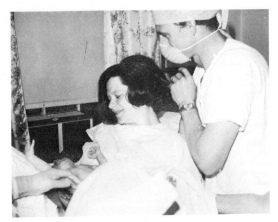

fig. 11-15 A job well done. Mother and father see their son at close hand for the first time. (*Photos in Figs. 11-9, 11-11, 11-12, 11-13, and 11-15 from Manchester Memorial Hospital's homelike birth and bonding room, Manchester, Conn.*)

nursing intervention during the third stage Once the newborn's condition is seen to be stable, the nurse assists the physician with the care of the new mother, still in a critical stage of labor. At this stage, the nurse should:

1 Assess the mother's condition and phase of labor:
    a Take vital signs as directed by the physician
    b Observe for signs of placental separation:
        (1) Uterus rises in globular shape as it contracts
        (2) Umbilicus cord lengthens through vagina
    c Assess condition of fundus
2 Assess condition of newborn:
    a Apgar score at 5 min
    b Appearance and behavior
3 Take appropriate nursing action in assisting physician. These may include:
    a Directing the mother to push to help expel the placenta

    b Administering medications, as directed. *Oxytocin* or *methergine* or both are sometimes given to stimulate uterine contractions and minimize blood loss.
4 Maintain a supportive and safe environment for the new parents. If appropriate, the nurse gives the baby to the parents to hold (Fig. 11-16). If the parents have to wait until the completion of this stage to hold the infant, the baby should be in sight and the mother assured that she will hold it shortly.
5 Evaluate nursing intervention.

fourth stage

During the hour after placental delivery, the physician repairs the episiotomy and any lacerations that may be present, using a local anesthetic. The physician observes the mother's general condition, particularly in regard to bleeding. The placenta is examined, to be sure that it was delivered intact and that no parts remain in the uterus which would interfere with the important uterine contractions that control bleeding.

fig. 11-16 Mother needs an opportunity to "claim" her baby by touching and holding.

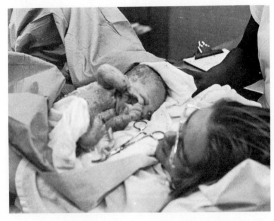

mother's reaction Soon after delivery the mother manifests *physiologic reactions*. She often becomes chilled and may tremble. She is tired and may be very hungry and thirsty.

If the mother is not given the opportunity to hold her baby, she experiences a strong feeling of deprivation and loss. Most progressive hospitals see to it that this opportunity is provided to diminish the sense of loss and increase her feeling of well-being.

More and more women are requesting to breast-feed immediately after delivery. The infant's sucking reflex is very strong at this point; nursing also seems to create strong maternal bonds with the infant, an important aid to the newly delivered mother (Figs. 11-17 and 11-18).

nursing approach The nurse's primary responsibility remains the observation of the mother's physical condition. The nurse removes the woman from stirrups, carefully removing her legs simultaneously, makes her comfortable, and observes her for bleeding.

In providing for the mother's physical comfort, the nurse has an opportunity to provide her with significant gestures of human caring.

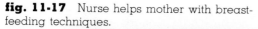
fig. 11-17 Nurse helps mother with breast-feeding techniques.

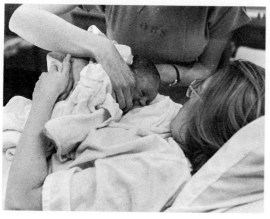

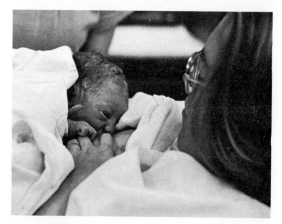
fig. 11-18 Newborn may lick the nipple or nurse vigorously immediately after birth.

summary of nursing intervention in immediate recovery period

1. Assess mother's condition
   a. Vital signs
   b. Fundal firmness
   c. Amount of vaginal bleeding
   d. Bladder distention
   e. Appearance and state of mind
2. Assess condition of newborn if it remains with the mother during this time. Be sure warmth is maintained.
3. Take appropriate nursing action:
   a. In *delivery room:* remove soiled linen, adjust delivery table, and remove both legs from stirrups simultaneously; provide mother with a covering and sterile perineal pad; give a sponge bath and clean gown
   b. In *recovery area:* provide warmth and cleanliness for mother and simple nourishment for both parents; encourage parents to verbalize; allow parents to remain together; facilitate mother-infant bond if newborn remains with mother, encouraging touching, "en face" position, and fondling
4. Evaluate nursing intervention

Table 11-1 provides a summary of the stages of labor.

table 11-1

LABOR SUMMARY

phase	technique	coach
latent: prodromal *Duration:* 0 to many hours *Contractions:* Mild, 30–40 s long, 20–5 min apart, irregular. *Work:* Early effacement. Show; membranes "leak" if they break. *Mood:* Excited, ambivalent.	Conserve strength. If at night, nap; if daytime, keep busy at light activities. Bland diet as permitted. Small amounts of sweet liquids. Experiment with position.	If at home, help with organizing household, assist general relaxation.
latent: early *Duration:* Nullipara, 8.6 h to 20 h* Multipara, 5.6 h to 14 h* *Contractions:* Moderate, 30–45 s long, 10–5 min apart, more regular. *Work:* Effacement and dilation to 4 cm *Mood:* Talkative, comfortable.	Conserve energy. Call doctor; emphasize degree of comfort. Take clear fluids as permitted. As necessary: Use *controlled relaxation* For control: *Rhythmic chest breathing,* (1) slow rate, 8 breaths per minute, (2) modified rate, 16–20 breaths per minute.	Time contractions and note progress every hour. Support her efforts. Help with relaxation. Monitor breathing techniques.
active: accelerated *Duration:* Average 2 to 3.5 h for both Nullipara at 1.2 to 3 cm/h Multipara at 1.5 to 5.7 cm/h *Contractions:* Strong, 50–60 s, 5–3 min apart. *Work:* Dilate 4–8 cm *Mood:* Very busy, concentrated; intense. If membranes break, contractions increase in strength.	Conserve energy. For control: *Controlled relaxation, combined breathing pattern— rhythmic chest/shallow* If necessary: *Shallow, accelerated-decelerated with contraction.* Usually go to hospital. Sips of water or ice chips, if allowed.	"Count down" contractions. Mouth rinses, cool cloth to hands and face. Touch; stroke arms and legs. Talk to her; encourage efforts. Remind: Labor intermittent. Monitor breathing.
active: transition *Duration:* 20 to 60 min of above time	*Controlled relaxation* *Shallow breathing:* pant-	Give specific directions. Insist on taking one

phase	technique	coach
Contractions: Erratic, intense, 60–90 s, 3–2 min apart *Work:* Dilate 8–10 cm. *Mood:* Irritable, discouraged, overwhelmed. *Physical sensations:* nausea, vomiting, chills, trembling, profusely sweating, pressure sensations, difficult to relax.	blow 3/1, 2/1, 1/1 as contraction demands. Rectal pressure: 1/1 pant-blow rhythm. Urge to push: Repeated blows. *Rhythmic chest breathing* between contractions.	contraction at a time. Remind her that baby is almost here. ENCOURAGE! Monitor breathing. If she uses repeated "blowing," summon doctor, R.N. Remain with her.
Special Considerations: *Hyperventilation:* Tingling, dizzy, light-headed, apprehensive, out of rhythm.	Rebreathe exhaled air between contractions. *Prevent:* Keep breathing light, rhythmic.	Monitor breathing. Correct technique—cadence, breathe with her.
Back labor: Strong discomfort in small of back; difficult to relax; contractions may be erratic; tension increases.	Get off back—lie on side. Focus on progressive relaxation throughout each contraction. Apply warm or cold compresses. Constant pressure to small of back.	Talk through contractions. Assist with techniques. Apply counterpressure. Stroke. ENCOURAGE!
second stage *Duration:* 20–60 min *Descent:* Nullipara 1.5 to 3 cm/h Multipara 2.1 to 5 cm/h *Contractions:* Rhythmic, strong, 90 s, 4–2 min apart. *Work:* Descent and birth of baby. *Mood:* Refreshed, sense of work. Cooperative. *Physical:* Vaginal fullness, pressure in rectum. Burning, stretching. *Episiotomy:* painless, "unzipped."	The harder the push, the better it feels. *Expulsion* technique. If instructed to stop pushing at birth of head, *pant-blow.*	Coach efforts: in, out/in, out/in, hold, relax key areas, push out (count slowly to 10), release air, in, hold (repeat above). Several deep breaths at end of each effort.

table 11-1
LABOR SUMMARY (*continued*)

phase	technique	coach
third stage *Delivery of placenta:* 10–30 min *Contractions:* Mod. strong. *Mood:* Thinking of baby. *Work:* Placenta expelled.	Push as directed. Enjoy baby.	Enjoy baby together. Praise wife.

* Duration includes entire latent phase (Friedman).

study questions

1 Using a labor you have observed, describe the nursing action used in establishing a calm and supportive environment for the mother and her coach on admission to the labor unit. Relate specifically to your nursing assessment of the mother. Discuss any additional intervention which may have been appropriate.

2 Women exhibit certain behavioral responses as labor progresses.
 a Describe the behavior of two women you have observed in labor, including both verbal and nonverbal behavior.
 b Compare this behavior to what is presented in the text.
 c Discuss appropriate nursing intervention
 d If the woman's husband was present, describe his reactions and intervention

3 Keep a log of your labor observations to describe the:
 a nursing assessment of the phase of labor and condition of mother
 b assessment of the fetus
 c nursing action you took
 d evaluation of your nursing interaction

bibliography

Castor, Constance R.: *Participating in Childbirth: A Parents' Guide,* 2d ed., Council of Childbirth Education Specialists, New York, 1973.

————, P. Hassid, and J. Sasmor: "The Childbirth Team during Labor," *American Journal of Nursing,* **73**(3): 444–447, 1973.

Farill, M. S.: "Adolescent in Labor," *American Journal of Nursing,* **68**:1952–1954, 1968.

Friedman, E. A.: *Labor: Clinical Evaluation of Management,* Appleton-Century-Crofts, New York, 1967.

————: "The Use of Labor Pattern as a Management Guide," *Hospital Topics,* **46**:57–59, 1968.

Kopp, Lois: "Ordeal or Ideal—The Second Stage of Labor," *American Journal of Nursing,* **71**(6):1140, 1971.

Loriner, A. B.: "Danger Signs in the First Stage of Labor," *Hospital Medicine,* **6**:115, 1970.

Oxhorn, H., and W. Foote: *Human Labor and Birth,* 2d ed., Appleton-Century-Crofts, New York, 1968.

Tryon, Phyllis: "Assessing the Progress of Labor through Observation of Patient's Behavior," *Nursing Clinics of North America,* **3**(2):315–326, 1968.

Whitley, Nancy: "Uterine Contractile Physiology: Applications in Nursing Care and Patient Teaching" *Journal of Obstetrics, Gynecologic, and Neonatal Nursing* **4**: 54–58, September–October 1975.

Willmuth, L. Ragon: "Prepared Childbirth and the Concept of Control," *Journal of Obstetric, Gynecologic and Neonatal Nursing* **4**:38–41, September–October 1975.

12

THE PROCESS OF RECOVERY

MARTHA OLSEN SCHULT

The period of time after a woman gives birth until her recovery 6 or 8 weeks later is known as the *puerperium,* derived from the Latin words *puer,* "child," and *parere,* "to bring forth." The two major occurrences of the puerperium are *involution* and *lactation.* The goals of physical care in the puerperium are three-fold:

To prevent infection of the bladder, breasts, and uterus

To promote healing and the return to normal of the pelvic structures and perineum

To establish successful lactation if this is the desire of the woman

Involution involves the return of the pelvic reproductive structures, particularly the uterus, to their prepregnant size and position. *Lactation,* the other phase of the puerperium, begins after the delivery of the baby and can extend well beyond the 6- to 8-week period. If a woman chooses not to breast-feed her infant, lactation can be suppressed or inter-rupted. Breast-feeding will be discussed in detail in Chap. 16.

THE UTERUS

At the time of delivery, the uterus weighs approximately 1000 g (2.2 lb). In 1 week it is reduced to one-half this weight, and by the end of the postpartum period, it weighs only 40 to 60 g (about 2 oz). The reason this organ can approximate its prepregnant weight and shape is that during pregnancy the *size* of the muscle cells increases while the *number* of muscle cells remains basically the same (Fig. 12-1). During the puerperium, the protein cytoplasm of the muscle fibers undergoes catabolic or autolytic changes. The products of this destructive process are carried off by the circulatory system and excreted as nitro-genous waste in the urine of the patient.

Immediately after delivery the very hard,

fig. 12-1 Postpartal descent of uterus into pelvic cavity. *(Courtesy of Carnation Company.)*

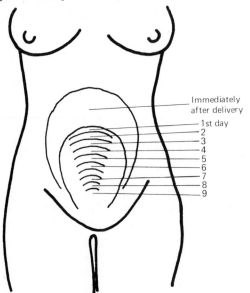

Immediately after delivery
1st day
2
3
4
5
6
7
8
9

round, contracted uterus lies between the umbilicus and the symphysis. Later the uterus rises to the level of the umbilicus or slightly above it. After the first postpartum day, the uterus begins its descent into the pelvic cavity. It diminishes quite rapidly in size, weight, and position until the tenth day, when it can no longer be palpated. At this point it is at or below the level of the symphysis pubis.

The uterus, throughout its descent, should remain firm and contracted in order to act as a tourniquet to prevent hemorrhage from the large blood vessels at the placental site. The uterus will contract on its own. However, oxytocics (drugs which act to contract uterine smooth muscle) are sometimes given to the patient following delivery to assist the uterus in this function. If the patient is to receive ergonovine maleate or methylergonovine ma-leate, the nurse must check the blood pressure prior to administration. These oxytocics have a vasoconstricting effect. In response to the sucking of the infant, breast-feeding also causes the uterus to contract, triggering oxy-tocin release from the posterior pituitary.

POSTPARTUM CHECK

After a period of observation in the recovery room, the patient arrives on the postpartum unit for the remainder of her hospital stay. This is a crucial time in the recovery process. To monitor this period, the nurse will check the following factors:

Fundus—position and firmness of the uterus
Lochia—type and amount of vaginal dis-charge
Perineum—check for bleeding, hematoma, episiotomy
Bladder—amount and time of voiding
Bowels—status and activity
Vital signs—reflection of postpartum ad-justment

Homan's sign—development of thrombophlebitis

Emotional state—reaction to experiences and to prospective parenting responsibilities

fundus

The palpation of the top of the uterus is called the fundus check (Fig. 12-2). It is done to determine the rate of descent and the position and condition of the uterus. The unit of measurement of descent of the uterus is in centimeters and is known as a *fingerbreadth*. Descent is measured and recorded in relation to the umbilicus. The fingerbreadth is the width of a finger, 1 cm (½ in), as it is placed horizontally on the abdomen at the height of the fundus. With *U* indicating the umbilicus, fingerbreadths are recorded in numbers. The usual rate of descent of the uterus is 1 fingerbreadth (1 cm) a day after the first postpartum day.

It is important for the nurse to keep an accurate check on the descent of the uterus. Any retardation of the process indicates a problem or complication.

1/U—The fundus is located 1 fingerbreadth above the umbilicus.

U—The fundus is at the level of the umbilicus.

U/1—The fundus is 1 fingerbreadth below the level of the umbilicus.

U/2—The fundus is 2 fingerbreadths below the level of the umbilicus.

Even though the patient may have received an oxytocic, it is still important to do the fundus check and determine the rate of descent.

With the change in pressure in the abdomen, the bladder easily becomes distended, pushing the uterus up and to the side. Because the uterus must be able to contract to

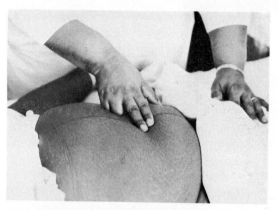

fig. 12-2 Measurement of descent of fundus in fingerbreadths. (*Photo by Ruth Helmich. Courtesy of Jamaica Hospital, Jamaica, N.Y.*)

stop bleeding from the placental site, a "boggy," soft uterus out of midline or above the umbilicus is an indication that the bladder is full and that bleeding will occur. Be careful not to knead or massage too vigorously because the uterus may become fatigued or overstimulated. Hemorrhage or undue pain may result. Check for the amount of bleeding and for the presence of clots or any other untoward symptoms. (See Chap. 22 for other causes of bleeding.) The following schedule suggests fundus checks for the first hours when danger of hemorrhage is greatest.

Every 10 to 15 min × 6 in recovery room; and then

Every 30 min × 6

Every 1 h × 3

Every 3 to 4 h for the remainder of the first day

A patient can be taught to check her own fundus and report to the nurse any changes. Involving the recovered patient in her own care is especially helpful when the unit is busy or short-staffed.

After the first 24 h, the fundus should be checked every 4 h the first postpartum day and once a shift every day thereafter. Any problems regarding the location or quality of contraction of the uterus would require more frequent checks.

procedure for complete fundus check

1 Explain reason for procedure to patient.
2 Screen and position patient.
3 Remove perineal pad and have her empty bladder, as necessary.
4 Lower the head of the bed.
5 Cup hand around the fundus. If firm, do not massage. If "boggy" or soft, gently massage in a rotating manner, and observe for passage of blood clots.
6 Cleanse perineal area, securing a fresh pad.
7 Assist patient to a comfortable position.
8 Chart findings. For example, fundus firm, 1/U, midline.

lochia

After delivery the decidual lining of the uterus sloughs off as a vaginal discharge known as *lochia*. This discharge includes blood, decidual tissue, epithelial cells from the vagina, mucus, bacteria, and occasionally membranes and small clots. The color of lochia is an indication of the progress of the healing of the placental site. At first the discharge is quite red and bloody. Frank bleeding occurs from the torn vessels of the placental site. As healing takes place and the lining of the rest of the uterus sloughs off, the discharge becomes more serous, contains leukocytes, and resembles menstrual flow. Then the discharge turns pale and diminishes. The first stage is termed *lochia rubra* (red), the second is *lochia serosa* (reddish brown), and the third is *lochia alba* (white) (Table 12-1).

Check the lochia whenever the fundus is checked. Record the amount on the pad—for example, scant, moderate, or heavy. Note the frequency of the pad change. If, in the early period after delivery, it is more often than every hour and the pad is saturated, the patient should be checked for causes of extra bleeding. Record any deviations such as odor, clots, or the absence of lochia. Save any large clots or pieces of tissue for examination by the physician.

When the postpartal patient is changing her own perineal pad and checking her own lochia, instruct her to notify the nurse or physician if she notices any of the following:

Bright red bleeding beyond the fourth postpartum day
Foul odor
Pain or discomfort in the lower abdominal area
Absence of lochia within the first 2 weeks of delivery
Clots or tissue in lochia
Bright bleeding recurring after lochia alba begins

table 12-1 lochia characteristics

rubra	serosa	alba
Bright red	Pink	Creamy-yellow
Bloody; small clots may be present	Pinkish-brown Serous	May be brownish
1–3 days postpartum	5–7 days postpartum	1–3 weeks
No odor or slightly "fleshy"	No odor, no clots	No odor or stale body odor

perineum

During delivery the pelvic muscles are greatly stretched, and usually cut by the episiotomy. It is most important that the area be kept as clean and dry as possible to prevent infection.

The initial perineal care routine is carried out by the nurse. When the patient is awake and alert she should be instructed in the following points:

1 Removing the perineal pad. Remove the pad from front to back so that the micro-organisms in the rectal area are not dragged across the vaginal opening.
2 Flushing the perineal area with warm water or a mild antiseptic solution.
3 Patting dry with paper wipes.
4 Securing the perineal pad snugly (to prevent its moving back and forth between the anus and the vaginal opening).

Inspect the perineal area daily by having the patient lie on the same side as her episiotomy, for easier viewing. Because of the edema of the tissue it may be difficult to see the episiotomy. Chart condition, whether sutures are intact, and any signs of inflammation. The episiotomy should heal in 7 to 10 days.

If the patient has pain in the perineal area, there are several ways to alleviate it:

1 Administer compresses, a heat lamp, or a sitz bath as prescribed by the physician.
2 Administer analgesics or local anesthetics, as ordered.
3 Advise the patient to rest on her side and to avoid standing for long periods of time.
4 Advise patient to relax and contract the perineal-pelvic muscles periodically to stimulate circulation and muscle tone (Kegel exercise).

Should the patient complain of severe pain in the perineal area, she should be checked for a possible hematoma caused by bleeding into the vaginal wall or vulva (see Chap. 22).

bladder

After delivery, the capacity of the bladder increases because of decreased intraabdominal pressure and the relaxed, stretched abdominal muscles. During the delivery period the bladder and urethra may be traumatized because of nerve damage or edema. Drugs and anesthesia during the labor and delivery may diminish sensitivity of the bladder or the alertness of the patient. Pain in the perineal area may cause a reflex spasm of the urethra. Psychologically, the patient may fear that voiding will be painful. Lack of privacy, inability to communicate with the nurse, and the discomfort of using the bedpan will all contribute to difficulty in voiding. The use of intravenous fluid therapy results in rapid urine formation, especially if fluids were given rapidly during immediate recovery. It is important that the patient void at least once and, more important, that she *empty her bladder* within 6 to 8 h of delivery to prevent:

Atony (loss of muscle tone of bladder)
Stasis of urine, predisposing to infection
Postpartum bleeding from obstruction of uterine descent

Methods used to determine the status of the bladder include checking oral and parenteral intake, checking output since delivery, and palpation of the uterus and bladder (Fig. 12-3).

After the nurse has determined that the bladder is distended or full, the patient must be assisted in emptying her bladder. Many methods have been used to help a patient void. Some of the following have helped:

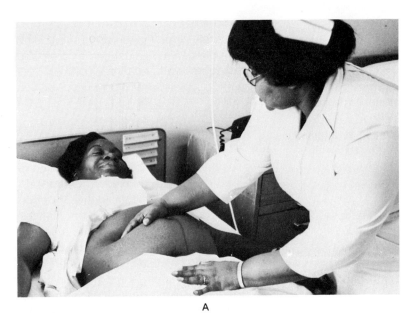

A

fig. 12-3 Postpartum bladder check. (a) A full bladder has displaced the uterus to the right. (b) After woman has voided, fundus is in midline and below umbilicus. (*Photo by Ruth Helmich. Courtesy of the Jamaica Hospital, Jamaica, N.Y.*)

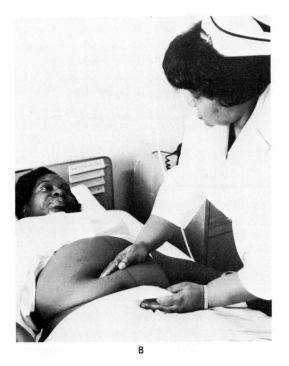

B

1 Have the patient walk whenever possible. Walking to the bathroom is normal and may trigger voiding.
2 If the patient is unable to walk, place her in a sitting position, either with a commode or on the bedpan.
3 Warm the bedpan and pour measured warm water over the perineal area.
4 Run the water faucet.
5 Provide for privacy. Give the patient fluids.
6 If the patient can walk, sitting in a warm tub often stimulates voiding. A sitz bath, especially the portable variety, may help.

Other methods that have been used to induce voiding are ice applications to the suprapubic area and hypnosis.

Early ambulation reduces the need to catheterize for retention. If the patient experiences difficulty in voiding, catheterization is done only upon the physician's orders. Catheterization is the *least* desirable method of emptying the bladder because of the possibility of contamination during the procedure. The meatus of the urethra may be edematous and difficult to locate. Explain the procedure to the patient, and drape her. Use a good light source and get some assistance if it seems necessary. If she is unable to void at all within 6 to 8 h of delivery, a Foley catheter may be inserted and left in place until edema or spasm has diminished.

After the first 24 h, when the patient is ambulatory, she generally requires little assistance in voiding. After the second day she may notice *polyuria* (frequent urination of large amounts). The change in hormonal levels of estrogen and progesterone leads to a diuresis during the intermediate period, when the excess body water and blood volume of pregnancy begin to diminish. An accurate record of intake and output is maintained until the patient is free of problems and the possibility of retention of urine, or residual urine in the bladder.

bowels

The abdominal muscles used in the act of defecation have been stretched and may be flaccid and ineffective in assisting with defecation. For this reason many patients experience difficulty in having a bowel movement in the early puerperium. Some of the means used to reestablish proper bowel function could include the following:

Exercise to tone stretched muscles
Early ambulation
Adequate diet
Adequate fluid intake

Some physicians order stool softeners or laxatives to assist the patient until she is able to resume adequate bowel elimination. Occasionally the doctor may order an enema to

eliminate straining or pain for the first bowel movement. A patient with hemorrhoids may require stool softeners, enemas, local medication, sitz baths, compresses, or suppositories to reduce pain and swelling and to assist with elimination.

vital signs

The vital signs are altered in the recovery period because of three radical changes in circulatory status: (1) removal of the placental bypass, (2) sudden change in intraabdominal pressure, and (3) the return to the system of 300 to 400 ml of blood which had formerly circulated to the uterine and placental tissue.

blood pressure Pressures may rise or fall during the immediate postpartum period. Factors effecting a rise in pressure are the physical exertion of labor, medications (particularly oxytocics), and the rapid infusion of intravenous fluids. Factors effecting a hypotensive response are the level of anesthetic or analgesic, the amount of blood loss at delivery, and the sudden change in intraabdominal pressure, which may allow blood to pool in the pelvic veins. It is important to compare pressures with baseline readings. The following schedule can serve as a guide for the frequency of vital signs in the recovery period.

Every 15 min × 1 h
Every 30 min × 6
Every hour × 3
Then every 4 h until stable
Then twice a day until discharge

pulse The pulse rate may become rapid and change in character before blood pressure drops to indicate hemorrhage. Fatigue may also elevate the pulse rate. An elevated pulse rate without any apparent cause may be an indication of infection or thrombophlebitis. Usually, pulse rates drop in the recovery period and may fall to as low as 60 beats per minute. During the postpartum period, pulse rates will slowly return to prepregnancy levels as body water and hypervolemia of pregnancy subside.

respirations Until the patient is fully reacted after delivery, respiratory rate should be checked. With the pressure of the enlarged uterus gone, she may breathe more easily, and respirations will return to normal rates quickly in the first few days. Analgesics and anesthetics may decrease respiratory rates, while hypotension and infection may increase them.

Temperature Dehydration, excitement, or fatigue may cause an elevation of temperature. Occasionally just after delivery, the patient may experience "chilling." This sensation lasts for about 10 to 15 min and has multiple causes, none of which are agreed upon. Various theories include: chilling resulting from exhaustion, change in intraabdominal pressures, and small infusions of fetal blood or amniotic fluid through the torn placenta. Simple supportive techniques provide comfort during this brief episode. Infection must also be considered, especially when there is a history of early ruptured membranes or hemorrhage, a traumatic labor and delivery, or preexisting infection. Unless there is an indication for more frequent checks, the schedule of temperature recordings should be q4h × 24 h, qid for 24 h after it is within normal limits, and then twice a day.

Although signs of postpartal infection are said to be an elevation of 38°C or more in 2 of the first 10 days, excluding the first 24 h, in reality, treatment will be begun as soon as it is observed that symptoms of infection are present. (See Chap. 25 for blood culture techniques and patterns of treatment.)

Homan's sign

The nurse should be aware of a simple procedure to detect the presence of thrombophlebitis in the postpartum patient. With the patient in a supine position, gently push down on the knee while the patient flexes her foot. Pain in the leg or the calf may indicate the beginnings of thrombophlebitis (see Chap. 23).

emotional state

Immediately after delivery the woman may experience elation and feel excited and "high" on the experience of giving birth and seeing her infant. She may talk excessively, asking questions over and over about the steps in the process. On the other hand, the fatigue generated by the process she has been through may tire her excessively, and she may wish only to sleep. The nurse must be sensitive to each individual and support whatever needs she expresses. Chapter 13 contains a complete discussion of these postdelivery moods.

REST AND SLEEP

Labor and delivery are strenuous, fatiguing activities. It may be difficult for the patient to rest after the excitement of the delivery, but the process of recovery is based upon adequate rest. Without sufficient rest and sleep her recovery will be retarded and she will become irritable, frustrated, and unable to cope with the situations around her, including the care of the new infant. Her need for rest cannot be overemphasized and must be a nursing priority. Nursing activities should be grouped and planned to interrupt the patient as little as possible.

After the first 24 h, at least half her day

should be spent resting in bed. If the patient finds it difficult to sleep in the hospital because of the noise, smells, and hospital routines, nursing intervention may be necessary. A back rub, a warm drink, conversation, altering the environment, or, as a last resort, a sleeping medication will promote a good night's rest. If the telephone is disturbing to daytime rest, it should be disconnected while the patient naps.

VISITORS

In the first 24 h the visitors are usually limited to the husband, the father of the child, or a member of the immediate family. Visiting time should be brief so that the patient can rest. Should she become lonely for visitors, encourage her to use the telephone to visit.

Depending on hospital procedures, usually the husband, parents, boyfriend, or other members of the family are allowed visiting privileges. Sibling visiting is a new development and a long-overdue change in policy (see Chap. 13). Visitors, although they are welcomed by the patient, can be exhausting.

DIET

One of the first needs of the newly delivered patient is for something to eat or drink. She has been without oral intake for several hours, and unless she has received intravenous fluids she is probably dehydrated. Replacement of fluids and electrolytes and the blood volume lost through diaphoresis and through the exertion and fluid loss of delivery are part of postpartal care. The patient requires adequate fluid intake to help her to void, to maintain a normal temperature, and to maintain adequate nutrition. With the exceptions below, the postpartum patient is allowed whatever she wishes to eat or drink:

The patient who is nauseated, vomiting, or not fully reacting because of a general anesthetic

The patient who must lie flat in bed because of a caudal or spinal anesthetic

The heavily sedated, drowsy, or unconscious patient

The diabetic, cardiac, or toxemic patient (or some other type of patient requiring a special diet)

Just after delivery the patient usually appreciates a cup of tea or coffee, preferably with sugar or honey. Encourage her to take fluids slowly to avoid nausea. Throughout her hospitalization the patient is encouraged to eat a well-balanced diet to assist her body in the healing regenerative process.

WEIGHT

At delivery the patient loses approximately 12 to 13 lb. This weight consists of the fetus, placenta, amniotic fluid, membranes, and blood. Contrary to what is generally believed, not all patients lose further weight during the first 8 days of the puerperium. In a study of 200 postpartum patients, Sheikh discovered that approximately 28 percent of the patients showed weight *gain* during the first 3 days after delivery.[1] Only 40 percent of the patients showed a weight loss. Breast-feeding patients lost significantly more weight than nonlactating patients.

A possible explanation might include the sodium- and water-retaining properties of the hormones used to suppress lactation. (The stress reaction of sodium and water retention and potassium loss found in postoperative patients may possibly explain the weight gained during the first week of the puerperium.) In any case, unless the patient gained excess weight during her pregnancy, she should return to her prepregnant weight by the end of the puerperium. If she gained excess weight, she may have difficulty losing it during the next few months. When weighing the patient, the nurse should check to see that she:

Has voided before being weighed
Is wearing a similar weight of clothing each day
Is weighed at the same time each day, usually before breakfast

DIAPHORESIS

Labor and delivery are strenuous activities, and many patients perspire freely during this time. In the body's attempt to rid itself of the extra tissue fluids accumulated during pregnancy, the patient may perspire profusely. Diaphoresis may also be caused by the hormonal changes in the body. Many patients experience nocturnal diaphoresis and awake during the night damp with perspiration.

It is important for the nurse to be aware of these physiologic reactions in order to reassure the patient that it is a normal body response and to provide comfort measures.

BATH

After the strenuous activity of labor and delivery, the patient, tired and perspiring, will probably welcome a sponge bath. The initial bath is given by the nurse either in the recovery room or on the postpartum floor. The patient may require special mouth care because of the special breathing techniques performed during labor and delivery or the drying action of scopolamine.

The patient may be drowsy and not reacting normally because of residual effects of analgesia or anesthesia. If the patient is not awake or alert enough when the nurse bathes her the first time, the nurse will have to teach her about the following hygienic care when she is alert:

1 Wash her hands. Then, with a clean washcloth, wash her breasts first. Start with the nipple and wash in a circular motion away from the nipple if she is breast-feeding.
2 Wash the rest of the body in the usual manner.
3 Use perineal care technique rather than a rough washcloth to cleanse the perineum.

Once the woman is ambulating without difficulty she is encouraged to take a shower. The emergency signal call-light should be brought to the attention of the patient. The nurse should carry an ammonia "pearl" in her pocket whenever she accompanies a newly delivered mother to a shower or sitz bath. Fainting is not uncommon.

Some physicians are encouraging their patients to take tub baths when a bathtub is available on the unit. They believe that immersion of the body in water is more effective in removing the lochia from the perineum and, particularly, from the folds of the labia. The warm water soothes the episiotomy, relieves the edema and soreness of the area, and soothes hemorrhoids if they are present. Water does not enter the vaginal canal, so there is no danger of infecting the uterus from this source. The nurse must accompany the patient for her first tub bath, to check on the cleanliness of the tub, to help the patient into the tub, and to acquaint her with the call-signal light should she need it. On subsequent days, the patient can shower or bathe on her own with assistance from the nurse as necessary.

AFTERPAINS

As discussed earlier, the uterus contracts and retracts in its descent into the pelvic area. In the primipara these contractions are generally painless. However, in the multipara or the patient whose uterine muscles have been stretched excessively, as in polyhydramnios, or multiple pregnancies, the uterus has lost some of its tonicity. For these patients the contractions may be painful. The pain usually subsides in 4 to 7 days. Mild analgesics are given as prescribed (see Chap. 20).

Lactating patients may be aware of the contractions when the infant nurses because of the sucking stimulus to oxytocin release.

BREAST CARE

During the prenatal period the patient has usually learned to wear a firm supporting bra and to cleanse her breasts daily. Especially when a mother is to breast-feed, these points should be reinforced. The nurse needs to check on breast condition daily for signs of infection, inflammation, or cracking or fissures of nipples. Be sure to touch the breast with clean hands only, after explaining to the patient why the inspection is done and how she can continue such a check during the recovery period.

The non-breast-feeding mother is usually given hormones to suppress lactation. Occasionally a woman may still experience engorgement, with the breasts becoming enlarged, hard, painful, and warm to the touch. The nurse can employ several measures to relieve the patient's discomfort:

1 Apply an ice pack to the breasts, as ordered by the physician.
2 Check that the woman is wearing a supporting bra or apply a breast binder.

3 Administer a mild analgesic as prescribed by the physician.

Nonlactating mothers should not pump the breasts to relieve engorgement because this only serves to stimulate further production of milk. Engorgement should diminish under these measures within 36 to 48 h (see Chap. 16).

ACTIVITIES

Just as early ambulation aids in bladder and bowel elimination, it also hastens the recovery of the postpartum patient. Ambulation stimulates circulation and helps to prevent thrombosis. It also helps the body to retain and regain muscle tone. The patient regains her strength sooner without harming her episiotomy or interfering with her vaginal discharge.

The patient should remain in bed until she is fully recovered from the effects of any analgesics or anesthetics she may have received. Unless otherwise indicated the patient should be out of bed initially 4 to 6 h after delivery for a short time with assistance, perhaps to the toilet. While she is in bed, raise the head of the bed and have her turn frequently, to assist in the draining of the lochia.

After the first day, the patient is allowed out of bed at will. However, nursing functions do not stop because the patient is now out of bed. The nurse's role as teacher, planner, and observer is necessary for the ambulatory patient as well. The nurse also sees that the patient rests, has an adequate diet, and does not stand for long periods.

exercise

The exercises the mother may have practiced during the antepartum period will be useful

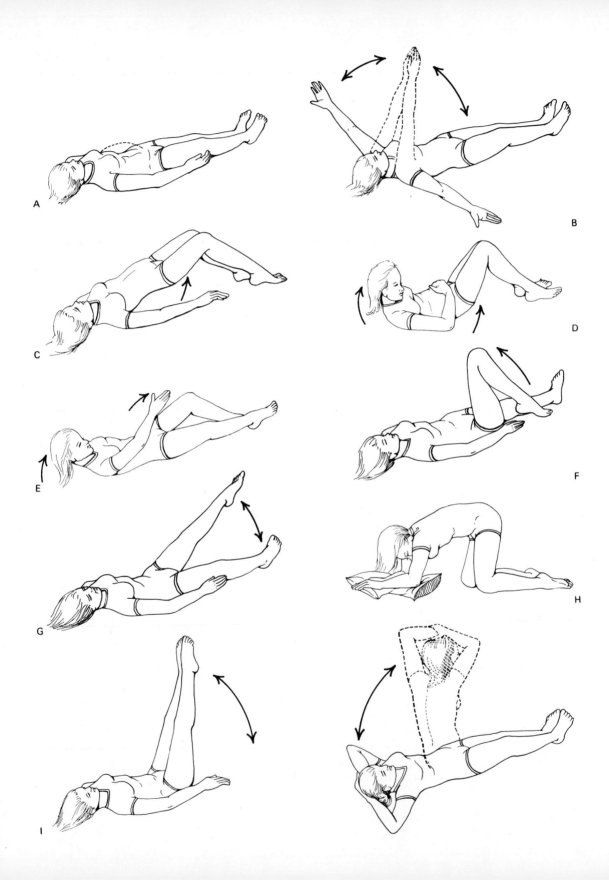

in helping the body and muscles regain strength and tone. Exercise promotes circulation and helps to reduce the possibility of thrombosis. The physician directs the program of exercise for the patient. The following schedule is suggested in the psychoprophylaxis method of preparation for childbirth (PPM) (see Chap. 9 for review and diagrams).

Day of delivery—Kegel exercise
Postpartum day 1 (P.P. 1)—Kegel exercise and pelvic tilt—bid
P.P. 2—Kegel exercise, pelvic tilt, abdominal isometrics, chest breathing
P.P. 3—Same as 2—add head tilt
P.P. 4—Same as 3—add back exercise-arch
P.P. 5—Same as 4—add modified sit-up

Additional exercises are illustrated in Fig. 12-4.

The postpartum period is a crucial time in the recovery process for the patient. The nurse must keep in mind the goals of postpartum care:

To prevent infection or hemorrhage
To promote healing
To promote lactation

Patients are discharged between the second and fifth days after delivery. Referrals are made for any woman who appears to be having difficulty in adjusting physically or psychologically to parenting and recovery goals.

study questions

1 Explain why a distended bladder should be prevented in the immediate postdelivery period.
2 What occurs during involution?
3 Write nurses' notes of the observations you make on a woman 12 h after delivery. What should her condition be if only a local anesthetic was used for a small median episiotomy and, assisted by her husband,

fig. 12-4 Postpartal exercises. Each exercise is to be repeated four times, twice daily, with a new exercise added each day.
(a) *First day:* Breathe in deeply; expand the abdomen. Exhale slowly, hissing; draw in abdominal muscles forcibly.
(b) *Second day:* Lie flat on the back with the legs slightly apart. Hold arms at right angles to the body; slowly raise the arms, keeping the elbows stiff. Touch hands together and gradually return arms to their original position.
(c) *Third day:* Lie flat on the back with the arms at the sides. Draw the knees up slightly. Arch the back.
(d) *Fourth day:* Lie flat on the back with the knees and hips flexed. Tilt the pelvis inward and contract the buttocks tightly. Lift the head while contracting the abdominal muscles.
(e) *Fifth day:* Lie flat on back with the legs straight. Raise the head and one knee slightly. Then reach for, but do not touch, the knee with the opposite hand. Alternate with the right and left hand.
(f) *Sixth day:* Slowly flex the knee and then the thigh on the abdomen. Lower the foot to the buttock. Straighten and lower the leg to the floor.
(g) *Seventh day:* Raise first the right and then the left leg as high as possible. Keep the toes pointed and the knee straight. Lower the leg gradually, using the abdominal muscles but not the hands.
(h) *Eighth day:* Rest on the elbows and knees, keeping the upper arms and legs perpendicular with the body. Hump the back upward. Contract the buttocks and draw the abdomen in vigorously. Relax, breathe deeply.
(i) *Ninth day:* Same as seventh day, but raise both legs at the same time, etc.
(j) *Tenth day:* Lie flat on the back with the arms clasped behind the head. Then sit up slowly. (If necessary, hook feet under furniture.) Slowly lie back.
(*Courtesy of R. C. Benson, Handbook of Obstetrics and Gynecology, 4th ed., Lange, Los Altos, Calif., 1971.*)

she delivered a 3400-g girl using prepared childbirth techniques?

4 Explain the expected pattern of weight loss for a woman who receives a lactation suppressant after delivery (refer to Chap. 20 as well).

5 Which exercises can be recommended for a woman in the first 4 days after delivery?

6 Be sure you can define the terms in this chapter, especially puerperium, lochia, Homan's sign, and Kegel exercise.

references

1 Ghulam N. Sheikh, "Observations of Maternal Weight Behavior during the Puerperium," *American Journal of Obstetrics and Gynecology,* **113**(2):244–250, 1971.

bibliography

Anderson, Edith H.: "Today's Parents and Maternity Nursing," in Betty S. Bergersen et al. (eds.), *Current Concepts in Clinical Nursing,* vol. 1, Mosby, St. Louis, 1967, pp. 355–364.

Clausen, J.: "Efficient Postpartum Checks," *Nursing '72,* October 1972.

Gruis, M.: "Beyond Maternity: Postpartum Concerns of Mothers," *American Journal of Maternal Child Health,* **2**(3):182, May/June 1977.

Hogan, Aileen I.: "The Role of the Nurse in Meeting the Needs of the New Mother," *Nursing Clinics of North America,* **3**:337–344, 1968.

Kleinberg, W.: "Counselling Mothers in the Hospital Postpartum Period: A Comparison of Techniques," *American Journal of Public Health,* **67**(7):672, July 1977.

Lozoff, B., et al.: "The Mother-Newborn Relationship: The Limits of Adaptability," *Journal of Pediatrics,* **91**(1): 1, July 1977.

Obrzut, L. A.: "Expectant Father's Perception of Fathering," *American Journal of Nursing,* **76**(9):1440, September 1976.

"The Postpartum Period," *American Journal of Nursing,* **77**(7):1170–1180, July 1977.

Rich, Olive J.: "Hospital Routines as Rites of Passage in Developing Maternal Identity," *Nursing Clinics of North America,* **4**:101–109, 1969.

Rubin, Reva: "The Neomaternal Period," in Betty S. Bergersen et al. (eds.), *Current Concepts in Clinical Nursing,* vol. 1, Mosby, St. Louis, 1969, pp. 388–391.

Salk, L.: "The Critical Nature of the Postpartum Period in the Human for the Establishment of the Mother-Infant Bond: A Controlled Study," *Diseases of the Nervous System,* Suppl., 110–116, November 1970.

Williams, Barbara: "Sleep Needs during the Maternity Cycle," *Nursing Outlook,* **15**:53–55, 1967.

13

THE FOURTH TRIMESTER

HILDA KOEHLER

INITIAL ADJUSTMENTS

New parents begin to come to grips with being a family at various points in their relationship—some during pregnancy, some at the birth of the baby, some at one of the visiting hours during the hospital stay. For first-time parents, the shift in thinking goes from "We're a couple," to "We have a child." For many it is not until the second child that the orientation becomes "We're a family!"

The first sensations after delivery vary from a matter-of-fact, "I'm relieved *that's* over!" to a mystical, triumphant sense of achievement. For women who actively participate in giving birth, a rush of maternal feeling may occur as the baby is born, with the mother reaching out her arms to enfold the baby (Fig. 13-1). If the baby is active, crying vigorously but becomes quiet in her arms or demonstrates a readiness to suck and nuzzles onto the mother's nipple eagerly, mother-child rapport seems to become more easily established.

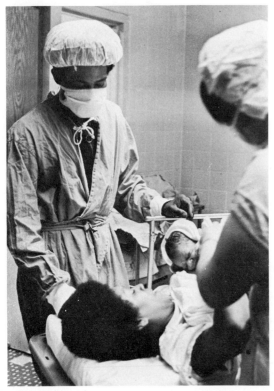

fig. 13-1 Mother holding baby on delivery table. (*Photo by Andrew McGowan.*)

On the other hand, especially to the woman who was not actively involved in the birth of her baby, the newcomer may seem like a very strange creature indeed, and a getting-acquainted period is in order. At first the mother may need to familiarize herself with the baby from top to toe, section by section, exploring with her fingertips in a tentative way (Fig. 13-2). Gradually she will feel more comfortable with the newcomer and will hold the baby close. Since practically all mothers-to-be expect that they will love their babies immediately when they see them, they are likely to be confused and feel guilty at feelings of strangeness and relative indifference in the presence of the little one. Reassurance that it can sometimes take 3 months or more after

the baby comes to begin really to feel like a mother can help ease the strain and start the first stages of this most intimate relationship. (Consult Chapter 17 for information on maternal-infant bonding.)

Most new parents need to know that a newborn baby tends to be very groggy, in a "twilight sleep," after initially being alert and active at birth. If a limp, uninterested, seemingly unresponsive baby is brought in to the mother several hours after birth, she may become anxious about the child's condition; in addition she may feel inadequate as a parent because she cannot rouse the child.

The mother's immediate energy level may vary from intense exhilaration and gaiety, especially in those who were "awake and aware" for the birth, to extreme fatigue and a need for restorative sleep. The nurse will find it therapeutic for the new mother to provide her with the opportunity to share her birth experience—and the nurse may find herself caught up in the mother's enthusiasm and joy.

An early visit with the baby's father, or another family member, is important. The visit should not be too long, though, because, whether or not she is aware of it, the parturient has worked very hard during labor, and she should be urged to try to rest at this point.

fig. 13-2 Mother exploring baby with fingertips. (*Photo by Andrew McGowan.*)

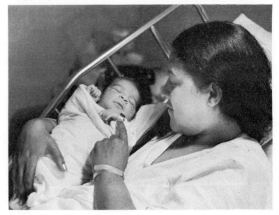

Usually these new mothers can only sleep in naps, anyway, many times reliving the childbirth experience during sleep or rehearsing it mentally in the drowsy state between wakefulness and sleep.

Prolonged, difficult labor or emotional/psychologic complications (for example, when a woman is not going to keep her baby or when there has been an abnormality) may lead her to retreat into sleep for a while. The exhausted new mother needs a milieu in which she can rest undisturbed. It will take a creative, watchful nurse to ensure this atmosphere in a busy hospital with its attendant "routines." Careful planning can minimize the number of times the new mother is disturbed for checking fundus, lochia, voiding, temperature.

If the new father is still present while the mother is resting or delayed in the recovery room, the alert nurse will be sensitive to his needs and suggest appropriate remedies if he seems to need direction. Providing refreshment or a listening ear or finding a place for him to rest undisturbed temporarily are services for which a new father usually is very appreciative.

TAKING IN–TAKING HOLD–LETTING GO

Reva Rubin has described three phases in the puerperium which help nurses to understand the behavior of new mothers and plan their care.[1] The first phase, *taking in*, lasts from 2 to 3 days and is marked by behavior which indicates that the mother is trying to absorb her new experience. She eats, she sleeps, she is concerned with the baby's eating and sleeping, and she is eager to verbalize to anyone ready to listen. The nurse can help her interpret what has happened, enabling her to integrate and make a cohesive whole out of her new status.

The second phase, *taking hold,* lasts about 10 days, and indicates that the new mother is now trying to take some initiative in her responsibility for herself and the infant. What she needs most is support and encouragement. Since she usually questions her competence to take charge of her own life and that of her infant, she may be overzealous in seeking advice and information. Organized teaching programs will be useful during the taking-hold phase—but the wise teacher/nurse will avoid the temptation to appear as having all the answers and knowing all the tricks.[2]

The third phase *letting go* signifies that the mother is ready to regard this new baby as truly a person separate from herself. Some women find this transition harder than others, for some derive great pleasure in considering the baby an extension of themselves.

Differing styles of maternity inpatient services are used throughout the United States today. They range from a rooming-in plan, in which the mother and father assume complete care for the infant, with professional help and guidance available as needed, to the standard central nursery, with the baby being brought out to the mother so that she may feed him only on a periodic basis. Somewhere in between is the flexible family-centered maternity care system, in which new parents participate in the baby's care as much or as little as they wish, with individual assessment made of both the baby and the parents' abilities by the professional staff and a planned educational program for new parents. Recently there has been an impetus, which springs from the expressed desires of parents, to have a "father's hour" in those institutions without rooming-in or family-centered maternity care plans. During "father's hour," the father can handle, play with, and perhaps feed his offspring, with supervision nearby (Fig. 13-3).

Whichever the situation, the nurse's support and anticipatory guidance can determine

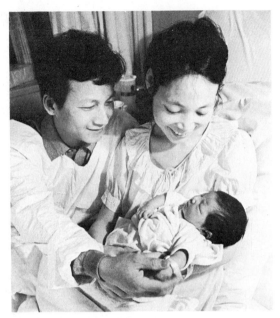

fig. 13-3 "Father's hour": participating in feeding time. (*Photo by Andrew McGowan.*)

POSTPARTUM DEPRESSION

In the intermediate postpartum period (frequently on the third day), there is a distinct possibility that the phenomenon called "after-the-baby blues" may occur. This period of depression can be quite frightening if it is not anticipated. It is thought to be caused by a combination of factors: losing the hormones of pregnancy, which disappear with the expulsion of the placenta; making general physical adjustments to return to the nonpregnant state; and dealing with the reality of the child's

fig. 13-4 Nurse teaching postpartum class on family planning. (*Photo by Nancy Goodman.*)

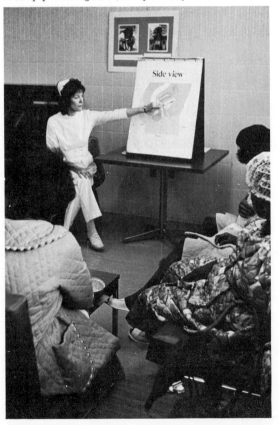

whether the adjustment period at home will be filled with anxiety and frustration or with an operational "Let's-learn-together!" approach, leavened with a sense of humor. If the same person is caring for both mother and baby throughout the course of the hospital stay, there are innumerable opportunities to fit teaching and anticipatory guidance into the natural pattern of care. In standard maternity care, a team plan is usually most convenient and effective, with the nursing care coordinator delegating responsibility to the team member most expert or willing to prepare new parents for home going. Depending on the skill and performance of the instructor, lecture/demonstrations, demonstrations returned by the mother or father, filmstrips/films/videotapes, and coffee-klatch discussions all have their place in helping new parents cope with their new 24-h-a-day, 7-days-a-week responsibility (Fig. 13-4).

truly being here. After-the-baby blues are usually short-lived—48 h at most. Typically, the attention of family and friends has swung from the woman, who enjoyed it during her pregnancy, to the baby. The baby's father may, without thinking, reinforce her feeling of decreased importance by putting his head into her room and saying "Hi! I'm going to go see the baby," and not returning until visiting hours are almost over. Obviously this does nothing for the mother's plunging self-esteem!

Some mothers, though they are relieved that they did not die in childbirth and profoundly grateful that the baby is normal, still have a certain amount of grieving to work through. This baby is simply not the "perfect" child they pictured in their fantasies. Some are exploring the impact which complete responsibility for the child will have on their lives. Others may be disappointed with their performance in labor; they may not have met their own expectations of how they should have acted. Changes in the mother's relationship to her spouse, other children, and possibly other family members may give general cause for apprehension.

If a woman begins to be increasingly irritable and anxious, with crying spells, insomnia, somatic complaints, and seclusiveness, the nurse should suspect that the patient has become one of those new mothers (statistically 1 in every 1000) who are unable to withstand these emotional burdens and who develop a psychosis. When a woman disclaims her baby or confides to a nurse that she doesn't like it or if she begins expressing antipathy toward her husband, the nurse should recognize the need for close observation and psychiatric referral.[3] Generally, the behavior changes indicating pathologic emotional disturbances arise in the first 6 weeks at home. (Some of these psychoses show symptoms during the antenatal period.) A woman who has had a previous mental disorder, with or without pregnancy, is the most obvious candidate for a postpartum psychosis, and the nurse should be particularly alert in such a case and responsive to the cues of depression (see Chap. 7).

GOING HOME

The first day home with a new baby is exciting, tiring, and bewildering (Fig. 13-5a, b). A sense of humor is invaluable. Even parents

fig. 13-5   Going home—a time for anticipatory guidance. (a) Father's turn. (b) Assuming new responsibility. (*Photos by Nancy Goodman.*)

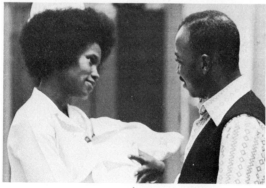
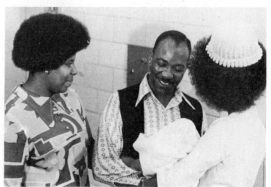

A   B

who have received a thorough orientation to infant care under the guidance of medical professionals are likely to have surprises in store. As Mann states:

> All people experience their babies uniquely. Taking an infant home after childbirth is a human experience so affect laden that it cannot be experienced vicariously. Touching this product of human intimacy, feeling its supplicating tenderness, responding to the urgency of its early bleating helplessness, coming to know its cycles of pain and pleasure, struggling with its phylogenetic heritage of animal needs and impulses, permitting it enough mastery in the external world to insure security while imposing enough limits so that it comes to know reality, these are performances which are necessarily spontaneous and immediate, and no educational procedure can be designed to soften the impact of their newness.[4]

Wuerger notes that:
Many young people are distressed when they are faced with the realities of infant care, and necessary changes in their life style. They've fantasied a cute, smiling, healthy, adaptable infant in their own image, and are presented with a stranger who cries, awakens them for feedings, produces a considerable amount of laundry, catches colds, and keeps them homebound. New parents must learn to know their child—his likes and dislikes, sensitivities, and sensory threshold. They must learn how to provide physical care, love and security, and stimuli for cognitive growth. It is important that they discuss feelings, share responsibilities for child care, and also budget time and resources for themselves.[5]

So those who have carefully schooled themselves for new parenthood, hoping, perhaps unconsciously, to enter the experience as "old hands" are likely to be disappointed. Nothing can totally prepare a parent for the experience of having a new baby but the experience itself.

Tissue recovery is fairly simple; recovery of the whole person, however, is much more complex and requires skillful nurturing. It must be understood that mothers need a chance for their own recovery before they assume full care of a newborn and other roles and responsibilities. Husbands often find that it is not their wives who have returned home, but a patient, and before much else can be done the mother and mate must be nursed back to full health. As a result of conflicting expectations in the postpartum period, there is always some feeling of alienation and resentment, with anger sometimes expressed. With mature partners, reconciliation occurs. Those who are less mature may harbor unexpressed feelings which will hinder family adjustment.[6]

Everyone will want to see the mother and child. But new parents should take caution to limit the number and kinds of visitors, especially the length of time visitors stay. The recovering mother and the newborn are particularly susceptible to infection, so any visitors with skin or upper respiratory infections should be asked to wait until they are well before they visit. The new mother should in no way do anything special to entertain the visitors, but, unless forewarned, she may find herself preparing meals for outsiders—and being exhausted! Signals should be arranged in advance between the mother and another family member, so that she may indicate when she is getting weary; the family then says a gracious but firm goodbye to the guests. If the mother does not get fully dressed for the first 2 weeks, visitors often are more considerate because they realize she does not have her usual level of energy.

HELP

Considering how physically weary new mothers are, and all the anxiety involved in having the complete care of a newborn when the baby is home, one of the most useful things a family can do is to arrange for housework help for the first few weeks at least. Dr. Spock says that if there are twins, the family should go into debt, if necessary, in order to ensure adequate domestic assistance.[7] Dana Raphael stresses the absolute necessity of a person she calls the *doula*, pointing out that almost all non-Western cultures ascribe the role of special assistant to an individual, usually female, who is available during pregnancy, delivery, and the newborn period; the doula teaches the mother how to manage and provides emotional support.[8]

Various sources are possibilities: agencies, family, neighbors; full-time, part-time, rotating help. Most needed is help with cooking, cleaning, shopping, and laundry. Actually, many of these thinngs can be done by new fathers—especially if homemade "TV" dinners are frozen in advance and a flexible schedule prepared which can be consulted after coming home. Many men arrange to take vacation when the baby comes home, which enables them to provide household care. There also are many men who find it very upsetting to leave the house for work, knowing they won't be back for several hours every day—they feel as if they are in some way deserting the family and not providing protection and support.

Mothers and mothers-in-law are most frequently called on to help; in most cases this works out well, but it is wise for the new mother to establish the ground rules ahead of time; otherwise she may find that grandmother is taking care of the baby and mother is doing the cooking, cleaning, etc. Conflict in styles of baby care between the novice mother and the experienced grandmother are an ever-present possibility; these often are focused on disagreements over how, when, and what the child should be fed. Grandmothers may also have a heightened sense of rivalry with their daughters or daughters-in-law, consciously or unconsciously seeking to confirm to themselves and their sons that they are still the experts. A frank discussion before the baby's birth can open the possibility for these feelings and attempts to minimize their destructiveness when the new mother most needs aid and reassurance.

Similarly, a baby nurse may be magnificently instructive and of real assistance to the family, or she may be possessive and tyrannical, scarcely letting the parents near the baby. Her role and functions should be agreed upon prior to employment.

Often overlooked are teenagers or senior citizens in the neighborhood who might be free to spend an hour or two just baby-sitting—listening for the baby, allowing the mother to sleep without having to keep one ear attuned for the baby's cry, or allowing her to go for a walk alone for a short time.

The Visiting Nurse Service is a frequently used resource, either because the new parents seek consultation, or because the professionals send a referral before the family is home. Referrals are especially important when there is a premature birth, when a teenager gives birth, or when there is an abnormality.

Some parents have the misconception that the visiting nurse will bathe the baby, prepare the formula, or perhaps check the house for dust. Being able to see the nurse as a helper instead of a policeofficer and as a consultant instead of a homemaker prepares the family for relating to the visiting nurse appropriately. The mother needs a nurse who can assess her lack of understanding and information and provide this information while conveying the impression that she views her as a concerned and potentially competent mother.[9] "All the technical knowledge is to no avail if the mother sits there and says, 'Yes, yes, I understand.' The only thing that she understands is that, if she says 'yes' to everything, the public health nurse will go away sooner than if she says 'no'."[10]

The following checklist has been found to be very useful. It was developed from the work of Richard and Katherine Gordon.

1   The responsibilities of parenthood are learned: *Get information.*
2   Get help from dependable friends and relatives.
3   Make friends with "experienced" couples.
4   Don't overload yourself with unimportant tasks.
5   Don't move soon after the baby arrives.
6   Don't be concerned with keeping up appearances.
7   Get plenty of rest and sleep.
8   Don't be a nurse to relatives and others at this period.
9   Confer and consult with your friends, family, and each other—*discuss your plans and worries.*
10 Don't give up outside interests, but cut down on responsibilities and rearrange schedules.
11 Arrange for baby-sitters early.
12 Get a family doctor/pediatrician early.[11]

JEALOUSY/RIVALRY

All previous relationships are open to jealousy when a new member joins the family—husband/wife, parent/child, master/pet. Open discussion is the primary means of minimizing jealousy.

husband/wife conflicts

Frequently the fathers of breast-fed infants may discover hostility toward the baby that surprises them, as expressed by one father who said, "Those breasts are mine, not that baby's!" Comprehending the facts intellectually is entirely different from being able to act without emotions interfering, however. An example of this is the new mother who remarked, "He knows I need rest, and urges me to take naps. But then he asks why his socks haven't been washed!"

If the new father participates in the care of the baby—and men are often far better at burping and quieting babies than women—jealousy is often sublimated through this sharing of responsibility. Unfortunately, cultural conditioning or fear of doing damage to the seemingly fragile newborn tends to make some men resist being included. Previous experience during a "father's hour" at the hospital, or in rooming-in or a family-centered maternity care unit, eliminates having to deal with the brunt of these feelings at home, away from professional encouragement and guidance. New mothers may need to be reminded to be sure to leave the new father alone with the child several times a week. He needs to develop his own special relationship with the baby, and her presence can interfere, particularly if she continually makes suggestions as to how to hold, handle, and relate to the baby (Figs. 13-6 and 13-7).

The birth of a son can be particularly stressful for a man who is unsure of his masculinity and his male role. In its extreme, this becomes a pathologic fear of closeness with the new, dependent male.[12] Added responsibility threatens the security of most husbands, but for some, a new son may be a real competitor.[13]

It is not uncommon for a new father's behavior to prompt jealousy in the mother and for the mother to begin to feel that he regards

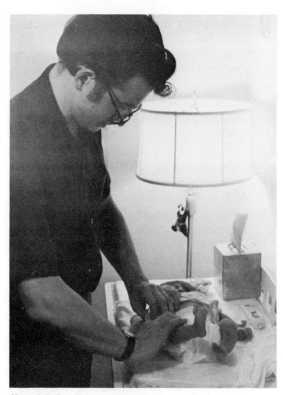

fig. 13-6 Father participates in baby care. (*Photo by John Young.*)

her primarily as the nurturer of his child rather than as his lover/wife. This feeling will be accentuated if he continually comes home from work to concentrate on the activity and behavior of the child, neglecting to relate to her as a person.

sibling rivalry

Other children are sure to be jealous of the new family member, the severity and manifestation of this emotion being peculiarly dependent on the age of the sibling. To the age of approximately 4 years, when the child's logic begins to be fairly reliable, the new baby is looked upon only and absolutely as

an intruder. Saying "We thought you were so wonderful we decided to have another child," to a 2-year-old is equivalent to a husband's telling his wife "I thought you were such a marvelous wife that I've decided to have another one. Here she is! I'm going to sleep with her one night and you the next."

Early, subtle involvement will help determine whether the older child(ren) will be an ally rather than a sulking, potential enemy. Dr. Kappelman[14] suggests the following:

preparation before the baby comes:

1   Include the child in activities related to the coming event, such as shopping, building, painting, redecorating.

fig. 13-7 Father and son get acquainted. (*Photo by John Young.*)

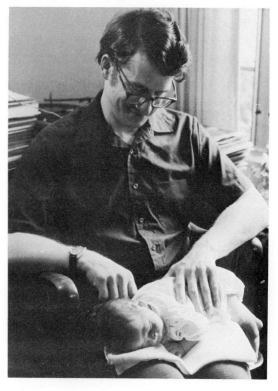

2 Plan with the child where she or he will stay during mother's hospitalization. If staying with a neighbor or relative, spending the night as a "dry run" in advance of the expected due date is a useful plan. (When mother returns as promised, this reassures the child that she or he had not been abandoned.)

3 Be aware that children can misinterpret things they overhear; parents should be matter-of-fact and positive about the impending hospitalization.

4 If the older child will be going into a new bed, make the transfer as early in pregnancy as possible.

5 If possible, begin toilet training well in advance of the new baby's arrival. Otherwise, delay toilet training until the older child has gotten used to the new baby and the attention given the new baby's bowel habits.

6 Consider buying (and wrapping) inexpensive items and storing them for later use when visitors arrive gift-laden for the newcomer. (Dr. Lee Salk cautions that unless handled wisely, giving the older child presents can emphasize materialism and not answer the child's need for caring and appreciation for his or her uniqueness as a special person.[15])

when the new baby arrives:

1 Try to understand that the older child needs to express continued dependency and need for attention. Explaining gently and frequently the positive aspects of "growing up" helps prevent regressive behavior.

2 When guests arrive with gifts for the baby, besides giving the older child the tucked-away surprises at intervals, let the child have the fun of pulling the wraps from the baby's gifts, especially if the child is 2 or 3 years old.

3 Consider giving the older children a special gift when the baby is brought home from the hospital, specifying this as the newcomer's "thank you" for making everything ready.

4 Remember that older children still need physical attention—snuggling, rocking, hugging. Often an older child will demand to be held during a feeding time, work out a way to do so, as this extra assurance helps convince the child that love can be expanded to fit two or three or more children.

5 Let the child "help" with the baby: this helps the child feel important. However, don't overdo it to the point that the older sibling feels like the baby's slave ("I'll never get to *play*, ever again . . .") (Fig. 13-8).

6 Alert other important people in the child's life—grandparents, friends—to be particularly sensitive to the child at this upsetting time. Prevent any anger or hurt that might get displaced on the baby.

7 If there is a change in the expected plan for the newborn, deal with the older child's fears kindly and realistically. For example,

fig. 13-8 Siblings. (*Photo by Karen Gilborn.*)

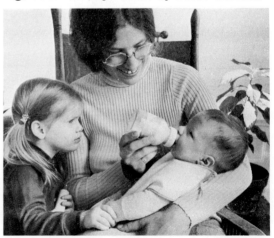

if the baby is premature, try to have a Polaroid picture to show to the older child.

8 Take advantage of books that express the message of the problems the older child experiences in living with the new arrival.

PARENTAL ROLES

Two obstacles are common to new parents as they seek to assume their new responsibilities. The first is a feeling of inadequacy, which can lose much of its devastating effect if a professional can remind them that they are not inadequate but merely inexperienced.

The second obstacle besetting new parents is the feeling of being trapped, followed by a feeling of resentment of the baby. Husbands often need help in understanding how claustrophobic and confining it can be to stay with a baby 24 h a day, 7 days a week. Good, thoughtful planning can eliminate much of this frustration in new mothers.

Mann lists the following as the most important and frequently played roles of parents:

1 Loving, cherishing, enjoying, caring for, giving
2 Observing, listening, inquiring, learning, understanding, accepting
3 Allowing, permitting, consenting, approving, encouraging, praising
4 Sharing, feeling with, playing with, working with, talking with, and even thinking with
5 Guiding, directing, controlling, requiring, leading, disciplining, socializing
6 Informing, teaching, demonstrating, explaining, helping set experience into a set of values and standards
7 Trying to prevent troublesome emotions, such as fear, anger, or hostility; and when these cannot be prevented, helping the child get rid of or manage them.[16]

Surely these are formidable responsibilities. Professionals should give all possible assistance to parents so that they may fulfill their roles smoothly—even if it takes the simple form of affirming their competence and goodwill.

INTERCONCEPTIONAL CARE

resuming sexual intercourse

Most obstetricians instruct new mothers that they should abstain from intercourse during the last few weeks of pregnancy and that nothing should go into the vagina until after the checkup 4 to 6 weeks postpartum; that is, "no douching, no tampons, and no sex." For the first couple of weeks after the baby is born, when the woman is having at least some lochia alba, following those instructions has traditionally been regarded as important to prevent infection. Usually, too, the episiotomy area is healing and tender. But when the episiotomy is healed and there is little vaginal discharge, the issue of whether to resume vaginal intercourse may become a priority. Although the couple may have been using other techniques of sexual pleasure, it may have been 2 or 3 months since the couple has enjoyed intercourse, and it is understandable that they want to resume that part of their relationship. Current opinion advocates counseling couples to return to coitus whenever they so desire. If the episiotomy site is tender, the position should be adjusted so that the shaft of the penis does not press directly on the posterior perineal area. Usually, intercourse tends to soften the scar and thus decreases problems in time.[17]

Women seem to divide clearly into two groups: those who are most eager to resume sexual intercourse and those who are completely uninterested. Frequently this subject is not discussed by any of the professionals who come in contact with the couple; but resuming intercourse certainly deserves as much attention as how to prepare formula!

If the woman is breast-feeding, vaginal secretions and lubrication may be greatly diminished because of the hormones that maintain lactation; water-soluble lubricants can be used to facilitate the comfort of love play and penetration. For some women, full, leaking breasts will be accompanied by a let-down reflex during orgasm. This may not only make the traditional position impossible but may also make for a very liquid experience if a towel is not used.

return of ovulation

Breast-feeding women are unlikely to ovulate for the first 9 weeks if they are giving the baby no other food, so that chances of conception are rare.[18] However, if one becomes pregnant, one is 100 percent pregnant, so contraception should be used.

If a woman is bottle feeding, the couple should know that she may ovulate before she resumes having periods, at 4 to 6 weeks. More and more women who plan to use contraceptive pills are beginning to use them on leaving the hospital. But not everyone is so protected.

contraceptive decisions and health maintenance

Women using contraceptive pills or an intrauterine device will receive a thorough physical examination each time they come for a follow-up visit, usually at least annually. Many women are tempted not to return for their postpartum checkup; they feel well and consider their chart's paperwork in order. The

nurse is in a key position to impress the mother that a postpartum examination is not simply "routine." Valuable data as to the woman's general well-being, as well as confirmation that the reproductive organs have resumed proper nonpregnant position and function, can set the woman's mind at rest, as well as give her family confidence in her ability to do her nurturing tasks. If conditions such as slight anemia or cervical erosions exist, they can be treated before they become major problems. At this visit, the effectiveness of the body-toning exercises that the woman should have been doing can be assessed and further instructions given as necessary. The nurse or the physician can teach or reinforce the necessity and method of breast self-examination and the wisdom of interconceptional health maintenance, including a Papanicolaou test.

In past years the health checkup was considered even more of a waste of time than the postpartum examination. But with the renewed emphasis on preventive medicine, plus the impact of the Woman's Movement, more and more women are taking advantage of gynecologic services before their condition demands a visit. With the expected coming of a national health care system within the next few years, women from all socioeconomic levels will use health maintenance facilities, not the least important of which is early prenatal care and complete postdelivery care.

study questions

1   In what ways do the hospital personnel work to support infant-parent bonding? How are fathers included?
2   What suggestions can you formulate to promote parenting skills while the couple is still adjusting to the thought of a new baby?
3   A 20-year-old primipara who was seemingly full of joy and enthusiasm on her first postpartum day greets you 24 h later with, "My mother is coming to help me for a month after I go home from the hospital!" What

phase of adjustment is she in at this point in recovery? What considerations would you explore with her?

4 The mother for whom you are caring had a very difficult forceps delivery, with some lacerations. How would her physical condition influence the counseling you would give her regarding sexual activity in the postpartum period?

5 What clues would alert you to anticipate the development of severe postpartum depression in any recovering mother?

6 Plan a discussion with a mother about how to reduce the impact of a new baby's arrival for her 3-year-old child.

references

1 Reva Rubin "Puerperal Change" *Nursing Outlook,* **9**(12):753-755, 1961.

2 Betty S. Bergersen et al., "Adapting Postpartum Teaching to Mothers' Low-Income Life-styles" in *Current Concepts in Clinical Nursing,* Mosby, St. Louis, 1969, chap. 27, pp. 280–291.

3 Elizabeth M. Seward, "Preventing Postpartum Psychosis," *American Journal of Nursing,* **72**(3):529, 1972.

4 David Mann et al. *Educating Expectant Parents,* Visiting Nurse Service of New York, New York, 1961.

5 Mardelle Wuerger, "The Young Adult: Stepping into Parenthood," *American Journal of Nursing,* **76**(8): 1283–1285, 1976.

6 Reva Rubin, "Maternity Nursing Stops Too Soon," *American Journal of Nursing,* **75**(10):1680–1684, 1975.

7 Benjamin Spock, *Baby and Child Care,* Pocket Books, New York, 1976.

8 Dana Raphael, "The Role of Breastfeeding in the Bottle Oriented World," *Ecology of Food and Nutrition,* **2**:121, 1973.

9 Rosalee C. Yeaworth, "Maternity Nursing—Challenging or Routine?" *Nursing Clinics of North America,* **6**(2):247, 1971.

10 Marguerite W. Bozian, "Nursing Care of the Infant in the Community," *Nursing Clinics of North America,***6**(1):93, 1971.

11 R. E. Gordon et all. "Factors in Postpartum Emotional Adjustments," *Obstetrics and Gynecology,* **25**(2): 158–166, 1965.

12 Arthur D. Coleman and Libby Lee Coleman, *Pregnancy: The Psychological Experience,* Herder and Herder, New York, 1971, p. 164.

13 Ibid., p. 165.

14 Murray M. Kappelman, *What Your Child Is All About,* Reader's Digest Press, New York, 1974.

15 Lee Salk, *Preparing for Parenthood,* Bantam, New York, 1974, p. 50.

16 Mann, op. cit., p. 102.

17 Ann L. Clark and Ralph W. Hale, "Sex During and After Pregnancy," *American Journal of Nursing,* **74**(8):1430–1431, 1974.

18 T. J. Cronin, "Influence of Lactation upon Ovulation," *Lancet,* **2**:422, 1968.

bibliography

Alfonso, Dyanne D.: " 'Missing Pieces'—a Study of Postpartum Feelings," *Birth and the Family Journal,* **4**(4): 159–164, 1977.

Bishop, B.:"A Guide to Assessing Parenting Capabilities," *American Journal of Nursing,* **76**(11):1784–1787, 1976.

Brown, M. S. and J. T. Hurlock: "Mothering the Mother," *American Journal of Nursing,* **77**(3):439–441, 1977.

Bergersen, B. S. et all.: "Adapting Postpartum Teaching to Mother's Low-Income Life-styles," in *Current Concepts in Clinical Nursing,* Mosby, St. Louis, 1969, chap. 27.

Bordon, D.: "Puerperal Psychosis" *Nursing Times,* **68**(20):615, 1972.

Boston Women's Health Collective: *Our Bodies, Ourselves,* Simon and Shuster, New York, 1976.

Clark, A. L. and Afonso, D. D.: "Mother-Child Relations. Infant Behavior and Maternal Attachment: Two Sides of the Coin" *American Journal of Maternal Child Nursing,* **1**:94–99, 1976.

Derthick, N.: "Sexuality in Pregnancy and the Puerperium" *Birth and the Family Journal,* **1**(4):5–9, 1974.

Donaldson, N. E.: "Fourth Trimester Follow-up," *American Journal of Nursing,* **77**(7):1176–1178, 1977.

Eckes, S.: "The Significance of Increased Early Contact Between Mother and Newborn Infant," *Journal of Obstetric Gynecologic and Neonatal Nursing,* **3**(4):42–44, 1974.

Edwards, Margot: "The Crises of the Fourth Timester," *Birth and the Family Journal,* **1**(1):19–22, 1974.

Fein, R. A.: "The First Weeks of Fathering: The Importance of Choices and Supports for New Parents," *Birth and the Family Journal,* **3**(2):53–57, 1976.

Greenburg, M. and Morris, N.: "Engrossment: The Newborn's Impact upon the Father," *American Journal of Orthopsychiatry,* **44**:520–531, July 1974.

Good, R. S.: "The Third Ear: Interviewing Techniques in Obstetrics and Gynecology," *Obstetrics and Gynecology,* **40**(5):760, 1972.

Heise, J.: "Toward Better Preparation for Involved Fatherhood," *Journal of Obstetric, Gynecologic, and Neonatal Nursing,* **4**(5):32–35, 1975.

Hurd, J. M. L.: "Assessing Maternal Attachment: First Step Toward the Prevention of Child Abuse," *Journal of*

Obstetric, Gynecologic, and Neonatal Nursing, **4**(4): 25–30, 1975.

Kennell, J. H. et al.: "The Mother-Newborn Relationship: Limits of Adaptability," *The Journal of Pediatrics,* **91**(1): 1, 1977.

Kitzinger, S.: *The Experience of Childbirth,* 3d ed., Penguin Books, Baltimore, 1972.

Klaus, M. H. and Kennell, J. H.: *Maternal-Infant Bonding,* Mosby, St. Louis 1976.

Ludington, S. M.: "Postpartum: Development of Maternicity," *American Journal of Nursing,* **77**(7):1171–1174, 1977.

Mercer, R. T.: "Postpartum: Illness and Acquaintance-Attachment Process," *American Journal of Nursing,* **77**(7): 1174–1178, 1977.

Millington, M. et all.: "For High-Risk Infants and Their Parents: Postnatal Discussion Groups and Well-Baby Clinics Operate in Storefront," *Journal of Obstetric, Gynecologic and Neonatal Nursing,* **4**(1):42–46, 1975.

Rath, P. G.: "Sibling Rivalry," *American Baby* **39**(4): 36–38, April 1977.

Ratsoy, M. Bernadet: "Maternity Patients Make Decisions," *The Canadian Nurse,* April 1974, pp. 42–44.

Reiber, F. D.: "Is the Nurturing Role Natural to Fathers?" *American Journal of Maternal Child Nursing,* **1**(6): 366–371, 1976.

Richardson, A. Cullen et al.: "Decreasing Postpartum Sexual Abstinence Time" *American Journal of Obstetrics and Gynecology,* **126**(4):416–417, 1976.

Rozdilsky, M. L. and B. Banet: *What Now?: A Handbook for Parents Postpartum,* Magic Machine, Seattle, 1972.

Rubin, R.: "Maternity Nursing Stops Too Soon," *American Journal of Nursing,* **75**(10):1680–1684, 1975.

Salk, L.: *Preparing for Parenthood,* Bantam, New York, 1974.

Shaywitz, S. E.: "Catch 22 for Mothers" *The New York Times Magazine,* Mar. 4, 1973, p. 50.

Smoyak, Shirley (ed.): "Parenting" *The Nursing Clinics of North America,* **12**(3):447–532, 1977.

Trien, S. F.: "Chasing Those Blues Away," *American Baby,* **39**(5):38–39, 1977.

14

ASSESSMENT OF THE NEWBORN INFANT

ELIZABETH J. DICKASON
BONNIE SILVERMAN

3

THE HEALTHY INFANT

During the first 28 days after birth the newborn infant experiences a number of adaptations to life outside the uterus. The first 24 h are the most critical, and adjustment becomes easier once the immediate cardiorespiratory changes have been accomplished. All supportive care for the newborn infant is based upon an understanding of these adjustments.

Assessment takes place during this period as well. The infant becomes identified as a specific, individual baby, with a unique inheritance and still unknown potential for growth and development. It is this potential which must be protected before birth, during birth, and after birth.

RESPIRATORY ADAPTATION

initiation of respiration

All infants are born in a slightly hypoxic state with a cord pH averaging 7.28. With additional distress during birth, the pH may be even lower, and spontaneous respirations may be delayed. This pH of 7.28 serves as one initial stimulus to respirations. Higher carbon dioxide levels and lower oxygen levels stimulate the respiratory center in the brain and activate aortic and carotid chemoreceptors. (The state of acidosis has been correlated with the Apgar score; see Table 15-2.) A near-normal acid-base state should be achieved by 1 h after birth if the infant progresses as expected.

A second stimulus is the squeezing of the thorax, which occurs during expulsion through the vagina. Intrathoracic pressures of 60 to 100 cmH$_2$O are created.[1] In response to this compression, just as the head emerges, 5 to 10 mL of amniotic fluid is expressed from the trachea and bronchi, thus clearing out the upper airways to allow easier filling with air. (Suctioning may remove more fluid.) The chest and abdomen recoil when the intrathoracic pressure is suddenly released at birth. As sudden expansion of the chest wall occurs, air is drawn deep into the pulmonary tree.

A third stimulus is the response of stretch receptors in the bronchi to the sudden change of pressure on first inspiration. Later, these same receptors respond to changes of pressure resulting from application of positive pressure in those cases where resuscitation is needed.

Finally, temperature changes, gravity, and the sensations associated with touching, handling, and suctioning the infant contribute to the initial respiratory responses. It is important for these stimuli to come into play, because any delay in the establishment of respirations will lead to further acidosis, and resuscitative measures will have to be initiated (see Chap. 29).

The first deep gasping breaths draw air into the lungs under an initial negative pressure of 40 to 45 cmH$_2$O, but after a residual volume is built up, a negative pressure of only about 5 to 7 cmH$_2$O is needed to exchange air. A residual volume is quickly built up in normal, nonstressed infants because only about half the inspired air is expelled with each early breath. Residual volume can be maintained because of the presence of the substance *surfactant*, a phospholipid of low surface tension which lines the alveolus and promotes movement of oxygen across the membrane. The presence of adequate surfactant allows the alveolus to remain open on expiration. (If each alveolus collapsed with each breath, the pressures to open it again would be just as great as those needed initially.) Surfactant is produced in increasing amounts during the last weeks of fetal life and should be quite adequate by the time a full-term infant is born. The lecithin/sphingomyelin ratio is one test used to assess maturity of lung function (see Chap. 27).

Lung fluid normally consists of secretion from fetal pulmonary capillary blood and some secretion from alveolar cells. After the chest compression of birth, the residual fluid which remains is removed in the early hours through the lymphatic circulation or is absorbed into the pulmonary circulation.[2]

maintenance of respirations

In the first 10 min, breathing patterns are quite irregular in rate, rhythm, and depth. Rates then assume an average of 40 to 50 breaths per minute, as lower pressures are needed to exchange air. Tidal volume assumes a level of about 15 to 20 cm^3. Respirations are still characteristically irregular in rate, rhythm, and depth but will become progressively more regular as the infant matures. A consistent rise above 60 breaths per minute is a sign of respiratory difficulty. Short periods of apnea are common in the early hours of adjustment. Although periodic breathing and short (<5 sec) apneic periods may be present in the early days of life, longer periods than these may be associated with illness or immaturity.

The respirations appear to be the result of diaphragmatic movement, with a slight drawing in at the lower rib margin. Any other use of accessory muscles of respiration, e.g., intercostal retractions, is a result of some difficulty in exchanging air and should be investigated (see Table 29-1). If marked irregularities in the respiratory pattern persist beyond the first few hours, the cause may be a state of continuing acidosis, birth injury, infection, respiratory distress, or depression of the respiratory center from the effects of maternal drugs during the transitional period.

CARDIOVASCULAR ADAPTATION

Before birth, about 10 percent of fetal blood circulates through the lungs to supply tissue oxygenation. When the baby takes its first breath and air is inspired, a number of changes take place. Alveoli open, pulmonary vascular resistance decreases, and there is a sudden increase in volume of flow through the pulmonary artery. In addition, after the initial deep breaths, circulation to the placenta ceases and pressures rise throughout the systemic system.[3]

High pulmonary vascular resistance has been present during fetal life. After the initial cardiovascular changes, vascular resistance continues to decrease and takes some time to reach the lower adult levels. In certain instances, the normal initial decline, followed by a continuing decrease in vascular resistance, does not take place as expected. Such continuing higher pressures are found when infants experience certain types of respiratory distress.[4]

Since blood will flow to the areas of least resistance, more blood should circulate to the pulmonary tissue because of this reduced resistance. After complete adjustment to extrauterine life is accomplished, the fraction of cardiac output going to the lung for oxygen exchange is proportional to that in the adult.

With access to inspired air, higher partial pressures of arterial oxygen (Pa_{O_2}) become possible in neonatal life than were possible in fetal life. In response to these higher oxygen levels and pressure changes, the ductus arteriosus (DA) constricts. (Substances such as the prostaglandins and bradykinin may also contribute to closure by stimulating smooth muscle constriction.) Functional closure of the DA is almost complete by 24 h unless episodes of hypoxia occur; under the stimulus of low oxygen tensions the DA can reopen and a shunt can be reestablished. Preterm infants with hyaline membrane disease are especially vulnerable to this reversal of blood flow.

With increased blood flow into the pulmonary circulation, a much higher flow must return from the lungs through the pulmonary vein (PV) into the left atrium. This flow serves to close the flap of the foremen ovale (FO), almost as if there were a "swinging trap door." Final anatomic closure does not take place for several months, but these mechanical pressures usually effect most of the closure soon after birth. Exceptions occur under the same conditions that keep the ductus arteriosus open. Obviously, maintaining adequate arterial oxygen levels is indeed important in early cardiovascular adjustment (Fig. 14-1).

As listed in Table 14-1, in most cases fetal structures change to become ligaments. However, the proximal parts of the umbilical arteries remain open as the internal iliac arteries, while the distal sections atrophy to form the lateral umbilical ligaments.

umbilical cord

The umbilical cord, with two arteries carrying deoxygenated blood from the fetus to the placenta and one vein carrying oxygenated blood from the placenta to the fetus, is no

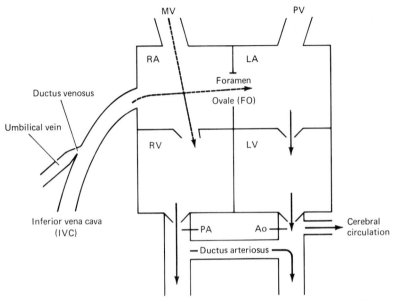

fig. 14-1 Diagrammatic scheme of fetal circulation. (*From M. H. Klaus and A. A. Fanaroff, Care of the High-Risk Neonate, Saunders, Philadelphia, 1973.*)

longer necessary. Clamping of the cord is done routinely, although the changes in circulation resulting from the first deep gasping breaths effectively reverse circulation pressures and stop flow to the placenta. Thus, in situations where sterile materials to clamp and cut the cord are not available, the newborn can remain attached to the placenta for a longer period without harm. (See "Emergency Delivery," Chap. 26.)

Within the first 15 to 30 s after birth, the squeezing associated with birth contractions has infused the infant with about 50 mL of blood. Controversy developed over whether it was better for the infant to have an additional amount of infusion, which is obtained by holding the infant below the level of the placenta for 2 to 3 mins and milking the cord toward the infant. Even though the newborn receives extra iron by this means, the extra hemoglobin may also increase bilirubin levels in the recovery period. Polycythemia, with hematocrit values over 65 percent, and hyperviscosity may also result. Opinion today favors a compromise, with less delay in clamping the cord, but with enough time (at

table 14-1 Anatomic changes in the fetal structures after birth

fetal structures	infant structures	range in which change is completed
Foramen ovale	Fossa ovalis	Several weeks to 1 year
Ductus arteriosus	Ligamentum arteriosum	Several weeks to 1 year
Ductus venosus	Ligamentum venosum of the liver	1–2 mo
Umbilical arteries	Lateral umbilical ligaments	2–3 mo
Umbilical vein	Ligamentum teres of the liver	2–3 mo

least 60 s) for the initial infusion.[5] In cases where iatrogenic problems or fetal distress result in a depressed infant who does not cry spontaneously, early resuscitation of course, takes priority. It may be important to note here that holding the infant above the placental level for an extended period may cause blood to leave the infant and pool in the placenta. Therefore with cesarean section, the infant should be held below the placental level before cord clamping.

Once the cord is clamped, it begins to dry. Within 24 h the Wharton's jelly will have hardened, and the cord appears like a shriveled, tough piece of skin. The clamp is removed once such dryness is evident. Further drying takes place over the first week, and the stump should separate from the skin level by about 7 to 10 days. A red, moist area may remain which will quickly scab over. (See Chap. 15 for the different methods of treating the cord.)

The cord stump will be raised 1 to 2 cm from the abdominal wall at first. It will become flatter and then in most cases will indent as the child grows.

cardiac function

Normal heart rate is between 110 and 160 beats per minute with some arrhythmia, especially when crying. During periods of quiet sleep, rates may be as low as 90, but during crying episodes, they may be as high as 180. In the term newborn in a resting state, any rate below 90 is considered *bradycardia* and any rate above 160 is considered *tachycardia*. Reference to an infant's heart rate in utero may help in the evaluation of its newborn rate. Pulse rates will drop in later infancy to between 110 and 130, and then by 1 year, rates will average about 100 beats per minute. Pulses can be palpated best at the elbow or groin or auscultated over the apex of the heart.

Blood pressure averages about 80/46 in a term infant, rising as infancy progresses to an early childhood level of 100/60. Cardiac output is about 55 mL/min. Blood volume averages 85 to 90 mL/kg in the first few days of life, decreasing to 75 to 80 mL by 2 months.[6]

The infant is born with about 80 percent of its hemoglobin as fetal hemoglobin (Hgb F), a type which has an extra ability to carry oxygen. Once oxygen is available from inspired air, adult hemoglobin (Hgb A) can bind to oxygen quite satisfactorily. Thus, hemoglobin F is not needed, and amounts gradually diminish over the first months of life. (Table 14-2).

In the first few days of the newborn period the hemoglobin levels are as high as 18 to 20 g/100 mL; they then fall to 16 to 17 g. The hematocrit ratio, from a high of 48 to 60 percent, falls toward 45 to 50 percent. Red blood cells are reduced from a level of 5.5 to 6 million per cubic millimeter to 4 to 5 million per cubic millimeter. All this hemolysis results in higher levels of unmetabolized bilirubin, one of the breakdown products of the heme fraction of hemoglobin. The catabolism of 1 g of hemoglobin yields 35 mg of bilirubin. Because of relative polycythemia, the newborn normally produces an average of 8.5 mg/kg of bilirubin per day, more than the healthy adult produces. In addition, there is deficiency of the enzyme *glucuronyl transferase* in the newborn liver. The immature liver is temporarily overloaded and is unable to metabolize the bilirubin into a form which can be excreted or recycled. Thus, all newborns are likely to show some elevation of serum bilirubin. Excess unmetabolized bilirubin (indirect, fat-soluble form) will result in a yellowish color which shows up first in the face and chest. The mean peak of about 6 to 8 mg/100 mL (dL) occurs on the third day of life for term infants. Since jaundice becomes clinically evident at 5 mg/100 mL, those babies who remain below 5 mg will not show signs of

table 14-2 Range of blood values in the fetus and newborn infant

	fetus (last trimester) or preterm infant of 1500–2000 g	term newborn weighing more than 2500 g (cord blood)	7 days later
Red blood cells (million/mm³)	4.5 to 6.5	5.5 to 6	4 to 5
Reticulocytes (%)	6	3 to 5	0 to 1
Hemoglobin [g/ 100 mL (dL)]	17 to 20 (90 to 95% Hgb F, 5 to 10% Hgb A)	17 to 19 (80% Hgb F, 20% Hgb A)	14 to 17
Hematocrit (%)	45 to 60 (others state: 53 to 65)	48 to 60 (avg. capillary blood 5 to 10% higher)	50
White blood cells (per mm³)		Up to 18,000	11,000 to 12,000
Blood volume (per kg)	100 to 108 mL/kg	85 to 90 mL/kg (higher if cord clamped late)	75 to 80 mL/kg by 2 mo
Platelets* (10³ per mm³)	290±70	310±68 (level below 150 is abnormal)	280±56
Prothrombin time* (seconds)	17 (12 to 21)	16 (13–20) Prolonged until 4 days, unless vitamin K given	Adult values by 1 week
Partial thromboplastin time* (seconds)	70±8	55±10	Adult values by 2 to 9 mo
Bilirubin [mg/100 mL (dL)]		1.8 to 2.0	After rising to 4 to 6 mg/100 mL, reduces slowly to adult levels of 1 to 2 mg/ 100 mL
pH	0.15 pH units less than maternal pH (fetal)	7.28 (rising to 7.34 to 7.45 soon after birth if no respiratory difficulty)	7.34 to 7.45

these slightly elevated levels. Normal adult levels, as well as cord levels, are 1.0 to 1.8 mg/mL. Treatment of infants with higher than normal levels is discussed in Chap. 29.

Iron released by the destruction of these erythrocytes is stored to be reused. When active production of red blood cells begins at 1 to 2 months, the infant will eventually need to receive additional iron in the diet or varying levels of anemia may develop. "Without supplemental dietary iron, the body stores of iron will be depleted sometime after two months of age (in the premature) rather than after four to six months of age as in the normal, full term infant."[7] Any supplementation before 2 months does not appear to be necessary, especially if the infant went to term and received maternal stores of iron.

table 14-2 Range of blood values in the fetus and newborn infant (*continued*)

	fetus (last trimester) or preterm infant of 1500–2000 g	term newborn weighing more than 2500 g (cord blood)	7 days later
Pa_{O_2} (mmHg)	35 (rises to 50 to 70 soon after birth)	35 (umbilical venous blood) (rises to 50 to 70 soon after birth)	50 to 70
Pa_{CO_2} (mmHg)	40 to 50 (35 to 40 after birth)	48 (50 to 55)	35 to 40
HCO_3 (meq/L)		17.5	19 to 22
Base excess		−4 to +4	−4 to +4
Glucose [mg/100 mL (dL)]	In utero reflects maternal levels 40 to 50 after birth Severe hypoglycemia when below 20 mg/100 mL (Others indicate that a value of below 40 mg/dL at anytime equals hypoglycemia)	Varies widely; average is 61 to 83 (cord) Severe hypoglycemia when below 30 mg/100 mL during first 72 h	45 to 115; quickly assumes adult range Hypoglycemia if below 40 mg/100 mL
Electrolytes Na (meq/L)	134 to 140 first day, depends on weight	147 to 149	147 to 149
K (meq/L)	5.6 to 6.4	7.8 (5.6 to 12)	5.9 (5.0 to 7.7)
Cl (meq/L)	100 to 105	103 (98 to 110)	103 (98 to 112)
Ca (mg/100 mL)	7.0 to 7.5 (preterm infant)	8 to 10 mg/100 mL or (4 to 5 meq/L) (hypocalcemia if below 8 mg/100 mL)	Imbalance can develop at 7 to 10 days
Mg		0.9 to 2.6 meq/L (depending on maternal level)	1.4 to 1.7

Source: Data from Stave, Smith and Nelson, Klaus and Fanaroff, and Korones.
*From W. E. Hathaway, "The Bleeding Newborn," *Seminars in Hematology* **12**:175, 1975.

RENAL ADAPTATION

Fetal urine is produced from the twelfth week of gestation, but independent renal function is not really necessary until birth. After birth, the kidneys assume the major role in excretion of waste products. Excretion and reabsorption of sodium, other electrolytes, and water has a fairly narrow range of adjustment in the early weeks of life. A glomerular filtration rate of 30 to 40 percent and a tubular secretion rate of 20 to 30 percent of adult values, plus lower reabsorption rates, are present at birth. Thus, during the neonatal period, less bicarbonate, sodium, glucose, amino acids, and phosphate can be reabsorbed. Urine is less concentrated, containing reduced amounts of urea and ammonia.[8] As a result, urine does not smell strongly and is light in color, with a low specific gravity. Specific gravity may be as low as 1.004, ranging to a maximum of 1.018. No protein should be excreted.

Renal function develops rapidly so that by the seventh day of life, glomerular filtration has increased to 50 percent of the adult rate,[9] and by 6 to 12 months the rate is relatively mature. Urinary concentrating ability depends on tubular reabsorption of water, electrolytes, and fat-soluble molecules from the renal filtrate. Mature ability to concentrate urine is generally achieved by 2 months of age in the preterm and somewhat earlier in the term infant. Maturation of tubular secretion occurs within 6 months.[9]

Sodium balance is a particular problem in the young infant. Formulas contain three times the amount of sodium in breast milk, and early feedings of solids may raise intake to ten times that of human milk.[10] As a result of these findings many baby food manufacturers have begun reducing the sodium content of their products (see Chap. 16).

Water balance is also less efficient than in the older infant. The newborn has a higher body water content (70 to 80 percent), with a daily turnover of 50 percent of extracellular water. Thus, imbalance in intake or output can lead to serious problems.

The amount of early urine formation depends partly on the time of cord clamping (as regulating blood volume), partly on the amount of retained body water, and partly on whether early feedings are instituted. In the first 48 h, the infant may form 30 to 60 mL of urine. Often the first voiding is just at delivery, in response to sudden chilling. Such a voiding must be noted, since the infant may not then void for a number of hours. In a recent study of 500 infants, all, regardless of gestational age, had voided by 24 h.[11] If no voiding has been observed by 24 h, the abdomen should be checked for distention just above the pubic bone and the infant seen by the pediatrician.

Voiding may occur as frequently as 10 or 15 times a day in the first month, frequency will then decrease as volume increases. By 2 months, 250 to 450 mL is being excreted daily.

minor variations

On occasion, urate crystals will be seen, leaving a pink-tinged "brick-dust" color on the diaper. These have no significance. In contrast, red blood cells in the urine will make urine appear brown; their presence may indicate renal damage. A baby under bilirubin lights may excrete higher levels of direct bilirubin, and urine may be darker and yellow-brown in color (for related problems see Chap. 29).

GASTROINTESTINAL AND METABOLIC ADAPTATION

The ability to suck and swallow develops during fetal life and is coordinated by 34 weeks. As early as the fourth month of life the fetus swallows amniotic fluid. Toward term, up to 500 mL a day is swallowed. The water is reabsorbed and returned through the placental circulation. Very small amounts of protein (similar to serum levels) are absorbed by the fetus, and the material remaining after digestion stays in the lower intestinal tract to become *meconium,* the first stool after birth.

The gradually maturing digestive functions prepare the infant for a diet of breast milk or modified formula. There is still a reduced ability to digest fats, but these functions quickly mature (see Chap. 16). The intestinal tract is sterile at birth and becomes colonized with bacteria by 48 h. During this initial period, vitamin K cannot be synthesized in the intestine, and levels may be low unless vitamin K is administered parenterally to an infant (see Fig. 15-4).

Certain other functions of the gastrointestinal tract are still maturing. The cardiac sphincter between the esophagus and stomach has less tone than it will later develop; therefore milk and air may be easily regurgitated (spit up) during or after a feeding. Regurgitation is discussed in detail in Chap. 18. The infant's position after feeding and the methods of feeding influence the amount of regurgitation.

stomach volume

The infant's stomach at birth can hold 30 to 60 mL but can expand to take about 100 mL by the end of the first week. The stomach empties rapidly in the right lateral position and in the prone position. It empties much more slowly in the supine or left lateral position.[12]

stool cycle

Meconium is sticky and dark green to almost black as a result of its constituents: bile pigments, fatty acids, mucus, blood, epithelial cells, and amniotic fluid. As the baby begins to ingest milk, the color, consistency, and frequency of the stools change.

Usually by the third postnatal day, the transitional stool appears as green-brown to yellow-brown; it is looser than meconium and contains some mucus. Subsequently, the breast-fed baby has stools which are soft, semiliquid, and yellow, possibly with a sour odor. In contrast, ingestion of cow's milk produces a firmer, paler stool. There is a characteristic, offensive odor to the stool of formula-fed babies.

The frequency of the stools depends upon the type and number of feedings. The number of stools each day may vary from one to eight in the young infant; later, one every other day may be within a normal range for a breast-fed infant. The color and consistency provide the clues to abnormality. Size of the feedings influences the consistency of the stools. Overfeeding can produce loose stools because the baby is unable to digest thoroughly all the milk forced upon it. Underfeeding may produce constipation and small, dark, stools.

metabolic function

The newborn grows rapidly, anabolic function exceeds catabolic function, and weight gain after the initial weight loss should assume a rate of 4 to 5 oz per week (see Chap. 16). The initial weight loss results from loss of retained body water (edema), first voiding and stool, and evaporative losses. Weight loss can be minimized by early feeding. The need for replacement fluids is higher in cases where known factors are contributing to weight loss, e.g., bilirubin light, radiant heaters, too warm an environment, or exposure for treatments without adequate protection.

Early weight loss is also associated with difficulty in feeding. Factors affecting the infant's ability to suck or swallow should be minimized, e.g., maternal analgesia, anesthesia in large doses, or a poorly instructed new mother who does not know how to coax a new infant to feed. Delayed feeding used to be the standard procedure, with the first feeding given by the nurse in the nursery at 12 to 16 h. This is no longer acceptable practice, and infants should be given sterile water within 4 to 6 h after birth. Breast-feeding babies should be put to the breast and then given supplemental water, plus water ad lib between the first few feedings until milk flow is established. Normal weight loss can range between 5 and 10 percent of birth weight; with these interventions, weight loss can be maintained near or below 5 percent.

Extra caloric requirements will result from increased muscular activity, such as crying for long periods, cold stress, diarrhea, or any stress requiring increased energy production. Some babies are more active than others and will use more calories. (See Chap. 16 for average protein, carbohydrate, and fluid needs.) Weight gain within normal limits usually indicates adequate provision of calories.

Liver function is somewhat immature, with delayed metabolism of certain substances. Function matures rapidly, so that by 2 to 3 months, levels are similar to those of an older infant. Delayed metabolism of drugs and bilirubin results from functional immaturity. Thus the younger the infant's gestational age, the more likely it will be that metabolism of drugs and other substances will be hindered.[13]

temperature control

The newborn infant is vulnerable to temperature extremes. Although provided at birth with a mechanism of *nonshivering thermogenesis* and the ability to increase metabolic rate remarkably, the infant cannot sustain such methods of heat production for extended periods. Without intervention, the infant can gradually become chilled, with core (rectal) temperature dropping rapidly to as low as 33.4°C (92°F). It has been noted that in the delivery room, a wet newborn can drop core temperature at a rate of 0.1°C per minute, while skin temperature falls at a rate of 0.3°C per minute. Unless quickly protected, it is obvious that in an air-conditioned delivery room with low humidity, the infant will soon suffer from *hypothermia*.

Having less fatty tissue than an older child, and with a large body skin surface in relation to body weight, the infant loses heat rapidly through the temperature *gradient,* the movement of heat in the direction of lower temperature. Since room air is usually cooler than body temperature, heat moves from the warmer body organs and muscles to the cooler skin, which is then further cooled by *radiation* (to a cooler solid surface not touching the body), *conduction* (to a cooler surface touching the body), *convection* (into cooler air), or *evaporation* (fluid becoming vapor on the body surface because of temperature or humidity differences).[14] Adjustments in the surrounding environment are necessary.

There is a very narrow range of environmental (ambient) temperature within which metabolic rate remains at a minimum. This narrow range is termed the *thermoneutral range:* the range of temperature within which body core temperatures can be stabilized by nonevaporative processes.[15] Such thermoneutral ranges differ for infants of different sizes, degrees of maturity, and states of illness or health. Extensive tables have been constructed for temperature regulation of high-risk infants (see refs. 4 and 8).

The core temperature thought most desirable for a full-term infant is 37°C (98.6°F), although the range of 36.5 to 37°C (98 to 98.6°F) is acceptable; below 36°C (97°F) is not acceptable. For the infant to maintain this temperature *without* exerting metabolic effort, an environmental temperature which maintains an axillary or abdominal skin temperature of 36.1 to 36.2°C (97 to 97.4°F) is desirable.

Hey suggests that for infants over 2500 g, environmental temperature should be in the range of 32 to 33°C if the infant must be nursed naked in a single-walled incubator. The addition of clothing, of course, decreases the need for such a warm environment. Nurseries should be kept warmer (21 to 24°C) than other recovery areas and should be free from drafts; cribs should be away from sources of heat such as sunlight or radiators.

The range in which a full-term infant can adjust is larger than the small thermoneutral range, but other mechanisms must be called into play.

methods of maintaining temperature The newborn cannot use temperature control methods used by older children and adults: shivering, changing body position, adding or removing warm clothes or coverings, drinking warm or cool liquids, or moving to a warmer or cooler environment. Until shivering thermogenesis becomes possible at 1 to 2 months, the newborn increases body temperature mainly by mobilizing stores of brown fat to gain kilocalories. The infant may also cry, increase movements of arms and legs, breathe faster, and utilize mechanisms of vasoconstriction.

brown adipose tissue All newborn mammals appear to be protected during the transitional period by the presence of a unique type of body fat, *brown adipose tissue* (BAT). Located, as shown in Fig. 14-2, in the neck, under the scapula, and around internal organs of the thorax and abdomen, brown adipose tissue produces heat by oxidizing fatty acids. The increased metabolism of fats uses oxygen and requires glucose for energy. In cases of chilling, if body temperature falls to 35°C, twice as much oxygen and glucose will be needed. If it falls to 33.4°C, three times the normal amount will be required.[16] Thus, kilocalories are used, and weight loss, hypoxia, and fatigue with acidosis will result if the condition is not corrected. As the infant matures and shivering thermogenesis becomes established, the amount of brown fat decreases, and the area becomes merely a lipid storage site (see Chap. 30).

fig. 14-2 Areas in which brown adipose tissue is located in the newborn: (a) Around organs, (b) subscapular area.

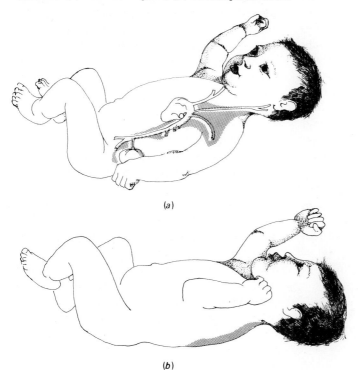

(a)

(b)

hyperthermia Hyperthermia occurs less frequently in the infant and is usually the result of iatrogenic factors. Excessive environmental temperature can cause a slightly higher temperature. Newborns who have had fluids withheld for treatments or those who have been neglected may show temperature elevation because of dehydration. Breast-fed infants may have a slight temperature elevation when fluid intake is low before the flow of milk is established. Bottle-fed infants who do not suck well because of poor feeding technique or residual effects of analgesia or anesthesia may also show signs of elevated temperature. Exposure to the bilirubin light or a radiant heater will sometimes increase insensible water loss and cause dehydration. In rare instances, fever may occur from central nervous system thermoregulatory disturbances resulting from brain injury or massive infection. In cases of infection, temperature is not usually elevated and instead may be low.

Symptoms (attempts at adjustment) are tachypnea, vasodilation (flushed skin), irritability, and sweating on face and palms. The newborn has poor ability to use other mechanisms to reduce heat and is dependent on observant caregivers for rescue.

Treatment of dehydration fever is, of course, to restore fluid balance by feedings of milk or water or by intravenous infusions. Environmental temperatures should be *slowly* adjusted downward; clothing can be loosened and extra blankets removed. Special care should be taken with machine regulation and placement of cribs so that radiant heat from sunlight or heating elements in the room does not add to the infant's temperature problems.

INTEGUMENTARY SYSTEM ADAPTATION

The newborn skin acts as a semipermeable membrane especially prior to full maturity, and capillaries can be seen through translucent epidermis in preterm infants. As the infant matures, the skin thickens, and hair follicles, sebaceous glands, and apocrine glands mature. Nails are well formed and will reach the fingertip by term, growing well beyond when the infant is postmature. Downey, fine hair may be present on forehead, shoulders, and back. This *lanugo* varies with parentage and gestational age; some infants have more extensive lanugo over face and shoulders than do others. Generally, the younger the infant, the more these areas are covered. The texture of scalp hair also varies as the infant matures. At first, hair is somewhat like lanugo, then it becomes thicker and bunches out from the head, and by 38 weeks it assumes a fine, silky texture.

At birth the infant's skin may be covered with *vernix*, a cheeselike mixture of sebaceous gland secretions and cast-off epithelial cells. The younger the infant, the more completely covered is the skin (Figs. 15-1 and 15-2). Vernix does not have to be removed from the skin; it serves a protective function in utero and also may lubricate the skin in the early hours after delivery. Although sweat glands are present, they function poorly in the immediate period after birth. Sweat can be seen only on a full-term infant's face and palms when body temperature rises.

skin color

Skin color changes with the infant's condition and can indicate problems with adequate functioning of the heart and lungs. Initially, the newborn shows some degree of cyanosis as a result of the hypoxia of birth. It is the rare baby who is delivered crying and completely pink. Within 1 min after birth the newborn should show a pink face and trunk, but it may have lingering blueness of the extremities. This early *acrocyanosis* is the result of venous stasis in the extremities and may be present as well in the tissues which have been subject to pressure of the cervix during labor. Later, acrocyanosis of the extremities may be attributed to chilling.

By 5 min of life, most babies are well oxygenated, with pink skin tone under whatever pigmentation they have inherited. Whenever any hypoxia occurs (Pa_{O_2} under 50), skin color will turn bluish gray. Thus, a color change will move from normal skin color in the direction of gray or blue. For a Latin baby with an olive or slightly yellow skin pigmentation, this means a gray undertone; for a brown-skinned baby whose normal lip color is gray-pink, color may deepen. For a baby with light, less-pigmented skin, the pinkish undertone may turn darker and bluer. Cyanosis may first be seen around the lips (*circumoral cyanosis*) and then extend to the face and trunk. Nail beds almost always appear bluish in any baby and are not so clear an area to observe such changes as they are in adults.

Melanocytes are limited in the first few weeks, so that infants whose parents are darker skinned may appear pale in contrast (Fig. 15-10). Depending upon hematocrit values as well, some babies appear very ruddy (polycythemia), while others are paler (lower hematocrit values). The nurse should note maternal pigmentation, as well as the cord blood reports, to assess skin color and changes fully.

Skin color can also indicate the status of temperature control. If the infant is overheated, flushing because of vasodilation will occur. If chilled, vasoconstriction with uneven areas will occur. This *mottling*, or *cutis marmorata*, is common in preterm infants because of immaturity of the vasoconstrictive processes but should be observed for while temperatures are checked (see back inside cover, Plate C).

skin turgor

The condition of the skin must be observed. Its elasticity, or *turgor*, is an important indi-

cation of adequacy of nutrition and hydration. The test is easily done by using the thumb and index finger to grasp the skin and subcutaneous tissue over the abdominal wall. By squeezing, releasing, and allowing it to fall back into place, the elasticity may be evaluated. The healthy skin will immediately return to its original place, and no residual impressions will be seen. Poor turgor is seen when skin remains suspended and creased for a few seconds after being released. Poor turgor suggests that the baby has been malnourished in utero or is presently dehydrated.

normal variations

Although variations on quality or color of skin may appear to be problems, many are considered normal minor variations. *Edema* may be present over the presenting part. Since the head is usually presenting, this edema is called *caput* (head) *succedaneum*. It subsides within the first few days after birth (see Fig. 14-7). Edema of the eyelids is common after a head-first delivery. Edema of the genitalia is common in both sexes, and it may be more pronounced in a baby after a breech delivery. Generalized edema is more difficult to recognize. The absence of wrinkles at the wrists and ankles is highly suggestive. If a finger impression can be left in the skin, the presence of generalized edema is certain.

Desquamation, or peeling of layers of skin on the trunk, palms, and soles, occurs primarily with full- and postterm infants. The more extensive the peeling, the later the gestation. Mothers often worry or spread thick lubricating ointments on their infants. Reassurance should be given that these agents will neither speed nor retard the sloughing of this outer portion of the skin.

Milia are epidermal cysts containing keratogenous material (Fig. 14-3). These "whiteheads" will open and disappear by themselves in the first few weeks of life. Because they are primarily present over nose and chin,

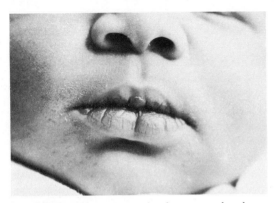

fig. 14-3 Milia (plugged sebaceous glands on nose and chin). Note newborn's mouth with sucking pads. (*Photo by Ruth Helmich. Courtesy of Booth Memorial Medical Center, N.Y.*)

parents may think they are pimples to be squeezed. A simple precautionary statement is usually helpful (see back inside cover, Plate D).

Milia are similar to *Epstein's pearls* in the mouth. These small, whitish cysts on gums or palate disappear quickly without treatment. *Miliaria* are clear vesicles on face, scalp, or perineum which indicate retention of sweat in unopened glands. They may persist in a high environmental humidity but will resolve normally within a few days of birth.

Erythema toxicum is seen very commonly (30 to 70 percent) in newborns. Reddish papules which may have whitish centers are found on the face, trunk, and thighs of a full-term infant. The erythematous areas will blanch on pressure.[18] A smear of the pustules and a Wright's stain will reveal eosinophils. The cause of this noninfectious rash is unknown, and no treatment is necessary (see back inside cover, Plate D). Contrasted to erythema toxicum are *petechiae*, which may result from increased intravascular pressure during delivery. These little petechiae, which do not blanch on pressure also cause a rashlike appearance.

birthmarks

At first glance, *mongolian spots* may be mistaken for bruising because of the bluish gray pigmentation of the deep skin layer. The gray areas appear over the sacrum and buttocks and may extend up the back and down the extensor surface of the extremities. This pigmentation is common (90 percent) in infants of Asian, southern European, African, and American Indian ancestry. The coloration spontaneously disappears by 4 years of age (see back inside cover, Plate C).

The "stork's beak mark," a *nevus simplex*, is a salmon-colored area of pigmentation at the nape of the neck, on the sacral region, and often on the eyelids and forehead (glabella). Such marks are common (30 to 50 percent) in lighter-skinned infants with northern European ancestry. These marks blanch on pressure because they consist of localized areas of capillary dilatation.[19] They, too, fade as the child matures, but they may turn a darker red when the infant cries.

The port wine stain, a *nevus flammeus*, is a more permanent, dark brown or purple mark made up of mature capillaries which have infiltrated the dermal layer. These do not disappear and often cause cosmetic difficulties. *Pigmented nevi* are groups of melanin-containing cells in the dermis. Occasionally, a hair follicle will also be present. These raised marks may shrink with the changing size of the infant and are usually not treated.

Later in the neonatal period, *strawberry hemangiomas* may appear. Beginning at 2 to 3 weeks, these small (1 to 3 mm), flat, red spots grow outwardly and become raised, with a texture like a strawberry. These may enlarge until about 3 months of age, at which time regression takes place. Parents must be instructed not to manipulate these hemangiomas. Any birthmark that is disfiguring or contains vulnerable blood vessels that might be injured is noted by the physician for follow-up. Other, less common marks will not be discussed in this chapter.

NEUROLOGIC DEVELOPMENT AND ADAPTATION

Maturity and the process of maturation in the infant has been studied extensively in the last decade. The development of neurologic characteristics follow a fairly concise timetable, and such a timetable is the basis of assessment of gestational age using neurologic criteria.

Maturity is correlated with the development of neural myelin sheaths. Myelinization begins by the sixth fetal month, with motor nerves developing before sensory nerves. Incomplete at birth, myelinization continues throughout the first year. "Myelinization is an orderly process in which the functionally allied system of neurons are synchronized in an orderly sequence and tempo."[20]

Once a nerve is completely myelinated, electrical impulses are conducted along the path without hindrance. Measurement of these conduction times indicates that the speed of transmittal increases in a linear pattern with age, unaffected by illness, muscle tone or sleep state.[21]

The brain has been protected during fetal growth by a more than adequate circulation and by "sparing" if intrauterine malnourishment occurred. The brain completes its growth in cell number by the fifth year but grows in weight until 15 years.[22] However, between birth and 1 year of age, the most rapid postnatal growth in cell number and size will take place. (Protein deprivation can have especially serious effect during this year.)

the head

The skull is made up of eight bony plates, connected by suture lines which represent the growing edge of the bones (Fig. 14-4). Fontanels, where suture lines meet, are "open," consisting of tough membrane rather than bone. Their presence allows for the rapid brain growth expected in the first year. The posterior and lateral fontanels will have *completely* joined by 2 to 3 months, and the anterior, by 18 to 24 months. The pulsations of the cerebral vessels may be felt through the anterior membrane. Normally, the fontanel should feel soft and flat. Persistent bulging and tenseness may indicate high intracranial pressure, as in babies with hydrocephalus or meningitis. A depressed fontanel may be indicative of dehydration and malnutrition. (Hold the baby in a sitting position to evaluate fontanels; this position permits more accurate

fig. 14-4   Anterior and posterior fontanels. (*Courtesy of Ross Laboratories, from "Mechanism of Normal Labor."*)

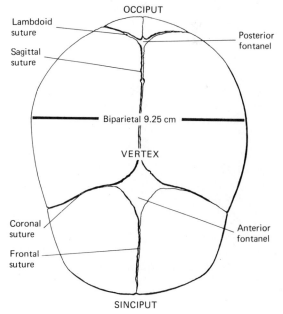

interpretation of palpation.) The head at birth is usually 1 to 2 cm larger than the chest diameter and should follow normal growth curves, as seen in Fig. 14-5.

fig. 14-5 Head circumference for the young infant. (*a*) Head growth last trimester (after Lubchenco). (*b*) Head growth in the weeks after birth (Harvard data).

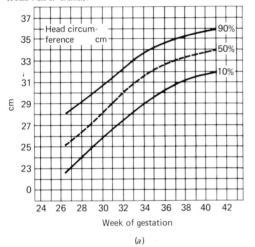

(*a*)

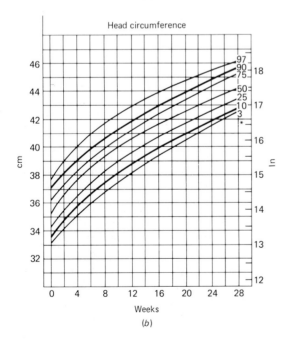

(*b*)

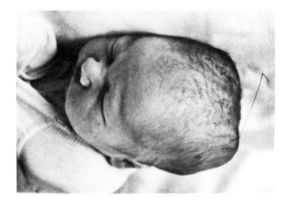

fig. 14-6 Cephalhematoma. (*Courtesy of Mead Johnson Company.*)

The most commonly occurring deviations from normal are caput succedaneum, cephalhematoma, and molding. All occur in response to birth pressures (Fig. 14-6).

Caput succedaneum is associated with pressure on the presenting part. Edema and some slight capillary bleeding develops over the area that has presented against a slowly yielding cervix. Edema feels spongy and crosses suture lines.

Cephalhematoma is caused by bleeding of ruptured blood vessels *between* the surface of a cranial bone and the periosteal membrane covering that bone. Therefore, it has a definite margin because the hemorrhage is confined by the membrane to the limits of the cranial bone. Points of difference are summarized in Table 14-3. The diagrammatic sketches illustrate the origin of bleeding in each condition (Fig. 14-7).

In contrast to caput succedaneum, cephalhematoma usually does not appear within the first 24 h after birth. Most authorities do not relate cephalhematoma to skull fractures. In one study, however, when systematic skull x-rays were performed on every baby with cephalhematoma, the fracture rate was 25 percent.[23] Because of extra bleeding, bilirubin levels may be higher.

table 14-3 Differential diagnosis: caput succedaneum and cephalhematoma

caput succedaneum	cephalhematoma
Present at birth	Appears usually 24 h after birth
May be seen on any part of infant's body that presented in labor	Seen only on the head, usually over parietal bone(s)
May cross suture lines	Contributes to hyperbilirubinemia
Decreases in size after birth	Never crosses suture lines
Fluid usually absorbed in 36 h	Increases in size before decreases
Is diffuse; pits on pressure	May persist for weeks
No treatment	Is circumscribed; does not pit
	Usually no treatment

Changes in the shape of the head, known as *molding*, allow the head to adopt to the changing diameters of the pelvic cavity. Both parietal bones move up, while the occiput moves down and in. There is no danger if the volume of the brain remains the same. Only in extreme cases can there be enough pressure on the brain tissue to cause internal hemorrhage or to result in a tearing of the *tentorium cerebelli* (Fig. 14-8).

Depending upon sleeping position, the soft skull bones return to normal shape within the first 7 to 10 days of life. During this period, placed routinely in the supine position, the infant will develop a flat occipital aspect. If the infant is placed prone with the head to either side, the head contour will assume the desired oval shape.

fig. 14-7 Comparison between caput succedaneum and cephalhematoma.

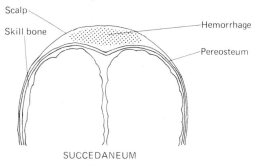

Scalp
Skill bone
Hemorrhage
Pereosteum

SUCCEDANEUM

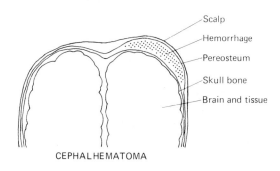

Scalp
Hemorrhage
Pereosteum
Skull bone
Brain and tissue

CEPHALHEMATOMA

sleep patterns

The newborn spends about 75 percent of the time sleeping, with little concern for day or night cycles. By 2 weeks, a more regular 24-h cycle is established, with night sleep longer and becoming longer still in the first few months.

Studies on infant neurologic maturation have shown that the time interval of these sleep states changes with increasing age (see Chap. 15). From term to 8 months, the infant increases an individual cycle by very little, 47 to 50 min, but more cycles will occur during night hours. (Later, cycles average about 50 to 60 min.[24]) The sleep cycle contains

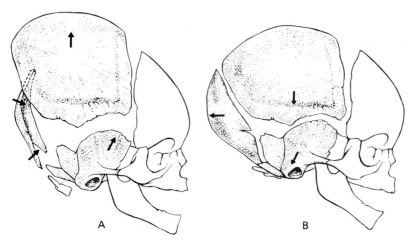

fig. 14-8 Molding during the birth process causes (a) overlapping and movement of cranial bones, (b) reexpansion of cranium on third day with return to normal positions. (*Courtesy of Mead Johnson Company.*)

active sleep, a transitional period, and then a period of quiet sleep. Active sleep may be a less mature state in the newborn.

Stern indicates that quiet sleep requires feedback and inhibitory mechanisms which develop with maturation. According to Stern, the length of active sleep in each cycle decreases markedly from 44 percent to 28 percent by 8 months, whereas quiet sleep increases from 37 percent to 56 percent by 8 months. (By the young adult period, active or REM sleep is about 22 percent and is 15 percent by the later adult period.[25])

Brackbill studies sleep positions of the newborn which appeared to promote or hinder sleep.[26] She found that the infant managed best in a prone position, with more sleep, less crying and movement and slower heart rates. Infants in the supine position cried approximately five times longer and slept 26 percent less than did prone babies. Such a practical research observation is useful to parents, who respond more positively to a rested, happy, alert infant than to a tired, fussy one. Continued crying can elicit extensive parental hostility as well. Finally, establishment of the day-night cycle of sleeping is important to parental rest and should be encouraged. Parents can work toward such a routine when they are given adequate information about infant sleep patterns.

testing for neurologic status

When questions arise from the initial neurologic evaluation for gestational age, a more thorough investigation is called for. An examination is done, especially when there is central nervous system depression secondary to trauma, metabolic disorders, or congenital malformation. The total extensive neurologic examination is usually performed by the physician. Tables are included here for reference, as part of the whole examination is included in initial scoring. The Brazelton scale must be performed by a trained clinician.

The Neonatal Behavioral Assessment Scale, designed by T. Berry Brazelton, is a tool that assesses an infant's ability to interact with its environment. It differs from other tools in several significant ways;

1 It emphasizes the effects the neonate has on the environment.
2 It recognizes that the physiologic adjustment which occurs during the transition to extrauterine life may leave limited energy for the activity of higher brain centers, and it therefore scores the infant's best response rather than its average response.
3 It recognizes the baby's state of consciousness as a vital parameter of neurologic assessment.
4 It recognizes the existence of cognitive and affective responses which are controlled by the newborn, whereas other tools evaluate primarily reflex activity.

The test consists of 27 behavioral items, each scored on a nine-point scale, and 20 elicited responses scored on a three-point scale. These demonstrate the infant's ability to shut off negative stimuli (to habituate), as well as to alert and orient to positive stimuli. The infant also will demonstrate ability to control states of arousal through self-quieting mechanisms such as hand-to-mouth action. It is postulated that without such self-controlling responses, the infant would be at the mercy of the environment.

To illustrate this point, examination of anencephalic infants reveals that the cortical function for such control is absent in these infants. They fail to habituate and become overwhelmed by the stimuli and may progress to physiologic shock. Immature infants also suffer from a deficit in cortical control and are not able to organize their own behavior efficiently to shut out negative stimuli. Brazelton postulates that the vasomotor and respiratory changes so often seen in small infants may reflect this inability.

Since self-control is necessary for the infant to be able to take in other stimuli, normal infants who seem to have little self-control will react with hyperactivity and/or excessive

sleeping. Disturbances in the mother-infant relationship can result if this situation is not recognized. If such problems are recognized before discharge, the mother can be oriented to such behavior and plan a structured environment with fewer stimuli for the baby.

The predictive value of the Brazelton scale is being investigated. At this time, it appears that an infant with good visual following and response to auditory stimuli who exhibits self-quieting behavior, even if other problems are present, may have a better long-term neurologic development than was previously thought. Continued investigation may reveal long-range prognostic uses for the scale.*

The basic neurologic examination is divided into several parts: overall observations, evaluation of cranial nerve function (Table 14-4), and evaluation of motor function and development reflexes (Table 14-5).

Overall observation should be done at the appropriate time when the infant is quiet and neither too sleepy nor too hungry. Warmth should be maintained. Observations of gross difficulties would include checking for symmetrical movement of all parts of the body and measurement of head circumference. Head size should be within normal ranges; infants with small heads (tenth percentile) or large heads (fiftieth percentile) and positive neurologic findings should be further evaluated.

Levels of responsiveness, sensory function and posture are all included in the initial overview. It is important not to tire the infant, and for that reason neurologic assessment may be divided into different sessions.

*For more information, the reader is referred to the small manual of instructions for use of the scale: *Neonatal Behavioral Assessment Scale,* Clinics in Developmental Medicine, #50, J. B. Lippincott Philadelphia, 1973. Usually a clinical training period is recommended before an examiner is skilled in administering the test with validity.

table 14-4 Examination of cranial nerves

number	technique	normal	abnormal
I Olfactory nerve	No way of easily evaluating this nerve in neonates is available at this time.		
II Optic nerve	Use a bright object held about 10 in from the infant's eyes. Move it from side to side.	Term infant can fix on and follow object 60°. Occular movements are not smooth or coordinated at all times.	No fixation or following.
III Oculomotor	Observe for ptosis (drooping of upper eyelid).	Neither lid droops.	One or both lids droop.
	Test the pupillary reflex by shining a bright light into the eye.	Pupil contracts approximately 1 mm after 31 weeks' gestation.	No response or a continuously constricted pupil (Horner's syndrome).
III Oculomotor IV Trochlear VI Abducens	Use the doll's head movements of the eyes to test for full range of motion.	Movement is not smooth constantly (Fig. 14-9).	Deviation from normal. *Nystagmus* (jerky lateral eye movements with or without stimulation) suggests seizure activity.
V Trigeminal	Chewing (masseteric) strength—evaluate strength of biting portion of the suck by placing a finger in infant's mouth.	Normal strength endures.	Weak, nonenduring.
	Observe for deviation of mandible when infant opens mouth.	No deviation.	Deviation laterally.
	Observe for facial weakness by stimulating one side with a pinprick.	Grimace on side stimulated spreads to opposite side.	No response on side stimulated. Response noted on opposite side only.
VII Facial	Evaluate facial symmetry at rest and with movement. Stimulate to cry and to suck.	Equal movement. Durable suck.	Marked weakness. Mouth will draw to the normal side. Ineffective sucking. Drooling.
VIII Acoustic cochlear division	Startle infant with a single loud sound. Be sure to avoid proprioceptive stimulus such as vibrations from banging the crib.	Moro reflex. Sudden change in behavior.	No response.
Oculovestibular division	Holding infant upright, examiner spins baby around several times.	Eyes deviate in direction opposite to spin.	No response.

table 14-4 Examination of cranial nerves (*continued*)

number	technique	normal	abnormal
IX Glosso-pharyn-geal X Vagus	Stimulate the gag reflex with a tongue depressor. Observe the movement of the uvula and muscles of palate and pharynx.	Symmetrical movement of the palate with uvula in midline.	No response or assymmetrical response. Deviation of uvula due to weakness of palate.
	Observe infant's ability to swallow. Listen to quality of cry.	Swallow strong. Clear strong cry.	Weak swallow. Hoarse cry with no history of intubation.
XI Accessory	Place the infant in the supine position. Extend head over the edge of table and turn side to side. Observe sternocleidomastoid muscle.	No masses. Symmetrical muscular development.	Shortening or hematoma of muscle.
	Sit infant upright and observe efforts to hold head erect.	Holds head erect several seconds.	Cannot right head.
XII Hypo-glossal	Observe for fasciculations (tiny tremors) of tongue at rest.	Tongue should be still, at rest.	Fasciculations at rest.
	Observe for atrophy of tongue. Note pull on nipple when sucking.	No furrows. Tongue is appropriate size. Strong hold on nipple.	Furrows of tongue. Tongue seems small. Easy to pull nipple out of mouth.

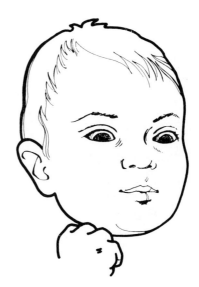

fig. 14-9 Doll's eye phenomenon. Apparently produced by lack of full integration of eye and head movements, this sign can be seen when the infant is lying supine and the examiner turns the head gradually from side to side. The eyes lag behind head movements. The test is uniformly positive from birth to 10 days; the phenomenon gradually disappears with the development of consistent fixation, at about 2 or 3 months. (*Courtesy of Mead Johnson and Co., Evansville, Indiana.*)

table 14-5A Evaluation of motor function

what to observe	normal	abnormal	cause of abnormal findings
Posture			
Resting posture	Flexion, even in sleep for first 2–3 weeks.	Hypotonia*—"frog leg posture."	Hypoxia, metabolic disturbances, e.g., hypoglycemia, hypothyroidism, hypermagnesemia. Down's syndrome.
Tone	Normal tone—some head lag, flexion at elbow and knee becomes extension when pulled to sitting.	Hypertonia—infant moves "as a block." No head lag, no elbow or knee extension when pulled to sitting.	Hypoxia, intracranial bleeding. Drug withdrawal.
Symmetry†	No difference between two sides of body or upper and lower extremities.	Tone increased or decreased from right to left or upper and lower parts of body.	Hypoxia, intracranial bleeding. Drug withdrawal.
Strength	Strong cry. Spontaneous movements. Resistance to painful or unnatural posture.	Weak cry. Lack of movement. Lack of response.	Hypotonia. Prematurity.
Movement	Smooth when opening and closing the hands, moving hand to mouth, kicking spontaneously.	Seizure activity tremors.	Hypoxia. Drug withdrawal.
Fascicula-tions (fine tremors)	None noted.	Fine tremors of fingers and toes at rest or during sleep; reduced spontaneous activity.	Hypotonia.
Spine			
Evidence of trauma to cervical area	Tonic neck reflex. Symmetrical Moro reflex.	Lack of response unilaterally or bilaterally	Erb's palsy = unilateral. Dislocation of cervical spine if bilateral.
Lumbosacral trauma	Normal appearance and reflexes.	Acute injury, bruising, mass in area, spinal shock, loss of knee and ankle reflexes.	Traumatic breech delivery.

*To demonstrate hypotonia when uncertain, note the position of the infant's head as the infant is placed back on the bed from a sitting posture. As the vertex of the head touches the bed, the infant with normal muscle tone will flex the head so that the weight of the head is on the occiput. A hypotonic infant will not be able to flex the head.

†Head should be held in midline when evaluating symmetry to avoid stimulating tonic-neck reflex.

table 14-5B Developmental reflexes

1 **Moro reflex**

Technique: Lift the head of the crib about 2 in and drop it. This method is less traumatic on the baby's back and neck than lifting the head and shoulders and dropping them. (Making a loud noise to elicit this reflex tests hearing.)

Response: Abduction and extension of the arms, extension of at least fingers three to five, followed by adduction and flexion of upper extremities. Lower extremities may be extended. Infant may startle and cry (Fig. 14-10a,b.)

Abnormal: Asymmetry = hemiparesis, fractured humerus or clavicle, brachial plexus injury. Sluggish = hypotonia

Disappears: After 4 months of age.

2 **Tonic neck reflex** (fencing position)

Technique: Turn the infant's head to the left.

Response: The left arm and leg will show extension and increased tone, while the right arm and leg will flex and show a decrease in tone.

Abnormal: The infant who is not able to break this posture a few seconds after it is elicited is exhibiting an obligatory response, which is abnormal.

Disappears: After 4 months of age.

3 **Stepping reflex**

Technique: Hold the infant upright and place one foot in contact with the bed.

Response: The leg in contact with the bed will extend while the other leg flexes (Fig. 14-11).

Abnormal: Hypertonic = both legs will be held in extension. Hypotonic = infant will not be able to bear any weight.

Disappears: 3 to 4 months.

4 **Palmar grasp**

Technique: Apply pressure to the palm of the hand.

Response: Flexion of the fingers and grasp of the object. This grasp is strong enough to allow the infant to be lifted from the bed by placing traction on the object (Fig. 14-12).

Disappears: Ten months.

5 **Plantar grasp**

Technique: Press your thumb to the infant's sole just below the toes.

Response: The toes should flex around your thumb (Fig. 14-13).

Abnormal: Absence of this reflex is seen in infants with hypotonia, spinal cord injury, or injury to the lumbosacral plexus.

Disappears: Ten months.

6 **Rooting reflex**

Technique: Touch the infant's cheek.

Response: Infant will turn head toward the stimulus and begin to suck.

Abnormal: Weak in infants with decreased alertness or in those who have just been fed.

Disappears: Six months.

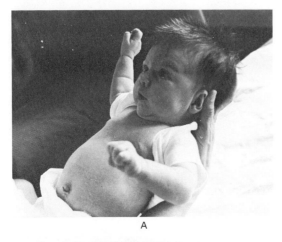

A

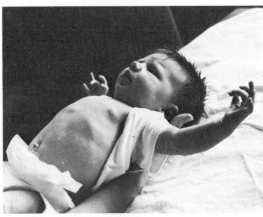

B

fig. 14-10 Moro reflex. (*a*) One position for checking the Moro reflex. (*b*) Arms begin to move toward the body; note finger position. (*Photos by Beverly Hemlock.*)

NEWBORN ASSESSMENT

The study of the newborn infant has progressed to the extent that it is possible to particularize each infant by his or her characteristics and early patterns of response. No longer can a person working in this health care setting say that infants are all the same. Indeed, part of the enjoyment of working with newborn infants is in the discovery of these unique characteristics. Of course, it takes

practice for the skill of newborn appraisal to be developed. In the following material, we recognize that some parts of the newborn examination are not usually performed by student nurses, and some of the abnormal findings are rare or at least less commonly encountered. To assist the student, therefore, the parts of the examination which should be left to more experienced personnel are printed in smaller type—there for the student to *read*, but not to *do*, until she or he has further opportunity to develop skill in the basic assessment steps.

The first step in appraisal is to obtain the history preceding the present time. Chapter 15 lists information which should be noted from the chart. The second step is to observe

fig. 14-11 Stepping reflex in 2-day-old infant. (*Photo by Mary Olsen Johnson, M.D.*)

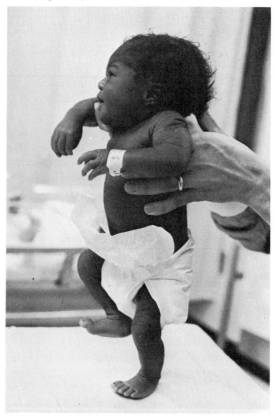

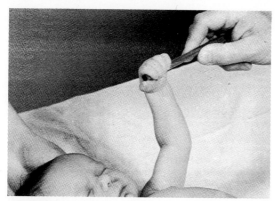

fig. 14-12 Grasp reflex. (*From the slide series "Neurological Examination of the Newborn." Courtesy of Kenneth Holt, M.D., London, England.*)

the infant at rest; to make an overall observation before disturbing the child by movement or touch. The third step is to assess cardiorespiratory function by observation and auscultation. Then measurements are taken and physical characteristics noted and compared with normal ranges. Finally gestational age characteristics are compared with charts, and age is evaluated in comparison with estimations made during prenatal and delivery care. In each category of the following step-by-step procedure, the technique of examination is described and both normal findings and the more commonly seen abnormal findings are listed. (If an unusual abnormal finding is included, it will be in small type, so that the student does not become overwhelmed with material.) The high-risk infant will be discussed in Chap. 29. When that chapter is studied, a review of the assessment procedures given here may be helpful.

overall assessment

Overall appraisal of the newborn is done to assess the infant's ability to adjust to extrauterine life and to identify any handicaps to that adjustment. An initial assessment has

been done briefly in the delivery room and again on admission to the newborn nursery. Newborn units differ in the amount of detail required, but increasingly, the nurse is the one assigned to do these initial appraisals. The nurse is expected to identify deviations from normal and to notify the pediatrician at once if any of these deviations appear to hinder the infant's recovery from birth. It is important not to delay this examination, since changes can occur in the first 24 h, and a baseline evaluation is important so that there is a point of comparison.

observations of adjustment to extrauterine life

The transition from fetal to neonatal life was described by Desmond and coworkers in 1963. The general pattern they described was determined from infants whose mothers had received rather heavy medication. Therefore, although the pattern may remain valid, the degree of difficulty in adjustment will certainly vary with the amount of analgesia or anesthesia received by the mother. New studies are needed to determine the validity of the

fig. 14-13 Plantar reflex. (*From the slide series "Neurological Examination of the Newborn." Courtesy of Kenneth Holt, M.D., London, England.*)

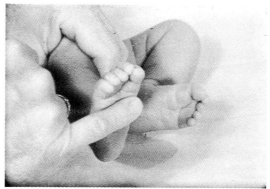

pattern for infants whose mothers did not receive any medication during labor and delivery.

Within the first hour of life, the normal term infant appears alert, cries lustily, and may suck vigorously. Heart rate is high, and respirations may be high and somewhat irregular. If there has been any intrauterine stress, hypoxia, or acidosis, the infant may have difficulty during this period and may need assistance.

The normal infant should meet its parents and experience the close handling, touching, and cuddling of these future caregivers. In turn, if allowed, the baby will look at the mother and father, appear very interested, and evidence interest in breast-feeding. Muscle tone is active, crying occurs only with unpleasant stimuli, and color will indicate a pinkish undertone, indicating adequate oxygenation. Nonmedicated infants may stay awake and alert for 1 to 4 or 5 h after birth. Medicated infants usually fall into the first sleep period within the first hour after birth and sleep for a longer period than do nonmedicated infants.

For both, the first sleep period usually includes a time of continued adjustments. If the environment has been supportive, temperature stability should be fairly complete by the time the infant awakes.

Once awake, each infant begins to establish an individual pattern of waking and sleeping. It is during this period that a more thorough assessment is in order.

Brazelton has described this first adjustment period based on extensive studies done to determine neurobehavioral responses. He identifies three periods: (1) the initial alert period after delivery, which lasts for varying periods of time; (2) a period of depression and disorganization, which lasts for 24 to 48 h in infants without medication or complications and for up to 4 days if the infant is affected by maternal medication; and (3) the

period of recovery to "optimal" function.[27] It is during this last period that neurobehavioral evaluations correlate well with tests at 30 days.

weight, height, and responsiveness The full-term infant ranges in weight from 2500 to 4000 g and measures 46 to 55 cm in crown-heel length (refer to Table 14-6). There will be good muscle tone in all extremities, and if any limb is extended, it should return to a position of flexion. There should be no signs of respiratory distress, although spontaneous crying is common. Even when alert, some children may have to be stimulated to cry by a short back rub, tweaking the hair, or a quick flick on the soles. The cry can tell something about the infant's responses. The pitch should be "normal," not high-pitched or whining nor weak or mewing.

Assessment of the skin is part of the overall appraisal of the newborn. The condition of the skin varies with maturity, state of nutrition, amount of vernix caseosa, activity, distribution and amount of fat, and hemoglobin and bilirubin levels. Skin appraisal will precede evaluation of individual parts of the body.

After the overall assessment has been completed, the rest of the examination is performed systematically. Although one usually proceeds from head to foot (cephalocaudally), it is usually best to begin with the assessment of the chest while the infant is quiet.

table 14-6 The average newborn in the United States

measurements	average
Weight	3400 g = 7.5 lb
Height/length	50 cm = 20 in
Head circumference	33 cm = 13 in
Chest circumference	30 cm = 11.75 in

Source: Maternal Nutrition and the Course of Pregnancy, Summary Report, U.S. Department of Health, Education and Welfare, Publication (HSM) 72-5600, 1971, p. 8.

skin

technique Observe skin color in natural light, as fluorescent light tends to mask true color. Blanch skin of the forehead or abdomen by applying finger pressure momentarily and observe the return of color. Be sure to examine the entire skin surface, including neck, inguinal, and axillary folds. Look for adequate skin turgor by gently pinching up a fold of skin on abdomen or thigh.

NORMAL Skin pigmentation ranges from pale to dark brown. Mucous membranes should have underlying pink tones, and no cyanotic changes should be seen with crying or activity. Acrocyanosis and mottling may be present early; later, these are signs of problems. Depending on maturity, vernix may be present, as well as desquamation and erythema toxicum.

ABNORMAL *Pallor* may be caused by chilling, anemia, infection, or shock; *jaundice,* by elevated bilirubin levels. *Circumoral cyanosis* and *generalized cyanosis* are results of respiratory distress, hypoglycemia, or cardiac disease and should not be present at any time. *Petechiae* may indicate low platelet count or be a sign of congenital infection. On the other hand, petechiae may normally be present if the cord has been wound around the neck (nuchal cord) or if there has been compression of a part during birth. Infants with intrauterine growth retardation may show evidence of recent weight loss and poor skin turgor. Skin may also be meconium stained in these infants. A difficult birth may result in forceps marks on cheeks, in ecchymotic areas, or in small lacerations. Skin lesions should be described in detail: *macules* (flat discolored areas), *papules* (red, raised areas), and *pustules* (small elevated areas filled with lymph or pus). Erythema toxicum should be differentiated from other skin lesions.

chest and lungs

technique Count the infant's respirations for a full minute and note quality. The chest should then be auscultated and quality of breath sounds noted (Fig. 14-14). The best place to listen is at the midaxillary line, but all lobes should be examined. Finally, measure the chest circumference at the level of the nipples and note placement and condition of nipples and areola.

NORMAL Respirations 30 to 60 breaths per minute, with symmetrical chest expansion. Scattered rales (sounds of moisture within the lungs) are considered normal during the first few hours after birth. After this, fluid should be absorbed. Chest circumference measures 1 to 2 cm less than head, and the chest appears small in relation to the abdomen. Nipples should be at midclavicular line; internipple distance should be measured and is plotted as a percentage of chest circumference. Size of areola should be 7 to 10 mm in diameter, but possible breast engorgement may make them seem larger. *Supernumerary nipples* (extra nipples) may be present without causing concern.

fig. 14-14 Listening for respiratory sounds. Note blanching of skin from slight pressure of stethoscope. (*Photo by Ruth Helmich.*)

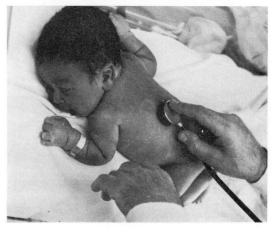

ABNORMAL Signs of respiratory difficulty: retractions, grunting, nasal flaring, other respiratory sounds, cyanosis and tachypnea, asymmetrical expansion of the chest, or increased anteroposterior diameter. (See Chap. 29 for more detail.) In addition, *decreased air entry* with absence of the breath sounds in a particular area of the lung is caused by obstruction of small airway with secretions (meconium), a collapsed area of lung, or pneumothorax. Respiratory distress is only a symptom and may be part of many syndromes involving the respiratory tract and other systems, e.g., sepsis, hypothermia, hypoglycemia, central nervous system damage, or cardiac malformations (see Chap. 29).

heart sounds

technique *Where to listen:* Auscultate the entire cardiac region in any order that works best for you. One pattern is to begin at the *apex,* found in the infant at the *PMI* (point of maximal impulse), which is the point on the chest where the pulse is best felt. The PMI is usually found at the midclavicular line. Work your way from the apex, up the left sternal border, toward the base of the heart. Then listen along the right sternal border; turn the infant over and listen between the scapulae. The fourth rib interspace on the left sternal border and the apex are especially important in the newborn.

What to listen for: S1 and S2 are the terms applied to the first and second heart sounds. S1 is heard when the *atrioventricular valves* (mitral and tricuspid) close. S2 represents closure of *semilunar valves* (aortic and pulmonary valves). The "lub-dub" sounds one hears are the S1 and S2 sounds, respectively. The time between S1 and S2 is systole; that between S2 and S1 is diastole. A good order to use in auscultating the heart is as follows: (1) listen and count rate for a full minute; (2) locate where in the chest the sounds are heard best, (3) differentiate between S1 and S2; and finally (4) decide if there are extra sounds other than S1 and S2.

Evaluation of abnormal heart sounds in the newborn is often difficult because an infant with congenital heart disease may have no murmur at all, while a normal infant may have an easily heard *innocent* murmur. This can occur because the turbulence in blood flow necessary to produce an audible murmur may not be present until the changes in systemic and pulmonic blood pressures occurring with transition to extrauterine life are completed. The nurse's role in this assessment is detection of abnormal findings and referral of these to the physician. *But,* until the nurse becomes proficient at auscultation, all findings should be verified by a competent associate.

NORMAL Heart rate should range from 110 to 160, but rates of 90 to 110 may be observed when the infant is at rest, just as a rate of 160 to 180 may occur during periods of activity. If a rate under 110 is heard, the examiner should stimulate the infant to cry, and the rate should rise. The pulse should be felt best at the apex. "Closeness" of heart sounds to the chest wall is a parameter that can be assessed accurately only after the examiner gains some experience. Evaluate S1 and S2. Each sound should be separate, and no extra sounds should be heard in the diastole, that is, between S2 and S1. An *innocent* systolic murmur may be heard as a short extra sound close to S1, but since it is not possible to tell if this murmur is truly innocent (functional), it should be referred to the physician. An innocent murmur represents a step in the transition from fetal to neonatal circulation. Repeated assessment and observation of other signs of cardiac distress are necessary before a diagnosis can be made.

ABNORMAL Rates of under 110 or over 160 that do not vary with activity or rest are suspicious. An infant with respiration distress, cold stress, hypoglycemia, hypocalcemia, or perinatal asphyxia can have abnormalities of cardiac rate. Infants with CNS damage or depression secondary to maternal oversedation can also have fixed heart rates. Scopolamine is especially known for its ability to cause tachycardia and lack of beat-to-beat variability, which can be seen if the neonatal heart is monitored with a system similar to that which is used for fetal heart monitoring.

A shift in location of heart sounds may be caused by *tension pneumothorax* (intrapleural air that causes a shift of the heart from its normal position, called *mediastinal shift*). This can occur secondary to aspiration of meconium (see Chap. 29), as a result of excessive pressures used to force gas into the lungs during resuscitative efforts, or as a complication of respiratory therapy. *Diaphragmatic hernia*, a condition in which the abdominal contents herniate into the thorax through a defect in the diaphragm (usually left sided), can also cause the heart sounds to shift from their normal position. In *dextrocardia*, a rare condition that may be harmless, the heart is found in the right chest. A decrease in intensity of the heart sounds may be caused by *pneumomediastinum* (air in the mediastinal space), which may lead to pneumothorax.

head

technique Observe the head from all sides for size, shape, and evidence of trauma. Palpate the head from the frontal bone along the suture line to the anterior fontanel and coronal suture. Then move along the sagittal suture to the posterior fontanel (see Fig. 14-4). Palpate the occiput and continue laterally to the parietal bones until the entire skull has been examined. Note the quality and distribution of hair as you palpate. Measure the head circumference from the forehead around the occiput at its largest point.

NORMAL Normal head circumference ranges from 33 to 38 cm at term, even in a small-for-

gestational age (SGA) infant, since in spite of intrauterine growth retardation the head and brain receives nutrition in preference to the rest of the body. Pressure during passage through the birth canal frequently causes molding of the head, with overriding coronal and sagittal sutures (Fig. 14-8). These can be felt as ridges and will realign within a few days. (Only if they are extreme will there be any adverse effect on the infant.) The anterior fontanel usually measures 1 by 2 cm and should be neither tense nor depressed. The posterior fontanel is usually *patent* (open). The anterior fontanel usually will close by 18 months; the posterior, by 2 to 3 months. Hair in a term infant has a silky quality and lies flat on the head. Fine, silky hair, *lanugo*, will be present on the forehead (Fig. 14-15).

ABNORMAL Abnormally small or large head circumferences in comparison with chest measurements may indicate microcephaly or hydrocephaly. Molding can make the circumference seem small in the first few days after birth; repeated measurement is necessary. Widely separated sutures are usually abnormal and may be associated with hypothyroidism. Cephalhematoma or caput succedaneum may be present. Lesions of the scalp may be developmental or iatrogenic in origin. Tiny lacerations associated with internal fetal monitoring and fetal scalp sampling for blood pH are common (see Chap. 27).

ears

technique Note the placement of ears by using a straight edge and visualizing a line between the pinna and the inner canthus of the eye (Fig. 14-16). Observe the configuration, firmness, and degree of incurving of the pinna. Examination of the canal and tympanic membrane (eardrum) soon after birth will often be obscured by vernix; this will be absorbed after the first day which will allow for visual-

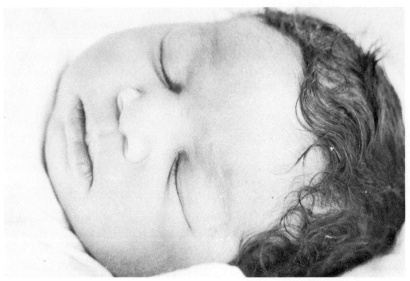

fig. 14-15 Lanugo on forehead. (*Photo by Ruth Helmich. Courtesy of Booth Memorial Medical Center, N.Y.*)

ization of the eardrum. (To examine the ear with an otoscope, pull the earlobe down and back. This part of the exam may be reserved for the pediatrician.)

NORMAL The ears should be placed symmetrically and be well shaped, without any

fig. 14-16 Placement of the ear in relation to the inner canthus of the eye. (*a*) Normal placement. (*b*) True low-set ear (*Courtesy of Mead Johnson Company.*)

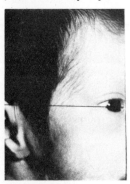
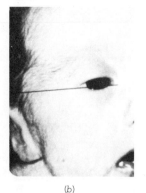

(a)   (b)

lesions or malformations. The eardrum should appear light, pearly gray, and translucent. The pinna should incurve appropriately for gestational age.

ABNORMAL *Skin tags* and *preauricular sinuses* can be innocuous or a sign of renal malformations. These extra pieces of skin anterior to the insertion of the ear and the small indentations anterior to the ear may occur with renal malformations because ears and renal organs develop at similar times in gestation. Some malformed ears are associated with chromosomal disorders (see Chap. 28).

eyes

technique While the infant is alert, observe ocular movements. Hold a light or red object 10 or 12 in from the eyes and try to get the infant to follow. (If the infant is not in an awake state, it may be impossible to induce it to open its eyes. Sit the infant at a 45° angle, and then raise and lower the head several times as one way of inducing opening of the eyes.) Observe for symmetry and size of the eyes, color of sclera and iris, and the presence of any deviations from normal. Note angle of slant from inner to outer *canthus* (corner where eyelids meet).

Now place the infant in the supine position and examine pupillary reflex by shining light first into one and then into the other eye. It may be necessary to recruit an assistant for this step. (In some nursery settings, this step is only done by the physician. Check with your instructor.) Note the red reflex, elicited by shining the light straight into pupil; a circular red area should be seen.

NORMAL In a state of quiet alertness, the term infant should be able to follow a bright object or a face horizontally for 180° and vertically for 30°. The infant's eyes may not move smoothly and in unison, however. The eyes should be equal in size and symmetrical in placement. The sclera is blue-white, and the iris is a darker or lighter slate blue/brown, depending upon parental eye color.

Pupillary reflexes appear at 30 weeks' gestation and should be equal. Small, salmon-colored patches (nevus simplex) may be present on the eyelids of a fair-skinned baby.

ABNORMAL There should be no exudate. However, with application of silver nitrate, a chemical conjunctivitis will occur in 90 percent of infants within the first 24 h.[28] *Subconjunctival hemorrhage* may appear as a result of the pressure on the infant's face during delivery. The sclera appears partially filled with blood. Such superficial hemorrhages are not dangerous and will be reabsorbed within a few weeks. Jaundice gives the sclera a yellow color, called *icterus*.

Infants with Horner's syndrome have ptosis (drooping eyelid) and a constricted pupil. This may be associated with Erb's palsy (brachial plexus injury). *Hypoxic-ischemic encephalopathy* resulting from asphyxia during birth may produce

diminished pupillary reflexes. An opaque density surrounded by red reflex is suggestive of *cataracts*. Mongolian slanting, *Brushfield's spots* (speckling of iris), and epicanthal folds (vertical folds of skin which cover the inner canthus) are signs of Down's syndrome (see Chap. 28). An antimongolian slant, sloping of the eyes downward from the inner to the outer canthus, is associated with chromosomal anomalies.

nose

technique Observe for nasal patency by passing a soft catheter through both nares. Note any discharge from the nose.

NORMAL The first step will have been done in the delivery room. *Do not* repeat it here. Some mucus discharge may be normal, causing the infant to sneeze in an effort to clear the passageway. Sneezing is not a sign of "catching a cold." Milia may cover the nose (see back inside cover, Plate D).

ABNORMAL Snuffles, a severe runny nose, may be present if the infant has congenital syphilis.

Choanal atresia (blockage of nasal passage) must be repaired surgically, for infants do not easily breathe out of their mouths.

mouth

technique While the infant is quiet, inspect the lips and mouth for external defects and symmetry. Place your finger near the mouth to note rooting and sucking reflexes. Put a clean finger in the mouth to test sucking and to palpate the hard and soft palates, gums, and tongue. Use a tongue blade to gently stimulate the gag reflex: touch the soft palate. Note the size of the tongue. When the child cries, note symmetry in movement of the palate and uvula (see back inside cover, Plate D).

NORMAL   Sucking and rooting reflexes should be strong and coordinated with swallowing. Gagging should be elicited easily. All movements of the mouth should be symmetrical. Mucous membranes should be pink and moist.

ABNORMAL   Weak or absent sucking and rooting reflexes may exist when the infant is depressed by maternal medication. *Facial nerve palsy* should be suspected if there is asymmetrical movement (best noted when crying). Check for forceps injury. Most obviously, there may be cleft lip or palate or both (see Chap. 29).

neck

technique   To properly visualize the anterior aspect of the normally short neck, extend it by placing one hand behind the neck and allowing the head to fall back slightly. Posteriorly, observe skin folds, hairline, and contour of neck. Palpate the clavicles and sternocleidomastoid muscle. Elicit tonic neck and head rotation signs.

NORMAL   The head should rotate almost to the shoulder in a term infant. The infant should be able to use neck extensors and flexors, bringing head up to a vertical position for a few seconds. (Fig. 14-17a, b).

ABNORMAL   Extra skin folds may appear as horizontal "rings" of flesh around the neck or as webbing (extra tissue at lateral aspects of neck). Webbing is a sign of Turner's syndrome (see Fig. 28-11). A sternocleidomastoid "tumor" may be felt as a mass at that muscle. It may be accompanied by *torticollis* if the muscle is contracted. Limited rotation of the head accompanies this condition. Congenital goiter is a rare condition accompanying maternal ingestion of antithyroid medications.

Finally, one or both clavicles may have been fractured during a difficult delivery.

abdomen

technique   Observe the abdomen for obvious defects. Observe the cord for color, amount of Wharton's jelly, and the presence of two arteries and one vein (such inspection should have been done in the delivery room and results charted on record). The rectum should also be inspected for patency if it has not been checked at birth. Gentle insertion of a soft rectal catheter can identify any problems. Auscultate for bowel sounds, which should be present a few hours after delivery.

Palpation of the entire abdomen is usually done by the pediatrician. It should be done at least 2 h after a feeding. The lower pole of the kidney can usually be felt if the lumbar region is supported from beneath the infant while the flank is palpated just under the costal margin, deeply to the spinal column. The liver is evaluated for size by palpation from the right iliac crest up to the right costal margin until the lower liver edge is felt to slip against the fingers. The liver should be found 1 to 2 cm below the right costal margin. The belly should feel soft, with some meconium-filled loops of bowel, felt as sausage-shaped masses. The kidneys and spleen should be smooth and firm. No masses should be present.

NORMAL   The abdominal wall should be free of any defects. The abdominal muscles may feel split longitudinally at the midline (diastasis rectii), a normal variation more common in black infants. The umbilical cord changes should be consistent with the age in days. The rectum should be patent, and meconium should be passed within 24 h after birth.

ABNORMAL   A single umbilical artery is a finding to alert the examiner to the possibility of congenital, especially renal anomalies. Meconium-stained cord is a sign of intrauterine stress; small, shriveled cords are seen

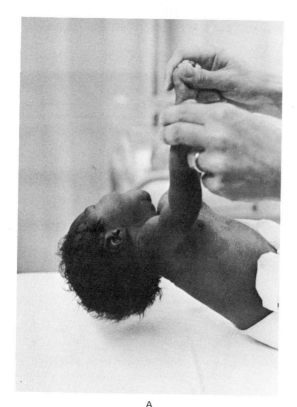 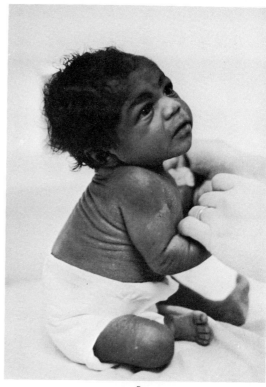

A   B

fig. 14-17   (a) Pulling to sit. (b) Sitting. Note head lag. (*Photo by Mary Olsen Johnson, M.D.*)

with intrauterine growth retardation. An umbilical hernia is not uncommonly found, protruding especially as the infant cries. An imperforate anus is a defect which should be suspected when the rectal catheter cannot be inserted or when no stool is passed. Other, more severe anomalies are discussed in Chap. 29.

back

technique   Hold the infant under the chest and lift horizontally, allowing the spine to arch. Observe for muscle tone and neck control. Place the infant in a prone position, observe for birthmarks and hair distribution over the shoulders. Run your fingers over the entire spine from neck to sacrum. Observe for dimple at base of spine, fatty pad, or hair tuft (Fig. 14-18).

NORMAL   Flexion and extension of spine should be smooth and regular. There should be no obvious defects noted by observation or palpation. Observe for mongolian spots and nevus simplex.

ABNORMAL   All abnormalities of the back are rare.

Meningomyelocele, herniation of the spinal cord and membranes through a midline defect, is an obvious defect found most often in the lumbar region (see Fig. 29-8). *Meningocele* is similar but

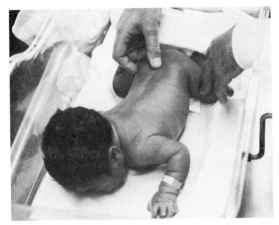

fig. 14-18 Newborn can lift head and turn it from side to side. (*Photo by Ruth Helmich. Courtesy of the Jamaica Hospital, Jamaica, N.Y.*)

involves only the membranes. Deformities associated with spinal anomalies are club foot, congenital dislocation of hips, and hydrocephalus. *Spina bifida occulta* is a defect which is less obvious but should be suspected when a small dimple, tuft of hair, or depression is found at the base of the spine.

extremities

technique Observe extremities for symmetry of movement, posture at rest, and any evidence of fracture, lacerations, or bruising. The hands and feet should be inspected for *polydactyly*, (extra digits), *syndactyly* (fused digits), *clinodactyly* (incurving digits), or absence of digits. Note condition of the nails. Note the degree and pattern of sole and palmar creases. Examine the feet for structural or positional deformities. (The latter may be passively manipulated past the midline and result from pressure in utero.) Elicit the Moro and tonic-neck reflexes to evaluate any damage to the brachial plexus as well as to evaluate overall neurologic status.

The physician usually examines for congenital dislocation of the hip by performing *Ortelani's maneuver*. The infant is placed in the supine position. The right side of the pelvis is fixed firmly to the mattress with the right hand. The fingers of the left hand are placed around the infant's left hip until the greater trochanter of the femur is felt. Using the left palm and thumb, the left femur is flexed onto the abdomen. If the hip is dislocated, a click may be heard and felt as the femur slips back into the acetabulum with the flexion of the hip. The right side is tested by reversing the hands.

NORMAL The extremities should move symmetrically, coming to a position of flexion when movement ceases. No evidence of trauma should be noted. There should be no deformities of the digits. Fingernails should come to the fingertip in a term infant. The feet should rest in a neutral position, and Moro and tonic-neck reflexes should be brisk and complete.

ABNORMAL Lack of movement of any limb should be investigated. Immature or depressed infants may return to a position of partial flexion, depending upon their condition. Duplication or absence of digits or limbs may occur as a single anomaly or in association with a syndrome. A simian crease (single horizontal palmar crease) is associated with Down's syndrome. Fractures may occur, especially during a difficult delivery of a large infant. There will be only unilateral responses to Moro and tonic-neck reflexes when *Erb's palsy* is found. In this brachial plexus injury, the affected arm is held adducted and rotated internally. It is caused by traction and lateral flexion upon the neck during delivery.

genitalia: female

technique The femoral pulses should be palpated during this part of the physical exam and their equality evaluated. The size of the clitoris and labia should be noted: these vary with gestational age. Configuration of the labia and presence of hymenal tag (small tag of mucous membrane extending from vagina) should be noted.

NORMAL The femoral pulses should be equal. In the term female, the labia almost completely covers the clitoris. There should be no fusion of the labia; hymenal tags may be found and are innocuous. A white mucous discharge, sometimes streaked with light pink blood (pseudomenstruation), is often present and is the result of withdrawal of maternal hormones. Labia may be edematous and darker than usual in response to birth pressures and maternal hormones.

ABNORMAL Ambiguous genitalia have characteristics of both sexes. In the female, fused labia, clitoral hypertrophy, and/or placement of the urinary meatus anterior to the clitoris are signs of sexual ambiguity. Causes of these malformations include disorders of the sex chromosomes or unusual amounts of androgens either formed by the fetus or taken by the mother (see Chaps. 28 and 29).

genitalia: male

technique Inspect the penis for correct placement of the meatus. Palpate femoral pulses. Then palpate the testes by blocking the inguinal canal with one finger while gently palpating the scrotum with a thumb and forefinger (Fig. 14-19).

NORMAL The meatus should be placed at the tip of the penis. Each testis should have descended into the scrotum to be palpated separately. Each should be smooth and freely movable. Changes in male genitalia which occur with gestational age should be equivalent to the infant's estimated age. Edema may be normally present in the first few days.

ABNORMAL *Hypospadias* is found when the urinary meatus opens on the ventral aspect

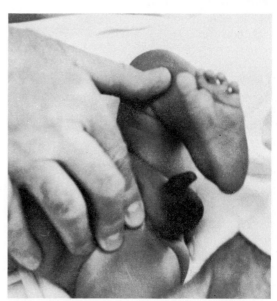

fig. 14-19 Examination for undescended testes. (*Photo by Ruth Helmich.*)

of the penis. In *epispadias*, the opposite occurs: the meatus is on the dorsum. An unusually small penis and bifid or split scrotum may actually be clitoral hypertrophy and fused labia. These findings call for more investigation before a sex can be assigned to the infant. *Neonatal torsion* occurs when one testis twists on its spermatic cord; this can produce infarction owing to lack of circulation. The scrotal skin appears darker on the affected side, and the testis feels irregular and fixed to the scrotal skin. Surgical intervention is necessary to prevent loss of the testis. *Hydrocele* is fluid in the scrotum and is found more frequently after a breech delivery.

EVALUATION OF GESTATIONAL AGE

The gestational age of the newborn infant is calculated in weeks from the LMP 2 weeks before conception (see Chap. 3). Prenatally, fetal age can be assessed by various indirect means, e.g. ultrasound and estimated size (see Chap. 27). After birth, physical examination of the infant can lead to a more accurate assessment of maturity. It is important to determine the maturity of the infant, for complications of the neonatal period vary greatly with the degree of maturity; premature and postmature infants have the most difficulty adapting to extrauterine life. Supportive treatment can be provided once it is recognized which handicaps might be present. Thus, every infant should have the benefit of this assessment, particularly since gestational age is usually related to weight at birth, but this may vary greatly.

Once gestational age is determined, it should be plotted against weight on the graph in Fig. 14-20. Then it can be seen if the weight is reflecting adequate intrauterine growth. Those infants who have appropriate growth

table 14-7 When should examination for gestational age be done?

Questionable menstrual history.

Infant born with less than 38 weeks or more than 42 weeks in utero.

EDD by LMP dates and ultrasound differ by more than 2 weeks.

Abnormal uterine growth.

Abnormal maternal weight gain.

The mother has a repeat cesarean section.

A primary cesarean section was done without labor.

Abnormalities in the neonatal adjustment to extrauterine life.

for gestational age (AGA) are those whose weights fall between the tenth and the ninetieth percentile. Deviations from expected weights are indicative of intrauterine conditions which have threatened the fetal well-being (Table 14-7).

Using statistics gathered over a 10-year

fig. 14-20 Neonatal mortality risk based on weight and gestation (Colorado data 1958–1968.) (*Reproduced with permission from Kempe Silver, and O'Brien (eds.), "Current Pediatric Diagnosis and Treatment," 2d ed., Lange, Los Altos, Calif., 1972.*)

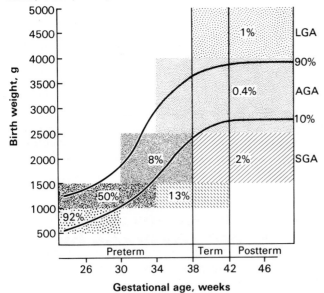

period at the University of Colorado Medical Center, Lubchenco et al. created a tool which allows easy postnatal assessment of intrauterine growth using parameters of both size and age. The determination of gestational age when plotted against birth weight on the graph in Fig. 14-20 classifies the infant in the LGA (large for gestational age), SGA, (small for gestational age) or AGA category.

LGA = over the ninetieth percentile for gestational age.

SGA = under the tenth percentile for gestational age.

AGA = between the tenth and the ninetieth percentile for gestational age.

large-for-gestational-age infant

Anticipation and early detection of conditions associated with deviations in intrauterine growth can reduce neonatal mortality and morbidity. One example is the identification of the LGA infant. Such an infant has an increased chance of being born of a mother with diabetes and may become hypoglycemic or hypocalcemic and have respiratory distress. The same infant may experience birth trauma as a result of its size but may really be premature in regard to lung maturity and neurologic development (see Chap. 29).

small-for-gestational-age infant

The SGA infant usually has been affected by one or more prenatal influences disturbing normal growth: (1) intrauterine malnourishment as a result of poor placental transfer of nutrients or unavailability of those nutrients because of poor maternal nutrition; (2) intrauterine infections or environmental teratogenic influences; and (3) congenital malfor-

mations serious enough to affect growth potential. An infant may be SGA in *any* category of maturity, and risk of complications in the neonatal period is high. (See Table 30-1 for detailed mortality rates in different weight and age groupings; see Fig 30-1.)

postmature infant

The postmature infant presents quite a different problem, and since such an infant is seen more often in the normal newborn nursery, some detail is included here. Postmaturity is defined as a gestational age over 42 weeks post-LMP, but the diagnosis cannot be confirmed until assessment has been completed. The causes for postmaturity are not known in the majority of cases.

The postmature infant appears unusually alert and attentive and is often described as "wide eyed." The infant may be SGA if chronic placental insufficiency was present, or it may be AGA, with a long, lean appearance as a result of recent weight loss. The skin is wrinkled and displays poor turgor. Desquamation is widespread owing to the total absence of vernix at birth. Typical newborn hair may be partially shed. Fingernails extend past the fingertips, as there has been extra time for growth in utero. Decreasing placental function with resultant hypoxia (chronic fetal distress; see Chap. 27) may have caused the passage of meconium. The amniotic fluid will then be stained with thick yellow-green material, and skin, nails, and cord may appear a greenish yellow. If the infant aspirated the meconium, the chest may appear hyperinflated (with an increase in anteroposterior diameter), and the abdomen may appear less distended than usual in the full-term newborn. The cord may be thin, with a decreased amount of Wharton's jelly. Genitalia appear mature, and many deep sole and palmar creases are evident. Unless there is neonatal distress, the infant's posture is hypertonic. When such infants have problems they are cared for in intensive care units.

scoring systems

Several attempts have been made to develop a system for assessment of gestational age that is easy to perform, is replicable by many examiners, and has a high correlation with actual gestational age. All involve observations of physical characteristics and a neurological examination. The two methods most often used are the Dubowitz score and the University of Colorado Medical Center examination based on research by Lubchenco and Brazie.

Dubowitz score   Research in 1970 by Dubowitz, Dubowitz, and Goldberg resulted in the creation of an exam using 11 physical and 10 neurological characteristics. A weighted score is used which has a 1.02-week error of prediction. The test is considered the most accurate assessment tool existing to date.[28] However, all 21 items must be investigated to obtain the score. In some cases, this complete procedure may add stress to an infant during the period of transition to extrauterine life. The score only gives the examiner a total assessment of gestational age and does not reveal select characteristics which may differ from the real gestational age as a result of an unfavorable intrauterine environment. Nonetheless, this work provided a foundation for the tools that followed. (The score is now used primarily in high-risk nurseries, and its use is illustrated in Chap. 30.)

University of Colorado, Lubchenco score   The Lubchenco method of assessment also uses physical and neurological criteria, but in a different way (see Fig. 14-21). The first part of the examination is performed in the first few hours after birth and requires little manipulation of the infant to yield a fairly accurate assessment of gestational age. The second part of the examination is done 24 h after birth, when the effects of maternal medication, birth trauma, and transition to extrauterine life have lessened. It is also best done 2 h after feeding, when the infant is neither too sleepy nor too hungry. This second aspect, a fairly complex neurological examination, needs to be performed only when a difference exists between the gestational age via maternal history and the gestational age estimated during the first part of the exam. However, the arm recoil and resting postures are two parameters included in the first part of the test which provides a good estimate of neurological development even in the early hours after birth.

This test provides for assessment with little manipulation. It also utilizes a chart citing the age of onset of each parameter, which can reveal uneven fetal development as a result of an unfavorable intrauterine environment.[29] Ranges are wide, however, and it may be difficult for a new student to interpret the sum of the variables. Therefore, the student should note that it is the trend which indicates age and not one item alone. Lubchenco states that "the estimation of gestational age is usually made by the nurse admitting the infant. The nurse gives each sign a gestational age, interpolating the age if necessary. If the ages assigned are fairly uniform, she records the clinical estimate as the observed mean, or gives the age as a range—37 weeks, or 36 to 37 weeks. If there are discrepancies . . . or if there is a clear difference between her assessment and the gestational age calculated from the mother's dates, she records both." Lubchenco goes on to state that infants who show such a discrepancy are classified as high-risk infants and should be observed more closely for additional problems.[30]

Since performance of the entire assessment may be impossible when the newborn is critically ill, the discovery of one physical or neurological sign that would correctly pinpoint gestational age would be ideal. However, uneven fetal development makes this discovery unlikely. Nicolopoulous et al. have determined that examination of the following nine physical signs yields a high (0.878) correlation with gestational age.[32] Use of these criteria alone provides for easy assessment of sick neonates. Although the use of the eight neurological criteria yields a lower correlation (0.850) and requires the examiner to disturb the infant, such criteria should be added when questions remain.

Physical criteria:
1 Skin texture
2 Skin color
3 Skin opacity
4 Lanugo
5 Plantar creases
6 Nipple form
7 Breast size
8 Ear formation
9 Ear firmness

Neurological criteria:
1 Posture
2 Square window
3 Dorsiflexion—foot
4 Popliteal angle
5 Heel to ear
6 Scarf sign
7 Head lag
8 Ventral suspension

Figure 14-22 (page 298) illustrates the record keeping necessary to summarize the course of newborn recovery. Lubchenco's method of assessment is given in detail in Tables 14-8 and 14-9 (pages 292–297).

Study Questions

1 Name four factors which influence the initiation of respiration at birth.
2 Describe why *surfactant* is essential.
3 Trace the changes in fetal circulation once respiratory function has been established.
4 Correlate the factors affecting weight gain or loss in the first 3 days of life; include renal function, blood volume, ambient temperature, and nutritional intake.
5 Describe at least four factors which affect the maintenance of a correct thermoneutral range for a term newborn.
6 What signs would indicate that a newborn was suffering hypothermia? What are the most common causes in the newborn nursery? In the home?
7 Describe the appearance of the following: vernix, acrocyanosis, desquamation, milia, miliaria, erythema toxicum, and petechiae.
8 Differentiate between caput succedeneum, cephalhematoma, and molding.
9 Observe three phases of an infant's sleep cycle. Describe sleep patterns to the mother and discuss ways of promoting a sleep routine once the infant is at home.
10 Note the lab results on a preterm baby, a jaundiced baby, and a postterm baby. Compare these with the readings in Table 14-2. (Remember to use your own hospital laboratory normals if there is discrepancy, as figures change according to lab techniques).
11 Practice assessment steps on a lab baby model before approaching a newborn. Note the sequence and the major observations first. Add subtle observations as your skill grows.
12 Note the nine physical criteria which correlate well for gestational age, and using only these check your assessment of several babies with those assessments done by fellow students.
13 Describe the differences between a postterm infant and a term infant in at least five ways.

Examination, first hours

Weeks of gestation

Physical findings		Findings across weeks 20–48
Vernix		Appears (20–21) · Covers body, thick layer (22–38) · On back, scalp, in creases (38) · Scant, in creases (40–41) · No vernix (44–48)
Breast tissue and areola		Areola and nipple barely visible, no palpable breast tissue (20–24) · Areola raised (35) · 1–2 mm nodule (36–37) · 3–5 mm (38) · 5–6 mm (39) · 7–10 mm (40–42) · ≥12 mm (46)
Ear	Form	Flat, shapeless (24–33) · Beginning incurving superior (34–35) · Incurving upper two-thirds pinnae (37–38) · Well-defined incurving to lobe (42+)
Ear	Cartilage	Pinna soft, stays folded (27–32) · Cartilage scant, returns slowly from folding (33) · Thin cartilage, springs back from folding (38) · Pinna firm, remains erect from head (43+)
Sole creases		Smooth soles without creases (25–31) · 1–2 anterior creases (32–34) · 2–3 anterior creases (35) · Creases anterior two-thirds of sole (36) · Creases involving heel (38) · Deeper creases over entire sole (43)
Skin	Thickness and appearance	Thin, translucent skin, plethoric, venules over abdomen, edema (29–33) · Smooth, thicker, no edema (34) · Pink (36) · Some desquamation, pale pink (40) · Thick, pale, desquamation over entire body (42)
Skin	Nail plates	Appear (20) · Nails to finger tips (33–34) · Nails extend well beyond finger tips (43+)
Hair		Appears on head (20–21) · Eyebrows and lashes (23) · Fine, woolly, bunches out from heat (30) · Silky, single strands, lays flat (38) · ?Receding hairline or loss of baby hair, short, fine underneath (44)
Lanugo		Appears (20–21) · Covers entire body (25–30) · Vanishes from face (34–35) · Present on shoulders (39–40) · No lanugo (45)
Genitalia	Testes	Testes palpable in inguinal canal (28–32) · In upper scrotum (37) · In lower scrotum (43)
Genitalia	Scrotum	Few rugae (32) · Rugae, anterior portion (37) · Rugae cover (40) · Pendulous (45)
Genitalia	Labia and clitoris	Prominent clitoris, labia majora small, widely separated (31–34) · Labia majora larger, nearly covered clitoris (37–38) · Labia minora and clitoris covered (43)
Skull firmness		Bones are soft (23–28) · Soft to 1 in. from anterior fontanelle (30) · Spongy at edges of fontanelle, center firm (35) · Bones hard, sutures easily displaced (38–39) · Bones hard (40) · Bones hard, cannot be displaced (43)
Posture	Resting	Hypotonic, lateral decubitus (22–23) · Hypotonic (28) · Beginning flexion, thigh (31) · Stronger hip flexion (33) · Frog-like (34) · Flexion, all limbs (36) · Hypertonic (39) · Very Hypertonic (44)
Recoil	Leg	No recoil (25) · Partial recoil (35) · Prompt recoil (40)
Recoil	Arm	No recoil (26) · Begin Flexion, no recoil (34) · Prompt recoil, may be inhibited (38) · Prompt recoil after 30 inhibition (41) · Prompt recoil (43)

Column scale (weeks of gestation): 20 21 22 23 24 25 26 27 28 29 30 31 32 33 34 35 36 37 38 39 40 41 42 43 44 45 46 47 48

Confirmatory neurologic examination

	Physical findings	Weeks of gestation (20–48) — findings
Tone	Heel to ear	No resistance → Some resistance (30) → Impossible (35)
	Scarf sign	No resistance → Elbow passes midline (34) → Elbow at midline (37) → Elbow does not reach midline (45)
	Neck flexors (head lag)	Absent → Head in plane of body (38) → Holds head (44)
	Neck extensors	Head begins to right itself from flexed position (33) → Good righting, cannot hold it (36) → Holds head few seconds (38) → Keeps head in line with trunk 40s (42) → Turns head from side to side (45)
	Body extensors	Straightening of legs (33) → Straightening of trunk (36) → Straightening of head and trunk together (43)
	Vertical positions	When held under arms, body slips through hands (29) → Arms hold baby, legs extended (35) → Legs flexed, good support with arms (38) → Head above back (42)
	Horizontal positions	Hypotonic, arms and legs straight (29) → Arms and legs flexed (36) → Head and back even, flexed extremities (38)
Flexion angles	Popliteal	No resistance → 150° (29) → 110° (33) → 100° (36) → 90° (39) → 80° (41)
	Ankle	45° (33) → 20° (37) → 0° (41)
	Wrist (square window)	90° (29) → 60° (33) → 45° (37) → 30° (39) → 0° (41)
Reflexes	Sucking	Weak, not synchronized with swallowing (27) → Stronger, synchronized (33) → Perfect (36) → Perfect, hand to mouth (39)
	Rooting	Long latency period, slow, imperfect (29) → Hand to mouth (32) → Complete (45)
	Grasp	Finger grasp is good, strength is poor (30) → Stronger (36) → Can lift baby off bed, involves arms (40) → Hands open (46)
	Moro	Barely apparent (26) → Weak, not elicited every time (30) → Stronger (34) → Complete with arm extension, open fingers, cry (37) → Arm adduction added (39) → Begins to lose moro (47)
	Crossed extension	Flexion and extension in a random, purposeless pattern (29) → Extension but no adduction (33) → Still incomplete (37) → Extension, adduction, fanning of toes (40) → Complete (45)
	Automatic walk	Minimal (31) → Begins tiptoeing, good support on sole (34) → Fast tiptoeing (37) → Heel-toe progression, whole sole of foot (40); A preterm who has reached 40 weeks walks on toes (43) → Begins to lose automatic walk (47)
	Pupillary reflex	Absent → Appears (30) → Present (42)
	Glabellar tap	Absent → Appears (33) → Present (38)
	Tonic neck reflex	Absent → Appears (35) → Present after 37 weeks
	Neckrighting	Absent → Appears (37) → Present after 37 weeks

Notes: A preterm who has reached 40 weeks still has a 40° angle (popliteal). A preterm who has reached 40 weeks walks on toes.

fig. 14-21 Clinical estimation of gestational age. An approximation based on published data. (*a*) Examination, first hours. (*b*) Confirmatory neurologic examination (24 h). (Adapted from Lubchenco, *Pediatric Clinics of North America* **17:**25, 1970. Reproduced with permission from Kempe, Silver, and O'Brien (eds.), "*Current Pediatric Diagnosis and Treatment*," 5th ed., Lange, Los Altos, Calif., 1978.)

table 14-8 Lubchenco exam: examination, first hours

physical findings

Weeks of gestation: 20 21 22 23 24 25 26 27 28 29 30 31 32 33 34 35 36 37 38 39 40 41 42 43 44 45 46 47 48

Physical findings	Description by weeks of gestation
Vernix	Appears (21–23) · Covers body, thick layer (24–37) · On back, scalp, in creases (38–39) · Scant, in creases (40–41) · No vernix (42–48)

Technique: Observe the amount and distribution of vernix.

Variables: Length of time that has expired since delivery. Vernix is often wiped away when baby is first dried.

Physical findings	Description by weeks of gestation
Breast tissue and areola	Areola and nipple barely visible, no palpable breast tissue (20–33) · Areola raised (34–35) · 1–2 mm nodule (36–37) · 3–5 mm (38) · 5–6 mm (39) · 7–10 mm (40–44) · ?12 mm (45–48)

Technique: Observe for the condition of areola and nipple, especially in a very premature infant. Palpate the areola and measure the diameter of breast tissue nodule in millimeters.

Variables: Engorgement of the newborn breast caused by maternal hormones which have crossed the placenta.

Physical findings		Description by weeks of gestation
Ear	Form	Flat, shapeless (20–33) · Beginning incurving superior (34–35) · Incurving upper two thirds Pinnae (36–38) · Well-defined incurving to lobe (39–48)
	Cartilage	Pinna soft, stays folded (20–33) · Cartilage scant, returns slowly from folding (34–35) · Thin cartilage, springs back from folding (36–38) · Pinna firm, remains erect from head (39–48)

Form
Technique: Observe the degree to which the pinna has become incurved, beginning from the superior edge to the lobe.

Cartilage
Technique: Fold the pinna in half and observe the return to its original position

Variables: Congenital malformation syndromes such as trisomy 18 and 21, Potter's syndrome, or others affecting renal development. This occurs because the ears and kidneys develop simultaneously.

Physical findings	Description by weeks of gestation
Sole creases	Smooth soles without creases (20–32) · 1–2 anterior creases (33–34) · 2–3 anterior creases (35) · Creases anterior two thirds of sole (36–37) · Creases involving heel (38–41) · Deeper creases over entire sole (42–48)

Technique: Observe the soles and note the number and depth of creases.

Variables: A black infant may have more sole creases than its 38- to 39-week age indicates.

Physical findings		Description by weeks of gestation
Skin	Thickness and appearance	Thin, translucent skin, plethoric, venules over abdomen, edema (20–32) · Smooth, thicker, no edema (33–35) · Pink (36–37) · Few vessels (38–39) · Some desquamation, pale pink (40–41) · Thick, pale, desquamation over entire body (42–48)
	Nail plates	Appear (20) · Nails to finger tips (33–41) · Nails extend well beyond finger tips (42–48)

Thickness and appearance
Technique: Observe for thickness, translucence, edema, *plethora* (ruddy color), vessels over abdomen, and *desquamation* (peeling).

table 14-8 Lubchenco exam: examination, first hours (*continued*)

Variables: Deeply pigmented skin can make this assessment difficult. Meconium staining of skin is seen frequently in postmature and SGA infants.

Nail plates

Technique: Observe for length of nails in relation to fingertips.
Variables: Total absence of nails (anonychia), partial absence, or dysplasia of nails occurs in several syndromes, such as Apert's syndrome and the trisomies.

Physical findings	Weeks of gestation																												
	20	21	22	23	24	25	26	27	28	29	30	31	32	33	34	35	36	37	38	39	40	41	42	43	44	45	46	47	48
Hair	Appears on head			Eye brows and lashes				Fine, woolly, bunches out from head										Silky, single strands, lays flat					?Receding hairline or loss of baby hair, short, fine underneath					

Technique: Observe the amount, texture, and distribution of hair.
Variables: Several syndromes, such as *Turner's syndrome* (XO), can cause variations in the quality and distribution of hair.

Physical findings	Weeks of gestation																												
	20	21	22	23	24	25	26	27	28	29	30	31	32	33	34	35	36	37	38	39	40	41	42	43	44	45	46	47	48
Lanugo	Ap-pears		Covers entire body											Vanishes from face				Present on shoulders				No lanugo						

Technique: Observe the amount and distribution of lanugo.
Variables: None.

Physical findings		Weeks of gestation																												
		20	21	22	23	24	25	26	27	28	29	30	31	32	33	34	35	36	37	38	39	40	41	42	43	44	45	46	47	48
Genitalia	Testes										Testes palpable in inguinal canal							In upper scrotum			In lower scrotum								
	Scrotum										Few rugae							Rugae, anterior portion			Rugae cover		Pendulous						
	Labia and clitoris											Prominent clitoris, labia major small, widely separated						Labia majora larger, nearly cover clitoris			Labia minora and clitoris covered							

Male

Technique: Palpate the testes for location. Apply gentle pressure over the inguinal canal to prevent the testis which you palpate from ascending through the canal.
Observe the amount of *rugae* covering the scrotum. These are deep, pigmented wrinkles in the skin.
Variables: Ambiguous genitalia can make the testes appear to be in the canal when they are in fact absent. The scrotum can appear immature when the testes are undescended.

Female

Technique: Observe the degree to which the labia covers the clitoris.
Variables: Ambiguous genitalia with fused labia and hypertrophied clitoris can appear to be immature male genitalia. IDMs have increased fat deposits, and genitalia may appear more mature. Conversely, an SGA infant may have decreased fat deposits causing the genitalia to appear less mature than the true AGA.

table 14-8 Lubchenco exam: examination, first hours (*continued*)

Physical findings	Weeks of gestation						
	20 21 22 23 24 25 26 27 28 29	30 31 32 33 34	35 36 37	38 39 40 41	42 43 44 45 46 47 48		
Skull firmness	Bones are soft	Soft to 1 in. from anterior fontanelle	Spongy at edges of fontanelle, center firm	Bones hard, sutures easily displaced	Bones hard, cannot be displaced		

Technique: Palpate the skull for firmness.
Variables: Malformations of the cranium and conditions which affect hypothyroidism.

Physical findings	Weeks of gestation							
	20 21 22 23 24 25 26 27 28 29	30 31	32 33	34 35	36 37	38 39 40 41	42 43 44 45 46 47 48	
Posture Resting	Hypotonic, lateral decubitus	Hypotonic	Beginning flexion, thigh	Stronger hip flexion	Frog-like	Flexion, all limbs	Hypertonic	Very hypertonic

Technique: Observe the position the infant takes while resting.
Variables: Maternal oversedation can cause hypotonia in a mature infant. Infants born with low Apgar scores can be hypotonic or convulsive. Hypoglycemia or hypocalcemia causes tremors at rest. Infants with trisomy 21 are hypotonic at term.

Physical findings	Weeks of gestation				
	20 21 22 23 24 25 26 27 28 29	30 31 32 33 34 35 36 37	38 39 40 41	42 43 44 45 46 47 48	
Posture Recoil - Leg	No recoil	Partial recoil	Prompt recoil		
Arm	No recoil		Prompt recoil, may be inhibited	Prompt recoil after 30 s inhibition	

Leg
Technique: Extend the leg for a few seconds and then let it return to its original position.
Variables: Maternal oversedation, periods of sleep in the newborn, and depression can cause a slowing of the leg recoil.
Arm
Technique: Extend the arm for a few seconds and then let it return to its original position.
Variables: Same as for leg recoil with the addition of Erb's palsy.

table 14-9 Lubchenco exam: confirmatory neurologic examination to be done after 24 h. (This part of the examination should be done about 2 h after feeding, when the infant is alert and not too hungry.)

Physical findings	Weeks of gestation				
	20 21 22 23 24 25 26 27 28 29	30 31 32 33 34	35 36 37	38 39 40	41 42 43 44 45 46 47 48
Tone Heel to ear		No resistance	Some resistance	Impossible	
Scarf sign	No resistance		Elbow passes midline	elbow at midline	Elbow does not reach midline

Heel to ear
Technique: Attempt to make the heel of one foot meet the same-sided ear by extending the leg. To test for this correctly, you must fix the pelvis to the mattress with one hand while extending the leg with the other.

table 14-9   Lubchenco exam: confirmatory neurologic examination (*continued*)

Scarf sign

Technique: Attempt to bring the infant's arm across the chest and around the neck until the elbow is as close to midline as possible.

Variables: Damage to the arm such as Erb's palsy or *arthrogryposis* (congenital muscular disorder with lack of active and passive movement in the extremities).

Physical findings		Weeks of gestation																												
		20	21	22	23	24	25	26	27	28	29	30	31	32	33	34	35	36	37	38	39	40	41	42	43	44	45	46	47	48
Tone	Neck flexors (head lag)													Absent						Head in plane of body						Holds head				
	Neck extensors													Head begins to right itself from flexed position				Good righting, cannot hold it	Holds head few seconds	Keeps head in line with trunk 40 s				Turns head from side to side					

Neck flexors

Technique: Grasp the infant's hands and attempt to bring the infant to a sitting position. Observe the degree to which the head is held in line with the trunk.

Variables: Trisomy 21 infants are hypotonic even when mature.

Neck extensors

Technique: Place the infant in a sitting position and observe efforts to lift the head in line with the trunk. A postmature baby can maintain this position and turn its head from side to side when placed on its abdomen.

Variables: Same as neck flexors.

Physical findings		Weeks of gestation																												
		20	21	22	23	24	25	26	27	28	29	30	31	32	33	34	35	36	37	38	39	40	41	42	43	44	45	46	47	48
Tone	Body extensors													Straightening of legs				Straightening of trunk				Straightening of head and trunk together								
	Vertical positions								When held under arms, body slips through hands							Arms hold baby, legs extended			Legs flexed, good support with arms										
	Horizontal positions								Hypotonic, arms and legs straight									Arms and legs flexed	Head and back even, flexed extremities		Head above back								

Body extensors: vertical positions

Technique: Hold the infant under the arms and note the degree to which it holds body straight. In the same position, note the stiffening or the attempts to support body with legs. Observe the degree of leg flexion.

Variables: Trisomy 21, drug-depressed infants. Infant too sleepy.

Body extensors: horizontal positions

Technique: Hold the infant under the chest in a horizontal position. Be sure hand is not over abdomen. Note the degree to which the infant can hold its head *even* with the back (Fig. 19-1).

Variables: Same as above.

table 14-9   Lubchenco exam: confirmatory neurologic examination (*continued*)

Physical findings		Values (weeks of gestation 20–48)
Flexion angles	Popliteal	No resistance (20–28); 150° (≈29); 110° (≈33); 100° (≈36); 90° (≈39); 80° (≈41)
	Ankle	45° (≈33); 20° (≈38); 0 (≈40); A preterm who has reached 40 weeks still has a 40° angle
	Wrist (square window)	90° (≈28); 60° (≈32); 45° (≈37); 30° (≈39); 0 (≈41)

Flexion angles: popliteal angle

Technique: With the infant on its back, try to extend the knee angle. The thigh may be against the trunk. This does not influence the result.

Variables: None.

Flexion angles: ankle flexion

Technique: Flex the ankle by attempting to make the superior aspect of the foot meet the ventral aspect of the lower leg (tibial surface).

Variables: None.

Flexion angles: wrist flexion

Technique: Try to flex the wrist by pressing down on the hand so that the palm can meet the forearm.

Variables: None.

Physical findings		Values (weeks of gestation 20–48)
Reflexes	Sucking	Weak, not synchronized with swallowing (≈27–30); Stronger, synchronized (≈32–33); Perfect (≈34–37); Perfect, hand to mouth (≈38–40); Perfect (≈42+)
	Rooting	Long latency period, slow, imperfect (≈27–30); Hand to mouth (≈32–33); Brisk, complete, durable (≈34–40); Complete (≈42+)

Sucking

Technique: A pacifier or clean finger can be placed in the infant's mouth to test suck reflex. Stimulated best with slight pressure near mid-tongue.

Variables: Infants with cleft lip or cleft palate.

Common variables for all reflexes: Depression owing to maternal oversedation, neonatal asphyxia/hypoxia, central nervous system damage, systemic disease (sepsis, respiratory distress syndrome, metabolic disorders) and hypoglycemia. Hypotonia often accompanies chromosomal problems.

Rooting

Technique: The infant will bring hand to face, turn toward hand touching cheek, and bring hand to mouth.

Variables: As above.

Physical findings		Values (weeks of gestation 20–48)
Reflexes	Grasp	Finger grasp is good, strength is poor (≈27–30); Stronger (≈32–37); Can lift baby off bed, involves arms (≈38–41); Hands open (≈46+)
	Moro	Barely apparent (≈22–26); Weak, not elicited every time (≈27–31); Stronger (≈32–33); Complete with arm extension, open fingers, cry (≈34–37); Arm adduction added (≈38–41); ?Begins to lose moro (≈46+)

Grasp

Technique: Place your finger in the infant's palm with some pressure. After the infant grasps it, try to bring the child to a sitting position using the strength of the grasp.

Variables: Erb's palsy.

table 14-9   Lubchenco exam: confirmatory neurologic examination (*continued*)

Moro

Technique: Lift the head of the bassinet 2 to 3 in and allow it to fall back (prevent any sound when the frame falls) This method assures that the infant's head and back are well supported by the mattress and yet will cause a sense of falling and thus startle. (Loud noises test hearing.)

Variables: Spina bifida, Erb's palsy.

Physical findings		Weeks of gestation																											
		20	21	22	23	24	25	26	27	28	29	30	31	32	33	34	35	36	37	38	39	40	41	42	43	44	45	46	47	48
Reflexes	Crossed extension								Flexion and extension in a random, purposeless pattern						Extension but no adduction		Still incomplete			Extension, adduction, fanning of toes					Complete				
	Automatic walk												Minimal	Begins tiptoeing, good support on sole				Fast tiptoeing		Heel-toe progression, whole sole of foot					A preterm who has reached 40 weeks walks on toes			?Begins to lose automatic walk	

Crossed extension

Technique: A painful stimulus such as a pinprick applied to one leg causes extension of the opposite leg in an attempt to remove the painful stimulus.

Variables: Spina bifida with neural involvement.

Automatic walk

Technique: Hold the infant in a vertical position and allow the soles of the feet to touch a hard surface (mattress of crib may or may not elicit this). Observe whether the infant walks on its toes alone or uses heel-to-toe progression.

Variables: Spina bifida with neural involvement (meningomyelocele)

Physical findings		Weeks of gestation																											
		20	21	22	23	24	25	26	27	28	29	30	31	32	33	34	35	36	37	38	39	40	41	42	43	44	45	46	47	48
Reflexes	Pupillary reflex		Absent								Appears					Present														
	Glabellar tap			Absent										Appears			Present													
	Tonic neck reflex			Absent							Appears					Present														
	Neck-righting				Absent											Appears			Present after 37 weeks											

Pupillary reflex

Technique: Hold the eyelids open with one hand while shining a light into the eye. The pupil will contract with the light (going from 2 to 3 mm down to 1 to 2 mm). This may be difficult to do without a helper.

Variables: Edema from birth or chemical conjunctivitis may hinder opening of eyes. Ptosis of lid is present with Horner's syndrome.

Glabellar tap

Technique: Tapping the infant's forehead between the eyes will cause both eyes to blink.

Variables: None.

Tonic neck

Technique: Turn infant's head to one side. Observe for "fencing position" with extension of same-sided arm and leg and flexion of opposite arm and leg.

Variables: As above, general reflex variables.

Neck righting

Technique: Place the infant in the prone position, face down. As a survival reflex, the infant will turn face to the side.

Variables: None except general variables above.

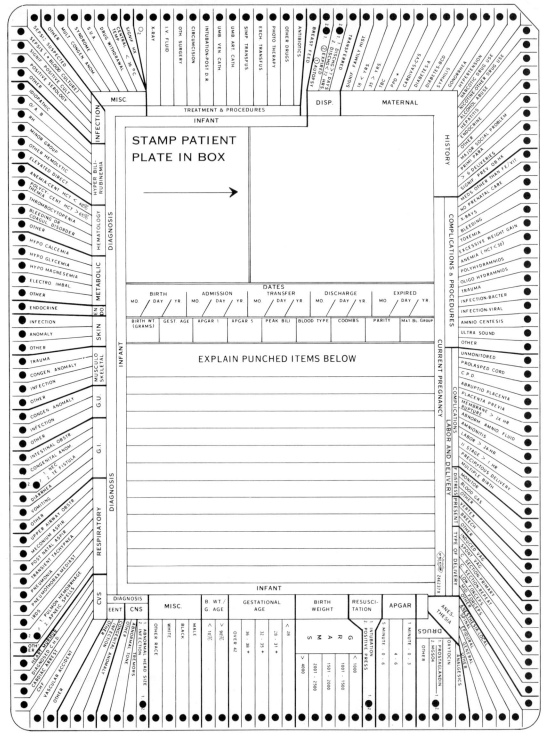

fig. 14-22 Record keeping to summarize course of newborn recovery. (*Courtesy of McBee Systems, Belleville, N.Y.*)

references

1   C. A. Smith and N. M. Nelson, *The Physiology of the Newborn Infant,* Thomas, Springfield, 1976, p. 122.
2   L. B. Strang, "The Lungs at Birth," *Archives of Diseases of Children,* **40**:575, 1965.
3   M. H. Klaus and A. A. Fanaroff, *Care of the High-Risk Neonate,* Saunders, Philadelphia, 1973, p. 236.
4   Ibid., p. 137.
5   Smith and Nelson, op. cit. pp. 232–237.
6   H. E. Evans and L. Glass, *Perinatal Medicine,* Harper & Row, New York, 1976, p. 157.
7   The Committee on Nutrition, "Nutritional Needs of the Low Birth Weight Infant," *Pediatrics,* **60**(4):519, October 1977.
8   S. B. Korones, *High-Risk Newborn Infants,* Mosby, St. Louis, 1973, p. 212.
9   E. Gladtke and G. Hermann, "The Rate of Development of Elimination Functions in the Kidney and Liver of Young Infants," in P. L. Morselli (ed.), *Basic and Therapeutic Aspects of Perinatal Pharmacology,* Raven Press, New York, 1975, p. 394.
10 H. E. Grupe, "The Kidney," in M. H. Klaus and A. A. Fanaroff (eds.), *Care of the High-Risk Neonate,* Saunders, Philadelphia, 1973, p. 257.
11 D. A. Clark, "Times of First Void and First Stool in 500 Newborns," *Pediatrics,* **60**(4):457, October 1977.
12 V. Y. H. Yu, "Stomach Emptying in Neonates," *Archives of Diseases of Childhood,* **50**:500, 1975.
13 Gladtke and Hermann, op. cit., p. 399
14 M. Johnson and J. Gash, "Transport of Neonates," *The Canadian Nurse,* May 1976, p. 19.
15 E. Hey, "Thermal Neutrality," *British Medical Bulletin,* **11**(1):69, 1977.
16 Klaus and Fanaroff, op. cit., p. 59.
17 D. Hull, "Temperature Regulation and Disturbance," *Pediatric Clinics of North America,* **24**(3):44, August 1977.
18 Evans, op. cit., p. 83.
19 Ibid., p. 82.
20 E. E. Crelin, *Anatomy of the Newborn Infant,* Lea and Febiger, Philadelphia, 1969, p. 24.
21 L. O. Lubchenco, *The High-Risk Infant,* Saunders, Philadelphia, 1976, p. 46.
22 Crelin, op. cit., p. 42.
23 N. Kendall and H. Woloshin, "Cephalhematoma Associated with Fracture of the Skull," *Journal of Pediatrics,* **41**:125, 1952.
24 E. Stern et al., "Sleep Cycles of Infants," *Pediatrics,* **43**(1):65, January 1969.
25 H. P. Roffwarg et al., "Sleep Patterns with Increasing Age," *Science,* **152**:604, 1966.
26 Y. Brackbill, T. C. Douthitt, and H. West, "Psychophysiologic Effects in the Neonate of Prone versus Supine Placement," *Journal of Pediatrics,* **82**:82–84, January 1973.
27 T. B. Brazelton, "Neonatal Behavior and Its Significance," in A. J. Schaeffer and M. E. Avery, *Diseases of the Newborn,* Saunders, Philadelphia, 1977, Chap. 3, pp. 37–53.
28 H. Nishida and R. M. Risenberg, "Silver Nitrate Ophthalmic Solution and Chemical Conjunctivitis," *Pediatrics,* **56**(3):368, September 1975.
29 L. M. S. Dubowitz, V. Dubowitz, and C. Goldberg, "Clinical Assessment of Gestational Age in the Newborn Infant," *Journal of Pediatrics,* **77**:1–10, 1970.
30 J. V. Brazie and L. O. Lubchenco, *Current Pediatric Diagnosis and Treatment,* 3d ed., Lange, Los Altos, Calif., 1974, p. 40.
31 Ibid., p. 61.
32 D. Nicolopoulous et al., "Estimation of Gestational Age in the Neonate," *American Journal of Diseases of Children,* **130**(5):480, May 1976.

bibliography

Akamatsu, T. J.: "Management of the Newborn," *Pediatric Clinics of North America,* **24**(3):660, August 1977.
Alexander, N. M. and M. S. Brown: *Pediatric Physical Examination for Nurses,* McGraw-Hill, New York, 1974.
Auld, P. A. M.: "Resuscitation of the Newborn Infant," *American Journal of Nursing,* **74**(1):69, 1974.
Avery, G. B. (ed.): *Neonatology: Pathophysiology and Management of the Newborn,* Lippincott, Philadelphia, 1975.
Boenisch, T.: "Biochemical Scoring," *Journal of Perinatal Medicine,* **2**(2):122, 1974.
Buist, N. R. M.: "Metabolic Screening of the Newborn Infant," *Clinics in Endocrinology and Metabolism,* **5**(1):284, March 1976.
Chard, M. A. and G. S. Dudding: "Common Skin Problems in the Newborn and Infant," *Issues in Comprehensive Pediatric Nursing,* July/August 1976.
Cook, L. N.: "Deviant Fetal Growth," *Pediatric Clinics of North America,* **24**(3):400, August 1977.
Desmond, M. M. et al.: "The Clinical Behavior of the Newly Born," *Journal of Pediatrics,* **62**:307, 1963.
Finer, N. N. et al.: "Ventilation and Sleep States," *Journal of Pediatrics,* **89**(7):100, July 1976.
Fredrickson, W. T. et al.: "Posture as a Determinant of Visual Behavior in the Newborn," *Child Development,* **46**(2):579, June 1975.
Hogan, G. R. and N. J. Ryan: "Neurologic Evaluation of the Newborn," *Clinics in Perinatology,* **41**(1):31, March 1977.
Hoppenbrowers, T. et al.: "Polygraphic Studies of Nor-

mal Infants During the First Six Months of Life: III. Incidence of Apnea and Periodic Breathing," *Pediatrics,* **60**(4):418, October 1977.

Lipsett, L. P.: "The Study of the Sensory and Learning Processes of the Newborn," *Clinics in Perinatology,* **4**(1): 163, March 1977.

Livingston, R., V. Crane, and L. C. Mims: "Clinical Assessment of Gestational Age," *Journal of Obstetric, Gynecologic and Neonatal Nursing,* **6**(6):7, November-/December 1971.

Lubchenco, L. O.: *The High-Risk Infant,* Saunders, Philadelphia, 1976.

Marcil, V.: "Physical Assessment of the Newborn," *The Canadian Nurse,* March 1976, p. 21.

Miller, M. E.: "Host Defenses in the Human Neonate," *Pediatric Clinics of North America,* **24**:43, 1977.

Nalepka, C. D: "Understanding Thermoregulation in Newborns," *Journal of Obstetric, Gynecologic and Neonatal Nursing,* **5**(6):17, December 1976.

Popich, G. A. and D. W. Smith: "Fontanels, the Range of Normal Size," *Journal of Pediatrics,* **80**:749, 1972.

Shaeffer, A. J. and M. E. Avery: *Diseases of the Newborn,* 3d ed., Saunders, Philadelphia, 1971.

Soloman, L. M. and N. B. Esterly: "Neonatal Dermatology. I. The Newborn Skin," *Journal of Pediatrics,* **77**(5): 888, 1970.

Stave, I.: *Physiology of the Perinatal Period,* Appleton-Century-Crofts, New York, 1970.

Vulliamy, D. C.: *The Newborn Child,* Churchill-Livingstone, Longman, New York, 1977.

Yao, A. C.: "Expiratory Grunting in the Late-Clamped Normal Neonate," *Pediatrics,* **48**:865, 1971.

15

NEWBORN INFANT CARE

JANET S. REINBRECHT

The transition from fetal to newborn existence is not necessarily uneventful. Although many babies make the transition to extrauterine life very easily, each newborn must be assessed individually. The baby needs to be observed closely to determine how smoothly and efficiently the adjustment has been made. The ultimate goal is *anticipatory* and *preventive* care. It is essential to know the stressors involved in the reorganization of the newborn's metabolic processes and the changes in the physiologic functions in order to prevent additional stress.

PRENATAL HISTORY

The following prenatal influences upon the intrauterine environment may compromise the newborn's potential for life.

1 *General health of the mother*, especially any maternal condition which might have

affected the fetal development, such as toxemia, Rh-negative blood type with rising antibodies, or a prediabetic effect. A medical disease may also compromise the fetal growth.

2 *Nutritional status* may be far more of an influence than presently credited. An anemia, even a mild one in early pregnancy, with a hematocrit value lower than 32 percent is hard to correct. A hematocrit value below 34 percent at the time of birth could be a liability, especially if the level has remained lower than 32 percent for weeks during either the second or third trimester.

3 *Chemical factors,* including sprays and drugs taken orally, inhaled, or rubbed on the skin. The dose and duration of exposure may influence the baby's progress.

4 *Gestational age,* which indicates the maturity of the fetus at various stages of development, indicating normal progress in functional maturity.

INTRAPARTUM HISTORY

The intrapartum period presents a different set of factors which may influence the transition of the fetus to life outside the uterus.

1 *Length and intensity of labor:* This may impair oxygen transfer across the placental membranes or cause fetal distress as a result of cord compression. Evidence of fetal response can be detected by changes in fetal heart rate and pattern and/or by meconium staining of the amniotic fluid. Causes of abnormal labor patterns and duration may be of fetal or maternal origin.

2 *Rupture of membranes:* The earlier the rupture, the more likelihood there is of severe molding and possible cephalhematoma, along with tearing of the tento-

rium cerebelli. In addition, there is danger of infection from prolonged rupture of membranes, too frequent vaginal examinations, or manipulations when the fetus is being monitored directly.

3 *Medications received during labor and delivery:* There is growing evidence that certain medications affect the behavior of the baby, interfering with reflexes and inhibitory responses.

4 *Type of delivery, including operative procedures* that could cause injury to the baby. If the mother was asleep for the delivery, it is important for her to see her child as soon as she awakes.

POSTDELIVERY INFORMATION

1 *Apgar score and specific behavioral responses at birth* that indicate the normalcy of the newborn's adjustment. These signs give an accurate picture of the immediate functioning of the heart and lungs (Table 15-1).

2 *Findings of the gross physical assessment in the delivery room,* so that the nursery personnel can compare the admission observations with the description given in the delivery room.

IMMEDIATE CARE AFTER BIRTH

The anticipated moment of birth has arrived. The event culminates many months of growth involving some hazards and potential problems. To assist the newborn in making a safe adjustment to extrauterine life, it is important to follow very basic principles.

1 Maintenance of an adequate airway
2 Provision of warmth and dry skin
3 Protection from injury and infection

clearing the airway

At birth the newborn will be held with the head slightly lower than the feet at the level of the mother's perineum. In this position the mucus, blood, and any amniotic fluid that may be present will be able to drain away from the baby's upper respiratory tract. A soft bulb syringe should be in the delivery pack and used to gently remove any excess fluid, first from the oropharynx and then from the nostrils. When drainage is performed in this order, it is less likely that the baby will inhale the fluid (Fig. 15-1). If the newborn cries or begins to breathe immediately, this initial suctioning may be sufficient. However, the bulb syringe should remain near the baby. Additional mechanical means for resuscitation should be close at hand should they be necessary.

After the cord has been clamped and cut, the baby should be gently dried with a warm blanket, wrapped in a warm dry blanket, and placed on the mother's abdomen. The baby should be positioned with its head down about 15°, and this can be accomplished on the mother's abdomen. If the mother is not awake, the baby should be placed in a warm crib at a 15° Trendelenburg angle.

For most babies, respiration will be initiated within seconds to a minute after birth. Initially, the newborn may show some degree of cyanosis. At birth, respiratory effort and color are evaluated on the Apgar scoring chart. The score is taken at 1 min after birth, and the nurse is in a good position to make this evaluation. It can be scored again at 5 min to note changes, especially if the score was low at 1 min. The scoring system helps to assess the adequate functioning of the heart and

fig. 15-1 Oropharyngeal suctioning. (*Photo by Mary Olsen Johnson, M.D.*)

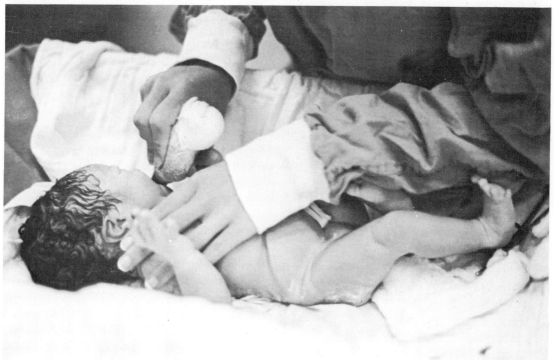

table 15-1 Apgar newborn scoring system*

sign		score		
Acrostic		*0*	*1*	*2*
A—Appearance	Heart rate	Not detectable	Below 100	Above 100
P—Pulse	Respiratory effort	Absent	Slow, irregular	Good, crying
G—Grimace	Muscle tone	Flaccid, limp	Some flexion of extremities	Active motion
A—Attitude (tone)				
R—Respirations	Reflex irritability	No response	Grimace	Cough, sneeze, or cry
	Color	Blue, pale	Body, pink; extremities, blue	Completely pink

Source: Used by permission of Dr. Virginia Apgar, 1974.

*If the natural skin color of the child is not white, alternative tests for color are applied, such as color of mucous membranes of mouth and conjunctiva, color of lips, palms, hands, and soles of feet.

lungs at birth (Table 15-1). It is by no means a diagnostic score for determining the presence or absence of anomalies. There is a correlation, however, with degree of acidosis present at birth (Table 15-2).

keeping the baby warm

Heat loss in the newborn occurs through evaporation, radiation, convection, and conduction. The immediate change from the warm intrauterine to the cool room environment increases the heat loss because the baby's skin is wet and evaporation takes place. The skin must be dried and the baby wrapped in a warm blanket to conserve the heat and restore the balance between heat produced and heat lost (Fig. 15-2).

In her study of neonatal heat loss, Phillips found that babies placed in their mother's

table 15-2 Correlation between Apgar score at 1 min and blood pH

Apgar score	pH
1 to 3	6.9 to 7.0
4 to 7	7.0 to 7.20
8 to 10	Over 7.25

Source: Adapted from P. A. M. Dawes, "Resuscitation of the Newborn," *American Journal of Nursing,* **74**(1):68, January 1974.

arms lost less heat in the first 5 min than was lost by babies put in heated cribs, whereas after 15 min, more heat was lost by the babies held by their mother than by those in cribs.[2] The room temperature contributes to the degree of loss in both situations. That is, the babies lost heat through radiation, heat being transferred from the baby's surface to the cooler surfaces in the environment.

The radiant heat loss has been overcome by encouraging skin-to-skin contact of the baby with its mother or father while the baby is covered with an oven-warmed blanket. An overhead radiant heater may also be used. The room temperature is such that the mother is comfortable in her hospital gown. In fact, the opposite effect may be produced at times, with the heat thus generated raising the baby's temperature above 99°F.

If the baby is to be weighed in the delivery room, the scale should be away from draughts; an overhead radiant heater would minimize the possibility of heat loss by convection as a result of air currents passing over the baby's skin. Similarly, loss via conduction can be minimized by having the surface warmed before placing the baby on it.

Keeping the baby warm must be a continued priority while caring for the newborn. An understanding of the principles of thermore-

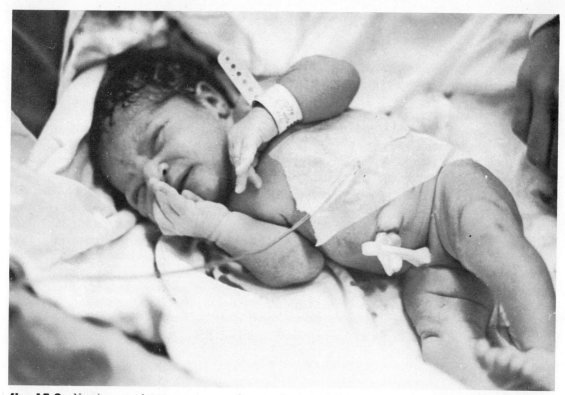

fig. 15-2 Newborn with temperature probe attached to abdomen to monitor temperature constantly. (*Photo by Mary Olsen Johnson, M.D.*)

gulation will influence the manner in which any care is undertaken so that the body heat may be preserved. The baby's ability to adapt to extrauterine life and establish normal respiratory patterns depends upon its being kept warm. Warmth also helps maintain an acid-base balance and helps stabilize the newborn's nutritional needs.

preventing infection and injury

The baby does not have protective skin flora at birth. This is important to remember because the newborn is exposed to a variety of bacterial agents. Abrasions from the forceps or fetal scalp monitor, as well as the wound at the tip of the cord stump, can provide entrance points for such agents. The newborn has passive immunity from the mother, but this immunity will not protect against the organisms encountered at the time of birth and immediately thereafter. Therefore, all supplies to be used in the care of the newborn must be medically clean. Hand-washing technique must be scrupulously practiced. The baby's body should be dried in the delivery room, and the face and head cleansed with sterile water and quickly dried. If the infant's temperature is below normal, any further cleansing can wait until it stabilizes. Even when the temperature is stable, the only other area to be cleansed regularly is the groin and perineal region after bowel movements and voiding. Unless other areas are soiled, they should be left untouched. The vernix caseosa may have a protective function, and there is no evidence to the contrary. It may also serve to conserve heat. This method of "dry skin care," that is, no abrasive soaps or hexachlorophene and limited early bathing, is recommended by the Committee on the Newborn of the American Academy of Pediatrics.[3]

The eyes are especially susceptible to infection, particularly to gonorrheal infection. The use of prophylactic ointment or eye drops is required by law in the United States. Some institutions continue to use the Credé treatment, which involves the instillation of a drop of 1% silver nitrate in each conjunctival sac. Hospital practice will determine whether the eyes are flushed with distilled water after the

eye drops. Other institutions use a broad-spectrum antibiotic ophthalmic preparation. Once the prophylactic medication has been instilled, the eyes begin to react; the lids may become slightly swollen and puffy, making it more difficult for the baby to open its eyes (Fig. 15-3).

Maintaining safety can require many forms of action besides preventing infection. The infant must be protected from all types of adverse influences because it is unable to do more than exercise protective reflexes.

Positioning is important to assist the infant's ability to handle secretions. If the mucus is excessive, the stomach may need to be aspirated to remove accumulated swallowed amniotic fluid (average amount, 10 to 15 mL).

fig. 15-3 Eye prophylaxis with erythromycin ointment. (*Photo by Mary Olsen Johnson, M.D.*)

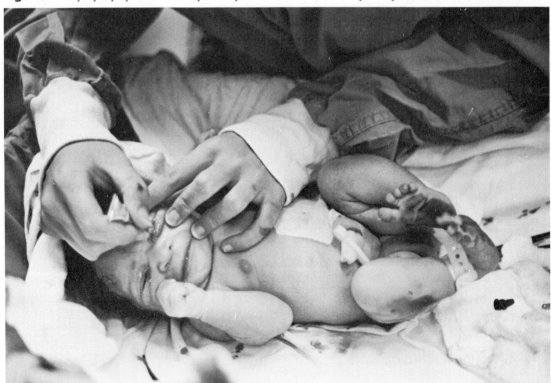

For a short while after the stomach contents have been suctioned, the infant should be placed on its abdomen with its head lower than its feet for postural drainage. Gentle patting over the lung bases will aid drainage. If any mucus remains in the mouth, the baby can be turned over for aspiration of the nasopharynx.[4] The newborn should not be left for long periods with the head down; although it prevents aspiration of mucus, such a position may contribute to increased cerebral edema. The head-elevated position allows for better expansion of the lungs with descent of the diaphragm. Finally, the infant should be placed on its side with the head slightly elevated. Observations should continue at 15-min intervals.

Protection from hemorrhage includes continued observation of vital signs, as well as observation of any abrasions, of the circumcision site, or of a cephalhematoma. A deficiency in coagulation factors is corrected by an intramuscular injection of vitamin K (0.5 to 1.0 mg) into the midanterior thigh (Fig. 15-4).

Such an injection can be administered either in the delivery room or upon admission into the nursery, since vitamin K factors are close to normal at birth but drop during the second and third day.

identification When the baby is separated from the mother after birth, the newborn infant must be protected by being identified before it is taken away (Fig. 15-5). This identification may be accomplished in the following manner:

1 Bracelets may be attached to the baby's wrist and ankle. The information on these bracelets is identical to that on the mother's bracelet. The bracelets contain the mother's full name, the baby's sex, the time and date of birth, and a code number.

2 Some hospitals also fingerprint the mother and footprint the baby on a special form that remains with the baby's chart. After this procedure, the baby's feet should be

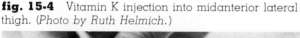

fig. 15-4 Vitamin K injection into midanterior lateral thigh. (*Photo by Ruth Helmich.*)

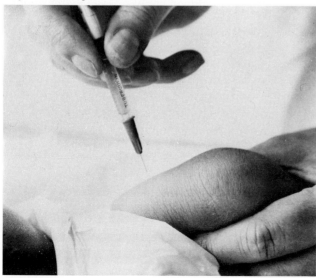

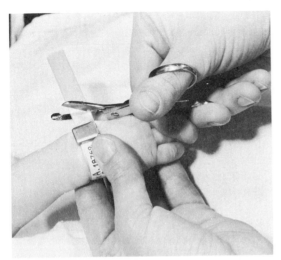

fig. 15-5 Attaching arm band. (*Courtesy of Hollister, Inc.*)

cleaned with oil, taking care to prevent chilling (Fig. 15-6).

bonding Because of the importance of bonding in the earliest possible period after birth, it is recommended that these prophylactic measures be delayed long enough to allow the baby a quiet and peaceful adjustment to the strange environment. When such a time of bonding is possible, for example, when the mother is not under anesthesia, the baby will probably look intently at the parent. Such gazing by both parent and child is considered an important part of the bonding process and will be hindered if eye prophylaxis has been done first or if the baby is upset. The baby's face and head should be washed with sterile water to remove any mucus or blood, and then the infant should be given to the parent to hold. Being warmly held in the arms of a parent will minimize the amount of disturbing stimulation in the first hour after birth. In fact, for some newborns the quiet atmosphere eliminates any need for techniques such as the warm bath suggested by LeBoyer. The beginning of the parent-child

relationship needs time for exploration for the interaction to develop into an ongoing relationship which will provide reciprocal satisfaction. Usually the baby will be transferred to the nursery after bonding has been completed and the baby has fallen asleep. Should the baby be transferred with the mother to the recovery room, she must be alert enough to continue to maintain heat control and hold the baby securely. If she is breast-feeding, this period is an excellent time to begin. The sucking reflex will be strong immediately after birth, and the feeding will help to stimulate uterine contractions as well.

transfer to the nursery

When the baby is admitted to the nursery, it is important for the delivery nurse to report the previously mentioned pertinent information to the nursery personnel. This information includes the type of labor, the length of each stage, the type of delivery (anesthesia, forceps), Apgar scores, and the general condition of both mother and baby. During the passage of the baby through the vagina, maternal secretions may have entered the baby's gastrointestinal or respiratory tract. If membranes are ruptured 12 to 24 h before labor, some infants may have swallowed amniotic fluid containing flourishing bacteria. Another part of the report would include any treatments given, such as the Credé or vitamin K injection, and a double check that the identification bracelet contains the same data as appears on the chart. Finally the nurse should check that both the treatments and the report given are recorded.

TRANSITION

The cycles of transition have not been thoroughly studied. An early report by Desmond and others indicated that there were activity

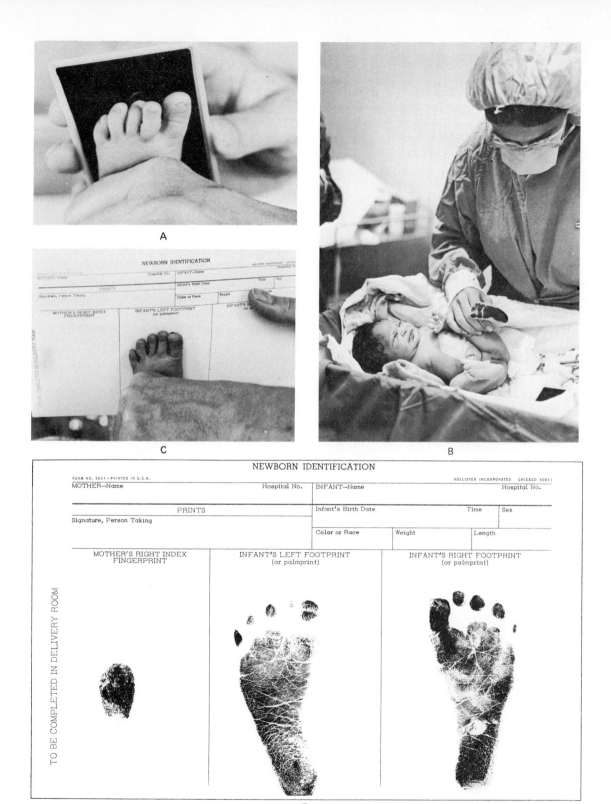

fig. 15-6 Identification process. (*a*) Footprint pad. (*b*) Inky foot. (*c*) Printing. (*d*) Mother's right index fingerprint.

and rest cycles which followed a pattern of postnatal activity peaks in the first and fourth to fifth hours of life, with sleep periods following these peaks times. It is well documented that the fetus has periods of wakefulness and sleep, and this pattern continues into the newborn period.

The term *state* has been used to describe the level of consciousness or responsive arousal. Prechtl et al. proposed five discernible states:

1. Regular or quiet sleep—eyes closed, respiration regular, and no movement.
2. Active or REM (rapid eye movement) sleep—eyes closed, but with rapid eye movement, irregular respiration, and no gross movement.
3. Quiet wakefulness—eyes open; no gross movement.
4. Active wakefulness—eyes open, gross body movement, but no crying.
5. Crying, fussing—eyes open or closed, and crying.[5]

The need for a transitional description to cover those occasions which do not fit neatly into the other five states has led to the term *indeterminate*. In the newborn, the REM sleep is characterized by small muscular twitches and irregularity in respirations, along with an increase in the respiratory rate.

On the first day of life, the newborn was found to have more periods of wakefulness than on the fifth day. On that first day, the pattern seems to consist of longer periods of active wakefulness and fussing, with regular sleep occurring in shorter periods, followed by decreasing amounts of REM sleep and quiet wakefulness. These facts are important to understand, especially for mothers who are discharged early, since the newborn sleep patterns will vary during most of the first week.[6]

The nurse can be alert to these states and

discover the individual variation that Brazelton emphasizes. Prenatal and perinatal factors may influence these behavioral states, such as bilirubin level and/or an inherited disorder. In assessing the newborn's functioning, the nurse notes whether the baby demonstrates the full range of states and whether they seem to be of appropriate frequency and duration. The nurse should also note how easily a change of state can be induced, perhaps by just a change in position. The parents should also be made aware of these observations. Including the parents in this assessment helps them become attuned to their baby's unique pattern of response. In this way, adjustments at home can become more pleasurable and less traumatic.

INITIAL CARE AND ASSESSMENT

Although the baby may have appeared to make a satisfactory adjustment at the time of birth, close observation is important in the next 6 to 8 h. When the mother is fully awake and holding her baby in these first few hours, her body heat will help to maintain the baby's body temperature. However, a crib in the nursery must be warmed prior to the baby's transfer if coming directly from the delivery room.

Individual supplies for each infant are stored in a crib unit and may include:

Mild soap
Shirts and diapers
Crib covers, sheets, and blankets
Lubricant
Individual thermometer or a disposable paper thermometer
Cotton balls in a covered container or paper wipes
Towel and washcloth

Additional equipment from a central area will be utilized for the admission procedures:

Alcohol or Betadine wipes
Capillary tubes
Hemosticks
Ophthalmoscope
Otoscope
Stethoscope
Syringes, needles of various sizes
Paper tape measure, disposable
Tongue depressors
Culture swabs for cord, nasopharyngeal, or stool cultures

The pediatrician may perform a complete physical examination soon after the baby arrives in the nursery or may not see the infant for a day or two. Meanwhile, the nurse should perform an assessment, disturbing the infant as little as possible, and record the findings in a systematic way. Planned assessment can provide essential clues to potential trouble and thus provide for the initiation of immediate intervention.

systematic observations

Each person caring for the newborn should make a systematic evaluation of the baby's appearance and behavior. A description of the newborn characteristics has been provided in Chapter 14. Observations made with a systematic outline will assure accuracy and reliability (Fig. 15-7). For the newborn, time is measured in the number of hours since birth. The practice of carefully adhering to an outline at specific times may reduce neonatal mortality and morbidity. Relationships between prenatal and intrapartal management and that of the baby's condition might become more apparent.

A record of these observations is essential if the baby's health is to be progressively assessed. It is *dangerous and irresponsible* to assume that a baby is developing normally when there is no record of any observations having been made. Be specific, concise, and consistent so that observations can be a guide for planning what action should be taken if there is an indication for intervention. For example, if the temperature is taken because the baby's extremities appeared blue, note the reason, the time of the temperature check, and the action taken in response to the findings. Follow through with another evaluation of the action taken.

provision for warmth

The importance of maintaining the balance between heat production and heat loss cannot be overemphasized. The heat loss is greater from radiation and convection than from evaporation under most newborn situations. Temperatures are higher where the delivery setting is warmer and the mother is able to continue to keep the baby immediately after birth in skin-to-skin contact. When cooler environments cause a drop in temperature, it may take as long as 4 h, with the infant placed in a warm, controlled environment, for temperatures to return to the thermoneutral range.

A word of precaution for newborns who are exposed to radiant heat warmers and phototherapy lamps: There is danger of insensible water loss. Although the mechanism by which nonionizing radiant energy can cause an increase in insensible water loss may not be well known, prevention of the loss is important. The rise in ambient and body temperature under heat lamps increases the skin blood flow. The loss of water may result from evaporation in order to dissipate the heat, because the environment is warm but the humidity is too low. To minimize the water loss, care must be taken to maintain a stable temperature around the baby and to monitor the skin temperature so that the exposure to the heat lamp may be terminated. Limitation of the

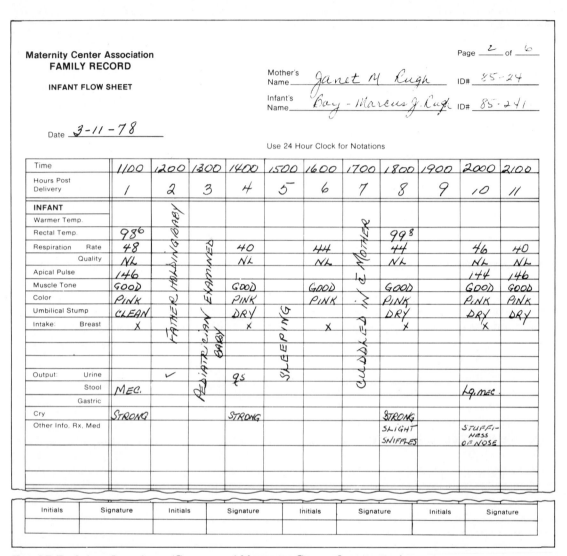

Maternity Center Association
FAMILY RECORD

INFANT FLOW SHEET

Page 2 of 6

Mother's Name Janet M Rugh ID# 85-24

Infant's Name Boy - Marcus J. Rugh ID# 85-241

Date 3-11-78

Use 24 Hour Clock for Notations

Time	1100	1200	1300	1400	1500	1600	1700	1800	1900	2000	2100
Hours Post Delivery	1	2	3	4	5	6	7	8	9	10	11
INFANT		FATHER HOLDING BABY	PEDIATRICIAN EXAMINED BABY		SLEEPING		CUDDLED IN ē MOTHER				
Warmer Temp.											
Rectal Temp.	98^6							99^8			
Respiration Rate	48			40		44		44		46	40
Quality	NL			NL		NL		NL		NL	NL
Apical Pulse	146									144	146
Muscle Tone	GOOD			GOOD		GOOD		GOOD		GOOD	GOOD
Color	PINK			PINK		PINK		PINK		PINK	PINK
Umbilical Stump	CLEAN			DRY				DRY		DRY	DRY
Intake: Breast	X			X		X		X		X	
Output: Urine		✓		qs							
Stool	MEC.									Lg. mec.	
Gastric											
Cry	STRONG			STRONG				STRONG			
Other Info, Rx, Med								SLIGHT SNIFFLES		STUFFINESS OF NOSE	

Initials	Signature	Initials	Signature	Initials	Signature	Initials	Signature

fig. 15-7 Infant flow sheet. (*Courtesy of Maternity Center Association.*)

time under these lamps and careful monitoring of the fluid intake of these babies are essential procedures to control any possible loss.

protection from injury and infection

The newborn has no immunity to pathologic organisms in the environment of the hospital or any other institution outside the parents' home. Therefore, the personnel must be extremely conscientious in hand washing before handling babies and between caring for one after leaving another. Thorough scrubbing of hands and nail beds is essential on entering the nursery. Washing in tepid water is less likely to cause excessive dryness. Removal of as many organisms as possible from the hands and forearms lessens the number that can be transmitted to the delicate and often bruised skin of the baby.

Along with hand washing, the personnel should be encouraged to practice preventive health measures. Often, personnel shortages hinder staff members from taking sick time when suffering from upper respiratory tract infections, skin rashes or lesions, or sore throats. Staff members need to rally to one another's support to encourage that proper care be given to each staff member. The parents will be grateful for the consideration and can be of help by assisting in the care of their baby.

cord care Since the use of hexachlorophene was rejected, there has been no single method recommended for cord care. The end of the cord stump is an open "wound" capable of being colonized with bacteria. Nursery protocol varies, but currently three methods seem acceptable: (1) no treatment except exposure to air to hasten drying; the diaper is folded below the cord to promote drying; (2) a local application of triple dye (a mix of brilliant green, proflavine hemisulfate, and crystal violet), which turns the cord and adjacent skin a dark purple; (3) a local application of alcohol or other antimicrobial agents.[4] Hand washing and careful cleansing after diaper changes may be as effective a preventive measure as the last two methods. In the event of infection, a hexachlorophene bath may be used, but it must be a 3% solution or less and be thoroughly washed off the skin.

Maintaining a separate, clean unit of equipment and layette for each baby assures protection from cross-fertilization of organisms. Bathing, as well as careful cleansing at diaper changes, keeps the baby clean *and* provides an excellent opportunity for a thorough assessment of appearance and behavior. In addition, the bath is an excellent time for parent teaching. Learning through participation in the baby's care will enhance the

parents' confidence in their natural capabilities.

ONGOING ASSESSMENTS

vital signs

Assessment begins with observations related to background knowledge of the normal newborn (Chap. 14) and factors influencing the baby's present status. The nurse's evaluation of all the findings provides the basis for decision making. The progressive stabilization of vital signs and body functions with the initiation of a feeding pattern, whether breast or bottle, indicates that supportive care is sufficient to help the baby make a smooth adjustment to the demands of the new environment. On the other hand, it may be evident that tests should be taken to determine what treatments are needed to assist the newborn in addition to the supportive care. Whichever decision is made, there must be follow-up observations and analysis to determine the appropriateness and effectiveness of the action. Thus, observation, evaluation, intervention, and/or maintenance supported with reassessment provide the process for continuous, safe, and efficacious health care.

temperature An initial rectal temperature should be taken to determine the amount of assistance the newborn will need to maintain or recover a normal core temperature. The baby's normal range lies between 36.7 and 37°C (98 to 98.6°F) after hospital deliveries.

When taking a rectal temperature, lubricate the end of the thermometer with lubricating jelly before insertion. Turn the baby to a side-lying position so the anus can be visualized, and gently insert the thermometer until resistance is felt. (The tip of the bulb should be just inside the rectum, no more than 1.5 cm past the anal opening.) Keep the thermometer in place as long as is required by the type of instrument—some register within 30 s, others by 2 to 3 min (Fig. 15-8).

The initial temperature is always taken rectally to check the patency of the anus as well as the core temperature. After this reading, until stable, axillary temperatures are usually taken every 1 to 2 h to avoid traumatizing the rectal mucosa and unnecessarily stimulating defecation. Remember that an axillary temperature usually records 0.8 to 1.0°F below rectal reading or 0.4 to 0.5°C less than core temperature. Once stabilized, temperatures are routinely taken every 12 h in nurseries. However, once the infant has adjusted to extrauterine life, there is minimal value in using the temperature as a guide to the baby's well-being.

It is important for the parents to know how to take the baby's rectal temperature. Be sure they know before they leave the hospital, but also help them to understand the importance of observing the baby before depending upon the thermometer. Behavioral changes are much more indicative of health, e.g., lethargy, irritability, fretfulness, sleeplessness, and poor sucking reflex, which decreases interest in feeding. These symptoms suggest the possibility that a temperature check may be important, showing either hypothermia or hyperthermia. The composite picture is important to report to the physician.

respirations Although the normal range of respirations lies between 30 and 60 breaths per minute, the average is around 40 breaths per minute. The rate and rhythm are easily influenced by stimuli and will vary with the baby's activity such as crying and feeding or during various levels of sleep and wakefulness.

The respirations of the normal newborn are almost entirely abdominal and quiet. Care must be taken to keep the baby warm while trying to observe the respiratory rate. The rate may be very irregular in the first few hours but will then stabilize. Always count for a full minute, as there are different rhythms within a given 15-second period.

Since the respiratory movements of the newborn are accomplished by the coordination of the diaphragm and abdominal muscles, there is little thoracic activity. Consequently, respiratory movements may be inhibited if pressure is put upward on the diaphragm. For this reason, care should be taken when positioning the baby. By slightly elevating the head of the crib there will be better expansion of the lungs with descent of the diaphragm. If the baby is left in the Trendelenburg position, the abdominal organs could put pressure on the diaphragm. This would be especially true after feedings. Teach the mother the proper position in which to place the infant after feeding (see Chap. 14, stomach emptying time).

pulse The changes in the heart rate reflect the activity of the baby. These variations relate to the states of sleep or wakefulness of the baby. The deeply asleep baby may have a heart rate as low as 90 beats per minute. An average pulse rate may be between 120 and 130 beats but may jump to as high as 160 to 180 beats per minute when the baby is very

fig. 15-8 Taking rectal temperature. (*Photo by Ruth Helmich.*)

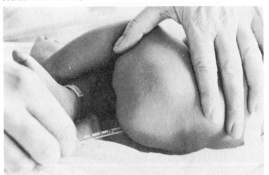

active or crying. These changes can occur rapidly; thus, care should be taken not to startle the baby nor to overstimulate it while trying to locate the sound. It helps to warm the bell before placing it on the baby's chest. Keep the stethoscope under a blanket in the warm crib until ready to use it. And keep the baby well wrapped.

color, cry, activity

Of more value than objective vital signs is the overall "look" of the baby. The state of the baby is reflected in its color, cry, and activity. Once the nurse has "tuned in" to normal newborn function, it will be possible to sense shifts in these three characteristics almost intuitively. "This baby just doesn't look right" is how the feeling is expressed. Such subtle overall changes can easily be seen by the parents, and they should be informed that the pediatrician wishes to know about these shifts in activity as well as the temperature readings. These changes are the infant's body language to inform the caregivers that it does not feel well.

Finally, as listed in Chap. 14, the formal initial assessment of adaptation to extrauterine life should be followed up by gestational age assessment in the first 24 h and neurologic assessment after 24 h if questions have been raised about actual gestational age. Since the infant will continue to change rapidly, an examination prior to going home may elicit data which had been missed. Evaluation will, of course, continue in well-baby follow-up or during the home visits by the community health nurse (see Chaps. 18 and 19).

initiating assessment

The bath provides both an opportunity for the application of the assessment process by the nurse and a time to encourage parent-infant relationship. When possible, include at least the mother in the preparation of equipment for the bath as well as the actual bathing. She will learn to save her own energy by having everything ready and handy. In addition, she can conserve the baby's heat by cutting down on cooling interruptions.

Whatever technique for bathing you teach, begin with the face. Start with clear, warm water and wash the eyes, wiping from the inner to temporal (outer) canthus. Note any discharge or inflammation. The use of one cotton ball or a separate corner of the washcloth for each eye will prevent spreading of possible infection from one eye to the other. Early detection and reporting of discharge may prevent irreparable damage through early initiation of treatment.

If the baby cries during the face washing, watch for symmetry of the facial muscles. Slight facial paralysis may be evident after some traumatic forceps deliveries. Improvement may be seen from day to day. If forceps were not used, other causes will have to be explored by the physician. Note the pitch of the cry, and the baby's behavior at the time of crying, e.g., whether it cries while frantically sucking or straining or whether the body remains limp and motionless.

Deep cleansing of the baby's ears and nose with swabs should be discouraged. A wick can be made from a piece of cotton dampened and then twisted into shape. What cannot be reached with this soft probe is not to be pursued! Further observation of the head can be performed while washing the baby's hair. It is important to wash the hair to prevent the development of cradle cap. After wetting your hands, put just a drop of soap on them and lather the hair. As you run your hand over the hair, you can feel the shape and molding. Be especially alert for any changes, since the last evaluation, in a cephalhematoma. Is it increasing or decreasing in size? If the mother has noticed this bump, explain the cause and care to her. Test the tension of the membranes over the fontanels and encourage the parent to feel and be less fearful of the soft spots.

You can observe the eye movements as you gently pat the hair dry. You may observe that the baby seems to focus upon one spot. More is known today about the baby's ability to see and its interest in bright colors. If you are in white the baby may prefer looking at the mother, who may be dressed in more interesting colors. If you move an object past the baby's face, note whether it follows the object. The baby's hearing is very acute, so do not distract the baby's attention by talking at the same time you are testing the vision.

Of course, the baby is not likely to become really "dirty" while in the nursery or in the mother's room—thus the concept of early "dry skin care." However, the folds of the neck, the axillae, and the creases of the arms, wrists, and clenched hands may become messy from milk or lint or even bowel movements on rare occasions. If left indefinitely, dried milk or lint could cause irritation to the baby's sensitive skin. Therefore, in addition to regular bath times, the folds of the baby's neck and arms should be cleansed after each feeding or regurgitation.

The baby can be kept warm while the face and head are being washed. If the water has cooled, this is a good time to warm it before continuing the bath. With the warm water ready you can now remove the shirt and diaper. Again, use your hands, soaping them and rubbing down the baby's arms and hands rather than soaping the washcloth. In this way, you are able to test the infant's muscle tone. Compare the reflex responses to those on the initial evaluation. This includes noting the symmetry, the vigor or lack of it, the amount of resistance to manipulation, and the type of response to stimulation. Poor responses may indicate a deterioration of the newborn's neurologic status. The legs can be tested in the same way. Wash gently and then rinse thoroughly with the washcloth to prevent irritation to the skin from residual soap. Describe accurately the condition of the skin; indicate the location of any abrasions, rashes, dryness, peeling, mottling, cracking, and bruises. The color of the skin should be observed for indications of jaundice (Chap. 14).

When the baby is quiet, watch the *chest movements* for synchronism and the movements of the intercostal muscles. Describe the respiratory rate and observe the regularity of these respirations for possible periods of apnea. If *breast engorgement* is present, note the degree and whether there is any discharge predisposing to infection. If the baby is quiet enough, check the pulse and compare it with the last recording. See Chap. 29 for symptoms of respiratory and cardiovascular abnormalities.

Since the newborn's breathing is mostly abdominal, you can observe the general appearance of the abdomen as you wash the torso, which, like the extremeties, should be washed with your hands. Note the symmetry from side to side and any distention or tension. Be conscious of the appearance before and after voiding. Palpate the suprapubic region for incomplete bladder emptying. Other masses are more likely to be found in the intestinal region. If any abnormality is suspected, consult with the physician for immediate evaluation to prevent irreversible damage as well as to correct the existing condition.

After carefully rinsing and drying the torso, check the *umbilical cord*. It is important to note the changes in the cord which have been described in Chap. 14. Be knowledgeable of the standing orders available to guide your action when you find indications of infection, such as inflammation of the skin around the cord, discharge from the base of the cord, or an odor. If there is very slight oozing at the base of the cord stump, without signs of infection, the mother can be taught to apply an alcohol sponge to the site of the moisture to help the drying process. Avoid applying the alcohol to the skin, as it has a drying effect that will exacerbate the already dry skin. The cord care may vary from institution to institution but the basic principle underlying the technique is the same. You must keep the cord clean and dry. Asepsis must continue after the cord separates and until the navel is completely healed. That is why a sponge bath is given until there is no longer any scab on the naval.

Dress the baby in a warm, clean shirt and proceed to cleanse the pubic area. In females, the labia minora appear unusually large because the labia majora are underdeveloped. The vaginal discharge is mucoid and may be slightly tinged with blood in the first week of life. As in the adult female, care must be taken to prevent the introduction of any contaminants into this rich media which can support rapid bacterial growth.

Gently cleanse the vulva with a single swipe from front to back with each cotton ball. It may take several days to remove the vernix caseosa from between the labia. A little cleansing with each diaper change is better than prolonged rubbing at one time. In the cleansing process, one should apply the principle of wiping from the front to the back, from the cleanest area to the least clean, even when there is no stool. Extra care is required to keep any excess feces from spreading toward the vagina. Cleanse the groin area and turn the baby on her abdomen to thoroughly cleanse the buttocks and folds in the back.

The genitalia of male infants vary in size. The swelling of the scrotum will decrease in the first week, although at times there may seem to be excess fluid. Cleansing of the area includes washing the scrotum and the glans of the penis. However, the foreskin should not be forced. An adequate cleansing of the smegma around the glans can be accomplished by gently moving the skin so that the opening is visible. The amount of foreskin varies and should remain loose. If the boy is not going to be circumcised, the mother must learn how to cleanse the penis. It is important that she realize the danger of forcing the retraction of foreskin, since it may tighten and cut off normal circulation. It may be several months before the foreskin can be easily retracted.

The groin and buttocks of the baby should be inspected for possible skin irritation resulting from feces or urine. If clear water removes the stool completely, that is fine; the area should then be thoroughly dried by patting gently. Sometimes a little oil may be used to remove the last signs of stool. It should be used sparingly so as not to leave a film upon which bacteria may grow.

elimination

urine Record the frequency, color, and presence of crystals. Since newborns do not excrete fluids and chloride efficiently the urine may become concentrated and dark yellow if the infant is dehydrated. This is another reason for *not* withholding fluids from the baby in those early hours after birth. Frequently the first voiding may occur at birth because the baby's bladder is full at that time. Adequate hydration will produce six to eight wet diapers daily in the first week of life. If it has not been noted and there has been no record of voiding in the first 24 h you will want to palpate the bladder as suggested above and reexamine the penis for any external evidence of obstruction.

stool Progressive changes in the baby's stool are indicative of the baby's general health status and intestinal functioning. *Meconium* is sticky and black-green to almost green in color. After the baby is started on milk feedings the color, consistency, and frequency of the stools will change. Record the color, consistency, and time of elimination to indicate the frequency and pattern of change. (Some color changes and differences in color and consistency, as a result of the type of milk ingested, are illustrated on the inside back cover in Plate D.)

If the stools appear green, this fact should be noted so that it can be determined if a new pattern is developing. A watery green stool is of concern because it may indicate that the baby is contracting an intestinal infection. Naturally, the physician should be notified immediately. In the meantime, the nurse must observe for other signs of infection and protect the baby from further exposure. The baby should be carefully isolated so as to prevent the cross-colonization with other babies. Attention to any sign of diarrhea must be acted upon immediately because dehydration can lead to deterioration of the baby's condition in a matter of hours. Other signs of infection are pallor, no interest in feeding, and hypoactivity, such as no response to the bathing process.

Because newborns are very susceptible to skin irritation, the baby requires appropriate dress for the environment. After the bath, dress the baby to fit the environment. Heat rash around the neck and groin may develop very quickly even when the baby has been too warm only briefly. Therefore, it is important to dress the baby appropriately while trying to keep the room temperature fairly constant. Disposable diapers are likely to keep the buttocks warm enough to develop a rash. Cleansing the buttocks with clear water and then drying and exposing them to the air for short periods may help clear up most rashes quite quickly. When the buttocks are being exposed for healing, a cover over the crib may prevent heat loss and an ordinary lamp nearby may be enough to keep an even heat around the baby.

weight

Compare the weight at birth with the daily weights (Fig. 15-9). The significance of the weight is in relation to the feeding schedule. However, there is no advantage in weighing the baby before and after feedings. The expected weight loss of 5 to 10 percent in the first week is based upon the general practice of starving the baby in the first 6 to 8 h of life or longer without any justification. If the baby is put on a demand feeding, the loss in the first 3 days will be less. A gain over birth weight has been noted early in newborn nurseries whenever demand feeding is encouraged from the first hours after birth.

provision for nourishment

The baby's physiologic hunger is a more reliable guide to needs for nourishment than artificial schedules imposed by hospital routine. Breast-fed babies may require more frequent feedings because they can digest the breast milk more easily. The earlier the feedings are begun, the more likely that a balance will be established between intake

fig. 15-9 Careful guarding of baby during weighing. (*Photo by Ruth Helmich.*)

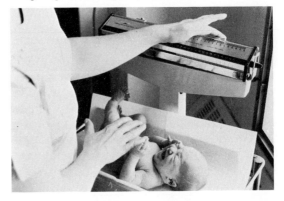

and elimination. The baby should have the full benefit of the *colostrum.* It is known to contain immunoglobulins which protect the baby's gastrointestinal tract from infection. It is of utmost importance that the baby be fed exclusively at the breast for complete protection to be achieved. Besides the freedom from gastrointestinal infections, there is a reduction in respiratory tract infections, and antibodies to polio virus are present in colostrum and breast milk. From birth, the newborn, is best protected against infection if put to the breast as soon as the baby starts sucking.

The important observations during feeding time are the strength of the suck, the ease of swallowing, the amount and type of regurgitation (i.e., if the milk comes up gently or with great force). If the baby appears unable to swallow or if the milk is regurgitated immediately, it is necessary to check for structural anomalies. No time should be lost, and the nurse may be the one to pass a catheter into the stomach. Because the catheter may curl in the esophageal pouch, a small amount of air (1 to 2 ml) injected into the catheter will help in making the diagnosis. The nurse listens over the stomach to hear if the air has passed into the stomach. If no sound is heard in the stomach, notify the physician. Tag the baby's crib with a "DO NOT FEED" sign to prevent other personnel from attempting to feed the baby until further diagnosis can be made.

The baby and mother will both have a satisfying interaction when each is most comfortable in temperature and position (Fig. 15-10). Help the mother into the most relaxed position, with a well-supported back, comfortable perineum, and freshly washed hands. Likewise, the baby needs to be dry and warm but not too warmly wrapped as to be more interested in sleep and cuddling than in nursing. If the baby is really hungry, sucking and rooting for food will be evident. Help the mother to recognize the difference between the sucking of hunger and that which is for comfort. If the mother is relaxed and comfortable, she will be able to convey this calmness to the baby, and the baby's response to the experience is more likely to be a pleasurable one.

circumcision

The medical explanation for the need for circumcision is that there may be a narrowing of the foreskin which obstructs urination, a condition called *phimosis.* However, this is rather rare, and continued practice of circumcision relates mainly to cultural and religious beliefs. The Committee on Fetus and Newborn of the American Academy of Pediatrics reported in 1971 that there were no valid medical indications for circumcision in the neonatal period.

During the prenatal period, the question of circumcision should have been discussed with the parents. They need information about the benefits and the hazards of circumcision at this age.[7] Since it is an operative procedure a parent must sign an operative permit. If the parents have not discussed this procedure prior to the birth of their boy, the nurse needs to take time to listen and provide information upon which they can make their decision.

For the Jewish baby, there will be a ritual circumcision on the eighth day after birth. Some *mohels* require the bilirubin to be no higher than 8 mg before they will perform the circumcision. If the infant is still in hospital, the ceremony can be arranged there. Many families from the Near East and the Orient or parts of Europe do not practice circumcision.

Other reasons for not circumcising the baby may be that the parents do not want to hurt the baby or feel that this early trauma may affect the infant's psychologic development.

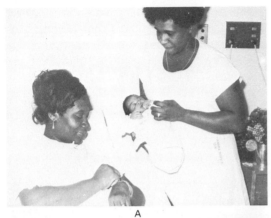

A

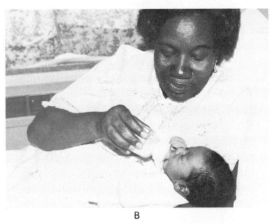

B

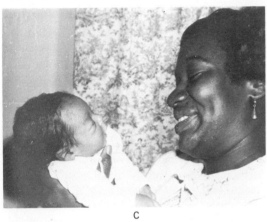

C

fig. 15-10 The critical nursing function of helping to establish a satisfying feeding pattern. (a) Identifying mother and baby by band number. (b) Checking that the mother's position is comfortable. (c) Allowing time for mother and baby to get acquainted. (*Photos by Ruth Helmich. Courtesy of Jamaica Hospital, Jamaica, N.Y.*)

When it is not a cultural preference but rather an emotional response, it is important for someone to explore the psychosexual implications of refusing the procedure with these parents. As the child grows, it will be the parents who will continue to teach him self-care. They must be comfortable with this responsibility and provide a wholesome atmosphere about the cleansing process. One may attempt to assess their maturity, to some degree, by their ability to think through later years.

Because pain may be less intense during the first few weeks of life, it appears to be an opportune time to perform the operation. Indeed, the best time is after the first week of life because the danger of hemorrhage from low prothrombin levels decreases. The blood-clotting factors are developing and the hematocrit value is usually down to a normal level.

The operation consists of surgically removing the foreskin of the penis. Cleaning of the glans is made easier, which lessens the danger of developing an infection when there is a lack of washing facilities. With good bathing habits, however, there should be no greater infection in uncircumcised than in circumcised males.

The operation is a sterile procedure requiring sterile gloves, a sterile field, instruments, gauze, wipes, draping towels, petroleum jelly dressings, and a solution for prepping the skin. The Gomco clamp helps to minimize the bleeding and to prevent the removal of too much foreskin. After the operation, a gauze strip soaked in petroleum jelly is wrapped around the penis (Fig. 15-11). It is important to watch the site for signs of postoperative bleeding. Later, if there is no bleeding and

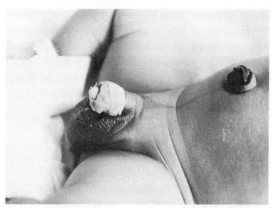

fig. 15-11 Petroleum jelly gauze dressing is kept on circumcision for 24 h and then removed (Gomco method). (*Photo by Ruth Helmich.*)

the gauze strip begins to come off, it may be removed. The major concern is to keep the penis clean and fairly dry. Frequent diaper changes, with the diaper attached loosely, will help to keep the nurse alert to possible bleeding and may "feel good" to the baby. The method using the Hollister plastibell is illustrated in Fig. 15-12. The plastic ring re-

mains in place for 3 to 4 days until healing takes place and then it falls off into the diaper. Parents should be informed that there may be additional problems with this method.[8]

MEETING THE BABY'S PSYCHOSOCIAL NEEDS

Past research has shown that infants in institutions must have loving human contacts to survive. A clean, warm environment and food do not satisfy the emotional needs. The baby is a person with remarkable capabilities of response and interaction, including visual, auditory, and vocal responses. The baby cries, and the caregiver attempts to detect the meaning of the communication. It helps to describe the baby's response to any intervention. The sooner the caregiver responds, the more quickly will the baby be quieted. The act of picking up a crying baby and placing it over one's shoulder will usually soothe the baby temporarily by increasing its visual field and

fig. 15-12 Circumcision. (*a*) Using Hollister plastibell. (*b*) Suture around rim of plastic controls bleeding. (*c*) Plastic rim and suture drop off in 7 to 10 days. (*Courtesy of Hollister, Inc.*)

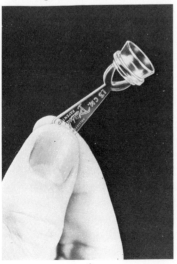

A

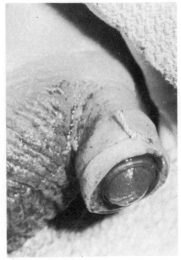

B

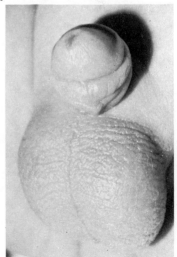

C

thus stimulating alertness to the surroundings and arousing a sleepy baby more fully. It is believed now that this proprioceptive-vestibular stimulation occurs when the baby is lifted and results in the change in the behavior of the baby and a readiness for interaction with the caregiver (Fig. 15-10c).

When the baby's initiation of interaction results in being picked up and becoming more alert, there is social exchange on a level which is understandable to the newborn. Thus the baby can provide the initial stimulation for social interchange. Eye contact further encourages a verbal response from the adult, and the baby can keep the conversation going by rhythmic body movements. This capacity to interact nonverbally with the talking adult in turn encourages parental verbal response and commendation. The presocial smile and reflexes are interpreted as recognition of the offered affection (see Chaps. 17 and 18 for further discussion).

FACILITATING THE PARENT–INFANT RELATIONSHIP

Because hospitals have focused upon setting up routines which help prevent infection and improve assessment and treatment of the newborn, the importance of the mother–infant relationship has often been ignored. More evidence is being found to link family disturbance and child abuse with the separation of the newborn from the mother in the immediate postdelivery hours and days.[9] Recognition of this so-called critical period should encourage immediate maternal contact with her baby. Then, perhaps, we will see a decrease in such disturbing parent-child relationships.

Most assuredly, the nurse can assist the parents to have more opportunities to interact with their baby. As the parents begin to perform caretaking acts for their baby, they begin to establish a bond which reinforces the response between child and parent. The breast-feeding experience, initiated in the delivery or recovery room and continued on the baby's demand, not only provides both comfort and nourishment as well as protection from infection for the baby but also provides a feeling of physical well-being for the mother as well as enhancing maternal affection.

By including the mother in a relaxed and nonrigid routine, she will be less likely to be fearful of handling her baby and more responsive to her baby's style of communication. It is believed that within 3 to 10 days the baby can demonstrate preference for its mother's voice, smell, and appearance. When the mother is relaxed, the unique parent–infant relationship has a better chance to grow.

The father also needs to be given many opportunities to handle and converse with his baby. Because breast-feeding and childbearing are the exclusive privileges of the mother, it is important for fathers to be given every chance to participate in other caregiving activities as early as possible. For this reason, the father should be allowed to spend time with his awake child that does not include feeding. Whenever possible, encourage private sessions between babies and their father. Unwrapping the baby may stimulate the parent to become curious and ask questions. Encourage touching and looking at specific features to assist in overcoming hesitancy and fear of harming the baby. A demonstration of how the baby grasps an extended finger helps to validate a comment about how strong the baby is or demonstrating how to pick up the baby will lessen the idea most parents have of the extreme fragility of a newborn (Fig. 15-13). We must remember that each person has to have the freedom to establish a relationship in his or her own way *and* within his or her own timing.

Privacy with the baby allows the parents to become uninhibited in their efforts to reach out to the baby. Continuation of these efforts to meet the needs of the baby depends upon the parent's feeling that the baby is responding and desires the exchange of emotions to continue.

evaluating the quality of the initial relationship

When the atmosphere has been one of encouragement, self-expression, and participation, one is more apt to be able to assess the quality of the parent-infant relationship and the readiness of the parents to care for their newborn.

During the times when a parent is with the baby, the expressions of affection can be noted by the amount of cuddling, fondling, kissing, and/or talking that takes place. The positive statements of encouragement and admiration will confirm the overt action of fondling and indicate an acceptance of this child as distinct and unique. The specific attention to the behavior of the baby indicates a responsiveness to the baby's social overtures.

The nurse will have many opportunities to note the parents' behavior during a caregiving activity. Are they hesitant in reaching out to touch the baby, is one more aggressive than the other, and do they ask to take part? Do they seek more opportunities to be with the child or are they content to see it only when offered? What kinds of questions do they ask about how to care for the baby when they go home, or do they discuss who will take responsibilities?

When the parents have had the preparation for care of the baby before arriving in the hospital, the postpartum days before going home can be a time to reevaluate and test reality. It may be that a referral is indicated

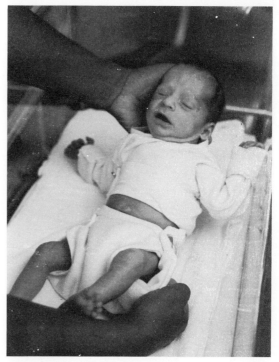

fig. 15-13 Hand placement for picking up infant.

for different reasons. The parents who seem to be hesitant and unsure of how to handle the baby may benefit from a visiting nurse to reassure and encourage the adjustment at home. On the other hand, the self-assured couple may appreciate the continued encouragement of the visiting nurse that what they had planned is workable, or perhaps they may ask for some suggestions in the home setting. In either case, it behooves the nurse to build on the strengths of the mother and father so as to free them to develop more fully their own capabilities. Figure 15-14 was developed jointly by Visiting Nurse Service of New York and Maternity Center Association to guide the VNS nurse in the home visit. The first column asks for the parent's initiated concern, followed by the nurse's assessment, and then the type of action taken.

BABY _____
(Name)

	Parents Had Questions		Problems Found		Instructions Given		Standing Orders Applied		Reinforcement Given		If YES, explain
	Yes	No	Yes	No	Yes	No	Yes	No	Yes	No	
Vital Signs											
Umbilicus											
Head											
Eyes											
Chest											
Skin											
Jaundice											
Elimination— Stool											
Elimination— Urine											
Genitalia											
Crying											
Reflexes											
Feeding— Breast/Bottle (circle one)											
Layette and Equipment											
Other (identify)											

fig. 15-14 Postdelivery Referral Form developed for follow-up visits. (*Courtesy of the Visiting Nurse Service of New York, 107 East 70th Street, New York, 10021.*)

PREPARATION FOR DISCHARGE

Preparation for the discharge of the mother and baby began with her admission. The provision for the participation in the baby's care will be a major factor in easing the transition from hospital to home. The assessment of the readiness for care at home has been the goal throughout her postpartum period. It is very important for the physical condition of the baby to be known to the mother at all times. When it is known that she will be discharged, the baby should also be ready. It can be a severe shock to the parents to be on the verge of getting ready to leave and then to discover that the baby's bilirubin level is elevated and the baby will have to stay another 24 h. It is better that the mother be told of this possibility so she can decide whether to stay in the hospital, especially if she is breast-feeding. In preparation for the discharge physical examination of the baby, therefore, it is wise to have all tests results available for the doctor to assist in making the decision to discharge or keep the baby for further observation and tests.

laboratory tests for the newborn

tests on cord blood The Coombs' test is performed to detect sensitized red blood cells in erythroblastosis fetalis and to identify antibodies in other syndromes. It does not define the blocking agent, but only that such an agent is present.

The direct method uses the serum of rabbits which has been immunized by human gamma globulin. The baby's Rh-positive cells in the cord blood may not agglutinate even though they are coated with Rh antibodies from the mother. But the addition of the rabbit immune antiglobulin causes agglutination to occur because the maternal antibodies are globulin.

If the results of the Coombs' test is strongly positive (+3 to +4) and there are clinical signs (weak sucking, lethargy, flaccidity, hypertonicity) and other laboratory findings (elevated bilirubin), an exchange transfusion is likely to be needed (see Chap. 29).

Blood type and Rh factor will be determined from the cord blood. In addition, in many settings, a test for serology to detect the presence of syphilis is done. Recently, testing for hypothyroid states is also being added.

urine tests Depending upon the nursery setting, a routine urinalysis may be obtained for each infant. In addition, for those infants who appear to be having some difficulty in adjustment or for those who have been subjected to the stress of maternal infection, a urine culture may be obtained.

cultures Cultures of the rectum, cord stump, and nasopharynx may be obtained routinely on admission, and before discharge certain of these may be repeated.

screening Screening for inherited diseases may be done on all infants before discharge, depending upon the length of the hospital stay. If the stay is short, these tests, which are dependent on milk intake, are done in the pediatrician's office. Most tests for metabolic screening do not become valid until there has been sufficient ingestion of milk. Particular tests can be done on infants from high-risk populations (see Chap. 28).

screening for cystic fibrosis Recently, a test strip that detects elevated levels of albumin in meconium has been developed. The first meconium stool is tested by inserting the strip into the meconium and then placing the strip in a test container holding six drops of water. As water is absorbed onto the strip, the color changes to deep blue if the test is positive. The pediatrician and parents are then alerted for the follow-up testing.[10]

screening for phenylketonuria Mandatory screening for phenylketonuria (with an incidence less than cystic fibrosis) was initiated on the discovery that a missing amino acid enzyme resulted in brain damaging levels of phenylalanine. To be at all effective, PKU testing must be done *after* several days of adequate milk intake. Otherwise, testing is inaccurate. Infants of susceptible populations should be retested at the first pediatric visit.

additional tests Using the same blotting paper soaked with heel stick capillary blood, other metabolic screening tests are now being included (see Fig. 15-15).

referrals and home plans

Planning for assistance at home is important. The kind of help required depends more on the parents' needs concerning housecleaning and meals than with the actual baby care.

At some time during the postpartum period, if prenatal arrangements have not been made, plans for *medical supervision* of the baby need to be discussed. If the parents plan to have a private physician, contact will be made with the office to arrange the first pediatric visit and establish contact for *emergency* or telephone contacts for reassurance. If the plan is for use of a well-baby clinic, the right office should be notified so that an appointment may be made. The *referral* form for the Visiting Nurse Service can be made out in advance so that early contact may be made with the family (Fig. 15-14; see Fig. 19-1). The financial cost of the service should also be discussed (see Chap. 19).

The baby's needs should have been thoroughly explored during the several days the mother has been in the hospital. Alerting her to the changes which she may notice in the baby after arriving home will prepare her and prevent any panic. The sleeping-feeding pattern may alter from the one that seems to have

fig. 15-15 Lab slip for metabolic screening. (*Courtesy Moore Business Forms.*)

INBORN METABOLIC ERRORS SCREENING

PATIENT:
Name:
Address:

Birth Date | Birth Weight | Date of Spec.

HOSPITAL (Name and Address):

PHYSICIAN:

	WITHIN ACCEPTABLE LIMITS	FURTHER TESTING ADVISED
PHENYLALANINE	☐	☐
LEUCINE	☐	☐
METHIONINE	☐	☐
HISTIDINE	☐	☐
GALACTOSE URIDYL TRANSFERASE	☐	☐
ADENOSINE DEAMINASE	☐	☐
HEMOGLOBIN SS	☐	☐

SATURATE ALL CIRCLES COMPLETELY

been established in the hospital as the *baby adjusts to a totally new environment*. Use the newly learned skills of the parents to suggest that they will be able to cope and explore ideas they may have of dealing with prolonged crying, quiet wakefulness, and emergency situations such as choking or vomiting.

Assisting the parents to recognize the normal appearance and behavior of their baby will help make them aware of the way to assess the baby's well-being. The following basic factors will indicate that their baby is progressing in a healthy manner:

1 Color: a clear, pink-tinged skin most of the time
2 Muscles which are resistant to straightening, both arms and legs, palmar grasp
3 A vigorous kick when awake
4 A lusty cry as an expression of feelings
5 An eager sucking response to the nipple when hungry
6 Normal stools
7 Periods of rest and sleep

When the mother has been with the baby almost constantly, as with rooming-in facilities, she will know her baby's cry from any other baby and will be able to pick out her baby from others. Nevertheless, the *identification bands* of mother and baby must be checked as they are being discharged. Of course, this is an especially important step when the mother has not seen her baby often or if the baby is being discharged to legal guardians.

homecoming The more the parents have been involved in caring for their newborn, the more welcome the idea may be to them of taking full care of the infant. A meaningful relationship will have been established, and homecoming will be less of a frightening experience.

study questions

1 What major goals govern the nursing action in the deliveryroom and nursery? Illustrate the application of these goals in (a) the physical examination, (b) weighing the baby, and (c) preparation for circumcision.
2 Discuss three examples of how to protect the newborn from injury in the home. List your recommendations for parents to prevent infection in the home.
3 How can the parent-infant relationship be enhanced? Give three examples and explain why each is important.
4 How does the father's relationship with his baby differ from that of the mother?
5 When you observe a delivery, be sure to assign your own Apgar score to the infant and compare it with the one noted on the chart. Why is there a temptation to assign a higher score than is really present? Discuss this problem with your instructor.
6 Write a brief descriptive paragraph about a newborn's adaptive process to extrauterine life.
7 Describe the laboratory tests done routinely for a newborn in regard to timing, reason, normal readings, and signs of deviation from normal.
8 Describe routine medications used for the neonate in regard to action, dosage, and undesirable side effects.
9 Find an opportunity to work with a new mother on a demonstration bath. Outline for yourself the points of teaching that could be covered during that period.
10 If a parent inquires about the value of a circumcision, how would you respond? What home-going teaching would be necessary if the circumcision was done on the morning of discharge?
11 What clues should the nurse recognize as indications of parents' readiness for discharge?
12 Note the needs for referral and planning for discharge in at least one primigravida. What resources are available in your community?

references

1 J. W. Scanlon, "How Is the Baby?: The Apgar Score Revisited," *Clinical Pediatrics*, **12:**61, 1973.
2 C. Phillips, "Neonatal Heat Loss in Heated Cribs and Mothers' Arms," *Journal of Obstetric, Gynecologic and Neonatal Nursing*, **3:**11, November/December 1974.
3 American Academy of Pediatrics, Committee on the Fetus and Newborn, "Skin Care of Newborns," *Pediatrics*, **54**(6):682, December 1974.

4 J. Roberts, "Suctioning the Newborn," *American Journal of Nursing,* **73:**63, January 1973.

5 H.F.R. Prechtl et al., Behavioral State Cycles in Abnormal Infants, *Developmental Medicine and Child Neurology,* **15:**606, October 1973.

6 Binzley, State: Overlooked Factor in Newborn Nursing, *American Journal of Nursing,* **77**(1):102, January 1977.

7 J. M. Perley, "Avoiding Circumcision Complications," *Contemporary OB/GYN* **10**(3):77, September 1977.

8 W. F. Gee, and J. S. Ansell, "Neonatal Circumcision. A Ten-Year Overview: With Comparison of the Gomco Clamp and the Plastibell Device," *Pediatrics* **58:**824, 1976.

9 P. deChateau, "The Importance of the Neonatal Period for the Development of Syncrony in the Mother-Infant Dyad—a Review, *Birth and the Family Journal,* **4**(1):11, spring 1977.

10 W. T. Bruns, T. R. Connell, J. A. Lacey, and K. E. Whisler, "Test Strip Meconium Screening for Cystic Fibrosis," *American Journal of Diseases of Children,* **131**(1):71, January 1977.

bibliography

Adamsons, K.: "The Role of Thermal Factors in Fetal and Neonatal Life," *Pediatric Clinics of North America,* **13:**599, 1966.

Affonso, D.: "The Newborn's Potential for Interaction," *Journal of Obstetric, Gynecologic, and Neonatal Nursing,* **5**(6):9, November/December 1976.

Anderson, G. C.: "The Mother and Her Newborn; Mutual Care Givers," *Journal of Obstetric, Gynecologic and Neonatal Nursing,* **6**(8):50, September/October 1977.

Committee on Environmental Hazards: "Infant Radiant Warmers," *Pediatrics,* **61**(1):113, January 1978.

Dahm, L. S. and L. S. James: "Newborn Temperature and Calculated Heat Loss in the Delivery Room," *Pediatrics,* **49:**504, 1972.

Desmond, M. M. et at.: "The Clinical Behavior of the Newly Born," *Journal of Pediatrics,* **62:**307, 1963.

Gerrard, J. W.: "Breast-Feeding: Second Thoughts," *Pediatrics* **54**(6):757, December 1974.

Kiernan, B. and M. A. Scoloveno: "Fathering," *Nursing Clinics of North America* **12:**481, September 1977.

Klaus, M. H. and J. H. Kennell: *Maternal-Infant Bonding.* Mosby, St. Louis, 1976.

Lozoff, B., G. M. Britenham, M. A. Trause, J. H. Kennell, and M. H. Klaus: "The Mother-Newborn Relationship: Limits of Adaptability," *Journal of Pediatrics,* **91**(1):1, July 1977.

Nalepka, C. D.: "Understanding Thermoregulation in Newborns," *Journal of Obstetric, Gynecologic and Neonatal Nursing* **5**(6):17, November/December 1976.

Pierog, S. H. and A. Ferrara: *Medical Care of the Sick Newborn,* Mosby, St. Louis, 1976.

Sumner, G. and J. Fritsch: "Postnatal Parental Concerns: The First Six Weeks of Life," *Journal of Obstetric, Gynecologic, and Neonatal Nursing,* **6**(3):27, May/June 1977.

16

INFANT FEEDING

BEATRICE LAU KEE
JANE WILSON

The infant in the first year of life undergoes the most rapid period of growth outside the fetal period. It usually triples its birthweight and increases in length by 50 percent by the first birthday. Nutrients provided for the infant must meet the demands of this rapid growth as well as maintain the health of the tissues.

The food intake of young children is to provide for their rapid linear growth and increase in weight. Their nutritional needs are influenced also by the maturation of their gastrointestinal tracts and by the changes in muscle development and coordination.

The gastrointestinal tract takes time to mature. Structurally, the stomach is small and the intestinal motility fairly rapid, causing the stomach to empty within 2 to 2½ h at first. Later the infant can go 3 to 3½ h without symptoms of hunger. Enzyme development is not yet fully mature, so that the infant's ability to digest certain foods is hindered. Sucking, swallowing, and gag reflexes must be coordinated, allowing the infant to suck about 10 to 12 times a minute while breathing 35 to 40 times a minute. Quite an intricate task!

METHODS OF FEEDING

In the United States, more than three-fourths of the infants are still fed by bottle rather than by breast milk, but there is a trend back to breast-feeding, especially among educated middle-class women. When cow's milk was first introduced for infant feeding, the main concern was to provide bacteriologically safe milk. Now, advocates of bottle-feeding are concerned with altering the cow's milk to resemble the nutrient composition of human milk, since most authorities agree that human milk is the best source of nutrition for human newborn infants.

Many factors contributed to the decline in breast-feeding over the last 40 years, and these same factors are now beginning to affect lactation practices in developing countries. First, advertising methods promoted the use of cow's milk, in the form of evaporated milk or as modified formula, as being healthier for babies. Use of these formulas did indeed free mothers from the demands of lactation, which was an important advantage when women had to return to the urban work force soon after delivery. Second, effective family planning methods substituted for lactation as a method of birth control. Third, the availability of a safe, acceptable substitute assured the mother that she was not depriving her infant of essential nutrients. Finally, there was the feeling that in an age of new fashions and rapid changes, women who breast-fed were somehow old-fashioned.

Today, although the woman who does not choose to breast-feed can be assured of a safe substitute in the modified formulas which are available, the superiority of human milk is generally more widely recognized. Nurses need to be familiar with the advantages and disadvantages of each choice and be able to teach the woman about the method she chooses for her baby.

No matter which milk is used in early infancy, fresh cow's milk in a cup and semisolid foods are gradually added to the diet as the infant becomes able to digest this milk and to swallow without sucking. When teeth develop, muscle coordination has reached a point at which the child is able to assist in feeding.

If infant feeding is based on maturation processes, questions about timing of new foods are easily answered. The nutritional adequacy of an infant's diet can be evaluated by making various observations. A steady increase in weight, length, and developmental ability to perform age-related tasks will show that the child is well nourished. Healthy tissues and normal amounts of subcutaneous tissue indicate good nutrition. Elimination should be normal, and the child should have a good balance of rest and activity.

NUTRIENT NEEDS

one to six months

The nutrient needs of the newborn infant are based upon the number of calories the baby requires to gain at the normal rate. The other nutrients, such as protein, minerals, vitamins, and fluids, are calculated in proportion to the caloric content of human milk. The infant receiving human milk regulates its own amount of intake, but the bottle-fed infant should be fed according to the figures for an infant from birth to 1 year of age found in Table 16-1.

calories The newborn infant from birth to 6 months of age requires 117 kcal/kg body weight, about 54 kcal/lb. To calculate the

table 16·1   Recommended dietary allowances for infants during the first year of life

	0 to 6 mo (0.0–0.5 yr)	6 to 12 mo (0.5–1.0 yr)
Weight	6 kg (14 lb)	9 kg (20 lb)
Height	60 cm (24 in)	71 cm (28 in)
Kilocalories	kg × 117	kg × 108
Protein, g	kg × 2.2	kg × 2.0
Fat-soluble vitamins:		
Vitamin A, IU	1400	2000
Vitamin D, IU	400	400
Vitamin E, IU	4	5
Water-soluble vitamins:		
Ascorbic acid, mg	35	35
Folacin, μg	50	50
Niacin, mg	5	8
Riboflavin, mg	0.4	0.6
Thiamine, mg	0.3	0.5
Vitamin B_6, mg	0.3	0.4
Vitamin B_{12}, μg	0.3	0.3
Minerals:		
Calcium, mg	360	540
Phosphorus, mg	240	400
Iodine, μg	35	45
Iron, mg	10	15
Magnesium, mg	60	70
Zinc, mg	3	5

Source: Adapted from *Recommended Dietary Allowances*, 8th rev. ed., National Research Council, National Academy of Sciences, Washington, 1973.

caloric need, multiply the weight in kilograms by 117, or the weight in pounds by 54. Thus, an infant weighing 3.5 kg would need 410 kcal each day.

protein   The amount of protein listed in the Recommended Dietary Allowances for an infant from birth to 6 months is 2.2 g/kg (1.0 g/ lb). To calculate the protein needs of an infant, multiply its weight in kilograms by a factor of 2.2, or its weight in pounds by a factor of 1. An infant weighing 3.5 kg will need 7.7 g of protein daily.

fluids   The amount of fluid needed by the infant depends on its caloric requirements. The infant needs about 1.5 mL for each kilocalorie, because the waste products of me-

tabolism, excreted through the kidneys, need adequate fluid in which to be dissolved. If the proportion of waste products from protein and calcium and electrolytes is too high in proportion to fluid output, the high renal solute load can be dangerous to the infant.

Fluid needs can also be calculated directly in proportion to the infant's weight. The infant should receive 165 mL/kg, (75 mL/lb). An infant weighing 3.5 kg should receive about 570 mL (19 oz) fluid a day.

If the nurse knows the caloric, protein, and fluid needs of an infant, it is then possible to determine how these nutrient needs can be met by the infant's diet. At 3 months of age, when the bottle-fed infant begins to receive additional foods in its diet, the milk intake may be no higher or may even be less than during the first 2 months. The breast-fed infant can receive milk exclusively until 6 months, at which time additional foods are begun.

six to twelve months

The Recommended Dietary Allowance for an infant from 6 to 12 months of age is 108 kcal/kg and 2.0 g protein per kilogram. The growth rate is slowing; thus the caloric and protein levels are diminishing. (If an adult weighing 55 kg received the caloric intake of an infant, the adult would take in 5940 kilocalories per day!) See growth charts in Table 18-1.

obesity

Recent studies have found that the incidence of obesity is higher among formula-fed infants than breast-fed infants. It seems to be easier to force an infant to finish the bottle even when he is not hungry than to overfeed an infant with breast milk. A mother who breast-feeds has only the awareness that the infant is satisfied and therefore does not coax him to drink more.

Obesity is an excess of adipose tissue in the body. In early childhood when body cells multiply rapidly, overfeeding will cause excessive formation of fat cells. As the child grows, these fat cells will also grow in size. If obesity is corrected by diet, the fat cells can only shrink in size; they will never disappear. To prevent obesity in adulthood, it is best to prevent it in early childhood.

Skim milk or 2 percent milk should not be given during the first year of life. If infantile obesity is a problem, the mother should be advised to dilute the formula or milk to lower the concentration of calories.

malnutrition

Malnutrition is defined as faulty nutrition, implying either under- or overnutrition, in any degree. However, this term is most commonly used to refer to severe undernutrition. Undernutrition, an inadequate supply of any of the basic nutrients to the cells, can occur as a result of primary or secondary deficiencies. A primary deficiency refers to a lack of food or nutrient intake. A secondary deficiency results from the inability of the body to digest, absorb, or metabolize nutrients from normal amounts of ingested food.

An example of a primary deficiency is infantile scurvy, which occurs when citrus fruit juices or other sources of vitamin C are not given to the infant. Secondary malnutrition may result from celiac disease, parasitic or bacterial infection of the gastrointestinal tract, or intestinal obstruction. The underlying cause of malnutrition must be discovered and corrected if possible before adequate nutritional intake will be effective.

Although undernutrition is not now a major health problem in the United States, the nurse may see some severely malnourished infants in the hospital. Their diagnoses may range from malabsorption syndrome, nutritional failure, failure to thrive, or marasmus. In countries where protein foods are scarce, kwashiorkor may be a major problem.

Marasmus, severe undernutrition of calories, is usually a secondary deficiency in the United States. It is sometimes referred to as "failure to thrive." Marasmus is usually found in younger children and is characterized by gross underweight and retarded growth, with atrophy of subcutaneous fat and muscle mass. The skin is wrinkled and has poor turgor. Body temperature will be below normal, as metabolism slows and body fat is metabolized. Diarrhea and vomiting are common, quickly upsetting fluid and electrolyte balance.

Kwashiorkor, protein deficiency, is found especially in poverty areas of the world and usually becomes evident after weaning. The basic lack of protein foods in the diet is too often accompanied by parasitic intestinal disease, which further complicates recovery. The most obvious signs of kwashiorkor are enlargement of the abdomen and depigmentation of skin and hair. Growth is retarded, and muscular atrophy, liver enlargement, mental apathy, and lethargy are found. Since brain growth is so rapid during the first years of life, protein malnutrition will prevent a child from developing to his or her potential.

BREAST-FEEDING

anatomy and physiology

The breasts, or mammary glands, are two accessory organs of reproduction located on each side of the anterior chest wall. In the adult, they extend from the second to the sixth or seventh rib and laterally from the sternum to the anterior axillary border. Although the size and shape vary a great deal among individuals, generally they are dome-shaped and have an average weight of 100 to 200 g. During lactation, they increase two to three times in weight.

These glands are composed of adipose, glandular, and fibrous tissue and are separated from the ribs and chest muscles by connective tissue. They are supported by bands of fibrous tissue called *Cooper's ligaments.* The glandular tissue radiates out from the nipple, forming 15 to 20 lobes. Spaces between the lobes are filled with adipose tissue, and the lobes are connected by fibrous tissue. Each lobe is divided into smaller lobules, which contain many *acini,* the acini constituting a layer of epithelium richly supplied with capillaries. The various elements of the milk are formed in this layer. Out of each lobule comes an excretory duct, the *lactiferous duct,* joining into a single main channel that becomes enlarged near the nipple to form a reservoir, the *sinus lactiferous* (Fig. 16-1).

The lactiferous ducts open at the tip of the nipple. The nipple, composed of fibromuscular tissue, is small, pigmented, and cylindrical. It may be flat or may project outward for a few millimeters, and it becomes erect on stimulation. The circular pigmented area around the nipple is called the *areola.* Many sebaceous glands, known as the *tubercles of Montgomery,* secrete fatty substances that lubricate and protect the nipple tissue.

changes during pregnancy

Feelings of fullness and tenderness in the breasts are among the first signs of pregnancy. The following are the changes most noticeable after the second month of pregnancy:

The breasts increase in size (some almost double in size).
The nipples become erect and prominent.
The areola becomes larger in diameter and more darkly pigmented.
The blood vessels enlarge, and darker bluish veins can be seen under the skin.
The tubercles of Montgomery become enlarged and more noticeable.
A thin, yellowish, watery fluid, *colostrum,* can be expressed from the breasts from about the fourth month on.

All these changes are brought about by the two major hormones of pregnancy, estrogen and progesterone. Estrogen is responsible for general breast and milk duct growth; progesterone causes the maturation of the lobular-alveolar system. The secretion of milk is inhibited during pregnancy by high levels of these two hormones. When estrogen and progesterone blood levels rapidly decrease after delivery of the placenta, the luteotropic hormone (LTH), also called *prolactin,* is released from the anterior pituitary gland to begin the production of milk (Fig. 16-2).

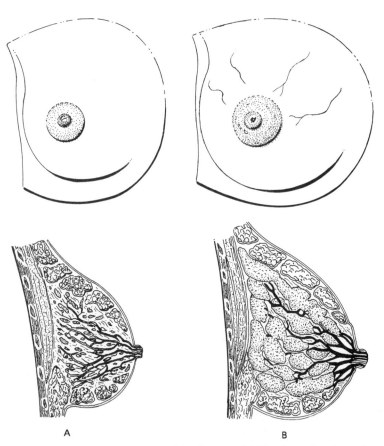

A   B

fig. 16-1 (a) Cross section of the breast. (b) The lactating breast.
(Courtesy of Ross Laboratories, Clinical Education Aid No. 10.)

mechanism of lactation

When the infant is put to the breast, the sucking stimulus at the nipple transmits nerve impulses to the spinal cord and brain, causing release of oxytocin from the posterior pituitary gland. Oxytocin stimulates the anterior pituitary gland, which released LTH, which in turn stimulates the production of milk. Oxytocin also causes contraction of the acini, forcing milk expulsion into the ducts. The sucking of the baby during nursing draws the milk out of the lactiferous sinuses. The whole process is called the *letdown reflex* or the milk-ejection

reflex. (Fig. 16-3). Some mothers may actually feel it as a tingling sensation; others feel nothing. Usually the first outward sign of the letdown reflex is the dripping of milk from one breast as the baby nurses from the other. The reflex may be triggered when a mother hears her baby crying or just sees the child, particularly before a feeding. The letdown reflex can be inhibited by pain or emotional stress in the mother.

Oxytocin, released as a result of the sucking stimulus, also causes the uterine muscle to contract strongly. For the first few days after birth, mothers will often complain of uterine cramps while they are breast-feeding.

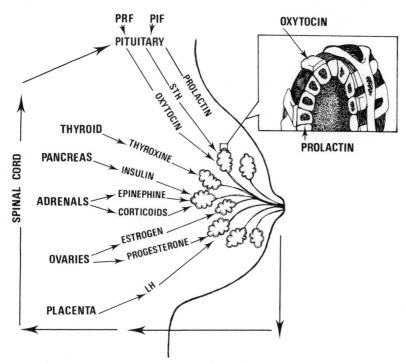

fig. 16-2 Hormonal influences on lactogenesis (*From C. S. Catz and G. P. Guiacoia, "Drugs and Breast Milk," Pediatric Clinics of North America, **19**:153, 1972.*)

maternal nutrient needs during lactation

In order to breast-feed her infant successfully, the mother must eat appropriate foods in adequate amounts in order to produce milk as well as to maintain her health (Table 16-2). The recommended dietary allowances for lactation[1] are determined in proportion to the amount of milk produced each day, the average being 850 ml (see Table 6-1).

calories For every 100 mL of milk which the mother produces, she should consume about 130 kcal over and above her usual baseline caloric intake. An average yield of 850 mL milk provides 650 kcal to the infant. Thus, calories from the mother's food intake can be converted to breast milk calories at 80 percent efficiency. The maternal fat which is stored during pregnancy can also provide 200 to 400 kcal each day for up to 3 months of lactation. Therefore an additional 500 kcal is needed to provide for lactation and the gradual restoration of normal body composition. After the mother loses the stored maternal fat and resumes her normal weight, she should increase her caloric intake to 750 calories over and above her usual baseline caloric intake.

protein Human milk contains an average of 1.2 g protein in 100 mL of milk. Assuming that the average production is 850, with maximum amount of 1200 mL, protein needs just for lactation are considered to be about 15 g daily. A margin of safety is considered in the allowances because protein quality varies in

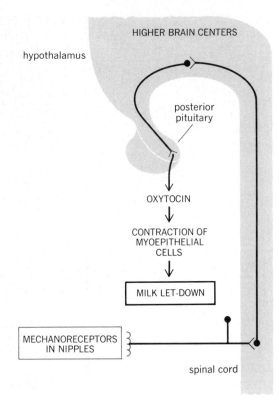

HIGHER BRAIN CENTERS

hypothalamus

posterior
pituitary

OXYTOCIN

CONTRACTION OF
MYOEPITHELIAL
CELLS

MILK LET-DOWN

MECHANORECEPTORS
IN NIPPLES

spinal cord

fig. 16-3 Sucking reflex control of oxytocin secretion and milk letdown. (*From A. Vander, et al., Human Physiology, McGraw-Hill, New York, 1970.*)

foods. To be completely safe, an allowance of 20 g protein over the normal intake is recommended daily during lactation.

vitamins and minerals An additional intake of calcium is recommended during lactation. Drinking two extra cups of milk over the baseline requirements will meet the calcium recommendations for lactation. If the mother finds that she cannot drink that much milk, the nurse should work with her to discover what milk-based foods she could include. An addition of 1000 IU of vitamin A is recommended. This need can be met by adding dark green and deep yellow vegetables daily to the diet. Recommendations for

table 16-2 Suggested meal plan during lactation

food	amount
Milk	4 cups
Meat and meat substitutes	5 oz daily, 2 to 3 servings
Vegetables, fruits Include:	4 servings
Dark green or yellow	1 serving daily
Vitamin C source	1 serving daily
Bread or cereal	4 or 5 servings
Fluids	6 to 8 cups daily in addition to milk

iron and for vitamins C and D are the same as for pregnancy.

fluids If 850 mL milk is produced by the lactating woman, she should receive at least that amount of fluids over and above her normal intake. The two extra cups of milk needed to meet the calcium needs will provide about half these fluid requirements.

other foods Additional foods to make up caloric requirements should be wholesome, not nonnutritional foods like sugar, candy, soda, and foods with high fat intake.

A mother will often ask if there are any foods which should be omitted during lactation. Some sources recommend that she refrain from chocolate or spicy foods because they might affect her milk and thus the infant. There seems to be no physiologic reason for avoiding these foods as long as she receives other adequate nutrients in her diet.

The nutritional quality of human milk has no direct relationship to the nutritional status of the mother. The composition of mature human milk varies among women of similar backgrounds, in the same woman from one time of day to another, and in the same woman from one breast to another. If the mother is breast-feeding one infant who gets the full amount of milk she produces, these changes of quality are not significant. If the nutritional intake of the lactating mother is not adequate, the *total quantity of the milk produced is decreased,* rather than the *quality.*

cost Breast milk is not free milk. The cost of lactation is related to the cost of additional foods that the mother needs during lactation. If the mother can choose economical foods to meet her additional nutrient needs, the cost of breast-feeding can be comparable to formula-feeding.

the process of breast-feeding

When the baby is brought to its mother for the first feeding, she may be truly overwhelmed with feelings of wonder and joy, mixed with those of tremendous anxiety over her responsibility for such a helpless, tiny creature. She needs not only emotional support but also positive, clear instructions on how to manage breast-feeding. Even if she does not ask, the nurse should be prepared to spend time with the mother for the first feeding, to help her handle her baby, and to help start the baby nursing. The mother will also need privacy while breast-feeding to enable her to relax so that the letdown reflex can effectively function.

positioning The mother should nurse her baby in the position most comfortable for her. If she has had a cesarean section or is sore from the episiotomy, the side-lying position may be most comfortable. If the mother chooses to nurse while sitting up in bed, a pillow can be placed under the baby so that she does not have to hold the child completely. Some women are comfortable in the tailor-sitting position; others prefer to sit in a straight-back or rocking chair. The mother should support her breast with her free hand, holding the breast just above the areola be-

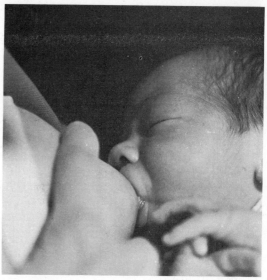

fig. 16-4 Note position of right hand. (*Photo by John Young.*)

tween her second and third fingers so that the breast does not press against the baby's nose and hinder breathing (Fig. 16-4). The whole of the areola should be in the baby's mouth so that the milk reservoirs above the nipple are compressed by the baby's lips (Fig. 16-5). Sucking only on the nipple will express no milk and will cause sore nipples.

fig. 16-5 The proper positioning of the infant's mouth on the breast. (*Courtesy of Ross Laboratories, Clinical Education Aid. No. 10.*)

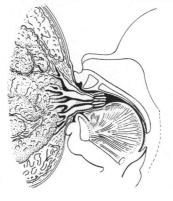

The nurse should show the mother how to use the baby's natural *rooting* reflex (Fig. 16-6)—a slight touch on the baby's cheek will cause the child to turn in that direction and open its mouth to take the nipple. This reflex needs to be understood, because if the mother touches any part of the baby's face while holding its head, the baby will keep turning its head in the direction of the touch and will become confused and frantic when it does not find the nipple.

The baby's sucking causes a strong suction, which should be broken before taking the baby from the breast. The mother can press down on the breast, thus letting air into the baby's mouth, or place a fingertip into the corner of its mouth and gently press it open (Fig. 16-7).

bubbling All babies swallow some air while sucking and thus need several opportunities to burp during and after a feeding. Babies can be bubbled halfway through the feeding or when they appear to slow down. (Figure 16-8 illustrates methods of holding an infant to bubble it.) During burping, small amounts of undigested milk may be regurgitated with the air. Mothers usually call this "spitting up." Regurgitation is caused by air swallowed during sucking and also by the fact that the cardiac sphincter at the entrance of the stomach is not fully closed in newborn infants. (An infant who regurgitates frequently can be placed on its right side with its head and trunk in an elevated position or placed in an infant seat for 15 or 20 min after a meal.) (See Chap. 18.)

feeding schedules Babies should be fed when they express hunger. Unfortunately, most hospitals still adhere to a 4-h schedule, even though early breast-feeding is best on a 2- to 3-h schedule. Rooming-in allows for self-regulatory demand feedings. Breast-feeding is much more easily established in such a situation. Night feedings are important in the

fig. 16-6 Rooting reflex. (*Photos by John Young.*)

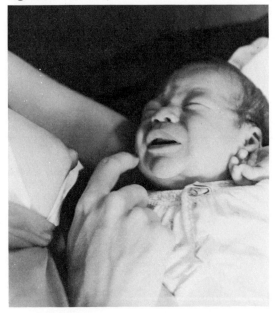
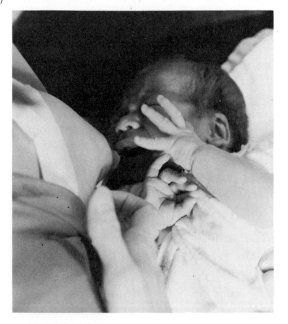

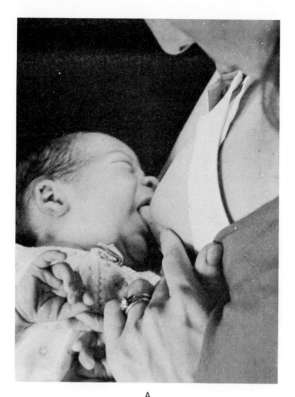 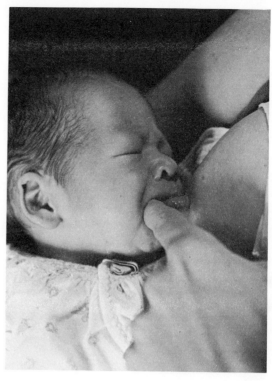

A   B

fig. 16-7 (a) Grasping nipple. (b) Releasing suction after feeding. (*Photos by John Young.*)

hospital. Many mothers who are bottle-feeding their infants request to sleep while the baby is fed in the nursery, but the lactating mother must carry on her frequent feedings to get lactation well established.

Feedings the first day are limited to about 5 min at each breast. The time period is increased slowly, so that by the time milk replaces colostrum on the third or fourth day, the nursing time is about 15 min. Extended sucking causes sore nipples, and since most of the milk is taken in the first 10 min, any extra time is for emotional satisfaction for mother and baby.

Once feeding is established, the most important principle in breast-feeding is to *empty at least one breast* at a feeding. Alternate

breasts should be used to start each feeding; a safety pin can be placed in the bra strap at the end of the feeding to remind the mother which breast to start with at the next feeding (Fig. 16-9). Complete emptying causes a fresh influx of milk, whereas partial emptying inhibits new production.

success at home In the 2 to 3 days that the mother and baby are in the hospital, breast-feeding is usually only tenuously established. In the hospital the mother may have the support of the hospital staff and the assurance from others that her baby is doing well. When she goes home, she may be very much on her own and may lose confidence in her ability to feed her baby. Feelings of

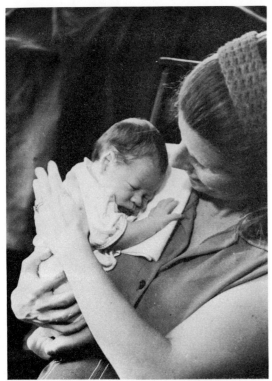 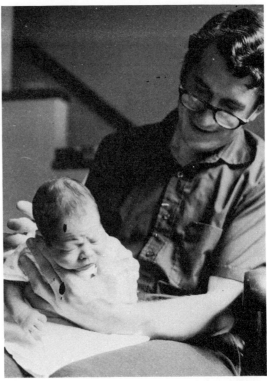

fig. 16-8 Two ways of bubbling the baby. (*Photos by John Young.*)

self-doubt may be fostered by relatives and friends who have not breast-fed and question if the baby is getting an adequate supply.

Before the mother goes home, the nurse should instruct her on several points, as anticipatory guidance. The mother should be instructed about the physiology of the letdown reflex and the need for emptying the breast at a feeding. The factors that diminish the milk supply can be discussed: fatigue, poor nutrition and inadequate fluid intake, and anxiety. If, in concern, the mother gives a supplemental bottle of formula, the breast-feeding process is due to fail, as the baby will take a bottle nipple more easily than the breast. Lack of the stimulation provided by enough sucking to empty the breast will decrease the supply, and the cycle of normal production will quickly cease. Of course, after breast-feeding is thoroughly established, the mother may use a bottle for a feeding when she is out of the house for dinner or a visit. She will become uncomfortable, perhaps, but the baby will be well fed, and the milk supply will not be hindered.

The mother should be made aware of books containing information on breast-feeding, and she should be informed of organizations that can be helpful to her. The Visiting Nurse Service is available in many areas: if the nurse assesses that the mother will need further support at home, she should make a referral.

common feeding problems

sore nipples Sore nipples are very common; they are most likely to occur in fair-

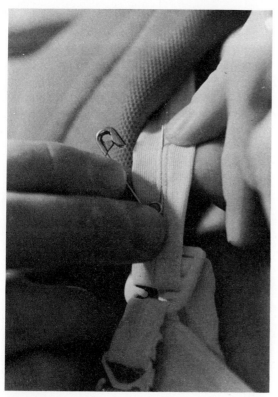

fig. 16-9 Pin is used as reminder of which side to begin next feeding.

skinned women and in those who let the baby suck too long at first. Soreness usually starts about the third postpartum day and may be present in one or both of the nipples. The nipple will look cracked and sore and may begin to bleed. Treatment consists mainly of keeping the nipple dry by exposure to air; the mother should be instructed to leave down the flaps of the nursing bra and to wear a loosely fitting gown to allow the air to circulate. The doctor may order short periods of heat-lamp treatment to promote fast healing. Topical medications such as lanolin or Massé cream help to relieve soreness. Preparations containing alcohol are excessively drying and painful and should not be used.

Nursing should be done for short, frequent periods so that the breasts do not become engorged. To relieve the pain and enable the letdown reflex to function, many doctors recommend an analgesic approximately ½ h before feeding. If the pain is severe, a nipple shield can be used: the mother holds the shield over the breast and the baby sucks the rubber nipple.

engorgement *Engorgement* of the breasts occurs to some extent with all nursing mothers as lactation begins, but it is most common with the first baby. It begins with tenderness and distension which result from the first formation of milk in the acini and a rush of blood and lymph to the tissues. The breasts become hard, hot, and heavy and feel lumpy. If the newly formed milk is not removed, the flow becomes obstructed and the breasts become red, swollen, and extremely painful. This swelling flattens the nipple, thus compounding the problem of nursing.

If the amount of engorgement appears to be only moderate, some milk should be hand-expressed just before feeding, making the nipple and areola softer and easier for the baby to grasp (Fig. 16-10). If the mother is experiencing pain and tension, an oxytocin spray administered nasally can be used to assist her letdown reflex. In addition, taking a hot shower just before feeding will stimulate circulation. After the baby has finished nursing, the breasts should be completely emptied by hand. When engorgement is severe, a firm binder or bra will give support between feedings. Discontinuing breast-feeding is an extreme measure and should never be necessary if the nurse is alert and the mother has been taught how to recognize and relieve engorgement.

Severe engorgement can be prevented to a large extent by frequent feedings whenever the breasts begin to feel full. One breast should be emptied at every feeding by massaging the breast as the baby nurses. The mother should be encouraged to tell the nurse whenever her breasts feel overfull; she can

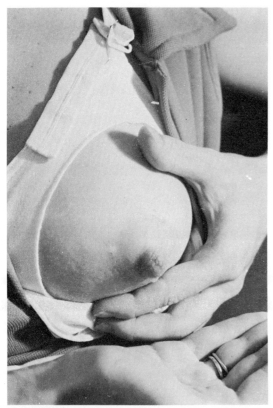

fig. 16-10 Expressing milk. The thumb and forefinger are placed on either side of the nipple at the edge of the areola. Thumb and finger are squeezed together, with care being taken not to slide down toward the nipple. The hand is rotated so that all the milk ducts are reached. Note the nursing bra. (*Photo by John Young.*)

then feed the baby or express her milk by hand until she feels comfortable.

With early discharge from the hospital, engorgement is likely to occur after the mother and her baby have returned home. Postpartum teaching becomes very important at this point.

mastitis *Mastitis* is an infection in the breasts, most commonly caused by *Staphylococcus aureus*. It results from entry of the bacteria through a cracked or sore nipple and

occurs most often in the third or fourth week post partum. The symptoms are an elevation of temperature, an increased pulse rate, and pain in the breast. Pain and swelling become localized in one area of the breast and then spread as cellulitis to the surrounding breast tissue. In some cases an abscess may form.

Treatment consists of administration of antibiotics and analgesics, and rest for the mother. The breasts should be supported with a firm bra. The application of ice packs will help to relieve the pain and swelling. A deep abscess may require needle aspiration or incision and drainage. Before the advent of antibiotics, mastitis was an indication to stop breast-feeding. This is no longer necessary. Continued breast-feeding will reduce engorgement and contribute to a quick recovery. With early treatment, symptoms should be gone within 24 h.[2] (See Chap. 25.)

contraindications to breast-feeding

chronic illness Chronic illness in the mother is the main contraindication to breast-feeding. Diseases such as tuberculosis, kidney impairment, cardiac insufficiency, or severe anemia already place enough stress on the mother.

Acute illness or infection during the postpartum period may also lead to a temporary or complete cessation of breast-feeding. Unless contraindicated by her physician, the mother's wishes should be followed. To maintain a flow of milk during her illness, a breast pump may be used. The infant would be given a premodified milk formula for the duration of the illness.

pregnancy Breast-feeding should be discontinued if the mother becomes pregnant again. Ovulation begins again in the nonlactating woman about 36 days after delivery, with the first menses occurring regularly following the woman's usual pattern. When the mother is lactating, the probability of ovulation during the first 9 weeks is nearly zero, according to Perez,[3] but it may occur any time after that even though the woman continues breast-feeding. Because ovulation is unpredictable, and women vary widely, lactation should not be considered an effective method of contraception beyond the first 6 to 8 weeks after delivery.

jaundice   In fewer than 1 percent of breast-feeding mothers, a factor is secreted in milk which seems to inhibit the reduction of bilirubin to a more water-soluble, more easily excretable form. The result is an elevated level of indirect bilirubin in the infant, usually beginning after 4 to 5 days of life (see Chap 29). The physician will usually prescribe extra water for the infant and, if the bilirubin level continues to rise, may ask the mother to discontinue breast-feeding for 3 or 4 days. By the second week, the infant should be able to metabolize bilirubin adequately and may be returned to breast milk. Such jaundice seems noninjurious; the condition is usually self-limiting. The mother who wishes to resume feeding may use a hand or electric pump on the breast while the infant is receiving formula.[4] Prevention of some jaundice may be possible by giving extra fluids to the breast-feeding infant in the first few days of life.

drug intake   Drug intake during lactation is not advisable, since most drugs in the maternal circulation will transfer across the breast-milk "barrier" into the milk. Effects and amounts are variable, however, depending on blood levels, time of ingestion, and metabolic fate of the drug once it reaches the newborn. Chapter 20 identifies factors for consideration and lists drugs which are not recommended for the lactating mother.

advantages of breast-feeding

immunologic advantages   The local antibody system produced at the epithelial surface in the human body (secretory IgA) is not present in the newborn until about 6 weeks of age.[5] Before the system is functioning in the gastrointestinal tract, large molecules may be absorbed into the circulation and may predispose the infant to allergic conditions either immediately or later in life. Food sensitivity (allergy) may often be a cause of eczema, diaper rash, vomiting, diarrhea, and upper respiratory symptoms. In addition, it has been estimated that 5 to 7 percent of all infants are sensitive to cow's milk.[6]

Human milk has low allergenicity and contains a factor promoting growth of *Lactobacillus bifidus,* which in the GI tract produces lactic and acetic acids. Such acids turn the stool acidic and provide additional protection against the growth of enteric infections. The bottle-fed infant has a more alkaline stool, which does not provide the same protective effect.

Specific antibodies available from human milk depend upon (1) the maternal level (titer) of antibody, and (2) the fate of the antibody protein in the digestive process. Recently, studies have demonstrated that antibodies to pertussis, staphlococci, *Escherichia coli,* and salmonella are not absorbed or destroyed in the GI tract but provide a protective effect against those organisms. In addition, if the woman has a high antibody titer against poliomyelits, the oral polio virus will be inactivated in the GI tract of the infant.[7] Beneficial effects against other diseases have not yet been completely studied.

psychologic advantages   Inherent in the process of breast-feeding is the stimulation of most of the senses. Close body contact allows the baby to recognize its mother's unique smell and feel and to hear the sound of her heartbeat; the visual *en face* position provides eye contact between mother and child. Those who bottle-feed or are substitute caregivers can provide most of these sensory stimuli just as well as the breast-feeding mother, especially if they understand the importance of feeding experiences in the growth and development of infants. The mother who understands that feeding should be a social time for play, exploration, and pleasure will not prop a bottle nor put the infant to bed alone with a bottle as a pacifier.

summary Breast-feeding has a number of advantages which, when explained to pregnant women, may influence them to use this method of providing infant nutrition.

1   The nutrients of human milk are in the right proportion for a human infant: there is a lower solute load and more unsaturated fatty acids; proteins/fats are more easily digested; and carbohydrate content is appropriate for growth.
2   There is protection against many enteric diseases and perhaps some respiratory diseases.
3   Allergic responses may be diminished in infants, especially if breast-fed exclusively until 6 months of age.
4   Cost and effort of formula preparation are unnecessary.
5   Problems based on poor sanitation, lack of refrigeration, or ignorance are avoided. Proper protein intake is available in diet-deficient countries.
6   A maximal opportunity to establish attachment with the infant is inherent in the process of feeding.
7   The tendency to overfeed and thus predispose the infant to obesity in later life can be avoided.

THE FORMULA-FED INFANT

There is little research to show that the bottle-fed baby in modern Western society fares any differently than the breast-fed baby.[8] Artificial formulas produced today are safe and, when used as directed, produce strong, healthy babies. The mother who chooses to bottle-feed her baby is not depriving her child, and she should not be made to feel guilty about it.

In contrast, in those areas of the world, where poor facilities for sterilization and inadequate refrigeration exist, a baby must be breast-fed to survive. Recently, advertising of formulas has created an impossible situation in such areas, for impoverished women have abandoned breast-feeding and yet cannot long afford commercial "feeds." The result is babies with severe malnutrition. In some cultures the standard diet is so unsuitable for infants that the mother must breast-feed for 2 or more years.

positioning Since most mothers in our society know something about bottle-feeding, the nurse might assume that a woman will feel comfortable giving her baby a bottle for the first time, and she may fail to give enough support and attention. The mother who bottle-feeds, as well as the one who breast-feeds, needs instruction on how to hold and burp her baby and how to recognize when the child has had enough.

The baby should be held closely, with its head in a slightly elevated position in the crook of the mother's arm, as in breast-feeding, so that the infant feels warm and secure while it feeds (Fig. 16-11). It is fairly common to see mothers or nurses, as they bottle-feed small babies, hold the baby out away from them on one knee with a hand behind the baby's head while the baby's arms flail around insecurely. The baby receives the milk but misses out on the comforts of cuddling.

It is much easier to hurry an infant through a bottle feeding. The mother should understand that food time must be as relaxed as possible. A baby needs the satisfaction of sucking, the socialization of being held and cuddled, and a mother who enjoys this time as much as the baby does. A mother does well to limit those who help her with feeding during the first few months so that the baby is not confused by multiple methods and styles of feeding.

bottle propping Consistency, socialization, and play are important aspects of feeding. In line with the findings on the importance of giving pleasure during feeding, the nurse should instruct the mother not to prop a bottle, for that would isolate the infant from contact with the mother. Infants should be fed *before* going to bed for naps or the night sleep for two reasons:(1) The taking of food should not be connected with separation from mother in a dark room. (2) Infants sucking slowly on milk as they lie flat in bed tend to get more inner-ear infections, as this position allows milk to enter the eustachian tube more easily. If the baby wants the security of something to suck on while going to sleep, the mother can provide a safely constructed pacifier.

feeding schedules A mother should be advised to feed her baby on demand, stopping the feeding when the infant is full rather than coaxing it to finish the bottle. Since newborn infants have a fairly rapid gastric emptying time, they will require six to eight feedings a day at intervals of 2 to 4 h. At 2 weeks of age, however, an infant should have progressed to needing only six feedings. By 2 months, an infant usually sleeps through the night and takes five feedings daily. By 6 months, the schedule includes at least four

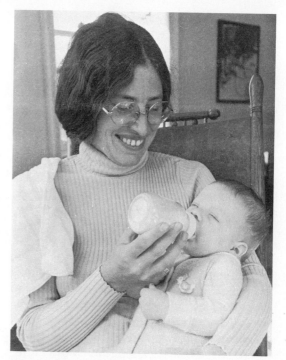

fig. 16-11 Satisfying a baby by bottle. (*Photo by Karen Gilborn.*)

milk feedings and three meals of strained foods.

content of formula

Cow's milk is the usual substitute for human milk, but it must be modified to meet the needs of the newborn human infant. Cow's milk is intended to provide for growth of calves, which grow to physical maturity at a more rapid rate than do humans. Because of the high ratio of casein to whey in cow's milk, the curd formed in the stomach is difficult for the newborn infant to digest. Boiling the milk changes the curd tension so that it is smaller and softer. Cow's milk is also more concentrated in protein and calcium and has less carbohydrate than human milk; therefore it must be diluted with water and have carbohydrates added to make it resemble human milk (Table 16-3).

The major nutritional differences between human and cow's milk are easily reconciled by the use of evaporated milk. Studies show that growth rates of infants fed evaporated milk are comparable to those of breast-fed infants as long as sanitary procedures are used to prepare and store the bottled milk. Today, the major nutritional concern for bottle-fed infants is the promotion of better digestion and absorption of cow's milk.

Fresh whole milk should not be given to a newborn infant because its gastrointestinal tract cannot digest the proteins and fats. In some cultures, fresh milk is a status symbol in newborn feeding, and mothers insist on using it. If they persist, nurses should instruct them to boil the milk before diluting it and adding sugar.

Condensed milk is canned milk with a large amount of sugar added. This is *not* suitable

for infant feeding, because the proportion of carbohydrates is too great. Infants fed on condensed milk become very obese before their first birthday. Obesity is a mark of health in some Latin cultures, and untutored mothers may feel very proud of their obese condensed-milk-fed infants.

Skim milk of any kind is not suitable for the first year of life because, if enough milk is given to provide the calories needed, the amount of calcium, protein, and electrolytes would be so high that the renal solute load would be too great for the infant. Skim milk has half the calories of whole milk because most of the fat is removed. Essential fatty acids are necessary to maintain the health of infants. Essential fatty acid deficiency is manifested by eczema-type lesions.

premodified milk formula Commercially prepared formula has had the butterfat removed and vegetable oils added to provide a larger proportion of unsaturated fatty acids. The exchange of vegetable oils for the butterfat provides a greater proportion of the essential fatty acids, especially linoleic acid, which is found in human milk. Milk is diluted to lower the concentration of protein and calcium, and lactose or dextrose is added to raise the carbohydrate level. Multivitamins are added. Some formulas have added iron and are used with infants with anemia or who had a low birth weight.

Premodified milks come in four different formats. Concentrated formula must be diluted with an equal part of water. Ready-to-use formula is sold in large cans, small (4-oz) cans, and prefilled disposable bottles. Because most hospitals send the mother home with a 24-h supply of disposable bottled formula, a new mother may think that that is the format she must use. The nurse must be sure to discuss methods of feeding and preparation of formula with the mother before she leaves the hospital. For the convenience of

table 16-3 Nutritional differences between human and cow's milk: Composition of human and cow's milk per 100 mL

nutrient	human milk	cow's milk
Calories	77	65
Protein, g	1.1	3.5
Fat, g	4.0	3.5
Carbohydrates, g	9.5	4.9
Calcium, mg	33	118
Phosphorus, mg	14	93
Iron, mg	0.1	trace
Sodium, mg	16	50
Potassium, mg	51	144
Vitamin A, IU	240	140
Thiamine, mg	0.01	0.03
Riboflavin, mg	0.04	0.17
Niacin, mg	0.2	0.1
Ascorbic acid, mg	5	0.1
Casein/whey ratio	40:60	82:18

Source: Adapted from B. K. Watt and A. L. Merill, "Composition of Foods, Raw, Processed, Prepared," *Agriculture Handbook,* No. 8, U.S. Dept. of Agriculture, Washington, D.C., 1963; and P. L. Pipes, *Nutrition in Infancy and Childhood,* Mosby, St. Louis, 1977.

disposable bottles, the cost becomes three or four times as much as the concentrated formula and much more than home-prepared evaporated milk formula.

The difference between the ready-to-use and concentrated formulas must be emphasized. The mother *must* add an equal amount of water to the concentrated formula to make it single strength. If not, the undiluted concentrated formula will increase the renal solute load and predispose the infant to tetany and hypernatremia.

As long as vitamins are given to babies receiving evaporated milk, there is no real difference in the growth rates of children whether they are breast-fed or given premodified or evaporated milk formulas. However, there are fewer fats in the stools of infants fed breast milk or premodified formula, indicating better absorption of essential fatty acids.

milk substitutes If the infant is found to be allergic to cow's milk, a formula of goat's milk or a soybean-based milk may be ordered by the physician. Formulas based on meat are also available. The substitutes have to be extensively modified to provide the necessary nutrients. They are available in drug and grocery stores and cost substantially more than standard formulas.

evaporated milk formula Canned evaporated milk has been used for many years. The process of evaporating and canning milk lowers the curd tension and makes the milk bacteriologically safe. It can be stored at room temperature and requires no refrigeration until the can is opened. It is fortified with 400 IU vitamin D per quart of reconstituted milk. Ideas on formula preparation differ, but evaporated milk must always be diluted with two parts of water, and sugar or corn syrup must be added for extra carbohydrates. Since water in most areas of the United States is considered to be essentially

safe, some pediatricians are recommending only medical asepsis in formula preparation; clean bottles and nipples and clean tap water mixed with milk fresh from a can. In these cases, where there is any question of poor refrigeration, contamination of bottles or nipples by flies, pets, litter, or other children, the mother should still be instructed in boiling bottles and nipples for the first 3 to 4 months and in preparing only one bottle at a time.

TERMINAL HEAT FORMULA PREPARATION The American Academy of Pediatrics Committee on the Fetus and Newborn continues to recommend the terminal heat method for preparing formula, in which heating is applied after the formula is bottled. This is often referred to as the "terminal sterilization method," although it is not technically sterilization. It is more properly called the *terminal heat method*.

Equipment needed:

  Baby bottles (heat-resistant type)
  Bottle caps or nipple covers
  Nipples
  Large kettle or bottle sterilizer with wire rack (if wire rack is not available, a clean cloth in the bottom of the large pot can be used)
  Saucepan or pitcher with a pouring lip
  Measuring cup
  Measuring spoon
  Long-handled spoon
  Funnel
  Bottle brush with stiff bristles and long handle
  Can opener

Procedure:

1 Wash hands.
2 Wash all equipment clean with hot soapy water, including the work surface. Use

brush to wash bottles; milk curd is hard to remove without a brush.

3   Wash top of can of milk and rinse well.
4   Measure the amount of water and formula into saucepan or pitcher. Stir with spoon.
5   Pour into bottles in prescribed amounts.
6   Put nipples and bottle caps or nipple covers on bottles, then loosen bottle caps.
7   Place bottles on wire rack or clean cloth in the bottom of the large pot. Add 3 or 4 inches water.
8   Cover the pot and turn on heat. After water in pot reaches boiling point, let it boil for 25 min. (In some areas, the local health departments may recommend that the boiling time be shortened because the water supply has been tested and found to be very pure.)
9   Turn off heat. With the cover on, let the entire pot cool slowly, undisturbed, until the entire unit is lukewarm. (The slow cooling of the formula prevents the milk from thickening, often a cause of clogged nipples.)
10 Remove bottles, tighten bottle caps, and place bottles in the refrigerator.

After each feeding the bottles and nipples should be rinsed and soaked in cold water. This will facilitate washing prior to the next use.

formula temperature   For many years, the formula was heated before being given to the baby. In hospitals, formula in disposable bottles is given at room temperature, and studies have been done on infants fed refrigerated cold milk. There is no difference in growth rates of infants fed formulas that are warm or cold. If the mother prefers to serve lukewarm formula, she should immerse the bottle in warm water just prior to the feeding. Warm milk is a good medium for bacterial growth, so it is wise not to let the formula

remain at room temperature too long. If the mother is in a location without refrigeration, she can mix one bottle of evaporated milk or premodified milk and feed it immediately. The opened can of milk should be covered and used within 1 day.

use of fresh whole milk   Some literature written by companies which produce infant formulas recommend that infants should not be given fresh whole cow's milk until 1 year of age. In reality, this may cause an economic hardship to families. Many pediatricians suggest that fresh whole milk can be given when formula-fed infants are 5 to 6 months old.

INTRODUCTION OF ADDITIONAL FOODS

Feeding an infant with a spoon involves a whole new system of swallowing. Until the third month when the tongue thrusting *extrusion reflex* disappears, this protective mechanism keeps him from inadvertently swallowing harmful foreign objects. Mothers observe this reflex as the baby appears to spit out any food offered by spoon (Fig. 16-12). The stimulus to swallow is triggered in the early weeks after birth by the touch of the nipple at the back of the tongue, as swallowing is intricately coordinated with breathing.

An infant pushing cereal or fruit out of its mouth in spite of mother's cooing and coaxing is not demonstrating a dislike of the taste. The spoon must be small enough to enter the mouth and touch the back of the tongue, and the cereal must be thick enough to be "wiped off" the spoon on the way out of the mouth.[8]

Studies have shown that infants most willingly accept cereal at 2½ to 3½ months, vegetables at 4 to 4½ months, and meats and meat soups at 5½ to 6 months. There seems to be no nutritional advantage in introducing foods on an earlier schedule. Although im-

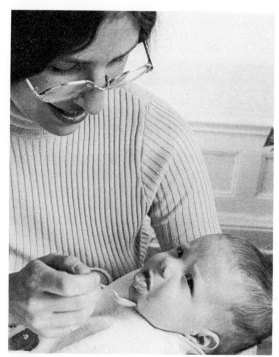

fig. 16-12 Spoon feeding while extrusion reflex is still present. (*Photo by Karen Gilborn.*)

weaning

A baby can be successfully weaned when it can (1) grasp with both hands, (2) reach, and (3) sit well. Babies will often lose interest in breast-feeding after 7 or 8 months; others will continue longer. The mother who is breast-feeding can wean directly to a cup. A bottle-fed baby will often hold on to the night bottle until well into the second or even third year. The baby gets satisfaction from sucking, and it will do no harm if only a small amount of milk or juice is given. To begin weaning the baby, the mother should put a small amount of milk in the bottom of a shallow, sturdy, flat-bottomed cup. A training cup with two handles is ideal. The baby will tip it over, bang it, and suck on it as part of the learning process. Each baby differs in its adjustment to drinking from a cup. The amount of milk consumed may decrease until the baby gets used to drinking from a cup (Fig. 16-13). Juices and water can be offered from a bottle to give the baby adequate fluids during the transition.

fig. 16-13 Baby using weaning cup. (*Photo by Mary Olsen Johnson, M.D.*)

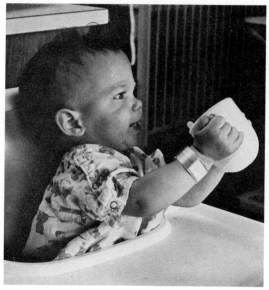

patient mothers often ask the pediatrician to begin at 3 or 4 weeks, it is best to follow the physiologic pattern of gastrointestinal maturation.

Some physicians feel that early introduction to a mixed diet enables the infant to adjust to a variety of foods at an earlier age. There seems to be no nutritional advantage to this practice.

By the time infants are 6 or 7 months old, they are usually eating foods from each of the four basic food groups. As they mature, the texture changes from strained to mashed or chopped foods. Puddings, toast, teething biscuits, and bite-sized pieces of cooked vegetables and fruits are added gradually. By the first birthday most infants are weaned for meals from the bottle to a cup, although they have "comfort" from bottles well into the second or third year.

commercially prepared foods

Commercially prepared strained foods have been subject to many criticisms. Ingredients are added to improve flavor (the manufacturer always visualizing the mother tasting a bite and telling the baby that it tastes good) and to stabilize the product. The nutritional benefits of additives are questionable.[9] Fruits and fruit juices are sweetened with sugar, which not only adds nonnutritional calories but also develops a desire for sweet foods in the infant. Salt is added to many foods. Since infants are not born with an awareness of how salty or sweet a food should be, these flavors begin to be learned in the very early months after birth. The role of sodium sensitivity in individuals with hypertension in later life does not support the use of excess salt in baby foods. Some companies have now voluntarily stopped using salt and sugar in their baby foods.

Since most infants in our society continue to be fed commercially prepared foods, the nurse can advise the mother to wean the infant to lightly seasoned, chopped table foods as soon as the child's digestive tract permits it. Other mothers will be willing to prepare puréed foods for their infants by using a blender, sieve, or food grinder (Fig. 16-14).

fruit juice and vitamin C By 3 to 4 weeks of age, especially if evaporated formula is used, it is necessary to supplement the food intake with ascorbic acid, because vitamin C is lost in the pasteurization process. Premodified milk has multivitamins added; human milk contains a small amount of vitamin C.

Orange juice is a good source of vitamin C. If there is any problem with sensitivity to orange juice, grapefruit juice may be used. Pineapple, apple, and prune juices are not as good sources of the vitamin but can be

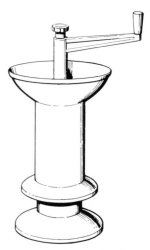

fig. 16-14 Mothers find a food grinder very convenient when feeding an infant at home or away from home. Cooked meats, vegetables, or fruit are placed in a container in the inner part of the grinder. The outer portion is placed over it. As the lever is turned, the food comes through to the top and can be spooned to feed the infant. This device is small, portable, and easily cleaned.

used later when the baby is taking a variety of foods and fruits.

If fresh fruit is used, it should be washed before the juice is extracted and strained. If canned juice is used, the top of the can should be washed before opening. The juice should be diluted in half when first introduced. After a few days this is not necessary; the amount is slowly increased over 2 or 3 weeks until the baby is accepting 2 oz of undiluted juice each day.

fruits Cooked, strained fruits may be prepared by mashing them with a fork or using the blender; or they may be purchased as baby food. Popular fruits are apples, peaches, pears, or apricots. The mother may start with a choice of any of these.

cereals When cereal is first introduced to infants, it is best to add a little formula to make the consistency very thick. Some mothers, to speed the meals, will add cereal to the formula. If that is done, a larger hole in the nipple or a cross-cut nipple must be used. Rather than continuing this practice, as soon as feasible the mother should teach the baby to eat from a spoon. When fruits and cereals are added to the diet, it is no longer necessary to continue the use of sugar or corn syrup in the evaporated milk formula, as these foods provide the extra carbohydrates.

vegetables Strained vegetables are added to the diet after the baby learns to accept fruits and cereals. Fresh, frozen, or canned vegetables (the mildly flavored ones such as peas, carrots, and green beans) may be puréed in the blender or sieved. Commercially prepared strained vegetables can be used until the infant is about 6 months old, at which time mashed or junior foods can be introduced.

eggs Cooked egg yolks are usually given to the infant before meats are introduced. The egg yolk should be cooked over hot water until the yolk is thickened but not hard because the protein of cooked eggs is more easily digested. Raw eggs should not be given to children because of the danger of salmonellosis, always a possibility in uncooked eggs. Egg whites are not usually given in the first year because infants do not tolerate the albumin in their immature gastrointestinal tracts or may have an allergic reaction.

meats Infants may be given canned strained meats or meats strained at home. Lamb, chicken, liver, and beef seem most easily digested. To prepare meats at home, the mother should use tender, lean meat. Scrape a little lean, raw meat and cook it at a low temperature with *little water*. A blender or grinder could also be used to purée cooked

meat. If fish is used, the mother should be sure it is mildly flavored and boneless. When the child is over 6 or 8 months old, canned fish such as tuna or salmon can be used if the oil is drained off.

conclusion

The timetable for introduction of foods varies from region to region. Remembering that for many years, infants did not begin on additional foods until well near their first birthday, the mother should not compare and contrast her pediatrician's choice of schedule with her neighbor's. The mother may feel pressured by advertising or may feel that she has to buy the most expensive product, as equaling the best. The nurse can instruct the mother to follow the growth patterns of the child and to:

Ensure that formula is prepared and stored in a medically aseptic way
Provide adequate fluid intake for the infant, especially during hot weather
Introduce one food at a time to test for response
Give vitamins and add foods as the pediatrician prescribes
Correlate development with the infant's ability to participate in feeding itself
Provide the baby with stimulation, pleasure, and play while being fed
Enjoy her infant during the whole feeding process

study questions

1 How many calories are recommended for a 2-month-old infant who weighs 5 kg?
2 How many ounces or milliliters of fluids are needed for this infant each day? If five feedings are given, how many ounces or milliliters are in each bottle?
3 If a 6-month-old infant is gaining weight too rapidly, how should the mother adjust the baby's milk intake?
4 What is the difference between marasmus and kwashiorkor?

5   How many extra calories should a lactating woman consume (1) before weight returns to normal? (2) after weight is normal?
6   Plan a 1-day menu for a lactating woman.
7   List the nutritional advantages of breast-feeding.
8   How do premodified commercial formulas differ from fresh cow's milk?
9   At what age can fresh cow's milk be used for infant feeding and why?
10 At what age does the infant need foods other than milk? In which order should they be introduced?
11 Plan to teach a mother who is bottle-feeding how to achieve the same satisfaction that a breast-feeding mother achieves. (Include schedule, sensory input, bonding, and formula content in your plan.)
12 Which disadvantages of formula-feeding can be overcome by correct instruction?

references

1   National Research Council, *Recommended Dietary Allowances,* 8th ed., National Academy of Sciences, Washington, D.C., 1973.
2   D. Theberge-Rousselet, "The Treatment of Mastitis in Nursing Mothers," *The Canadian Nurse,* March 1976, p. 32.
3   A. Perez, "First Ovulation After Childbirth: The Effect of Breast-feeding," *American Journal of Obstetrics and Gynecology,* **114**:1041, 1972.
4   M. Gartner and M. Hollander, "Disorders of Bilirubin Metabolism," in N. Assali and R. Brinkman (eds.), *Pathophysiology of Gestation,* Academic Press, New York, 1972, vol. III, chap. 8.
5   B. J. Oseid, "Breast-feeding and Infant Health," *Clinical Obstetrics and Gynecology* June 1976, p. 157.
6   S. R. Halpern, et al., "Development of Childhood Allergy in Infants Fed Breast, Soy or Cow Milk," *Journal of Allergy and Clinical Immunology,* **51**:139, 1977.
7   Oseid, op. cit., p. 155.
8   S. O'Grady, "Feeding Behavior in Infants," *American Journal of Nursing,* **71**(4):736, 1971.
9   A. Anderson and J. Fomon, "Commercially Prepared Strained and Junior Foods for Infants," *Journal of American Dietetic Association,* **58**:520–526, 1970.

bibliography

Adams, C. F.: "Nutritive Values of American Foods," *Agriculture Handbook,* No. 456, U.S. Dept. of Agriculture, Washington, D.C., 1975.

Brewer, T.: "Nutrition and Infant Mortality," *Pediatrics,* **51**:1107, 1973.

Brown, C.: "Breast Feeding in Modern Times: A Review," *American Journal of Clinical Nutrition,* **26**(5):556, 1973.

Castle, S.: *Complete Guide to Preparing Baby Foods at Home,* Doubleday, Garden City, N.Y., 1973.

Countryman, A.: "Hospital Care of the Breast-fed Newborn," *American Journal of Nursing,* **71**:2365–2367, 1971.

Dialogues in Infant Nutrition **1**:2, July 1977; and **1**:3, October 1977 (publication for Mead Johnson Laboratories).

Dickey, R. P., and S. C. Stone: "Drugs That Affect the Breast and Lactation," *Clinical Obstetrics and Gynecology,* June 1976, p. 95.

Fomon, J.: *Infant Nutrition,* Saunders, Philadelphia, 1974.

How the Nurse Can Help the Breast-feeding Mother, La Leche League International.

Infant Nutrition, Medcom 1972 (monograph for Wyeth Laboratories).

Jelliffe, D. B.: "Unique Properties of Human Milk, *American Journal of Medicine* **14**(4):133–136, 1975.

MacMahon B., T. M. Lui, and C. R. Lowe: "Lactation and Care of the Breast: A Summary of an International Study," *Bulletin of WHO,* **42**:185–194, 1970.

Nutrition in Pregnancy and Lactation, Report of a WHO Expert Committee, Tech. Rep. Ser., no. 302, World Health Organization.

Piper, P. L.: *Nutrition in Infancy and Childhood,* Mosby, St. Louis, 1977.

Slattery, J.S.: "Nutrition for the Normal Healthy Infant," *American Journal of Maternal Child Nursing* **2**(2):105–112, 1977.

Stokan, R. E.: "The Right Formula for the Right Infant: Making Sense of Infant Nutrition," *American Journal of Maternal Child Nursing,* **2**(2):101–104, 1977.

Stone, S. C., and R. P. Dickey: "Management of Nursing and Nonnursing Mothers," *Clinical Obstetrics and Gynecology,* June 1976, p. 139.

Watt, B. K., and A. L. Merill: "Composition of Foods, Raw, Processed, Prepared." *Agriculture Handbook* No. 8, U.S. Dept. of Agriculture, Washington, D.C., 1963.

services for patient education

La Leche League International
9616 Minneapolis Avenue
Franklin Park, Ill. 60131

International Childbirth Education Association
Supplies Center   or   Box 22
1414 NW 85th Street   Hillside, N.J. 07205
Seattle, Wash. 98117

17

PSYCHOLOGICAL DEVELOPMENT IN THE FIRST YEAR OF LIFE

PHILIP E. WILSON

How does the new baby display the psychological and emotional qualities by which we know that she or he is "human"? Is the baby aware of love, hope, justice, pride, envy, guilt, disgust, and anger? The newborn's humanity lies in the potential to develop all these feelings—the human emotions—and to act upon them and control them.

It may be difficult to imagine what is in the mind of a newborn, and yet consistent observation with accurate recording of what infants do and how they react at different ages has given us much insight and evidence from which we can construct what the infant perceives, knows, and begins to understand.

In seeking understanding of the psychology of the first year of life, the following questions need to be answered: By what means do infants begin to comprehend the world around them? Can infants begin to build relationships from birth? Why is one consistent relationship so important? Why is separation so harmful to both mother and infant? How well does an infant's perceptual system work? Why do infants believe that they are the cause of everything that goes on around them? Why do infants feel that their mothers are a part of themselves and, later, that their mothers know everything they feel? Why do infants cry? What are the effects of adequate and inadequate mothering? As we seek to answer these questions, we will discuss the psychological processes and tasks of the first year.

ESTABLISHING THE MOTHER–INFANT BOND

Nothing is more important to the new mother and new baby than their relationship and the necessity of having that relationship understood by the helping professionals who surround them. Basic to the psychology of infancy is the psychology of the mother–infant unit. Human infants are obviously totally dependent for a length of time, which separates them from even those animals whose young have a dependent period. But what is often overlooked is the psychological importance of that long period of dependence. While the neonate's physical dependence is obvious, the depth of the infant's psychological dependence is subtle and all too often brushed aside by hospital procedure and routine.

The process of mother–infant bonding is the basis for the relationship between mother and child. This relationship is, in turn, the basis for the necessary interdependence required for good psychological and physical development of the infant. What is of absolute importance is the establishment of an extremely close relationship in which the infant's dependency can flourish. Each must be bonded to the other. The infant must be bonded so that he or she can feel totally dependent on the mother. The mother must be bonded to her infant so that she is able and willing to give the enormous outlay of time and energy required by the new infant and so that this giving is done with pleasure. Usually the new mother is very aware, through her positive feelings, of her half of the mother–infant unit. She is intensely interested in her child. The process of bonding is also important for fathers, and as more fathers take over more traditionally maternal roles with their infants, the process of close bonding between them will increase in importance. It does not matter whether this happens with the mother or the father. Although in our culture it is usually the mother who assumes the close nurturing position with the newborn, it is important to encourage the attachment of both parents (see Fig. 17-1).

The mother's first spontaneous response to her new baby is usually a mixture of joy and relief. Her very positive exuberant feelings about the birth of her baby and the completion of the birth experience itself combine with her maternal feelings to bring about the bonding process. Pregnancy has given the mother 9 months to consider what it will be like to be a mother—to have a baby. The birth experience is the final task to be accomplished. Whether the birth experience has been easy, with the mother well prepared physically and psychologically, or difficult, or even traumatic, relief and pleasure will be a part of the mother's immediate feelings. If the experience has been easy, then the immediate positive feelings will also come easily. If the experience has been difficult, the mother will need to be cared for as she begins to shift her attention from herself to her new baby. In either case, the bonding process should be aided, not hindered, by the professional staff. The mother's first pleasure and touching responses to the infant are responses of great psychological value and need to be appreciated as the basis for a strong mother–infant relationship which will assure the normal psychological growth and development of the infant.

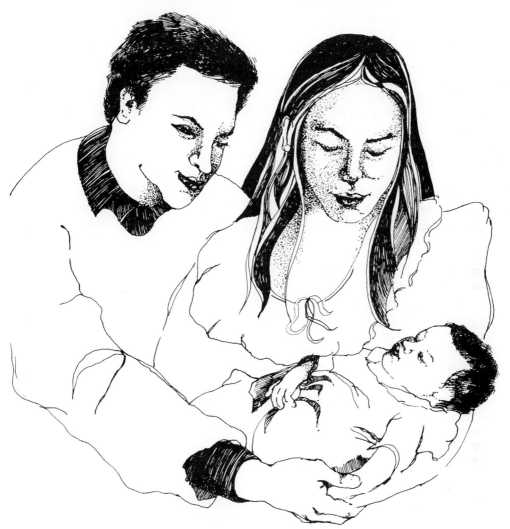

fig. 17-1   Early parent–infant contact. (*Drawing by Patricia Rodriguez-Lovink.*)

Many things can be done by the professional staff to promote the bonding process. Every effort should be made in the delivery room to allow time for the mother and father to meet their infant. The first spontaneous desire to hold the baby and to touch the infant's fingers is extremely important. The mother should have enough time with her new baby so that she is able to explore the infant and his or her reactions, cuddle the baby, and, if desired, begin the breast-feeding process. The father should share in this time with the mother and hold his new baby on his own. Delivery room staff members have the responsibility of seeing that this all-important psychological process of bonding is allowed to take place by giving the parents the time and encouragement they need. Interestingly,

Klaus has noted that some emotional bonding to the infant even takes place among the staff witnessing the delivery[1] (Table 17-1).

There is a fine line between helping and encouraging a new mother to be more involved and comfortable with her new baby and taking over by entering the dyad between the mother and the baby. New mothers, especially, may need help in recognizing that their baby is responding to them or "likes them" when the infant is indeed unresponsive just after the birth experience. Such situations need to be explained to the mother for just exactly what they are: a new baby who is too tired to respond but who desperately needs and "loves" the mother.

The importance of mother–infant bonding has been even more dramatically stated recently by the well-known Scottish psychiatrist and psychoanalyst R. D. Laing.[2] He stated, "I believe that the mother-baby relationship must be preserved during and after birth." He goes on to emphasize that "there is a critical period of the first 72 hours following birth. This is just the right time for bonding, when the mother's natural desire is to have her baby and when the baby needs the mother." The deep importance of Laing's beliefs comes with his conclusions: "It is the shattering of the bonds that is a precondition of insanity. The mother-child interaction is most significant. The disruption of bonding can be one of the causes of schizophrenia in later life."

The first days immediately after the baby's birth are perhaps more important to the establishment of the mother's relationship with the baby than the baby's with the mother. They both need time to gaze at each other, to touch and explore. The mother needs the assurance that she can meet the infant's needs. If the baby can remain with her continually from birth, her positive feelings of coping and the continual expression of caretaking help to assure the formation of a fulfilling relationship.

Separation of the infant from the mother

table 17-1   Seven principles in the process of attachment

1   "There is a sensitive period in the first minutes and hours of life during which it is necessary that the mother and father have close contact with their neonate for later development to be optimal.
2   "There appear to be species-specific responses to the infant in the human mother and father that are exhibited when they are first given their infant.
3   "The process of the attachment is structured so that the father and mother will become attached optimally to only one infant at a time. Bowlby (1958) earlier stated this principle of the attachment process in the other direction and termed it *monotropy*.
4   "During the process of the mother's attachment to her infant, it is necessary that the infant respond to the mother by some signal such as body or eye movements. We have sometimes described this, 'You can't love a dishrag.'
5   "People who witness the birth process become strongly attached to the infant.
6   "For some adults it is difficult simultaneously to go through the processes of attachment and detachment, that is, to develop an attachment to one person while mourning the loss or threatened loss of the same or another person.
7   "Some early events have long-lasting effects. Anxieties about the well-being of a baby with a temporary disorder in the first day may result in long-lasting concerns that may cast long shadows and adversely shape the development of the child (Kennell and Rolnick, 1960)."

Source: From Marshall H. Klaus and John H. Kennell, *Maternal-Infant Bonding*, The C.V. Mosby Co., St. Louis, 1976, p. 14.

causes her to repress her maternal feelings, because of the frustration experienced at not being able to express these maternal desires. A prolonged separation immediately after birth, because of illness or immaturity in the infant, or infection and poor recovery in the mother, will interfere with the establishment of the maternal-infant bond.[3]

The subtleties around the process of breastfeeding give a clear example of how separation interferes with the development of the mother's relationship with her new baby. Breast-feeding comes as another step in the process of holding and handling the new one. Nervousness and fears are overcome when the mother can capitalize on her initial positive emotional response to her infant, but this response can be utilized by the mother only if she has early consistent contact with her infant. The mother and baby both must go through the *process* which leads up to the baby's taking the nipple and beginning to breast-feed. The mother needs to have ample opportunity to acquaint herself with her child and to present the breast in an unhurried and relaxed fashion. The infant also must go through the process of connecting the "rooting" reflex to the actual nipple he or she is looking for. All infants look for or "root" for the breast, but even with this instinctual reflex working, it takes time—trials and errors—to work out the pattern for breast-feeding. The nursing staff also has the opportunity of teaching the mother about breast-feeding in the optimum setting, if the mother and baby are consistently together.

If the baby is brought to the mother only on the hospital's nursery schedule, then the mother and baby do not have the leisurely opportunity to go through the handling process which leads up to breast-feeding.

Any hospital routine which separates mothers and their infants, unless for real medical need, is requiring the mother to shut off her feelings like a water tap. Each time the infant is taken away, these feelings are in part repressed, and fears and doubts are magnified in the baby's absence. Put in this position, the mother feels that she has to prove herself in the time allotted to her. The mother should never have to feel that she is competing with the hospital staff about the care or needs of her own baby. Instead, she must be reassured that they are there to help and to instruct her as necessary. She should never have to feel that she is scheduled according to the hos-

pital's time clock but should be able to request her infant for a visit or be able to choose a rooming-in plan in order to care for the infant at all times.

The nurse's role is one of supporting the new mother as her relationship is established with her infant. Supportive teaching is especially important so that the inexperienced mother becomes confident in using her own instinctive responses in caring for the child. The importance of all the mother's natural responses to her new baby is underscored by the well-known British pediatrician and psychoanalyst D. W. Winnicott.[4] He feels that the best mothering comes from the mother's natural response to her baby and not from what she has read or learned. Indeed, he feels that her learning by reading or by being told about being a mother may inhibit her natural instinctual responses to her baby. If the mother lacks knowledge in a specific area, the nurse will need to fill in the gap in the mother's understanding. The same is true in helping the inexperienced mother in such things as beginning to breast-feed. But in doing any of these things the nursing role is to aid the mother to do them, not to take over the mother's role, taking the experience and the infant away from the mother.

DEVELOPMENT OF THE INFANT'S PERCEPTUAL SYSTEM

During the first few days of life, an infant experiences first "perceptions" of the world and begins to develop many of the basic feelings on which all other experiences will be built. Initially, the infant does not have a fully developed sensory system, and perceptions are not received with the same intensity, clarity, or meaning that they later will be, but the system does operate and begins to provide the initial input to the infant's mind.

Because all of these perceptions are new to the infant, with the exception of some sounds, motion, and perhaps the sensation of closeness which are experienced in utero, a receptive framework has not yet been established for understanding or giving meaning to perceptions. At birth the infant begins to look around, responds to soothing sounds and motion, and reacts to pain and discomfort by screaming. Although the perceptual system provides only limited input[5] and even fewer meaningful perceptions at the time of delivery, it is a mistake to minimize the importance of these earliest perceptions. The French obstetrician LeBoyer has pointed out how our modern medical techniques and routines have been unnecessarily cruel by disregarding the infant's ability to feel and the impact of discomfort and pain on the infant. It is important that these earliest experiences be as soothing as possible and that the earliest perceptions be reassuring and not flood and overwhelm the infant with anxiety or pain.

Positive, comforting early experiences, along with repetition, continuity, sameness, and routine of the *mothering experience*, are the infant's building blocks for developing an internal framework which allows the child to make use of his or her perceptions. With continuity of mothering and repetition, perceptions are organized into the earliest memories. The significance of each memory develops through the gratification of the experience. Because of the routine and physical gratification involved with feeding, its significance is great and is organized into memories of satisfaction and pleasure. These memories then make feeding even more important. Sensations in the infant's mouth and stomach while feeding are of such intense gratification that they become the unconscious symbolic essence of feeling satisfied and thus become the basic feeling of satisfaction throughout the infant's later life.

The sensory system parallels the development of all the body's voluntary systems. Initially uncontrolled and unrefined, the motor reflex system is immature in human infants and requires physical maturation and experience in order to develop. In the same way as the infant gains experience, the perceptual system develops, giving the child more usable material and thus making it possible to select perceptions on a voluntary basis. As the systems develop together, the infant can more clearly understand the world and effectively react to it. Thus, although the infant receives sensory input readily, ability to interpret accompanies maturation.

tactile and motion perception

Perceptions of motion and touch are perhaps the most important of all sense impressions for the new infant. Rocking and other motion are sensations of equilibrium that are sensed in the inner ear. The awareness of motion is already acute at birth, having been present for months in utero. Infants respond with pleasure to rocking and other motion, as well as to tactile sensations of warmth, closeness, and snugness.

visual perception

The infant's initial visual impressions are unfocused, and every object is strange, unfamiliar, and without meaning. Objects and faces float in and out of view and come into focus as if by magic. Since everything is new and only somewhat significant, visual stimuli must be moving, bright, or flashing in order to capture the infant's attention. Robson feels that the mother's eyes in particular have both the stationary location and the brightness to be initially noticeable and to quickly achieve special importance.[6] At birth, the neonate can easily follow a moving object held near the eyes. Eye-to-eye staring of mother and new child is frequently observed and seems to be gratifying to both (see Table 17-2).

Gazing, really "looking," develops gradually. Soon after birth a baby begins to pick out single objects from the whole clutter of stimuli available.[7] Typically the infant will stare transfixed at something like a picture on the wall, not seeing the picture itself, but fixing on the square shape which is seen as a single object of contrasting color. By 12 to 29 weeks, the infant is inspecting his or her hands and focusing on objects further and further away. Newer research is constantly

indicating that the infant perceives more than previously realized and at an earlier age.

sound

Many sounds are at first filtered out during infancy. However, Laing believes that a baby responds to music.[8] Usually infants react to soothing hums and frightening bangs, but they also respond to higher tones and are sometimes startled by deeper male voices. Other sounds are just part of the background and are meaningless to the infant. Sounds gradually gain significance and meaning

table 17-2 Early visual awareness

age		response
Newborn	Can perceive changes in light intensity and movement	Protective blinking; ability to follow bright object to midline if 6 to 8 in from eyes; doll's eye phenomenon may be present (see Chap. 14)
5 to 6 weeks		Able to fix gaze on an object if 12 to 24 inches in distance and patterned (interesting)
6 to 8 weeks		Ability to follow objects is well established if still kept close to eyes
3 to 5 months		Visual and tactile links rapidly developing (see-touch-grasp); begins to inspect hands; focusing distance increasing
6 to 10 months	Macula now well developed, for fine discriminations	Visual following of an object now present in all directions; depth perception increasing, becoming interested in small objects; visual alertness high, but looking may inhibit other responses
12 months		Can perform visual function tests at 10 ft (3 m)

Source: Adapted from Kenneth Holt, *Developmental Pediatrics*, Butterworths, London, 1977.

when they are associated with caregivers, food, and pleasure. The mother's voice is important from the beginning as a pleasant background to feeding and as a contact with the mother when she is close but not touching her baby. Groundwork for verbal ability begins to be developed long before words appear, and many observers feel that infants whose mothers spontaneously talk to them tend to begin speaking earlier than infants who are not exposed to such sounds (see Table 17-3).

The ability to listen and to discriminate among sounds is an important task to be undertaken in the second 6 months of life. The closer the infant is to the sound, the easier it will be to discriminate. A child on the far side of the room may be able to hear the mother's voice but may not be able to distinguish meaningful speech sounds[9] (see Table 17-4).

smell

Many individuals report remembering their mother's distinctive smell, even into adult-

table 17-3 Normal speech and language development

age	speech	language
1 mo	Throaty sounds	
2 mo	Vowel sounds ("eh"), coos	
2½ mo	Squeals	
3 mo	Babbles, initial vowels	
4 mo	Guttural sounds ("ah," "goo")	
7 mo	Imitations of speech sounds	
10 mo		"Dada" or "Mama," non-specifically
12 mo		One word other than "Mama" or "Dada"
13 mo		Three words
15–18 mo	Jargon (language of the infant's own)	Six words
21–24 mo		Two- to three-word phrases
2 yr	Vowels uttered correctly	Approximately 270 words; use of pronouns
3 yr	Some degree of hesitancy and uncertainty common	Approximately 900 words, intelligible 4-word phrases
4 yr		Approximately 1540 words, intelligible 5-word phrases or sentences
6 yr		Approximately 2560 words; intelligible 6–7-word sentences
7–8 yr	Adult proficiency	

Source: By permission from C. H. Kempe, H. K. Silver, and D. O'Brien, *Current Pediatric Diagnosis and Treatment*, 4th ed., Lange Medical Publications, Los Altos, Calif., 1976.

hood. The newborn's sense of smell soon allows the baby to become keenly aware of his or her own mother's odor and to use this like all other perceptions of the mother: to provoke memories of the satisfying experiences which make up the "image of mother." In recent research, MacFarlane has shown that within a period of 6 days, an infant can distinguish his or her mother's breast from the breast of another mother by smell alone.[10]

"I AM THE CENTER OF THE UNIVERSE"

Each infant believes that he or she is the center of the world—all activity revolves around the infant's needs and wishes, everyone else exists to do the infant's bidding. Simply, there is nothing more central to an infant than the infant's own existence.

Infants are preoccupied with their own needs and believe that in some magical way the outside world is connected to their inner world. They believe that they cause everything to happen and that everything which goes on round them and every person, especially mother, is an extension of themselves. If mother's face appears above the crib, it is because the infant magically caused it to appear.

Infants believe that they are magically connected to their mothers, and this is their first understanding of a relationship. For instance, during the interval of crying which immediately precedes his late night feeding, baby Scott believes that his mother feels everything that he himself feels and is therefore able to know exactly what Scott needs and wants. From Scott's viewpoint, if his stomach hurts he feels it and his mother feels it, and that is why his mother comes and changes and feeds him. To Scott, his mother is as much a part of him as his stomach is. After all, he does not know yet how his stomach works and assumes

table 17-4   Hearing responses in infancy

age	response to sound
4–5 weeks	Occasional reflex turning of eyes in direction of sound origin
4 mo	Consistent turning of head toward side of sound; widening of eyes; quiet, listening attitude (audiovisual link important)
6 mo	Turns toward sound but recognizes it below eye level first, then above eye level
10 mo	Can locate sounds precisely, especially if meaningful; can screen out insignificant noise

Source: Adapted from K. Holt, *Developmental Pediatrics,* Butterworths, London, 1977, p. 148; and M. P. Dow and H. K. Silver, "The ABCD's of Hearing: Early Identification in Nursery, Office and Clinic of the Infant Who is Deaf," *Clinical Pediatrics,* **11:** 563, October 1972.

that it belongs to him. He makes the same assumption about his mother and everything else—they are extensions of himself.

Infants are totally dependent; all their needs must be met by their caregivers. Infants are also totally dependent upon their parents to introduce them to the world and to allow them to perceive the world as a place of gratification and relative harmony, with frustrations, but with hope of relief from tension as well. If parents are not able to allow this dependency to flourish during this period, a child may learn to perceive the outside world as a place of hostility and indifference, hopelessly frustrating.

Child studies have shown that continuous loving contact between infant and mother provides stimulation and gratification for the infants which has a positive observable effect on their physical and psychological development (see Fig. 17-2). Loving, stimulating contact in the amounts required for normal child development is only available to newborns if they have a relationship established with their mother. If the mother–infant bond has not been allowed to develop or has been

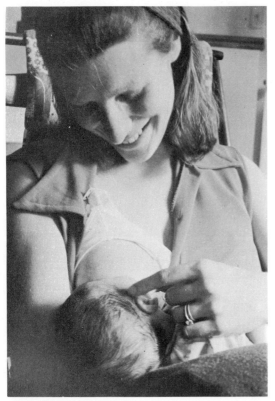

fig. 17-2 Feeding time brings satisfaction to mother and infant. (*Photo by John Young.*)

overcome her own inner emotional distance from her child as well as her baby's withdrawal and inner emotional distance from her. Mothers and babies who have to start their relationship late do not experience the first bloom of their love relationship. Making up for this gap or late start in the relationship can be arduous work, since unresponsive babies are not as gratifying to their parents and, because they are unresponsive, are not played with as much as a responsive child. This, of course, exacerbates the problem.

Salk has pointed out that the child is stimulated and gratified through cuddling and simple play.[11] The child responds and begins to subtly "understand" the personal warmth the mother transmits through her body and tender gestures. The child directs initial small and then growing amounts of attention toward the outer world, through gratification of his or her needs (see Fig. 17-3).

What happens if there is not adequate gratification of needs and adequate outside stimulation? Without parents who gratify and stimulate, the infant concentrates only on unmet inner needs, particularly the demands of hunger. Left for long periods without per-

emotionally or otherwise interrupted, the newborn will not receive the optimal amount of loving, growth-producing outside stimulation. If the mother–infant relationship has not been established in the hospital or if the mother has been either literally separated or is emotionally separate from the newborn, psychological development will be delayed and emotional barriers caused by the separation will have developed. A new mother might be emotionally separate from or unavailable to her new infant either because of a psychological trauma at the time of birth or because of the mother's adjustment problems at having a new baby and being faced with the demands of motherhood. The mother trying to establish a late relationship with her infant will have to

fig. 17-3 A big stretch after eating. What is the infant feeling or thinking? (*Photo by John Young.*)

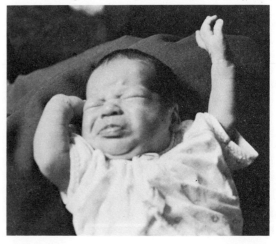

sonal contact, or left to cry it out when either food or other forms of attention would reduce discomfort, the infant learns not to expect anyone to satisfy these needs. As a result, the baby can develop *autistically.* The child will be totally self-involved to the exclusion of the outside world.

why the infant cries

All crying in infants is a response to their need to *discharge tension.* The infant who wakes up in the night for a late feeding does not cry to attract mother's attention, but cries to discharge immediately the tension which has built up in the baby's nervous system from hunger spasms or other causes. This discharge is accomplished through the motor reflex system of crying. As infants grow and mature, they develop more sophisticated motor reflex systems. Babies cry because they have needs which cause tension, and for no other reason. Since they feel they magically communicate with mother and that she automatically "knows" their every need, then crying does not need to be done to attract attention or communicate, but only to release tension.

However, some parents feel that an infant is "after" attention, is deliberately disturbing them, or is in some way plotting against them. The infant's crying may interfere with sleep so much that the parents become angry and feel the child is deliberately crying to get even with them. These feelings are simply the parents' feelings, not the child's. Babies cry often at irregular and interfering times. But they cry out of their needs; they have no ability to develop any other motive, especially one of revenge. If a baby cries excessively, the parents should discuss it with their pediatrician (see Chap. 18). Possibly, the condition can be helped, or possibly the parents will have to tolerate having the household upset by their new arrival. Whatever the case, it

should be made clear that the baby is not punishing them.

the perception of feeling

While developing a relationship with mother, the infant is learning the way the mother *feels* toward him or her. Later on as the ability to perceive and remember develops, the infant will remember particular things about their relationship but initially will only reflect and remember mother's *feeling* tone. If a child has an adequate mother who can provide the necessary emotional atmosphere, then the early impressions are of warmth, tenderness, comfort, and the satisfying milk that mother gives. If the child has an inadequate mother who is unable to provide a healthy emotional tone, then the early impressions are of isolation, frustration, coldness, and as a result, "undesirable" milk. Even food can be given in such a way as to make good milk *seem* bitter.

Even at a very early stage, unhealthy mothering can greatly affect the child's development, because the feelings at this stage will be carried the rest of the child's life. Because basic feelings are so essential to personality makeup, adults who have not had a satisfying infancy have the mark of infancy always with them. Some children continue to be "babies"—to act in babyish ways—until they reach adolescence. In adolescence, they either do not rebel at all or overreact and become destructive in their desire to be independent. As adults they are very dependent and cling to friends, their spouses, or parents. Thus, it is necessary first for infants to have relationships. That is most basic. Then the healthier the person is to whom they relate, the healthier their development will be (Fig. 17-4).

Melaine Klein,[12] the British child psychoanalyst, believes that in the early development of children, parents are internalized by chil-

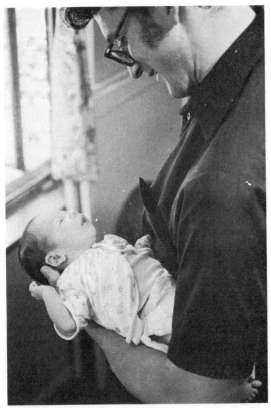

fig. 17-4 Security with father, too. (*Photo by John Young.*)

dren and taken within themselves like little people or *inner objects* living inside of them. These *inner objects* are either bad or good and continue within the growing infant the feeling states of parental figures that predominated in their relationships from infancy through the early years.

THE PSYCHOLOGICAL TASK OF SEPARATION

The *beginnings* of the psychological task of separation and individuation is one of the major psychological tasks undertaken in the first year of life. The process begins while the baby is completely physically dependent on

the parents and still believes that in some way he or she and the mother are attached. After the child's first birthday, the unquenchable need to explore drives the child toward independence. By the age of 2, the child has begun to rebel, armed with the word *no,* which is fired at anyone in range. In the third and fourth years, the child's understanding greatly expands, and he or she is capable of much more independence. Normally, this theme of individuation and separation is again the major developmental concern years later in adolescence. People who have not been allowed to develop normal independence because of overprotective parents will stay concerned their entire lives with the psychological tasks of individuation and separation, as is shown by those who never "cut the apron strings."

Margaret Mahler's major work, *The Psychological Birth of the Human Infant,* presents descriptive research about the first phase of human development.[13] Her theoretical schema begins when infants are 4 to 5 months old, and it follows the separation-individuation process through its normal course, concluding when the child is 3 to 3½ years old. (Although this chapter deals only with the first year of life, it must be recognized that this developmental task extends well beyond that period.)

Prior to the fourth and fifth months, Mahler believes that total dependency on the mother exists, with the infant feeling that he or she is connected to the mother. The infant only becomes ready to separate if dependency needs have been met and satisfied. Thus a healthy dependence leads to a healthy beginning for separation-individuation.

differentiation

In the early months, the infant's perceptual system is focused inwardly, with needs, discomforts, or pleasures dominating attention. Such inward orientation is the beginning of the infant's body awareness. However, a change soon begins to occur in the orientation of this perceptual system. There is a shift to a greater awareness of the outside world. Mahler has termed this shift *hatching*. Initially in the hatching process, it is likely that an infant can distinguish the separateness of two objects outside of him- or herself before being able to distinguish the fact of separateness from the mother. It has been observed in this point of development that babies display a new look of awareness.

experimenting with separation

Around 6 months of age, another shift begins to be noticed: the beginnings of experimentation with separation. Instead of the baby just molding into the mother, a detailed body exploration of the mother begins. The baby begins to look intently at mother, pull her hair, put food in mother's mouth, or stand, straining and pulling away from mother. The infant begins to break away from being a passive lap baby. On the floor, a baby at this phase usually plays right at the mother's feet.

checking back Around 7 to 8 months of age, the infant moves away from mother's feet and begins to engage in a checking-back pattern. Observers have consistently noted how these infants will visually check back on the mother's presence. At this time, these babies also begin to do comparative scanning, scrutinizing things and faces, taking ever greater notice of the environment outside their own bodies.

stranger reactions Mahler has raised a point not often noted when separation anxiety is discussed. She points out that this phase of development is marked as much by curiosity as by anxiety. Therefore, Mahler uses the term *stranger reactions* or stranger anxiety. Although every infant between 8 and 10 months of age may react to a stranger with initial anxiety, curiosity may be a more fre-

quent reaction if the infant earlier has been allowed a good dependence relationship. If the infant has had a frustrating relationship earlier, then a more abrupt 8-month anxiety is observed, and the period of anxiety reaction seems to be prolonged.

practicing

The second phase of the process of separation outlined by Mahler is called *practicing*. Although this period naturally overlaps with the preceding phase of differentiation, it continues through until the middle of the second year (16 to 18 months). The phase is based almost entirely on the newly found skill of locomotion. The infant's ability to crawl and explore alone and then to walk upright has enormous psychological impact. There is consolidation of body differentiation and a development of all the voluntary muscular systems, especially locomotion. All this takes place still within the bond of the infant's relationship to the mother. The developing infant maintains a physical proximity to mother in the midst of exploration. The child frequently returns to touch mother or be hugged, only immediately to go off again. This is a kind of emotional refueling—a touch at home base—but during this phase the child wants, needs, and achieves a new degree of distance, with some *disengagement* from mother. Often one can hear a mother say during this period that she has "lost" her baby.

The practicing phase ends at approximately 16 to 18 months. Two other stages follow: rapprochment and consolidation of individuality with the beginnings of object constancy. *Rapprochment* is marked by the growing child's need to be separate and to have distance from mother, together with the periodic need to "refuel." In contrast to the practicing phase, the toddler leaves the mother for longer periods of time.

The last phase, *consolidation of individuality* and the beginning of object constancy, marks the development of the child's own individuality and the internalization of a positive inner representation of the mother.

help for parents

Nurses need to be prepared to help parents negotiate some of the difficult problems involved in separation during the first year. Within the normal routine, the child suffers enough mini-separations and frustrations to develop a certain degree of tolerance, but long, unprepared-for separations must be handled with great understanding. Occasional separation with a familiar baby sitter can add the sense that life is not perfect, but not consistently terrifying either. Parents who use a totally strange baby sitter or who sneak out of the house when their baby is not looking, sabotage the child's beginning attempts at handling anxiety. Separation, like anything else, should be handled openly. It is better for a child to cry over the parents' leaving when they straightforwardly wave and say "bye-bye," than when the child misses them and vainly searches the house for them. If mother is going to have to leave her baby or young child, the person (including father) who will be substituting for her should spend time beforehand with the child to build some familiarity.

Should an infant under 1 year of age have to be hospitalized, it is just as important for the mother to be with the child then as it is when the child is older.

AN EXAMPLE OF CROSS-CULTURAL MOTHERING PATTERNS

In different cultures, basic mothering patterns vary greatly and offer alternative methods for consideration. In particular, one mothering pattern of the Kikuyu tribe of central Kenya in East Africa stands out as strikingly different from Western styles. Infants and babies are almost at no time put down, either to sleep or for any other reason, but rather are consistently carried, usually tied on their mothers' backs, and therefore are rarely deprived of physical contact with their mothers. The reasons for this are simple. Traditionally, in a Kikuyu hut there is no "nursery." Baby's bed is that part of mother's bed between mother and the wall. Because of the excellent weather and agricultural tasks of the household, much of the day is spent outside, not inside. The child has no problem in adapting to sleeping on mother's back; being quite used to riding around *in* mother, the child has no new feeling when riding *on* mother. This continuation of a pleasurable, relaxing, known experience in the midst of a world of unknown experiences offers security.

The question which may be raised here is who really has the advantage—infants who sleep in their own room, in a beautiful crib, surrounded by cuddly teddy bears, or those who sleep feeling the warmth and motion of the mother's back? The first situation is the outgrowth of a highly materialistic society. The other is still part of a highly personal society where only now the emphasis is shifting from living things (people, cows, sheep, crops, etc.) to material things (money, radios, cars, etc.). The traditional Kikuyu mother is using her own warmth and physical contact as a part of her relationship to her child. Western society tends to be much more "hygienic" and materially oriented, perhaps to the detriment of the development of physical and emotional relationships. To have a relationship there must be *contact*. There is a tendency to intellectualize the meaning of "contact," but in fact it necessitates large amounts of time spent together—the mother and the baby getting the "feel" of each other.

One method to provide more physical contact has been tried in our society by mothers who use the cloth carriers (for infants and babies) to carry their babies around the house (Fig. 17-5). Use of such a carrier makes it very easy to put to sleep an infant who is satisfied but a little uppity; the mother simply puts the child in the carrier and gets on with her duties. By the time the dishes are done, baby is asleep and can be easily lowered into the crib.

THE INFANT WITHOUT A FAMILY: COMMENTS ON FOSTER CARE AND ADOPTION

Many infants do not become a part of the families into which they were born. These infants are placed in either adoptive or foster homes. For a variety of reasons, many parents are unable to care for or bring up a child to whom they have given birth. The reasons for the parents' or mother's inability to care for the child are as widespread and varied as the situations and personalities of the people themselves. Some parents or individual mothers recognize that, given their circumstances, they are inadequate to care for a baby or raise a child, at least at this time in their lives. Other mothers, because of social pressures, problems of drug addiction, or mental illness, either give up or abandon children. But, of course, there are many reasons other than those why children are given up either temporarily or completely.

fig. 17-5   A front carrier for babies from 1 to 24 months old. (*a*) With young infant. (*b*) Diagram of how to attach carrier. (*Courtesy Baby, Too, A and B House, Gilbertsville, New York.*)

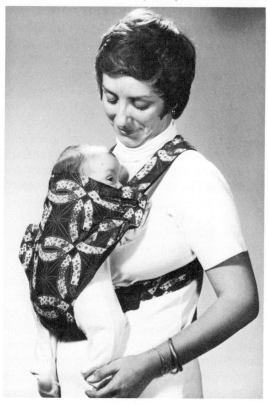

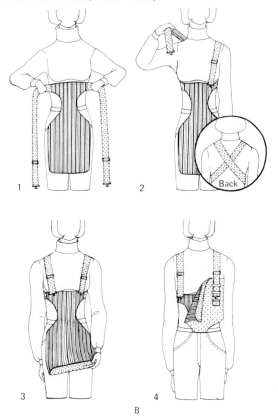

A

B

For a mother to recognize that she is unable to care for and raise a child because of whatever circumstances and to plan so that the child will be provided with good parents, requires great maturity and courage. Such an individual needs the understanding and support of the nursing staff with whom she will deal at the time of delivery and immediately after.

The infants who go into either adoptive or foster home placement frequently remain in the hospital nursery longer than other infants. The nursing staff has a special responsibility to these children, as to those who are left longer because of medical reasons, to supply the missing personal attention, warmth, and comfort that an enthusiastic and loving mother would normally provide. Even in a brief stay, the infant faces the risk that all infants who are institutionalized face. Although all their physical needs may be met, they have great need for psychological stimulation in the form of tender and playful handling. Studies have shown that infants in institutions without personal contact, given adequate food and comfortable but unstimulating surroundings are retarded in their physical and psychological development, and in extreme cases may even die.[14]

Nurses who establish some type of relationship with an infant risk their own feelings of attachment to the child. Nurses who have gone through the experience of extending themselves to an infant left for several weeks in the hospital have suffered with their own normal feelings of separation and loss and must grieve when the infant has had to leave. Although these feelings are painful, normal signs of separation, they are also the proof that the infant has had the giving relationship that will help to approximate a normal experience.

Some children who leave the hospital will go into adoptive homes. *Adoption* is the legal placement of a child with suitable adoptive parents to whom the state gives full responsibility for the child, with the child becoming an actual legal member of the family. Adoption requires either that the child's biologic mother has voluntarily given up her legal rights to the child or that a court has terminated her rights, usually on the basis of abandonment. After a period of placement, usually 1 year, the adoption is legally finalized in the courts, and in most states a new birth certificate is issued showing the adoptive parents as the only parents. At this point, there is *complete protection* against removal of the child from home because of claims to the child made by another party. Once the child is adopted, the adoptive parents are entirely responsible for the child's life, as in a natural birth. Adoption assures the child of having continuing family relationships throughout his life. These relationships can begin as soon as the infant leaves the hospital, sometimes 1 or 2 weeks after birth, but possibly later.

Other babies leave the hospital's nursery for foster homes. If the biologic mother chooses not to give up her rights to the child and remains at least somewhat interested in the child so that abandonment cannot be proved (even though possibly the biologic mother can in no way care for the child herself, for whatever reasons), then the child is placed in a foster home. Often foster care is used for children who could be adopted but for whom adoptive homes are difficult to find because the children are older, of a minority race, have medical problems, etc. *Foster care*, then, is defined as a method of child care in which the child is placed with a family which is given major responsibility for the child's care. Legal responsibility for the child is assigned to a state agency or a state-licensed private agency. Foster homes are usually administered directly through these agencies. Foster parents are paid a monthly rate through the agency or the child's expenses plus medical and other expenses. A social worker is assigned to each home to give professional assistance in the raising of the children. The social worker works with the biologic parent toward resolution of the uncertainty of the child's status by proving abandonment, voluntary surrender of the biologic mother's rights to the child, or return of the child to the biologic mother.

The distinction, then, between a child who can be placed for adoption and a child who is placed in a foster home for extended care is usually a legal one. The child must be "free" for adoption, which means that there is no parental claim to the child. Biologic parents may voluntarily surrender their rights to the child by signing affidavits stating that this is their wish. Or biologic parents can be sued in court and have their rights to children severed. The judicial system of many states have in the past favored the "blood bond" over the "psychologic bond" that the child has to the family with whom he or she lives, but this appears to be changing. Complete abandonment of the child by his biologic parents constitutes the one consistent grounds on which the courts of the various states usually sever parental rights.

If the biologic parental rights remain intact while the child lives with a foster family, then many psychologically damaging conflicts are intrinsic to the situation. The foster parents find it difficult to commit themselves totally to the child because of the possibility that the child will be removed from their home to be returned to biologic parents. The child at first does not understand the situation and then is confused by the burden of two sets of parents (one set of which the child knows as his or her "real" parents but whom in fact are hardly known); later the child is in conflict because of the uncertainty of not knowing where his or her identity and allegiance really lie. Finally, the biologic parents are also frequently in conflict over the situation, torn between their own feelings of guilt over not being able to

take their child and their sense of inadequacy produced by a combination of all the reasons which have made it impossible for them to care for their child themselves.

The foster care situation is difficult from the foster parents' viewpoint because the legal uncertainties make them insecure in their feelings of love for their foster children. Many foster parents who commit themselves fully to children placed in their care suffer agonizing loss when the child is removed from their home. Even for the child who remains in the foster home, there can be deep emotional conflicts around such matters as visits from the biologic parents. Foster parents must be unusually strong parents to be able to reach out to the child and explain the very mixed feelings which are involved in this situation.

The present trend in the legislative and judicial systems is to give the children themselves and their foster parents more rights in court.[15] Presently, children, even infants, are being assigned their own lawyers to protect their rights and to guarantee that the best possible living situation is available to them in terms of both their psychological and physical development. Every state has its own laws concerning foster care, but as an example of progressive legislation, New York State has given foster parents who have had a child in their home for 2 or more years the right to a hearing prior to the removal of the child from the home for any reason. This is a step toward protecting the *psychological bonds,* the delicate, fragile feelings of relationship, between the foster child and foster parents. Foster care needs to be further restructured legally to guarantee that the "psychological parents" of the foster child will have the fullest possible opportunity to develop normal family relationships and—most important—that the child will have the fullest opportunity to feel that he or she is a secure and wanted member of a family.

Many states also now have *subsidized*

adoption for foster parents who cannot afford to adopt a child who has been their foster child. Subsidized adoption means that the state will continue to provide foster care payments to such a family. Such payments are usually subject to an annual review of the adoptive parents' income.

Compared with other forms of child care, foster care is the most excellent way devised by our society of taking care of the child who cannot be brought up by the biologic parents. In a foster home, a child relates to a complete family and has the possibility of close relationships on an individual basis. Even in the present legal situation, it is possible for a child to enter a foster home immediately after birth and to remain as a member of the family throughout childhood and adolescence, although, unfortunately, this usually does not happen. The infant who enters a foster home will be able to relate to one consistent mother with whom he or she can form the comforting, satisfying, and stimulating relationship which every baby must have in order to be able to go on to more mature levels of psychological development.

study questions

1 Why is the understanding of the mother-infant bond so basic in infant care?
2 How can medical routine interfere with the process. Observe, in your clinical setting, ways in which bonding is promoted or inhibited by hospital practices.
3 Identify the ways in which the "mothering" function can be carried out by either parent or by another significant person in the new baby's life.
4 What is the meaning of bonding?
5 How much can the infant perceive at birth?
6 Which senses does the infant use prior to birth?
7 How does routine contribute to the formation of memories?
8 In what ways is it theorized that the infant feels "I am the center of the universe"?
9 List at least three reasons why it is important for the infant not to be frustrated in the first 4 months of life.
10 After a mother has been separated from her infant, give two reasons why it may be difficult to reestablish a relationship right away.
11 Why do infants cry?
12 What psychological phase must precede separation-individuation for it to be successful?
13 In what practical ways can a parent help a young child accept periods of separation?
14 Is it a positive sign that the nurses grieve when a baby who has had an extended nursery stay is discharged?
15 What support is necessary for parents when their infant has had an extended nursery stay?
16 Note the basic differences between foster care and adoption.
17 Study Fig. 17–1. Describe the "body language" of mother, father, and baby. What feelings do you think may be present?

References

1 M. Klaus and J. H. Kennell, *Maternal-Infant Bonding,* Mosby, New York, 1976, p. 14.
2 R. D. Laing, *New York Times,* January 15, 1978, p. 48.
3 N. Klaus, et al., "Maternal Attachment: Importance of the First Postpartum Days," *New England Journal of Medicine,* **280:**460, 1972.
4 W. Winnicott, *The Child, the Family, and the Outside World,* Penguin, Middlesex, Eng., 1964, p. 9.
5 R. Spitz, *The First Year of Life, a Psychoanalytic Study of Normal and Deviant Development of Object Relations,* International University Press, New York, 1965, p. 36.
6 K. S. Robson, "The Role of Eye-to-Eye Contact in Maternal Infant Attachment," *Journal of Child Psychology-Psychiatry,* **8:**13–25, 1967.
7 B. L. White, *Human Infants' Experience and Psychological Development,* Prentice-Hall, Englewood Cliffs, N.J., 1971, p. 16.
8 Laing, op. cit.
9 K. Holt, *Developmental Pediatrics,* Butterworths, London, 1977, p. 156.
10 J. A. MacFarlane, *The Parent-Infant Interaction,* Ciba Foundation Symposium 33, Elsevier, Amsterdam, 1975, p. 137.
11 L. Salk and R. Kramer, *How to Raise a Human Being,* Random House, New York, 1969, p. 12.
12 H. Guntrip, *Personality Structure and Human Interaction,* International University Press, New York, 1961, pp. 234–245.
13 M. Mahler, F. Pine, and A. Berman, *The Psychological Birth of the Human Infant,* Basic Books, New York, 1975.

14 J. Bowlby, *Child Care and the Growth of Love*, Penguin, Baltimore, 1965.
15 J. Goldstein, A. Freud, and A. J. Solnit, *Beyond the Best Interests of the Child*, Free Press, New York, 1973, pp. 37–39.

Bibliography

"Adoption—Some Answers to the Doctor's Dilemma," *Contemporary OB/GYN*, **1**(1):10, January 1972.

American Academy of Pediatrics: *Adoption of Children*, 3d ed., Committee on Adoption and Dependent Care, Evanston, Ill., 1975.

Bowlby, J.: "Nature of a Child's Tie to His Mother," *International Journal of Psychoanalysis*, **39**:350–373, 1958.

Brazelton, T. B.: *Infants and Mothers*, Delacorte, New York, 1969.

————: "Anticipatory Guidance," *Pediatric Clinics of North America*, **22**:533, 1975.

Boulette, T. R.: "Parenting: Special Needs of Low-Income Spanish-Surnamed Families," *Pediatric Annals*, **6**(9):95, September 1977.

Fraiberg, S.: *The Magic Years*, Scribner, New York, 1959.

Greenberg, M., and N. Morris: "Engrossment: The Newborn's Impact Upon the Father," *American Journal of Orthopsychiatry*, **44**:(4)520, July 1974.

Harrison-Ross, P.: "Parenting the Black Child," *Pediatric Annals*, **6**(9):605, September 1977.

Kennell, J. H., and A. Rolnick: "Discussing Problems in Newborn Babies with Their Parents," *Pediatrics* **26**: 832–838, 1960.

Lipsitt, L. P.: "Sensory and Learning Processes of the Newborn," *Clinics in Perinatology*, **23**(3): March 1977.

Lozoff, B., G. M. Brittenbarr, M. A. Trause, J. H. Kennell, and M. H. Klaus: "The Mother-Newborn Relationship: Limits of Adaptability," *Journal of Pediatrics*, **91**(1):1, July 1977.

Maurer, D., and P. Salapatek: "Developmental Changes in the Scanning of Faces by Young Infants," *Child Development*, **47**:523, 1976.

Smart, M. S., and R. C. Smart: *Infants*, Macmillan, New York, 1973.

Waters, E., L. Matas, and L. A. Stouge: "Infants Reactions to an Approaching Stranger," *Child Development*, **46**:348, 1975.

"Why Babies Cry," *Journal of American Medical Women's Association*, **31**(7):271, July 1976.

Zimmerman, Beverly McKay, "The Exceptional Stresses of Adoptive Parenthood," *Maternal Child Nursing*, **2**(3): 194, May 1977 (annotated bibliography).

18

WELL BABY CARE

JANE CORWIN REEVES

Maternal care does not begin when a woman becomes pregnant, nor does it end when she takes her infant home from the hospital. It is a process which effects changes within her and within the family throughout life, but especially during the next 12 months.

Nurses are functioning in a new role in well baby clinics and in private pediatric offices across the country. They are essentially making four basic nursing judgments: (1) This baby is well. (2) This baby is sick but can wait to see a doctor. (3) This baby is sick and needs to see the doctor immediately. (4) This baby is sick and I will treat it. The emphasis of this chapter is on wellness and includes such things as growth and development, assessment, intervention, stimulation, safety, and common problems of infants.

ASSESSMENT SKILLS

The two most important nursing tools are the eyes and the ears. Observation of what is happening will help give the nurse an accurate assessment of the baby and the relationship between the mother and her infant. Henry K. Silver, M.D., has said that once professionals begin to touch, they often cease to use their eyes and their ears. Look at the baby. Is the baby happy, sad, fussy, solemn, crying, jolly? Is he or she fat, thin, sturdy, pale, rosy, well nourished? Does the baby look healthy? If not, why not? How old does the baby appear to be by size and activity? Look at the mother. Does she appear happy, sad, frightened, apathetic, frustrated, tense? Do you see a corresponding tension response in the infant? Look at the relationship between the mother and her baby. Observe the mother's "body language." How does she hold the baby? Does she grip tightly or hold the infant loosely? How does the mother respond when the baby cries or disregards her verbal commands? Are her commands reasonable for the infant's age level?

Accurate observation requires concentration. Listening is also a deliberate art that is difficult to master. It takes a conscious decision to concentrate on verbal and nonverbal cues. The nonverbal messages are sent through posture, facial expression, tone of voice, gestures, and by things omitted from usual interactions. Developing rapport must be part of any mother-infant observation, for defensiveness and fear can hide important information from the nurse. Process, not exact content, is of supreme importance.[1]

WELL CHILD MANAGEMENT

Health supervision visits are recommended every 2 months for the first 6 months of life, beginning at 4 weeks, and every 2 to 3 months during the last half of the first year. These visits can be handled by the nurse except for one or two scheduled with the physician. The visits correspond to the immunization schedule, and the spacing should be adapted to the needs of the infant and the parents. Alpert suggests late afternoon or evening appointments so that both parents can participate in the health care visit. Working mothers also find this time more convenient.[2]

The workup contains five basic components: "A verbal gathering of information (history taking), a look at the child (physical examination), interpretation of all laboratory findings, an impression based on all the objective and subjective information gathered, and a plan of action including both counselling and interpretation of this information to the patient."[3]

OBSERVATION BASED ON GROWTH AND DEVELOPMENT

Silver defines growth and development as follows:

> *Development* signifies maturation of organs and systems, acquisitions of skills, ability to adapt more readily to stress, and ability to assume maximum responsibility and to achieve freedom in creative expression. *Growth* refers to a change in size resulting from the multiplication of cells or the enlargement of existing ones.[4]

Everything that nurses do in assessment is based on principles of development and growth. An understanding of the normal ranges of growth and development is a basic tool for the nurse in comparing each child with others (see Figs. 18-1 and 18-2). Wide variations are possible, and skill in interpreting differences will come as experience is gained with many infants. Brazelton, in *Infants and Mothers,* has made an interesting comparison between the "average" baby, the "quiet" baby, and the "active" baby. He states

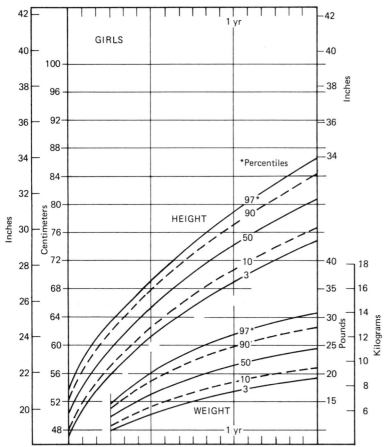

fig. 18·1 Height and weight for girls (Harvard data) 3, 10, 50, 90, and 97 percentile ranges. (*From Kempe, Silver, and O'Brien (eds.), Current Pediatric Diagnosis and Treatment, 4th ed., Lange, Los Altos, Calif., 1976.*)

that each new mother must find her own special baby. Each is "stuck" with the other's unique ways of reacting. He further states that the idealized suggestions of authorities may be entirely wrong for a particular mother and child. Nurses working in cultural situations that are different from their own must avoid the pitfalls of an authoritative approach based on textbook ideals and yet must be able to bring some clear suggestions to the mother when problems are observed.[5]

In a prospective, comprehensive analysis

of individuality in behavior from infancy onward, "The New York Longitudinal Study of Child Development," Thomas et al. defined nine categories of reactivity or temperament: activity level, rhythmicity or regularity, adaptability to change in routine, approach or withdrawal as a characteristic response to a new situation, level of sensory threshold, positive or negative mood, intensity of response, distractability or persistence, and attention span. It was found that children showed distinct individuality of temperament in the first

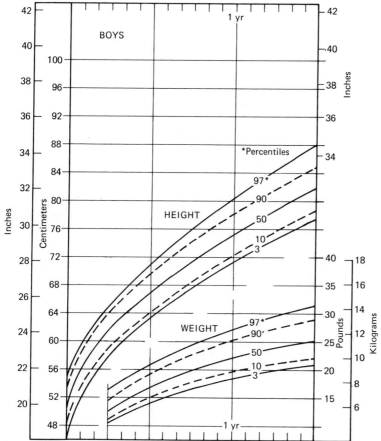

fig. 18-2 Height and weight for boys (Harvard data). (*From Kempe, Silver, and O'Brien (eds.), Current Pediatric Diagnosis and Treatment, 4th ed., Lange, Los Altos, Calif., 1976.*)

weeks of life, independent of parental handling or personality.[6] Environmental circumstances were found to heighten, diminish, or modify behavior. Table 18-1 lists characteristics of the three groups identified.

The basic principle is well stated by Silver:

Development and growth are continuous dynamic processes occurring from conception to maturity and take place in an orderly sequence which is approximately the same for all individuals. At any particular age,

however, wide variations are to be found among normal children which reflect the active response of the growing individual to numberless hereditary and environmental factors.[7]

The focus of development is at the center of the head and trunk and moves downward and outward, cephalocaudal and proximaldistal. Development also proceeds from the general to the specific; gross, large muscle functions are present before the finer abilities

table 18-1 Children are born different

Easy children: 40%
 Positive mood
 Regularity of body function
 Low or moderate intensity of reaction
 Adaptability
 Positiveness in a new situation

Slow to warm up: 15%
 Low activity level
 Tendency to withdraw from new stimuli
 Slow adaptability
 Somewhat negative mood
 Low intensity of reaction

Difficult: 10%
 Irregularity of body function
 High intensity of reaction
 Withdrawal in face of new stimuli
 Slow adaptability

Mixture of above attributes: 35%

Source: Adapted by Jeanne B. Brown in "Infant Temperament: A Clue to Childbearing for Parents and Nurses," *American Journal of Maternal and Child Nursing,* July/August 1977, p. 231, from Thomas, et al.

of the hands and fingers. When development is normal, one period prepares the infant for the next milestone. The newborn's aimless movements become more specific as the infant learns to take an object and then to use the pincer grasp of thumb and forefinger around a cereal flake or raisin. The infant rolls over before sitting alone, learns to pull to a stand before cruising, stands alone well before walking alone. Each child should be evaluated for growth and development at each well baby visit.

Denver prescreening developmental questionnaire (PDQ)

The Denver PDQ is a brief, valid, *prescreening* questionnaire used to identify those individuals who should be more thoroughly screened with the Denver Developmental Screening Test (DDST). For any given child, only the age-appropriate items are to be completed from the total group. If the parent reports that the child cannot perform most of the items, the child is referred for the DDST. Only approximately 30 percent of all children prescreened with the PDQ will require further screening. If the PDQ is used at the recommended ages (3, 6, 9, 12, and 18 months and 2, 3, 4, 5, and 6 years), it will serve as an ongoing log of the child's developmental progress. The questionnaire is included in the DDST packet.[8]

Denver developmental screening test

Frankenburg and Dodds formulated the Denver Developmental Screening Test[9] as a tool which can be used to pick up developmental lags. Some developmental problems can be corrected by introducing new experiences into the infant's world, but sometimes lags indicate something more serious. For instance, the baby who does not turn to the sound of a voice or respond to the bell by the age of 5 months may have a serious hearing problem.

Cautions in the use of the DDST by nurses are given by Roberts.[10] The tool is for preschool screening only, and its validity rests there. However, nurses have used it in a variety of ways—to alert parents and students to the dynamics of child growth and development, for stimulation needs in any one area, for referral, and for evaluation of follow-up. The tool should not be adapted, and its purposes should be kept clear. Frankenburg adds that it is not an intelligence test but a screening instrument to determine whether the development of a particular child is within the normal range (Fig. 18-3).

instructions for use Generally, in the first year the test utilizes the nurse's observation skills, rather than giving verbal direc-

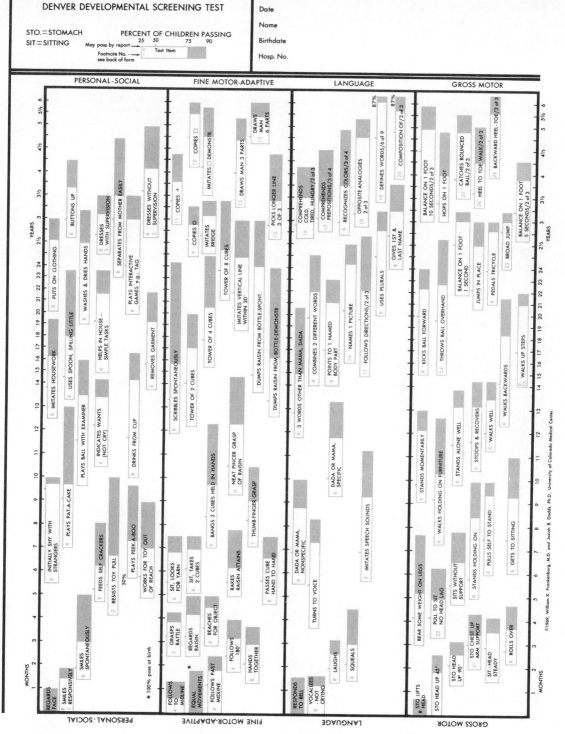

fig. 18-3 Denver Developmental Screening Test (continued on page 378).

1. Try to get child to smile by smiling, talking or waving to him. Do not touch him.
2. When child is playing with toy, pull it away from him. Pass if he resists.
3. Child does not have to be able to tie shoes or button in the back.
4. Move yarn slowly in an arc from one side to the other, about 6" above child's face. Pass if eyes follow 90° to midline. (Past midline; 180°)
5. Pass if child grasps rattle when it is touched to the backs or tips of fingers.
6. Pass if child continues to look where yarn disappeared or tries to see where it went. Yarn should be dropped quickly from sight from tester's hand without arm movement.
7. Pass if child picks up raisin with any part of thumb and a finger.
8. Pass if child picks up raisin with the ends of thumb and index finger using an over hand approach.

  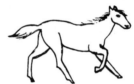 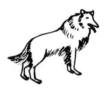

9. Pass any enclosed form. Fail continuous round motions.
10. Which line is longer? (Not bigger.) Turn paper upside down and repeat. (3/3 or 5/6)
11. Pass any crossing lines.
12. Have child copy first. If failed, demonstrate

When giving items 9, 11 and 12, do not name the forms. Do not demonstrate 9 and 11.

13. When scoring, each pair (2 arms, 2 legs, etc.) counts as one part.
14. Point to picture and have child name it. (No credit is given for sounds only.)

 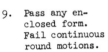 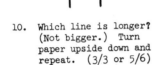 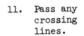 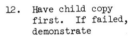

15. Tell child to: Give block to Mommie; put block on table; put block on floor. Pass 2 of 3. (Do not help child by pointing, moving head or eyes.)
16. Ask child: What do you do when you are cold? ..hungry? ..tired? Pass 2 of 3.
17. Tell child to: Put block on table; under table; in front of chair, behind chair. Pass 3 of 4. (Do not help child by pointing, moving head or eyes.)
18. Ask child: If fire is hot, ice is ?; Mother is a woman, Dad is a ?; a horse is big, a mouse is ?. Pass 2 of 3.
19. Ask child: What is a ball? ..lake? ..desk? ..house? ..banana? ..curtain? ..ceiling? ..hedge? ..pavement? Pass if defined in terms of use, shape, what it is made of or general category (such as banana is fruit, not just yellow). Pass 6 of 9.
20. Ask child: What is a spoon made of? ..a shoe made of? ..a door made of? (No other objects may be substituted.) Pass 3 of 3.
21. When placed on stomach, child lifts chest off table with support of forearms and/or hands.
22. When child is on back, grasp his hands and pull him to sitting. Pass if head does not hang back.
23. Child may use wall or rail only, not person. May not crawl.
24. Child must throw ball overhand 3 feet to within arm's reach of tester.
25. Child must perform standing broad jump over width of test sheet. (8-1/2 inches)
26. Tell child to walk forward, ⟨⟩⟨⟩⟨⟩➤ heel within 1 inch of toe. Tester may demonstrate. Child must walk 4 consecutive steps, 2 out of 3 trials.
27. Bounce ball to child who should stand 3 feet away from tester. Child must catch ball with hands, not arms, 2 out of 3 trials.
28. Tell child to walk backward, ◄⟨⟩⟨⟩⟨⟩ toe within 1 inch of heel. Tester may demonstrate. Child must walk 4 consecutive steps, 2 out of 3 trials.

DATE AND BEHAVIORAL OBSERVATIONS (how child feels at time of test, relation to tester, attention span, verbal behavior, self-confidence, etc,):

fig. 18-3 (continued) Denver Development Screening Test. (*From William K. Frankenburg, and Josiah B. Dodds, University of Colorado Medical Center.*)

tions for infant responses. Involving the mother in the test is one way of recognizing her unique contribution and provides a good opportunity for teaching. The parent must participate if the child refuses interaction with the observer. The parent also participates by reporting behavior (R = passes test according to report of parent) (see Fig. 18-4).

Begin the evaluation by drawing a line through the chart at the chronologic age (for a premature child, subtract the number of months premature from the chronologic age). Administer pertinent items—the footnotes give specific directions. The significance of the test lies in the comparison of the child with his or her own development as the months go by and in a comparison of the child with the norms demonstrated on the bar graph. Each marking on the bar means that a certain percentage—25, 50, 75, or 90 percent—of the age group had a successful performance. If the child does not pass what 90 percent of his or her peer group passes, it is considered significant and reportable.

During the test, the nurse can explain how the baby develops and how the mother can help. She can ask what the baby is doing that is new. She can talk about what is normal for the baby's age and what the mother should watch for over the next month or so. The nurse should explain what the test shows. For instance, an infant low in social development may not be getting enough stimulation.

STIMULATION, TOYS, CLOTHES, AND SAFETY

stimulation

The changes in growth and development are more rapid in the first year of life than in any single year thereafter. The "helpless" newborn is not a passive entity but is continuously

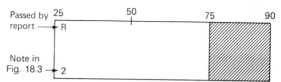

fig. 18-4 DDST bar graph. R - passes on basis of mother's report; 2 - footnote number; shaded areas indicate the ages at which 75 to 90 percent of children can pass the test item. Failure to perform an item that can be done by 90 percent is significant and should be reported.

monitoring and integrating experiences. It has been found that from birth to 2 months of age, infants focus on objects 6 to 8 inches away. Eight inches is just the distance of a baby's outstretched arm, which is one reason that hands are the first playthings. The crib can be decorated with bright pictures or a few cards with painted geometrical designs or faces. Ribbons tied to wrists or a mobile made up of various colors of balloons offer the infant moving objects to watch. The introduction of one or two objects at a time is better than the overstimulation of a completely decorated crib.

Newborns would rather watch people than things, and parents need to be encouraged to hold, touch, rock, talk, and sing to their new baby. They need to know that although the baby is not yet able to understand what they say, the child will enjoy the sound of their voices and begin forming the language he or she will speak the following year. An infant seat, a blanket on the floor, or a front or back baby carrier will allow a variety of positions, the enjoyment of being with the family, and the stimulation of sound and activity.

toys

Educational toys are not necessary to proper development. Brazelton states, "The suggestion that there is a *need* for educational toys is coming from the child experts. For a number of years psychologists have been pushing toward earlier cognitive, or intellectual stimulation, and the implication has been that parents must provide their infants with toys that will help them learn how to learn. This kind of pressure implies that parents cannot offer enough stimulation for their babies, that affectionate play and caring does not provide children enough necessary building blocks for the future."[11]

In the first year, most of what the child *needs* can be assembled from bits and pieces around the house. A cradle gym can be made by stretching a piece of elastic across the crib with metal measuring spoons, colored cellophane, a rattle, or squeaky toy. The objects can be changed periodically (Fig. 18-5). This same piece of elastic can be stretched across the back of a car or the back seat of an airplane. Alexander lists some homemade toys: various sizes of blocks can be made out of different sizes of milk cartons; tin cans protected by colored cellophane tape can become nesting boxes (6-oz juice can, soup can, 303 pear can, 2½-lb peach can).[12] Paper bags, aluminum foil, colored cellophane paper, clothespins (the old-fashioned kind) with

fig. 18-5 Homemade cradle gym over baby's crib. (*Photo by Mary Olsen Johnson, M.D.*)

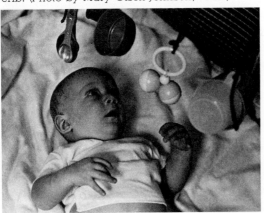

various containers to put them into, pots, pans, and lids, an old coffee pot, a ball or two, a cuddly teddy bear, a squeaky toy, a push-pull toy, and a few cloth books will provide much stimulation in the first year. The educational toys on the market are a nice addition if the family can afford them, but they are not essential to proper child development.

clothing and equipment for the nursery

Most books advise too much clothing for the layette and too much equipment for the nursery. Babies grow quickly, and so it is best to advise the mother to purchase shirts, rubber pants, blanket sleepers and stretch suits that are 6 to 9 months in size. Mothers tend to overdress their infants even in summer. Only one good outfit needs to be purchased, but often, this may be received at a baby shower. Second-hand shops and garage sales are invaluable to supplementing clothes, toys, and nursery equipment.

layette and nursery needs for the average family
Bedding: waterproof mattress, pads
   Three crib sheets
   One crib blanket
   One set of crib bumper pads
Furnishings: crib or cradle
   First 3 months: a basket, box, large drawer, or bassinet may be used
   After 3 months: a safe crib with narrow slats
   A storage unit for clothes
   A reclining infant seat
   A rocking chair, optional but very useful
   A diaper pail
Clothing: for the 1- to-3 month-old infant
   Four to six shirts
   Four nightgowns, kimonos, or stretch pajamas

Two pairs of booties or stretch socks
One sweater
Three to four dozen disposable diapers
    or washable diapers
Four waterproof pants
Cold weather: warm, windproof blanket,
    snuggly or snowsuit with cap, and mit-
    tens
Outside equipment:
    Lightweight stroller, with good back sup-
      port
    Cloth front carrier for small baby, back
      pack carrier after 4 months
    Safe car seat
    Diaper bag

safety

Accidents are always unexpected and, in retrospect, could almost always have been prevented. Accidents tend to increase with the mobility of the infant, but even a new baby can wiggle or flip off a table, bed, or chair. Most modern homes are fraught with hazards to the exploring infant. Often, before parents recognize dangers, the crawling baby is pulling up and cruising. Anticipatory guidance should be offered to the parents so that they have an opportunity to study the house before the baby begins to crawl. Table 18-2 correlates growth and development with stimulation of the baby and important safety factors. Some possible hazards include: open electric outlets, light cords, harmful cleaning products, medication in purse or on a bedside table, harmful objects carelessly discarded in a trash basket, small and/or sharp objects left around by an older child, a knife too close to the edge of a table, unguarded pools, water in bathtubs, stairs, poisonous plants, chipping paint, and toys with small parts.

In the latter half of the first year, the parents should purchase a bottle of Ipecac, an ounce of which can be obtained without a prescrip-

tion. The bottle can be stored where it is easily accessible, along with the telephone number of the poison control center, which should be called before giving the Ipecac. (Ipecac is given to induce vomiting, and for some poisons, vomiting is contraindicated.)

Lead poisoning is often associated with pica (the eating of nonfood items), as the child may eat plaster and paint chips. Parents need to be cautioned about this possibility in refinished crib furniture, toys, and old buildings. Crawling, teething infants need chewing experiences with nutritional finger foods, teething rings, and other surfaces that are harmless.

Automobile safety is a subject to be discussed at an early visit. It is important that the parents get into the habit of using a crash-tested device from the very first car ride. About 10,000 children under 5 years of age have died in automobile accidents in the last decade, not including the number of children permanently disabled.*

Babies can be taught to crawl backward down stairs. This is a safer procedure than relying solely on a closed gate. The process begins when the baby is 4 or 5 months old and wants to get down on the floor. Instead of placing the child on the floor, the mother should turn the baby on its abdomen and slide the child down feet first to the floor. If it is done consistently, the baby will automatically crawl down stairs feet first with only a little encouragement.

IMMUNIZATION

Active immunization of children provides an effective means of disease prevention and health maintenance. The schedule for active immunization given in Table 18-3 is recom-

*Automobile Safety Belt Fact Book, U.S. Government Printing Office, Washington, D.C., 10402.

table 18-2 Summary of development correlated with anticipatory guidance

age, months	development	stimulation	safety
1 (Fig. 18-6)	Smiles	Hold, smile at, talk to. Something to watch over crib: geometric designs and faces pinned over crib; change often; use one or two at a time.	Protect from falls. Flat, hard mattress, no pillow, blankets tucked in. Leave on side or abdomen after meals. Use approved car seat.
2	Coos, gurgles	Responds to voices. Talk and sing to infant. When awake, let baby be with people.	Strap into infant seat. Protect from falls.
3	No head lag; head up 90°	Responds to singing, talking, outdoors, people. Becoming sociable. Give hard and soft things to chew.	As above. Prop up infant to watch family activities.
4 (Figs. 18-7 to 18-9)	Reaches, laughs, kicks	Cradle gym over crib. Will play with small blocks, "squeeze toys," soft toys, rattles, teething rings. Play records, read nursery rhymes.	Keep small, sharp, dirty, harmful objects away. Make sure that toys contain only lead-free paint.
5	Rolls over	Allow more room. Put baby on floor or in playpen with toys. Play peek-a-boo, give paper to crumple, spoon to hold.	Protect from falls. Never leave alone in bathtub.
6	Sits alone	Can be put in high chair to eat. Likes to sit in laps. Needs lots of "lapping." Give pot lids, squeaky toy, big and little balls.	Does not sit securely. Fasten into high chair. Big enough to change to bigger car seat; check brands carefully. Get Ipecac.
7 (Fig. 18-10a,b)	Crawls	Needs freedom and room to crawl. Toys for the bath. Paper to scribble on. Cups to stack.	*Dangerous time:* Put detergents, bleaches out of reach; cover open light sockets; place cords out of reach; keep unsafe objects out of wastebasket; put gates on stairs. Baby can be taught to crawl backward down stairs.
8	Pincer grasp	Likes nesting boxes. Is happy picking up objects (Cheerios) from high-chair tray. Give spoon, cup at mealtime. Clothespin, containers, mirror.	Will pick up and eat the tiniest objects—pins, dust, pills.
9 (Fig. 18-11)	Pulls to stand	Sociable. Likes to be out of crib and playpen. Likes object constancy, peek-a-boo. First attempts at self-feeding.	Crib sides up. Turn pot handles in; take dangerous objects off tables.

table 18-2 Summary of development correlated with anticipatory guidance (*continued*)

age, months	development	stimulation	safety
10	Cruises	Needs people, blocks, pots and pans, and safe rooms. Likes pat-a-cake, cloth books, stacking toys.	Remove valuables from low tables. Check house for hazards.
11 (Fig. 18-12)	Stands alone	Pull toy, playing cards, lids to take off and put on. Likes to rip paper, put things in cabinets.	As above.
12	Walks*	Needs to hear something besides "no"—music, conversation, etc. Rolls ball back and forth. Likes to be read to.	Check yard, house, stairs for hazards. Watch baby.

*Note: Babies vary. It is perfectly normal for a baby to begin to walk at 18 months.

fig. 18-7 A 4½-month-old infant with good head control beginning to sit with a straighter back. (*Photo by Mary Olsen Johnson, M.D.*)

fig. 18-6 Social smile at 6 weeks of age.

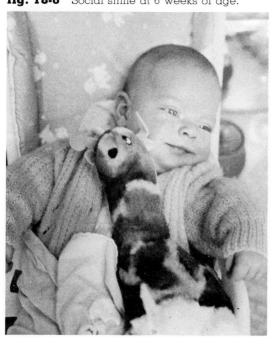

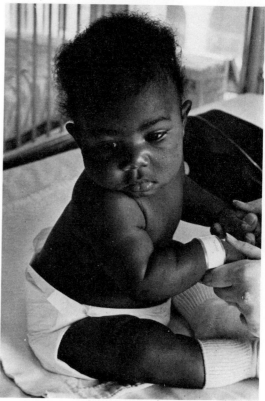

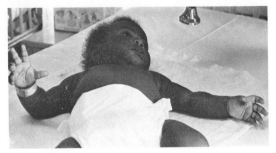

fig. 18-8 A 4½-month-old infant alerting to the sound of the bell. (*Photo by Mary Olsen Johnson, M.D.*)

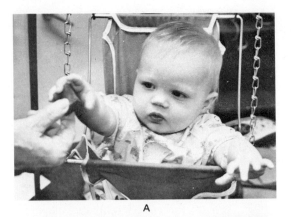

A

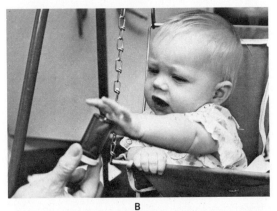

B

mended for healthy infants. It is intended as a *guide* to be used with any needed modification to meet the requirements of an individual or a group. Immunization is a dynamic field in which the continuing changes require constant evaluation.

The generally recommended age for beginning routine immunizations of normal infants

fig. 18-9 At 4½ months of age, this baby demonstrates item 21 on the DDST. He reaches for everything to put it into his mouth and lifts chest off the table with support of forearms.

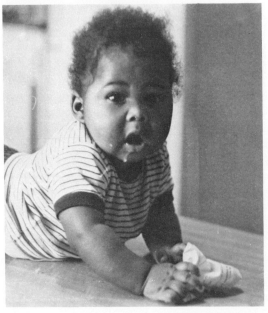

fig. 18-10 (*a*) At 7½ months of age, this baby reaches equally well with either hand but may still be palming objects. (*b*) This infant enjoys jumper, conversation, bright unbreakable toys, and mother. (*Photos by Mary Olsen Johnson, M.D.*)

is 2 months; the first vaccines given are diptheria and tetanus toxoid, combined with pertussis vaccine (DTP) and trivalent oral poliovirus vaccine (TOPV). Measles vaccine is most effective when given at or after 15 months of age because all the maternal antibody has dissipated by then.[13] If measles vaccine needs to be given by 6 to 12 months of age because of the prevalence of the disease, a repeat dose should be administered after the first birthday.

Parents should be fully informed about the

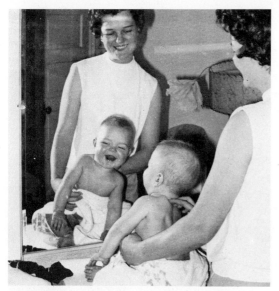

fig. 18-11 At 9½ months of age, bath time is a wonderful opportunity for playing with one's mirror image. (*Photo by David Dickason.*)

immunization proposed. They should know the antigens to be administered, the reasons for their use, and the associated reactions which might occur. Antigens should be injected deep into the muscle mass, preferably into the midlateral thigh muscle; caution should be used about the deltoid. The upper outer quadrant of the buttock is not used until the child is walking because the gluteus medius muscle is not well developed. In an older child, if injection is given in this area, it should be toward the ventrogluteal area. During the course of primary immunizations, each injection should be made at a different site (Table 18-3).

MINOR PROBLEMS OF THE FIRST YEAR

crying, fussiness, and colic

Most newborns cry about 2 h out of every 24. Some do it all at once, while others cry intermittently. Some infants show a fussy irritability which can lead to colic if not handled correctly. These babies are hard to satisfy and seem to reach a peak in demand for attention in the late afternoon or evening. Certainly the baby picks up on the fatigue, tension, and busyness of the parent at the end of the day.

table 18-3. Activities at pediatric visits

age, months	immunizations	tests	reviewed on each visit
1	Immunizations explained		Activity
2	DPT no. 1, trivalent OPV	Phenylketonuria	Sleep
3		PDQ explained and administered	Appetite Elimination Illness exposure
4	DPT no. 2, trivalent OPV		Allergies
6	DPT no. 3, trivalent OPV	Urinalysis, PDQ, hematocrit	Fainting Safety
9		PDQ	Stimulation
12		Tuberculin test, PDQ	Nutrition Next developmental changes

Source: Immunization Schedule, from *Report of the Committee on Infectious Diseases,* 18th ed., American Academy of Pediatrics, Evanston, Ill., 1977.

Note: DPT, diphtheria-pertussis-tetanus; OPV, oral polio vaccine: PDQ, Denver Prescreening Developmental Questionnaire.

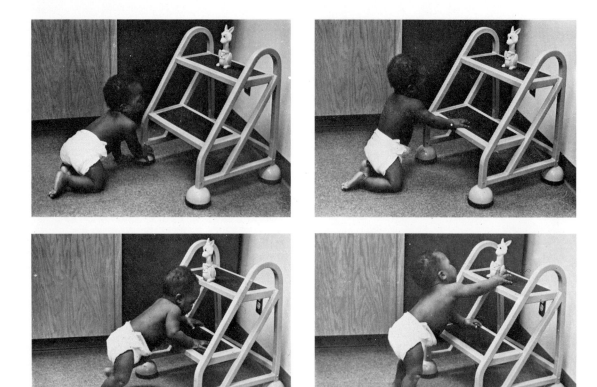

fig. 18-12 Watch out for the practicing 11-month-old baby—he can reach objects that may seem safely out of reach, and he is *determined*. (Photos by Mary Olsen Johnson, M.D.)

Parents of these infants might try an infant carrier, a swinging infant seat or bed, swaddling, a pacifier, a steady noise such as a vacuum cleaner, a ride in the stroller or car, a change in nipple, or more careful burping.

In colic, the pattern varies, but babies may cry for 4 or more hours without letup. They appear very much distressed after feeding, draw their legs up to the abdomen, and scream. The anxiety level, perhaps even hostility, of the parent adds to the problem of quieting the colicky baby.

Dr. Brazelton discovered early in his practice that half of his morning phone calls were about crying infants. He suggested many of the above activities, which would work at first but then quickly failed. He found that as parents became more worn out, the babies cried even more. Brazelton asked the parents to keep charts on crying, with the following results[14] (see Fig. 18-13):

1 Total crying usually did not amount to more than 2 h a day.
2 The more frantic the maneuvers a parent instituted, the more the baby cried.
3 If parents could allow for a certain amount of crying and interspersed their own quiet attempts to soothe the infant periodically, the crying settled down to 2 h each day.

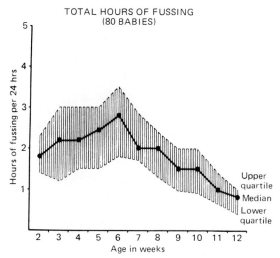

TOTAL HOURS OF FUSSING
(80 BABIES)

fig. 18-13 Results of experiences with 80 babies. (*Exerpted from the book Doctor and Child by T. Berry Brazelton. Copyright © 1976 by T. Berry Brazelton. Reprinted by permission of Delacorte Press/Seymour Lawrence.*)

4 The crying began to decrease by 7 weeks and by 10 weeks was just about gone.
5 By 12 weeks, the time of day formerly used for crying became the infant's most sociable period.

Armed with this information, Dr. Brazelton decided there is no easy solution to crying but that it seems to be a channel for the baby's energies, a time to let off steam, or an exercise period. He now encourages parents to try various methods of quieting the baby but not to get excited if they do not work. If they are able to relax, they do not add to the infant's tension.

There are a certain group of infants who respond to outside stimuli with unusual amounts of crying and motor activity. They cry longer than 2 h each day and are difficult to quiet. If the parents of these infants do not remain calm, the babies can end up crying for as much as 12 h a day. Follow-up studies on some of these overreactive infants show that they often grow up to be extremely intelligent—which may be of some encouragement to distraught parents.[15]

In 1970, an organization called Mothers Anonymous (now Parents Anonymous) was formed. Although called by different names in different locations, e.g., Parental Stress Hotline, COPE, CALM, it is a helpful resource for mothers who have crying babies.

the common cold

During the first year, infants can be expected to have one or two colds, although the problem does not usually begin until the baby is several months old. There is normally very little fever. The cold is usually characterized by sneezing, coughing, and a runny nose. If the baby looks sick, has a fever over 38.5°C (101°F), has any difficulty with respirations, has a bad cough or a congested chest, is refusing food, or is pulling at her or his ears, then the problem is more serious than a simple cold (Fig. 18-14).

To prevent frequent colds, babies should be kept out of crowds and away from other babies during cold, wet weather. This may be very difficult for the working mother, especially if she utilizes a day-care facility.

fig. 18-14 Position of infant during taking of rectal temperature. (*Photo by Mary Olsen Johnson, M.D.*)

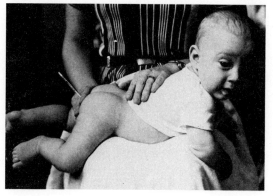

intervention Nursing intervention consists of the following:

1 Inquiry into dryness and warmth of the home.
2 Advising cool steam, by vaporizer or by holding the baby in the bathroom while running the shower.
3 Teaching use of bulb syringe to empty clogged nasal passages, especially before feeding and sleep (babies are obligate nose breathers).
4 Advising sufficient fluids in the form of juice, water, and milk.
5 Instructing to keep infant inside until fever is down for 24 h.
6 Plan telephone follow-up with mother, because frequent colds may be a sign of more serious streptococcal infections in this age group.

Spitting up/vomiting

Spitting up involves a small amount of liquid (which may look like a large amount when splashed on mother's dress) and is never a sign of abnormality. The cause is mechanical; milk comes up with an air bubble or when the baby is bounced after feeding.

Vomiting is the bringing up of a large amount of food, which gushes forcefully out of the mouth and sometimes from the nose. It occurs occasionally in most babies and is of no concern unless it is frequent. Vomiting may be caused by sucking on soft nipples or on nipples with holes that are too large; by eating too much and/or too often; or by a formula that disagrees with the baby. It could also be an indication of a bowel obstruction or a symptom of a generalized illness. In these cases, the baby will probably look sick, refuse solid food, or have other major symptoms such as repeated vomiting with every feeding, fever, or diarrhea (Fig. 18-15). *Note:*

Any time the nurse is concerned about the baby or the baby is presenting more than one major symptom, the physician's advice should be sought.

assessment The following questions will help to differentiate spitting up from vomiting:

1 How much is spit up (would it fit in a teaspoon, cup, or bowl?) When does it occur, how often, what color, and is it forceful?
2 Does the baby look sick?
3 Is the baby dehydrated? Is the baby's mouth moist? Is the baby passing urine normally? Color? Are the baby's stools hard or is there diarrhea?
4 Is the baby gaining weight normally?
5 Is the baby eating normally? A baby who wants to eat is less likely to be seriously ill.

intervention Instructions for the mother when the baby spits up.

1 Burp the baby well and more frequently.
2 Keep the baby in an upright position after eating—use infant seat.
3 Do not bounce the baby after meals.
4 Give solids with liquids, as spitting up decreases when solids are added.
5 Reassure mother that condition clears up when infant is walking.

Instructions for the mother when the baby vomits.

1 Instruct her to give no fluids or solids for 6 h other than Coca-Cola syrup every 15 min x 6, then ginger ale or 7-Up in small quantities, frequently.
2 Give no solids or milk for 24 h.
3 Ask mother to call back in several hours to report status.
4 After 24 h of no vomiting, the older baby

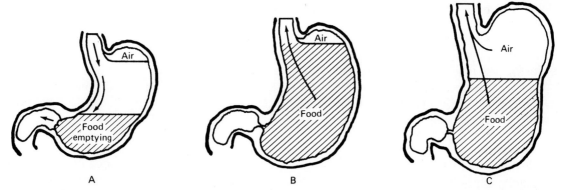

fig. 18-15 Regurgitation, vomiting, and stomach emptying. (a) Normal emptying of stomach, (b) overeating or overdistension, and (c) swallowing air while crying or nursing may cause regurgitation or vomiting. (*Courtesy of the Carnation Company.*)

can be started on a progressive diet of crackers, baked potato, toast, plain gelatin, soft boiled egg, skim milk, cottage cheese, cooked rice cereal, banana, apple sauce.

5 The younger infant must be seen by physician and then may be given an electrolyte formula such as Pedialyte, Vivonex, etc. for 24 h and then slowly restarted on breast-feeding or formula.

6 Refer to physician when there is:
   a Vomiting and fever or bulging fontanelle in an infant under 4 months;
   b Prolonged or persistent vomiting with dehydration;
   c Presence of blood or bile in the vomitus;
   d Vomiting with abdominal distention, localized tenderness or pain, or a palpable abdominal mass;
   e Vomiting with visible peristalsis or projectile vomiting;
   f Vomiting and a history or suspicion of ingestion of a drug or poison.

bowel movements

Each baby has his or her own pattern for bowel movements, and this pattern will vary with maturity and changes in diet. The stools of the newborn are described in Chap. 14. By the time an infant is 1 month old the bowel movements should be yellow and of pasty consistency. There may be a bowel movement with every feeding or only one every 2 to 5 days, as is characteristic of some breast-fed babies. Even when passing a normal stool, babies may pull their legs up, grunt, and get red in the face. This causes some mothers to think that their child is constipated.

As the baby grows and new foods are added to the diet, the bowel patterns, consistency, and color will change. Green vegetables may give looser, green stools, while beets may produce red stools. Whole milk can make bowel movements softer, firmer, more frequent, or less frequent. As the first year draws to a close, stools should be firmer, less frequent, and may have a routine pattern.

constipation

A constipated baby has hard, dry, infrequent stools. It often begins when a baby is switched from formula or breast milk to cow's milk. Great effort is required to pass the stool, producing anal irritation and fistulas. This results in the infant withholding the stool, which then aggravates the problem. Causes of constipation in the infant include: insufficient sugar in the formula, low fluid intake, starvation, prolonged vomiting spells, constriction, fissures, severe diaper rash, toilet training, and psychological problems. Constipation also can be a sign of Hirschsprung's disease or hypothyroidism.

assessment

1 Check the rectum for a fistula or constriction.
2 Determine the amount of fluid the baby is receiving.
3 Ask if fruits, vegetables, and whole-grain cereals are in the diet.
4 Determine if there has been a recent change to whole milk.
5 Ask about the routine pattern of elimination.
6 Discover if there have been any stressful changes at home.

intervention

1 Dilation of anal constriction can be done with lubricated fingertip.
2 Petroleum jelly or A&D ointment should be applied to fissure by the mother.
3 Work with the mother to increase liquids, fruits, vegetables, whole-grain cereals. Sometimes just the addition of prune juice (½ oz and increase gradually) will alleviate the problem.
4 For the younger infant, a temporary increase in sugar in the formula will help.
5 Work with mother and physician for correction of diaper rash. Teach mother diaper care if she appears unsure.

Between 6 and 12 months of age, the baby may be trying to hold the stool in, a developmental change that must be appreciated by parents. Caution the mother not to use a laxative, enema, or soap chips to stimulate a stool. The physician may want to order barley malt extract or a stool softener for a truly constipated infant.

diarrhea

Diarrhea is defined as more frequent bowel movements which become loose and watery. The causes can be viral or bacterial upper respiratory infection, streptococcal infection, too much sugar in the infant's formula, drugs (e.g., ampicillin, other antibiotics, and possibly oral iron compounds), allergy to milk or new foods, emotional stress, constipation with overflow, and finally, ulcerative colitis and regional enteritis. True diarrhea should be considered as a major cause of dehydration and/or acidosis. Within a few hours, the mother should report back on the results of the interventions.

assessment

1 Obtain description of onset, duration, frequency in the last 24 h, as well as amount, consistency, and color. Any solid material present?
2 Assess fever, vomiting, and solids or liquids taken in the last 24 h.
3 Estimate weight loss and moisture of mouth and skin as well as volume and concentration of urine.

intervention

1 Advise water, weak tea, flat 7-Up, or Gatorade.
2 24 h later—apple sauce, crackers, baked potato, banana, plain gelatin.
3 Third day—skim milk, cottage cheese, then to normal diet.

4 Yogurt or Lactinex granules may restore altered bowel flora when infant is on antibiotics.
5 Refer the infant to physician for any of the following conditions:
 a Bloody diarrhea;
 b Persistent, chronic, or prolonged diarrhea—more than 48 h with no improvement;
 c Diarrhea in an infant less than 4 months old;
 d Diarrhea with dehydration;
 e Diarrhea accompanied by high fever and vomiting.

rashes

Tender baby skin is very susceptible to irritation. Mild rashes are quite common, but sometimes rashes are a sign of illness. The resistance of the skin is lowered with fevers and systemic disease. Other symptoms to be noted are temperature elevation, feeding response, stools, and state of irritability. Any fluid-filled vesicles or pustules are serious and may indicate a staphylococcal infection, herpes simplex, or impetigo neonatorum.

cradle cap Cradle cap is a form of seborrheic dermatitis which results in yellowish oily scales on the scalp. There may be a rash on the forehead, cheeks, and shoulders. It can usually be prevented by scrubbing the scalp, including the soft spot, with soap and water at bath time. It is much easier to prevent than to cure. If it is present, suggest mineral oil rubbed into the scalp at bedtime followed by a shampoo with a medicated shampoo such as Selsen Blue the next morning. A fine-toothed comb can be used to loosen crusts. Most mothers wash the scalp superficially, being afraid of hurting the soft spot. The nurse can demonstrate on the back of the mother's hand to show what is meant by *firm* scrubbing.

If the condition persists, medication can be prescribed.

diaper rash (diaper dermatitis) With diaper rash, the skin becomes reddened and then breaks down because of chemical irritation by the urine and feces. Often occurring in infancy even though diapers are changed at reasonable intervals, diaper dermatitis can be treated best by gentle washing with soap and water and then exposure to the air. Before reapplication of diapers, a thick coat of zinc oxide or Desitin Ointment can be applied. The best prevention is to use plain water for cleansing after each stool or voiding and then to coat the perineal area liberally with plain petroleum jelly. Disposable, flushable diaper liners will help the diaper-washing problem so that strong detergents may be eliminated.

The mother needs to check the infant's responses to the type of detergent, bleach, or water softener being used. Double rinsing or using sodium borate in the wash or 2 cups of vinegar in the final rinse will help overcome irritating ammonia. Some babies with sensitive skin may not be able to tolerate plastic waterproof pants or disposable diapers. A change in diet may add a new element in the stool or urine that irritates the skin. If, after all these factors have been checked, the problem still exists, or if any ulceration occurs, call the physician.

heat rash (miliaria rubra) Some infants develop rashes when they are too warm. Face, neck, trunk, and diaper area are the first to break out with reddened pustules. Cooling the infant with a tepid bath or changing to lighter clothing will improve the rash. In winter, turning down the thermostat might eliminate the problem. Corn starch can be used sparingly in the creases around the neck and underarms. Commercial powders often have ingredients which augment the problem.

Monilia If the mother was infected with *Candida albicans* during delivery or subsequently develops such an infection, the infant may also become infected. The diaper rash will have well-defined areas with scalloped edges, a grayish hue, and an oozing wet look. Although *Monilia* usually manifests itself in the diaper area, it can also invade the mouth, where lesions appear in the form of white patches on reddened tongue and cheeks. The baby will characteristically begin to suck and then cry. It is easy to differentiate between milk curds and the lesions found in thrush because the former will come off easily when scraped by a tongue blade. Medication such as suspension of Nystatin is essential in the treatment and must be ordered by a physician.

sleep and sleep problems

The new baby sleeps between 20 and 22 h out of every 24, but a few babies seem to need much less sleep. It is important that the infant has her or his own place to sleep, preferably in a separate area. A new infant appears to feel more secure in a smaller enclosure such as a bassinette.

The pattern of sleep varies from month to month (see chap 15). Infants typically go through several cycles of semiwakefulness, with a period of deep sleep in the middle of each cycle. It takes sensitivity to know when to intervene or when the baby should go through this process undisturbed. The periods of semialert states are accompanied by noise and trials of new skills. For instance, the baby who has learned to turn from stomach to back may do so and not be able to get over again to a sleeping position. The baby who has learned to stand may cry because she or he cannot sit again, but most of the time the baby is able to get back into a conditioned position for sleep without intervention.

Problems about sleep upset parents who do not understand the developmental changes affecting the baby's pattern. At about 6 months of age, many infants begin to fuss about going to bed. This fussing results from the realization that mother leaves and yet is still available. It is an important milestone but hard to appreciate. Firmness and consistency are the keys to returning to normalcy as quickly as possible, for temporary sleep problems can easily become chronic ones to the detriment of the whole family. If the mother offers food or toys, her participation becomes part of the baby's sleep pattern, and the infant will incorporate these actions each night. Thus, patterns such as taking an infant into bed with the parents can become firmly ingrained.

The parents should be encouraged to spend a little extra time with the baby at bedtime. A firm "goodnight" indicates to the baby that they mean business. A workable plan is to stay out of the room for 20 min by the clock and then go back and tell the child he or she is loved but that it is bedtime. Then stay out for 30 min and repeat the process. The same plan can be instituted in the middle of the night, although very wakeful babies may appreciate a night light so they can see and play.

Teething may also present a problem, and a mild baby analgesic may help the child go to sleep. Illness can also set up patterns which need to be altered after the baby is well again. The author has found that most first mothers bend under the pressure of a crying infant. Neither the parent nor the baby gets enough sleep, which leads to chronic fatigue and irritability. Second babies tend to sleep better because mothers report that they are more easily able to tolerate the discomfort of a crying baby at bedtime.

teething

Eruption of teeth usually begins at 6 to 8 months of age for the lower central incisors, and at 7 to 10 months for the upper central incisors. Teething never causes high fevers, diarrhea, or ear infections, though it may predispose an infant to an infection. Parents will sometimes attribute an infection to teething and will not consider the baby to be sick. If a baby is having difficulty, a teething ring, dry toast, and plenty of fluid may help.

Suggest putting a metal spoon in the refrigerator to get cold or freezing a small amount of water in a teething ring, for chewing helps to numb the gums. Sometimes the physician will order paregoric for the gums, or "baby aspirin" at bedtime, so that both mother and baby can get some sleep.

Some babies take months to get a tooth through, and there seems to be a great deal of pain associated with it. It has been said that an adult would have a hard time tolerating this degree of pain.

Once the teeth are through the gums, there is no pain. It is suggested by dentists that the parent brush the new teeth with a soft terry cloth daily.

A delay in dentition may be part of the family history and therefore normal for the infant. Delayed dentition may also be associated with hypothyroidism, rickets, and some types of mental retardation.

thumbsucking

There is a picture of a 17-week-old fetus in utero sucking its thumb. Since most infants need to suck something, parents may need help to be more relaxed about thumbsucking. Sucking of thumbs and fingers is very common among babies who are contented at feedings and is not a reflection of inadequate parenting. The sucking seems to become a symbol of the pleasant situation, and an infant soon learns to reproduce this gratifying aspect of feeding. Some infants do not find their thumbs in the early months and will become quiet when offered a pacifier. Encourage the parent

to help the baby switch to thumbsucking at about 3 months of age. Pacifiers get lost at night, thumbs do not.

T. Berry Brazelton has studied babies in his own practice, using mothers as observers, and has discovered that sucking peaks between 3 and 7 months of age.[16] As infants begin to use their hands to manipulate objects, extra sucking only takes place as they investigate their hands, as an aid to sore gums, or for comfort when tired or frustrated. Children can suck their thumbs without harm until their permanent teeth come in, about age 5 or 6. Prolonged bottle sucking may set up a pattern of tongue thrusting and so has a similar effect. Once the child starts kindergarten, peer pressure to stop thumbsucking is strong.

spoiling, limit setting, routines

Our adult lives are built around certain routines that help to give us structure and stability. Infants, too, need the structure and security of routine. After the first few weeks, either the infant or the parents are on some sort of schedule. Usually, there is a compromise in the adjustment period.

A few babies change their patterns with each developmental milestone and are so adamant that it is easier for both parents and infant if the parent does most of the compromising. Usually, eating, sleeping, bath time, and play will fall into a pattern. Eating and sleeping on schedule are especially important for a happy baby—and happy babies are nice to have around.

The problem of spoiling comes up very often. Some parents feel that holding babies will spoil them, and so they do not give enough love and affection. The baby who is held often is not necessarily spoiled. Babies need lots of "lapping." The spoiled infant is the infant who demands and gets attention when the parent is busy and does not want to hold the baby at that time. As the pattern repeats itself, the baby is learning how to manipulate the parent.

By 9 months of age, a child can understand what "no" means but does not have the ability to develop the necessary internal controls to prevent the next episode. Parents can reduce the use of the word *no* by doing two things: (1) Remove from the child's environment whatever they do not want the child to handle. (2) When the child is heading for a forbidden object or a source of danger, the parent can go and turn the child around while saying "turn around." If the parent then distracts the child with something that is fun, the young explorer will perceive the words as a positive command and will begin to respond to the words alone. At some point, it could save the baby's life.

intervention

1 Parents should decide together what is off limits.
2 They should agree on reasonable and appropriate discipline.
3 Consistency is the most important common denominator. When parents are not in agreement, or when punishment is inconsistent or too harsh, children become confused and do not know what is expected of them.
4 Even children under 1 year of age will test the limits to see if the parents are serious about them.
5 It is a sign of love to the child that the parent is willing to provide external controls. The infant does not have them innately but can begin the learning process before the end of the first year of life.

SUMMARY

What is gained in well child care is greater than the sum of its parts. Much of what has been said has more than an element of common sense. Well child care has a great deal to do with prevention of problems and helping parents to cope better with the changes in their baby. The stress has been on interaction with the mother, because she is the one who usually brings the baby in for well baby visits; however, the whole family is involved in the healthy development of an infant. As more and more neighborhood clinics and health centers open across the country, the nurse will play an increasingly important part. The nurse can add a dimension of concern and creativity in helping families adjust to the arrival of a new member (Table 18-4).

study questions

1. What are the four basic nursing judgments a nurse should be able to make about an infant who appears to be ill? What are the nurse's main tools?
2. In every well baby visit, what activities should take place?
3. Be able to explain the immunization schedule to an inquiring mother.
4. Using growth and development as a basis, instruct the mother on:
   a. Stimulation needs of the infant,
   b. Measures to maintain safety,
   c. Sleep patterns.
5. Take a common problem of the first year of life and plan a teaching outline for the mother. Describe for yourself the steps in nursing assessment/interventions.
   a. Spitting up vs. vomiting
   b. Constipation vs. diarrhea
   c. Colic vs. normal crying needs
   d. Teething
   e. Upper respiratory infection and fever
6. Review at least three paperback books about parenting. Look at those found on racks in drug or grocery stores. How does the advice in these books sound to you? Which would you recommend to a new parent?

references

1. P. Chinn, *Child Health Maintenance*, Mosby, St. Louis, 1974, pp. 24, 25.
2. M. Green and R. Haggerty, "Ambulatory Pediatrics,"

table 18-4 Summary of teaching points at well baby visits

1 to 6 months	every visit
Discuss:	Sleep
Sleep patterns	Feeding, appetite
Breast-feeding, bottle-feeding	Elimination
How to start solids, new foods	Activity
Stimulation	Illness exposure
Safety	Allergies
Problems:	Immunizations
Teething	PDQ
Thumbsucking	
Spoiling	
Sibling rivalry	
Mother's adjustment and level of fatigue	

6 to 12 months	every visit
Discuss:	Sleep
Sleep patterns	Appetite
Feeding habits	Elimination
Weaning	Activity
Stimulation	Illness exposure
Safety	Allergies
New developments:	Immunizations
Different safety levels	PDQ
Limit setting	
Temper tantrums	
Pica	
Toilet training	
Tooth care	

in J. Alpert (ed.), *Infancy and Early Childhood*, Saunders, Philadelphia, 1977, Chap. 2, p. 393.
3. M. Brown and M. Murphy, *Ambulatory Pediatrics for Nurses*, McGraw-Hill, New York, 1975, pp. 1, 2.
4. H. K. Silver, "Growth and Development," in C. H. Kempe, H. K. Silver, and D. O'Brien (eds.), *Current Pediatric Diagnosis and Treatment, Los Altos Lange*, Los Altos, Calif., 1972, Chap. 2, p. 8.
5. T. B. Brazelton, *Infants and Mothers*, Dell, New York, 1974, p. xviii.
6. J. Brown, "Infant Temperament: A Clue to Childbearing for Parents and Nurses," *American Journal of Maternal and Child Nursing*, **2**(4):229, July/August 1977.
7. Silver, op. cit., p. 8.
8. *Instructions for Prescreening Test*, Ladoca Project and Publishing Foundation, Denver.
9. W. K. Frankenburg, "Denver Developmental Screening Test," *Journal of Pediatrics*, **71**:181, 1976.
10. Paula Roberts, Personal communication, Nov. 30, 1973.
11. T. B. Brazelton, *Doctor and Child*, Dell, New York, 1976, p. 222.
12. M. Alexander, "Homemade Fun for Infants," *American Journal of Nursing*, **70**:2557, December 1970.
13. S. Krugman, "Present Status of Measles and Rubella Immunization in the United States: A Medical Progress Report," *Journal of Pediatrics*, **90**:1, 1977.
14. Brazelton, *Infants and Mothers*, op. cit., p. 74.
15. Brazelton, *Doctor and Child*, op. cit., p. 175.
16. Brazelton, *Infants and Mothers*, op. cit., p. 113.

bibliography

Alexander, M., and M. Brown: *Pediatric Physical Diagnosis for Nurses*, McGraw-Hill, New York, 1974.

Battle, C. H.: "Sleep and Sleep Disturbances in Young Children," *Clinical Pediatrics*, **9**:675, November 1970. (Normal sleep patterns, sleep difficulties in infants and toddlers, and their management.)

Brown, M., and M. Murphy: *Ambulatory Pediatrics for Nurses,* New York, McGraw-Hill, 1975.

Carey, W. B.: "Simplified Method for Measuring Infant Temperament," *Journal of Pediatrics,* **77**:188, August 1970. (Infants 4 to 8 months of age.)

DeAngelis, C.: *Basic Pediatrics for the Primary Health Care Provider,* Boston, Little, Brown, 1975.

Goda, S.: "Speech Development in Children," *American Journal of Nursing,* **70**:276, February 1970. (Normal patterns, deviations.)

Hynovich, D. P.: *Nursing of Children: A Family Centered Guide for Study,* 2d ed., Philadelphia, Saunders, 1974.

Klaus, M., and J. Kennell: *Maternal-Infant Bonding,* Mosby, St. Louis, 1976.

————, T. Legar, and M. Trause: *Maternal Attachment and Mothering Disorders, a Round Table,* Johnson and Johnson, New Brunswick, N.J., 1975.

Morris, A. G.: "The Use of Well-Baby Clinic to Promote Early Intellectual Development via Parent Education," *American Journal of Public Health,* **66**:73–74, January 1976.

Murphy, M.: "The Crying Infant," *Pediatric Nursing,* January/February 1975, pp. 15–17.

Powell, K.: "Basic Principles of Immunization," *Pediatric Nursing,* **3**(5):7, September/October 1977.

Nelson, A. C.: "How Can You Stand the Crying?" *American Journal of Nursing,* **70**:66, January 1970. (Knowing the significance of cries; concern about baby who does not cry; eighth-month anxiety.)

pediatric nurse practitioners

Brown, M. S.: "Pediatric Nurse Practitioner. A Primary Manager of Well-Child Care," *Nursing '76,* **6**:70–72, July 1976. (Excellent article on function of PNP in a typical day, including where training programs are located.)

Hellings, P., M. Davidson, and C. Burns: "Education of the PNP: Present and Future," *Pediatric Nursing,* **2**(6):6, November/December 1976.

Pediatric Nurse Practitioners—Their Practice Today, American Nursing Association, Publication, 1975, pp. 1–56.

Storms, P.: "Just What Do You Do as a Pediatric Nurse Practitioner?" *Pediatric Nursing,* **2**(3):42 May/June 1976.

books to recommend to parents

Brazelton, T. Berry: *Infants and Mothers,* Dell, New York, 1974.

————: *Doctor and Child,* Dell, New York, 1976.

Fraiberg, Selma: *The Magic Years,* Scribner, New York, 1959.

"The Growing Child" (1 mo–6 yr), Information Monthly Service for the Young Family, Dunn and Hargate, 124 West 8th St., West Lafayette, Ind., 47902. (Monthly information on growth and development. Matches age of child, as birthdate is sent with order.)

19

HOME CARE OF MOTHER AND INFANT

JOYCE HANNA-NAVE

THE ROLE OF THE NURSE IN THE COMMUNITY

Returning home from the hospital is an event that is anticipated with both pleasure and some anxiety by most parents. The nurse working in a hospital unit tries to prepare the family for discharge by making a thorough appraisal of the physical health of mother and infant and by providing the parents with emotional support, anticipatory guidance, and opportunities to participate in the care of their infant. However, busy hospital units and shorter hospital stays—not to mention the alternatives to hospital deliveries which are becoming increasingly more common (e.g., home, office, or clinic deliveries)—may make it difficult for the hospital nurse to satisfactorily achieve these objectives.

To assure continuity of nursing care throughout the first month, many innovative approaches are being tried. The family may be encouraged to call the maternity unit if they run into problems, or the nurse who cared for the mother in the hospital may call the family during the first week at home. Sometimes the pediatric nurse visits the mother and baby in the hospital and leaves a telephone number where the nurse might be reached.[1-3]

This chapter explores the role of the nurse who visits the family in their home. It discusses how a referral is made and how the nursing process is used in planning nursing care for the family. The description of a home visit with a community nurse affords the reader an opportunity to observe a nurse integrate the basic nursing care principles learned so far. It is hoped that the reader will gain a better appreciation of what the first few weeks at home are like for the family. Finally, some of the more common questions concerning the utilization of community health nurses in maternity care are raised during an interview with a public health nurse.

making the referral

Nurses working in any setting should be familiar with the resources available in their community. In some communities, all babies are visited by a nurse from the local community health agency; in other communities, only mother and babies with problems or potential problems are seen. Many agencies publish guidelines to aid the hospital in making referral decisions. As a general rule, it is best to err on the side of overreferral than underreferral.

The nurse or physician makes the contact with the agency, giving a brief summary of the obstetric history and reason for referral. A sample referral form is shown in Fig. 19-1. The hospital nurse also explains to the parents that a nurse will be visiting to examine the mother and baby and to answer any of the parents' questions. Since parents may occa-

sionally interpret the visit as criticism of their ability to care for the baby, the explanation should be as matter-of-fact as possible. The home visit may be presented to the family as a "service."

the role of the nurse

Nurses who make home visits have a very important role. The mother and baby have been discharged (assuming a hospital delivery) from the protective and artificial hospital environment. If all goes well, they will not be seen by a health care professional for another 2 to 6 weeks. Their need for physical assessment, emotional support, and teaching does not end with their discharge from the hospital. Indeed, the entire first month is an extremely important time in the health of the mother and baby and in the adjustment of the family to a new member. Mothers are most receptive to professional help during the first week at home, after they have explored their resources and become aware of their concerns, but before they have found their own solutions. The nurse who visits in the home may be the only health care professional present during this crucial time.

using the nursing process

The nurse's role varies according to the needs of the family. How does the nurse decide what ought to be done in each home? Using the nursing process may help. The nursing process involves four major steps: (1) assessment, (2) planning, (3) implementation, and (4) evaluation of a *nursing care plan*. Let us discuss each of these steps before we observe the nurse using them during a visit.

assessment The nurse not only obtains information from the referral source but also learns to develop awareness and listening

HIGH RISK INFANT REPORT

Please send on infants born 5½ lbs. or less, 37 weeks
gestational age, congenital abnormality or other problem rendering infant high risk, **within 48 hours of birth.**

Send Report to:

Please have guardian sign before sending.

   **I give permission to release this information to the
   Division of Public Health Nursing. I understand
   that a Public Health Nurse may contact me.**

Signature _____ Date _____

Witness _____

Father's and/or Mother's Name_____
                                           Last Name   First Names - Mother   Father

Resident Address_____ Tel._____
                                Street   Town

Mailing Address, if different_____

Born: In Hospital (name) _____   ☐ Home

Date of Birth _____ Birthweight _____lbs. _____oz.   ☐ Not Weighed

Multiple Birth _____ Sex: Male _____ Female _____ Status: Good _____ Fair _____ Poor _____

Apgar score at 5 min. _____ Gestation_____

Congenital abnormality - diagnosis _____

Transferred to: _____ Infant death, Date:_____

Infant's Physician_____

Date_____ Signature_____ Tel. _____

                         Title _____

                                                                              HPHN-47   Rev. 777

fig. 19-1   Referral form. (*Courtesy Maine State Department of Human Services.*)

skills, to ask appropriate questions, and to make pertinent observations. All the nurse's skills will be needed to gain information about the community and its resources, the home, the physical status of mother and infant, and parental readiness.

ASSESSING THE COMMUNITY AND ITS RESOURCES
Each community, rich or poor, rural or urban, has its own unique characteristics. Some communities have a myriad of social agencies, while others have very limited facilities. In some communities, unofficial sources of help, such as close family or neighborhood ties, may be available; in other communities, one family may be socially isolated from the neighboring family. Lack of transportation may be a problem in a rural community; a deteriorating neighborhood may be a problem in

an urban community. It is the responsibility of each nurse to learn about the community and the resources available in that community. Most hospital social service departments maintain an up-to-date file of community resources and would be pleased to share their knowledge of the community. Other initial sources of information are nonprofit home health agencies and health or welfare departments.

ASSESSING THE HOME   The home environment has far-reaching effects on a baby's physical health and emotional and social development. It is often the area in which nurses feel they have the least amount of control. Yet if nurses are observant of problems in the home environment and are aware of community resources for help, it may be the area where

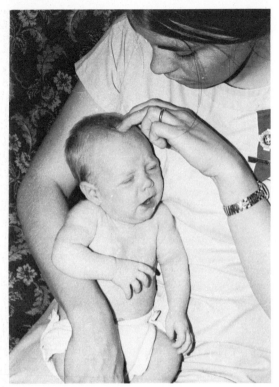

fig. 19-2 Checking anterior fontanel. (*Photo by Bill Nave.*)

they will see the greatest change. When evaluating the home, it is important that nurses not prejudge the family on the basis of their own standards and that they look for the effect the environment actually has on the baby and the family.

Temperature   The temperature of the environment may adversely affect a newborn. The environment is too cold if the newborn's skin is mottled, cool, or dusky, or if the baby is cyanotic around the mouth or extremities. The parents, especially if they are unfamiliar with the requirements of a cold climate, may need to be taught how to dress a baby warmly enough. However, even a warmly bundled baby seems to suffer cold stress in the chronically cold environment found in much substandard housing.

More frequently, you will find babies who are overdressed, especially during warm weather or in a room that is too hot or too dry. Sometimes babies are exposed to too much sun or are too close to hot stoves or radiators. Also, the environment may not be adequately humidified. Wood heat is especially drying. A pan of water on the radiator or wood stove will help humidify the air.

Infestation   Infestation of rats, mice, flies, and roaches occurs frequently in substandard and occasionally in good housing. Their source (garbage, holes in the walls, etc.) must be located and eradicated if possible; for this, the services of the board of health may be available. The family should be taught good sanitation practices, particularly proper food storage. Rats, which have been known to bite infants, and flies, which may carry disease, are more of a health hazard than mice or roaches.

Communicable disease, crowding   Since the newborn's resistance to communicable disease is low, the presence of an ill family member or the crowding of many people into small living quarters may be a health hazard. Parents should be advised to limit the number of people who care for the infant and to avoid taking the infant into crowded areas (stores, theaters, parties, etc.) until the child is over 6 weeks old and has developed more resistence to disease.

Safety   The neonatal period is an excellent time to begin discussions of safety, as the parents usually have many fears and concerns about their baby at this time. By observing the home environment for safety hazards and by listening for parental understanding of safe infant care practices, the nurse can decide which of the following safety principles need emphasis:

An infant should never be left alone—not even for a second—on a high surface. Arrangements for day care and baby-sitting should be adequate. Those caring for the baby should be mature and responsible. The baby should never be left alone in the house, in a car, or in a carriage.

If the family uses a car, the baby should always be appropriately secured in an approved infant car seat.

Every family should have a fire safety plan, and adequate fire exits should be available.

Nothing (jewelry, pacifiers on cords, etc.) should be worn around the infant's neck or wrist or ankles.

The crib slats should be less than 2⅜ in apart to prevent the baby from being strangled when older by locking his or her head between the crib slats. As the baby grows older, the crib sides should be high enough to prevent the child from falling out of the crib.

Baby rattles should not be small enough to choke the baby and should be constructed so that they cannot come apart.

The nurse offers guidance in anticipation of the baby's growing needs and is aware of the safety needs of siblings also (see Table 18-3)

Equipment Families are able to manage in the most difficult environments with the sparsest of equipment. Very little is *essential* for a newborn, and families with limited incomes should be discouraged from buying unnecessary infant supplies. Some equipment, however, is necessary. Refrigeration (or some means of keeping food cold), a tall covered pot, bottles and nipples, a bottle brush, and measuring spoons are essential for formula preparation. If the formula is prepared one feeding at a time or if one of the commercially prepared formulas is used, the family may get by with less equipment. If bottles need to be purchased, urge the family to buy the more easily sterilized glass bottles in the 8-oz size.

Diapers, shirts, and something in which to bundle the baby (blankets, sweater) are also essential. Infant clothes may be bought a size larger than that needed so they can be worn longer. The cost of disposable versus washable diapers may be computed with the family who wishes to choose the least expensive method (the family with a washing machine may choose cloth diapers as a less expensive alternative, but electricity costs should be recognized).

A newborn may sleep in a drawer or cardboard box temporarily. If income is limited, a full-size crib is a better buy than a cradle, as it will be utilized for a longer period of time by the child.

The nurse also evaluates the environment for the availability of adequate stimulation. These need not be expensive—a loving grandmother who sings to and rocks a baby is certainly as effective as an expensive baby swing, and a simple mobile may be made with bright-colored paper and string. Different babies have different requirements for stimulation, but the proper amount of stimulation is important to the infant's intellectual development.

Other family members Although nurses ostensibly visit the mother and infant, they are

fig. 19-3 Head measurement by nurse at home. (*Photo by Beverly Hemlock.*)

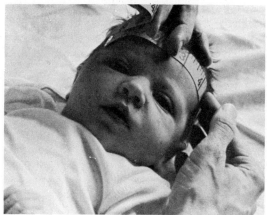

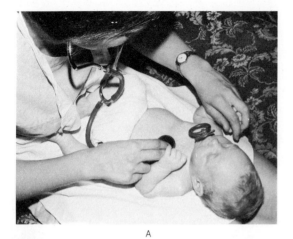

A

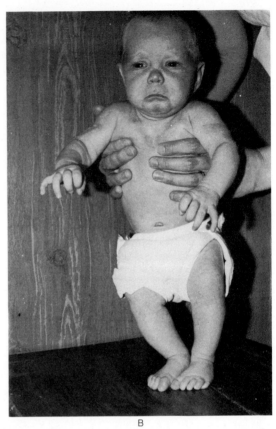

B

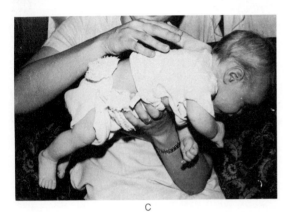

C

present in the home and often have an opportunity to observe the family as a unit. They evaluate the health needs of other family members. They observe the interaction among family members and the support or the problems they provide for the mother. They may then identify areas in which appropriate intervention is possible.

ASSESSING THE PHYSICAL STATUS OF THE NEWBORN The nurse's role in infant appraisal is extremely important. Although the infant has been screened for potential problems before hospital discharge, the entire first month of life remains hazardous. Changes occur rapidly in the newborn, and not all problems are detected before discharge. An illness which may be minor in an older child (such as diarrhea) may be life-threatening to a newborn. Serious disorders affecting an individual's entire future (such as congenital dysplasia of the hip) may often be corrected if detected during this period. Problems (such as dehydration) may appear after the infant has been home for a few days. Newborn appraisal is described in detail in Chapter 14. As you read the description of the home visit, notice how the nurse includes this important function during the visit. (See Table 19-2.)

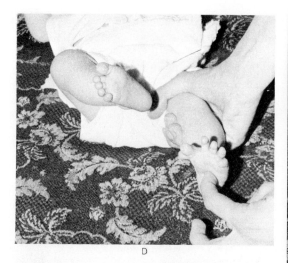

D

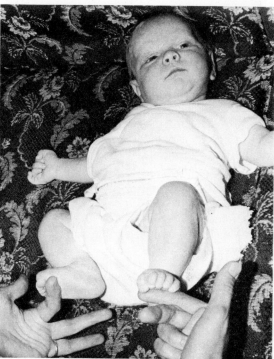

fig. 19-4 (a) Checking apical heart rate. (b) Eliciting stepping reflex. (c) Eliciting Landau response to check muscle tone. (d) Eliciting Babinski sign. (e) Plantar grasp. (f) Palmar grasp. (*All photos by Bill Nave.*)

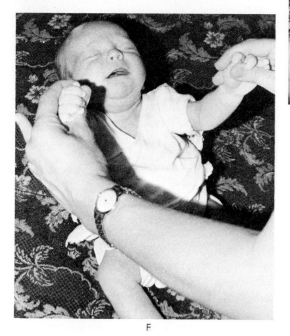

F

ASSESSING THE PHYSICAL STATUS OF THE MOTHER   Appraisal of the mother is also very important, for complications do arise at home. This evaluation is described in detail in Table 19-1 and in the nursing visit.

ASSESSING PARENTAL READINESS   Many people assume that parenting is instinctive and that new parents not only should know how to care for their baby but should also have appropriate maternal or paternal feelings about their baby. Actually, readiness for parenting differs in each individual. In the home visit to be described, notice how the nurse assesses the parent–child bond and the mother's previous experience with infants and how the nurse actively listens to the mother to gain a better appreciation of her readiness for parenting. From this assessment, the nurse identifies the needs which exist for learning and support.

developing a plan of care The second step of the nursing process is the development of a plan to meet the needs identified in the appraisal. Although the nurse asks similar questions and makes similar observations in each home, the nurse's services will not be utilized in the same way in every situation. In one home the need may be to help the parents gain a sense of balance after the disrupting event of having a baby. In another home, the presence of rats or lack of refrigeration may be the focus of concern, or perhaps the nurse may find that a baby with diarrhea is severely dehydrated and requires immediate medical attention. Thus the nurse's role varies according to the needs of the family.

It may be that problems perceived by the nurse are not seen as problems by the family and vice versa. In developing a plan of care, the nurse must feel free to respond to the agenda the mother brings to the visit—once her needs are met, she will more readily accept the nurse's suggestions.

Assessment and identification of problems usually take up the first visit. Before leaving the home, the nurse plans future visits with the mother to provide her with a certain amount of support and security—she can save up her questions for the nurse and will not feel alone in caring for her infant. The number and spacing of visits vary according to the situation. Usually, frequent, short visits during the first crucial days at home are most meaningful to the family. Later, the nurse records the observations made and develops the plan of care, based on the nursing care needed and the goals agreed upon.

implementation The third step in the nursing process is implementing the plan of care. In addition to the services given directly to the family, the nurse plays a strategic role in maintaining communication with the referring hospital and community agencies.

evaluation After each visit, the nurse should evaluate the care plan in light of any updated knowledge of the situation. Do these plans meet the needs of the family and the nursing goals? Are they practical and realistic? Is there a better approach to the problem?

ANECDOTAL RECORD OF A HOME VISIT

Mrs. Linda Murray and newborn daughter live in an older neighborhood in an apartment two stories above a busy coffee shop. Mrs. Murray's husband is a cab driver, and this was her first pregnancy. Apparently her pregnancy was normal, but her membranes ruptured 2 days past her EDD and she required intravenous administration of pitocin to induce labor. Labor lasted only 5 hours; delivery was normal, except that a small cervical laceration was sustained and an episiotomy was necessary. No anesthesia was used. After delivery, Mrs. Murray had had difficulty voiding and required a Foley catheter for 12 h. Her hemoglobin level was 11 g, and her hematocrit reading was 30%. She was given oral iron and a stool softener to take home. The baby, born 5 days earlier, was a normal, full-term, 6-lb, 10-oz girl. She is on a commercially prepared formula.

The nurse, Sue Holmes, made a mental list of the actions she should take based on this report—checking the lochia, episiotomy, pulse, blood pressure, energy level, voiding and elimination, and discussion of the proper use of medication. At an early visit, signs of mother–infant bonding should be noted and feeding and basic health care reviewed.

establishing trust

A young woman in a bathrobe poked her head out of the door—"Who is it?"

"I'm Sue Holmes, the nurse. I called you."

"I am glad to see you! Come in."

Sue put her public health bag down and took off her coat. "Well—so how is everything going for you?"

"Oh—so-so, I guess."

Mrs. Murray's reply alerted the nurse, for she knew that bringing home a new baby—particularly a first baby—creates tremendous upheaval for a family.

"Only so-so?"

Sue could see something was upsetting Mrs. Murray, but perhaps the new mother needed to establish trust in the nurse as someone who was knowledgeable and who would understand and accept her before she felt comfortable confiding the real problems.

Sue changed the subject by giving a brief description of the public health agency and the reason for the visit. She then directed her attention to the mother's physical status. With all the attention a newborn receives, Sue wanted her to know that her own health was considered important also. By asking about her pregnancy, labor, delivery, and postpartum experiences, Sue will not only gain a basis to guide her examination but also receive an impression of Mrs. Murray's perception of her experience.

self-esteem is important

"I was excited when I found out I was pregnant. So was my husband. I felt good—in fact, I worked up until the baby was born. They had to give me medicine to get the contractions started because my water broke and nothing happened. It hurt—I didn't think it would hurt that much. We took a course the hopsital gave so my husband could stay with me in the

delivery room, and I thought if I did the breathing right, I wouldn't feel anything, but I did. I guess I flunked the course."

Mrs. Murray's perception of her performance in labor and her subsequent lowered self-esteem are of concern because they affect not only her memories but also her confidence in herself for the tasks ahead.

"You know, the course prepared you for a normal labor with normal contractions, but contractions that are induced are much different and much harder to keep on top of. You didn't flunk at all—you just weren't prepared for an induced labor."

"Well, we did miss a couple of weeks—maybe that's when they talked about it." Mrs. Murray's face appeared relieved as she went on to discuss her delivery experience.

rest is important

"Anyway, I was exhausted after my baby was born, and because I had trouble urinating, I was awake all night. I didn't sleep very well in the hospital at all."

"Did you feel tired when you came home from the hospital?"

"I was exhausted. And I haven't slept too well since I've been home, either."

"You don't feel rested now?"

"I don't ever remember being so tired. I try to sleep, and after an hour or more I might fall asleep, but then the baby wakes me up."

"How many hours of actual sleep are you getting?"

Enough questions must be asked to obtain an accurate picture of the problem. Energy is required for physical recuperation, for adjustment to all the changes a newborn brings, for the initiation of new relationships, and for a general sense of well-being. Thus, probably the most important need of a new mother is for rest. The next step was to encourage a *gradual* return to normal activity.

"What kinds of activities do you feel you *must* do?"

"Well—feeding and changing the baby, of course. And laundry. And cooking, and dishes, and cleaning. . . ."

Sue looked about the apartment. It was sparsely furnished but spotlessly clean.

"Who do you have to help you?"

"Well," Mrs. Murray replied thoughtfully, "no one, really. My husband fed the baby last night, but he really doesn't help out much."

"Do you have relatives or friends that could help out?"

"No, my friends are all working, and my parents live 800 miles from here. My husband's mother lives in the city, but I wouldn't want to ask her. She doesn't think I can do anything right, anyway. She's dropped by twice to see the baby, but she wears me out. And we don't have any other relatives or friends that I'd feel right about asking. I can't afford to hire anyone."

"Well," Sue replied, "you know, most mothers find they tire quickly once they get home from the hospital and are able to care only for themselves and the baby. Do you think for a few days you could let things slide a bit so that you can get rested up, or would that only make things worse?"

"Is that like—like a doctor's order?"

"Yes," Sue laughed. "That's a nurse's order! For the next 2 days, you concentrate on getting rested and try to let everything else go."

"OK—I'll tell my husband you said that, and maybe he'll help."

physical assessment of the mother

"Now," said Sue, "I'd like to give you a brief checkup to make sure everything is progressing as it should" (see Table 19-1). She took Mrs. Murray's blood pressure (100/60) and pulse (98, regular and strong) and asked about the lochia. The mother reported changing pads every 4 h or so. "It seems a little heavier flow than yesterday, but the color was reddish-brown." Because of the increase in flow, the low blood pressure, and slightly elevated pulse, Sue checked the fundus and found it firm and U/4.

"Your flow is a little heavier than it should be, and you are slightly anemic, but everything else checks out fine. The flow usually increases when the mother takes on too much activity too soon, so I think your body is trying to tell you to rest a lot more. Your blood was checked in the hospital, and your hemoglobin and hematocrit were a little low, so that is another reason why you are feeling so tired. You were given some iron pills to take?"

"Yes, I'm taking them once a day. I'm also taking one of those stool softeners every day because of the effect the iron has."

"Does the stool softener work?"

"No problem. Since I've been home, they've been soft. I'm trying to drink fluids and eat foods with a lot of roughage so I won't need that softener."

"You had stitches—are they uncomfortable at all?"

"No problem."

"Are your breasts soft, comfortable, no cracking near the nipple?" Mrs. Murray nodded yes to each question. Mrs. Murray seemed knowledgeable and concerned about her health, so Sue didn't feel she needed to examine the lochia or breasts, as she often did. Sue asked about headaches, nausea, pain, burning on urination, pain in the lower extremities. Again, Mrs. Murray reported no problem.

"Well, except for the fact that you need more rest, it all looks pretty good. What questions do *you* have about your health?"

altered physical image

"Well—I suppose this sounds silly—but my husband is worried, too. My aunt gained 10

table 19-1 Postpartum evaluation of the mother's physical status

examination	observation	report or check
Lochia	Note the amount, color, or presence of a strong odor.	If there is any deviation from normal, check the *fundus*. Lochia may increase if the mother assumes too much activity too soon. If the flow is heavy, emphasize the importance of *rest* and check the *pulse* and *blood pressure*.
Episiotomy	If the mother has had an episiotomy, ask if the "stitches" are uncomfortable. If so, examine the perineum.	Look for and report any signs of infection.
Vital signs Pulse and blood pressure	Note the rate and quality. Note relationship to baseline pressure.	If rapid or weak, check the amount of lochia, the hematocrit value, adequacy of rest, presence of infection.
Temperature	This may be eliminated if there are no other signs of infection and if the mother has not been exposed to infection.	Look for other signs of infection—headaches, pain, nausea, burning on urination, pain in the lower extremities.
Breasts	Should be soft and comfortable. Look for signs of cracking or infection. Engorgement may occur after the mother returns home. If mother breast-feeding, evaluate nipple condition.	Look for signs of infection—check temperature. To ease discomfort of engorgement, see Chap. 16.
Elimination	The mother should have had a soft movement since delivery. Constipation is a frequent problem. Ask about voiding, frequency, and color of urine.	Dietary measures (fluids, roughage) and mild exercise should be tried before referring to the doctor for prescription for cathartic. *Prevention* of constipation is the goal.

lb with every baby, and my husband told me to watch out or I'd look like her. I tried to get back into my clothes, and they don't fit. And I still haven't lost what I gained when I was pregnant."

"You expected to get back to your normal weight and fit into your former clothes right away?"

"Of course. So did my husband. Why?"

"Well, most women don't lose *all* the extra weight right away—it may take 6 weeks or so. Did you learn any exercises in the hospital?" As Sue reviews exercises to strengthen abdominal and perineal muscles, she reflects on the importance of body image and the frequency with which she encounters this concern. And yet, it is a subject so often neglected by nurses!

nutrition

Mrs. Murray's concern about her figure allows Sue to raise the issue of proper nutrition, as she had planned. In order to gain a better understanding of how well balanced her diet is and whether nutrition education is needed, Sue does not ask directly, but uses open-ended questions, such as "What kinds of foods have you felt up to eating?" or "Do you feel up to preparing meals?" or "Do you sometimes just 'forget' to eat?" The answers to these questions serve as a guide for further discussion.

assessment of the infant

"What did you say you named your baby? Melissa?"

"Melissa Ann"

"What can you tell me about Melissa?" As Sue obtains a history about the baby, she looks for clues that an effective parent–child bond is developing. (See Table 19-3.) Sue is concerned that Mrs. Murray's acceptance and readiness for the parental role may be diminished by her exhaustion, the lack of available support in her environment, and also her anxiety over her body image and performance in labor.

"I usually examine the baby when I visit— just to make sure everything is OK and to give you a chance to ask questions about the baby, especially questions you might feel uncomfortable about asking the doctor. Let's look at Melissa together."

"Sure. I was kind of hoping you would."

Melissa was sleeping between two pillows on her mother's bed. She noticed that although the room was warm, the baby was not overdressed. "I'm so glad to see a baby who is dressed appropriately. Most mothers I see bundle their babies up too much in a warm room, but Melissa seems to be dressed just right. I'm sorry I'm going to have to pick you up, Melissa, you're sleeping so peacefully." Sue moved Melissa closer to the sunny window where the lighting was best. She maintained an alert concentration as she systematically examined Melissa, looking for evidence of congenital disorders and illness (see Chap. 14). Occasionally she had discovered slight deviations from normal in an apparently normal newborn during this appraisal. One of the most difficult tasks she faced was to determine the significance of an observation. She knew these deviations may represent an important clue to a serious disorder, but on the other hand, there is a tremendous range of normal variations in the newborn period, and the line between normal and abnormal is poorly defined. She was helped in making her decisions by a thorough understanding of the more common newborn problems (respiratory distress, feeding problems, umbilical infection, diarrhea, dehydration, thrush, skin rashes, etc.) and by her awareness that the further from normal the observation is, the more significant it is.

As she assessed the baby, she pointed out and explained minor variations she knew were frequently of interest to parents: "That little bit of bleeding is normal—baby girls pick up some of their mother's hormones and, often have a mini-menstrual period. It doesn't cause any problem, and it will go away in a day or two."

teaching

The mother interrupted. "See her strain like that? Should I give her prune juice or something?"

"Well, straining while having a bowel movement doesn't necessarily mean constipation. Have her stools been soft?"

"Yes"

"Does she work hard like that with every movement?"

"She seems to."

"You know, straining with every stool usually is normal, although sometimes it indicates the baby has extra gas. You might try bubbling her more than usual. Let me know if that helps."

"Also she has a diaper rash. I change her diapers a lot and rinse them well, and I put petroleum jelly and baby powder on it, but it doesn't seem to help."

Sue hesitated. She knew the petroleum jelly and powder aggravated the rash, but she also knew a ritualistic practice such as this served the purpose of giving a mother confidence in her skill. Her answer must not destroy this confidence but strengthen it, building on the already present strengths and knowledge.

"You certainly have done a lot of the right things—keeping the diapers changed frequently and rinsed well—and I see you aren't using rubber pants or disposable diapers—that's good. The best cure I know is air. If the room is warm like it is now, try taking off her diapers and letting the air get to the rash to heal it. Petroleum jelly is a good way to *prevent* a rash from developing, but once the baby has a rash, petroleum jelly keeps the air from reaching the skin, and powder clogs the pores.

"Usually the air treatment works. If not, we'll look into soaps and other possible irritants. But—see—it really isn't a bad rash. There are no blisters or sores or white patches, the skin is just a little red.

"You seem to know quite a bit about newborns. Have you had experience taking care of newborns before?"

"Well, I've done a lot of baby-sitting before . . . but not real tiny babies like this."

"Tell me, have you ever had an opportunity to learn how to take a baby's temperature?" Mary shook her head. "How would you like to learn—I'd like to show you."

"Well, I guess so. I guess I should know in case she's sick. The doctor would ask what her temperature was. I have a thermometer. It came in Melissa's kit from the hospital."

"Let's use Melissa's own thermometer. The temperature isn't a very reliable indication of illness in a newborn, but as Melissa grows, the doctor will probably want to know what her temperature is if she's sick."

After Sue showed her how to take the baby's temperature (see Fig. 18-14), she assessed Mrs. Murray's understanding of signs of illness in a newborn, when to call the doctor, and what to tell the doctor (see Table 19-2). Sue was aware that although a lot of information can be *taught* during one visit, it can only be *learned* in small doses. Information which is remembered and utilized by parents is that information which parents see as relevant, meeting *their* needs. Although Sue tried to follow the mother's concerns, she had her own agenda as well. She wanted to discuss safety and share with her some ways to save money on infant care supplies. In addition, it was important to emphasize returning for the postpartum exam and the well baby visits and to discuss immunizations, sexual relations, and birth control. Rather than overwhelm Mrs. Murray with too much information at once, she looked for clues to her present understanding of these areas and decided what information to save for the next time. Because Mrs. Murray had mentioned using Dr. Spock as a reference, Sue recognized that she did acquire information by reading.

table 19-2 Signs of illness in a newborn—when to call the doctor

The doctor should be called when:

The eyes, umbilical cord, or circumcision site is red or swollen.

The baby appears very lethargic or sleeps a lot.

The baby does not cry normally.

The baby is not eating well or vomits feedings.

The baby does not move all extremities well.

The baby's skin seems very yellow, even in sunlight.

The baby's stools are watery and frequent.

The baby has a stuffy nose and seems to have difficulty breathing (breathing very rapidly, more than 60 times a minute).

You notice anything unusual or have a vague, uneasy feeling that all is not well.

The doctor's telephone number is _____ .

Note: This list may be given to parents on discharge from hospital or by public health nurse.

Although Mrs. Murray may need to learn specific skills (taking a temperature, giving a bath, preparing a formula), in general, Sue was more interested in sharing information on what to expect of young infants than in giving advice on what a mother ought to do. For instance, infant crying or lack of crying is a common concern of parents.

"You were telling me Melissa cries a lot."

"Yes. Especially at night."

"At night—that doesn't sound very pleasant. How much does that interefere with your sleep?"

"Well, I get a couple of hours of sleep, and then she cries and wakes us both up. She fusses most of the night, and I never seem to get back to sleep again."

"What do you do when she cries?"

"I see if she's hungry, or wet, or needs to be bubbled or something."

"Does that help?"

"Well, sometimes. But usually she keeps on crying."

"That must be very frustrating. That must make you feel kind of helpless."

"It makes me feel like crying myself. I don't know what to do—my husband needs his sleep so he can go to work in the morning, so sometimes I give in and pick her up, but I'm afraid I'll make her into a spoiled baby."

"You are afraid that picking her up will make her spoiled."

"You know—like she'll think she can get her own way and be real bratty and all. Why, doesn't it?"

"Crying is the only way Melissa has to say she needs you. She probably can't think through *why* she's uncomfortable, but she is in distress and can't help herself feel better, so she cries. You carried her around for 9 months, and she heard your heart beating and your stomach gurgling and felt warm and cozy. Now she is by herself and not feeling cozy and cuddled, and its awfully quiet in the middle of the night. If she cries when she doesn't seem to need food or fresh diapers, and you hold her, she doesn't feel quite so helpless; she feels like she has some say in this strange new world—so she begins to trust this new world and to trust you. She feels more secure, and as she grows older, she is less demanding and more willing to do what you say because she *trusts* you to know what is best for her. Does that sound right to you?"

"Umm . . . yes . . . I never thought of it that way."

"You know, most parents don't expect anywhere near the crying that most newborns do in the early weeks. There are a lot of things you can try—I'll write these ideas down as we talk about them so next time you feel desperate, you'll have something to refer to! But if these ideas don't work, try to remember the baby isn't deliberately trying to upset you—she is just getting rid of tension. Maybe she likes the sound of her own voice! As a baby gets older, she begins to have a better idea of what is bothering her, and she'll cry a little differently when she is hungry than when she wants to be held, and it will be easier as time goes on to understand what she wants. So things *will* get better. But right now, I'm concerned about you. Is there any way for you to get away from the crying for an hour or so a day?"

"Well, I don't know. Maybe my mother-in-law or my husband could watch the baby. I'll have to think about it."

"Do you feel funny about leaving the baby?"

"Well, yes. I think a mother ought to be there."

"That's a very normal feeling. And a good feeling. But it's also important for the father to develop his own special relationship with his baby. And grandparents, too. You know, in the old days, when several generations lived in the same house, a new mother had much more support. Friends and relatives were there to help with the work and keep the mother company, and the father was nearby.

Today, the mother so often has to carry the burden all by herself, with no support from the outside."

feeding

Melissa was fussing. Her mother picked her up and held her *en face*, looking into her eyes. "Are you hungry? Huh? You want something to eat? It's been three hours since you ate last. Let me get your bottle ready."

Sue was glad she had the opportunity to witness a feeding. So many new parents had problems related to feeding—formula pre-pared incorrectly, nipple hole too large, nipple not inserted far enough into the baby's mouth, overfeeding, underfeeding. Observing a feeding was an efficient way to spot some of these errors before they became a major problem. Unusual problems, while feeding—choking, vomiting after every feeding, refusing feedings—might be a clue to a more serious disorder or a subtle sign that all is not well.

While preparing Melissa's bottle, Mrs. Murray mentioned how expensive the commercial formula was and said she planned to switch to evaporated milk next week. Sue, therefore planned to discuss infant formulas at the next visit.

fig. 19-5 Breast-feeding at home. (*Photo by Lester Bergman, in D. Vietor and M. McCutcheon, Care of the Maternity Patient, McGraw-Hill, New York, 1971, p. 493.*)

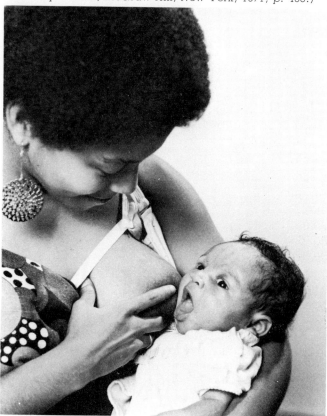

assessing the parent–child bond

As Mrs. Murray began to feed Melissa, Sue quietly observed the interaction between mother and infant. The initial concern that Mrs. Murray's exhaustion, nonsupportive environment, and low self-esteem might affect her relationship with Melissa was alleviated. She seemed able to establish contact with Melissa and seemed to be learning about her baby as a separate individual. She was comfortable in close physical proximity with Melissa, maintaining eye contact and the *en face* position (see Table 19-3). In order to obtain more information, Sue asked an open-ended question—"What have the past few days been like for you?"

listening: the pressures of the early weeks

"Well, I don't know . . ." Mrs. Murray hesitated.

"Is it what you expected?"

"No, it's *very* different. I thought having a baby was so normal, and I'd bounce right back and be able to do everything I used to when I was working. I was going to make sure my baby wouldn't interfere with our way of life. I'd schedule it so she'd fit right in, and I'd have so much extra time to do what I wanted. I was going to be a good mother and do everything just like you are supposed to, so she wouldn't need to cry, and I'd love her to pieces. All my friends would stop by and see how good I was to her and be real excited over how pretty she is, and I'd feel so warm and motherly and all."

"And it hasn't turned out that way?"

"No, it sure hasn't." A tear ran down her cheek. "It hasn't turned out that way at all. The baby keeps me up all night crying and fussing, and I can't seem to figure out what

table 19-3 Clues to difficulty in parent–child bonding

A The nurse will be alerted to potential problems in parent–child bonding if:
The mother is young or immature.
The mother must struggle against a nonsupportive or isolated environment.
The mother is beset by stress-causing situations in addition to the arrival of the new infant (e.g., poor environmental conditions, serious illness in the family, severe disappointment, rapid and repeated pregnancies).
The mother was separated from her infant for a prolonged period after birth (e.g., prematurity, maternal illness).

B The nurse will strongly suspect that there is a problem in parent–child bonding if:
The parent expresses inappropriate feelings in response to infant's crying (e.g., anger, frustration, helplessness).
The parent fails to express anything about the infant that she or he likes (i.e., the parent has not found in the infant a physical or psychological attribute valued in self).
The parent expresses unresolved feelings over a "dream" child. (e.g., disappointment over sex of infant).
The parent expresses mostly negative feelings about the infant (e.g., disgust over messy diapers or a perception that the infant is too demanding).
The parent expresses expectations of infant far beyond the baby's developmental potentials.
The parent fails to exhibit close, gentle, physical contact with the infant (e.g., holds infant away from body, plays roughly with infant, or avoids eye contact and the *en face* position).

she wants, and she wakes up my husband and he tells me to get her to stop crying, but no matter what I do, she cries. And I'm so tired, and I try to do everything I used to and make the house normal—you know, just like it used to be, and then everything goes wrong. I thought being a mother was supposed to give you a good feeling, but all I feel is scared and alone, and I wish I never decided to do this. I wish my mother were here. I don't know how to be a mother. I wish somebody were here. All of my friends are working, and it's so lonely, and I have to worry all by myself. When I was working, I could go off by myself and do my own thing. Now I'm trapped. Tied down to a tiny room and a fussy baby and no way to escape. And no money either. I feel like—like I'm doing all the giving and not getting anything back. I guess that sounds terrible. I guess I should be happy my baby is normal and healthy."

Sue sat quietly, trying to absorb and assess all the many feelings this new mother expressed. She was glad she had gained her trust so that she felt comfortable unburdening herself. Sue answered quietly and slowly, "May I call you Linda?"

"Yes, I'd like that."

"What you've said doesn't sound terrible—it sounds perfectly normal. Your feelings are real, and they are OK, and these are the same things every new parent feels.

"Bringing home a new baby creates a family crisis. When you are pregnant, you picture a cute, loving baby who somehow is grateful to you for bringing her into this world and giving her such good care. And you picture yourself calm and happy and feeling so fulfilled as a mother."

"That's what I thought."

"But in reality, you take home a stranger, who doesn't express her appreciation, doesn't fit right in to your style of living, and despite your best intentions, creates chaos. You find out you are more tired than you thought you'd be, and there's more work to be done than you anticipated, and you aren't quite up to all this.

"And when you're pregnant, you tell yourself you are going to be a 'good' parent; you are going to avoid the problems and mistakes of your parents or your friends—you're going to do things 'right'." Linda nodded.

"And then you find things don't happen that way for you. You find out the baby won't just do things your way—she's an individual, and *her* behavior affects *you*. There are no pat answers like you'd hoped; the information you got from your aunt or Dr. Spock doesn't apply. And then you wonder if your're going to be a failure, especially if you feel kind of clumsy caring for the baby. At least that's the way most parents feel. Does that sound anything like your experience?"

"You mean," ventured Linda hesitantly, "I'm not abnormal or anything?"

"You're OK. It's just that the first few weeks are very hard—especially for someone who really tries to do a good job, like you. You know, being a parent isn't so much an *achievement,* or doing things the 'right way', as it is a relationship that is developed slowly as both parent and baby get to know each other. Beginning relationships are difficult and take time to develop. As you get to know your baby, you may discover some things about her you don't like. Those feelings are OK; it doesn't mean you don't love your baby. All mothers don't enjoy all stages of childhood. You may find you don't enjoy newborns—that's OK, too. You may not have a lot of warm motherly feelings right away. It often takes time to develop, just like it does getting to know any new person."

"I feel better," said Linda with a sigh.

"That's great, because all the feelings you expressed are perfectly normal. You *are* doing all the giving and getting nothing in return. You *are* tied down and trapped, at least for awhile. It *is* lonely with only a fussy baby to keep you company. And it is especially difficult when you have to face all this alone all day, with no one to tell you what a great job you're doing, no one to share the responsibility. This is a whole new experience—most new parents feel like children themselves, and need 'mothering'. Sometimes this puts a lot of strain on a marriage.

terminating the visit

"Well, Linda, we've talked a lot. It's time for me to go. I *am* concerned about the baby's crying and your need for more rest."

"I'll try some of those suggestions you have about the crying. And I will try not to push myself the next couple of days."

"I'd like to plan another visit this week, and we can go over formula preparation and talk some more. Why don't you write down any questions that come up, and I'll try to answer them when I return."

When Sue returned next time, she would have a clearer picture of the family dynamics, find out what Linda found helpful in those pamphlets, check the baby again for things like thrush and dehydration and CDH (because limitation of abduction of the hips sometimes does not appear until the baby is 3 to 6 weeks old), and discuss well baby visits, birth control, and other points not raised at this first visit.

discussion

Nurses who visit the family in their own home have a role that is unique yet complementary to that of nurses functioning in the hospital setting. Visiting nurses continue the important observation, emotional support, and teaching tasks begun in the hospital. They also serve as valuable resource persons to the hospital personnel and to the physician, because they have been in the home and can assess and report on the home situation. They are aware of the resources of their community so that they can utilize these resources to better support the family. As the need arises, they become an advocate for the family in securing improved health care for the newborn and other family members.

During her visit, Sue utilized the nursing process. She made a thorough initial assessment of Mrs. Murray and Melissa. She and Mrs. Murray had agreed upon the primary goals of obtaining more rest and trying various methods of coping with Melissa's crying. During her next visit, Sue would evaluate how these goals were being implemented, and she and Mrs. Murray could revise these goals as needed.

THE INTERVIEW

To answer some further questions about the role of community nurses in maternal-child health, an interview has been arranged between the hospital-based nurse and the nurse in the community:

Hospital Nurse: "Can you tell me just which families should be referred to the community nurse?"

Community Nurse: "Every newborn baby and new mother should be visited shortly after going home, especially after mothers and infants have been discharged within a day or two of giving birth. In many communities, infants and mothers who are well when discharged are not seen by a health care professional until the routine checkup 4 or 5 weeks later. This practice continues in spite of the fact that the entire first month is such a precarious time of life for an infant. More than that, bringing home a new baby is a time of great adjustment and tension for the whole family. When given the right kind of support, the family can get off to a much better start. Think of the tension and concern the nurse can *prevent* by her presence and anticipatory guidance."

Hospital Nurse: "Are you saying that every family has a nurse visit?"

Community Nurse: "Unfortunately, no, not in most communities. Our society has not yet accepted the importance of the postpartum and neonatal period."

Hospital Nurse: "So how do you set priorities—who most needs a visit?"

Community Nurse: "Babies and mothers at risk because of their physical condition—premature babies, those with birth defects, or those that presented complications during labor—are usually referred. But babies and mothers who are emotionally at risk also need referrals. For example, hospital nurses who observe interactions between parent and infant indicating that a positive emotional bond is not taking place should refer these families (see Table 19-3). In some cases, such infants may develop emotional problems or are at risk of abuse or neglect. The hospital nurse should also be alert to mothers who must go home to a nonsupportive or isolated environment—mothers who do not have the support of husband or family, who have less than a high school education and a low income, who come under medical care late in pregnancy or not at all, and who may move shortly after discharge.[3] Many of our adolescent mothers fall into this category."

Hospital Nurse: "What about premature babies—they are often referred to the public health nurse—what do you do on those visits?"

Community Nurse: "If the nurse visits before the baby arrives home, she tries to help the parents deal with their fears and feelings. She may help a parent who had begun the grieving process when the baby's life was endangered to regain hope now that the baby is well enough to be sent home. She may encourage parents to talk about the pregnancy—perhaps the parent somehow feels responsible for the infant's early birth. She may give information and encouragement to the parent who fears the baby will not be normal or is extremely fragile and

vulnerable. A visit made after the premature infant arrives home is similar to any newborn visit. The nurse is not only aware of the feelings I just described, but she also is particularly alert for clues to difficulty in parent–child bonding. You see, parents of premature infants do not have the opportunity for the early close contact so necessary in forming an effective bond, and because of this, prematures run a much higher risk of becoming abused."

Hospital Nurse: "Do you see much child abuse?"

Community Nurse: "We try always to remain alert to the possibility, especially when we encounter parents who seem to have difficulty establishing a positive bond or parents who were themselves abused as a child. Of course, unusual burns, bruises, or scars found during the newborn appraisal should be further investigated, as well as infants who seem to be receiving insufficient or inappropriate care."

Hospital Nurse: "What if you do find an abused or neglected infant?"

Community Nurse: "Each community has its own system for reporting abuse, and nurses in any setting should be familiar with the resources in the community. Any injury to an infant is considered highly suspect, as true accidents in infancy are rare. When the nurse does find injury or neglect in an infant, she makes sure the infant is seen by a physician right away, shares her suspicions with the physician, and follows community guidelines to make sure the family receives the help it requires. Although the nurse expresses her concern about the baby with the family, she does not share her suspicions of neglect or abuse with them. She needs to be especially sensitive and nonjudgmental so that the parents begin to develop a sense of trust in the professionals who will be working with them."

Hospital Nurse: "Would a mother who was very depressed neglect her baby?"

Community Nurse: "The typical 'pospartum blues' seldom interfere with a mother's ability to care for her infant. The nurse visiting in the home can assess the degree to which depression is immobilizing the mother and interfering with baby care and can refer the mother for further help as necessary. Normal postpartum blues should never be ignored—by active, concerned listening, the nurse can discover some of the stresses contributing to the depression and work with the family to alleviate these stress factors." (See Chap. 13.)

Hospital Nurse: "Someone who lost a baby would be depressed—would these parents benefit from a home visit?"

Community Nurse: "The parent who gives birth to a stillborn child, who relinquishes a baby for adoption, who has a defective child, or whose baby dies after being brought home (e.g., crib death) should be referred to the community nurse. The hospital nurse or busy office nurse should be aware of just how supportive such a visit can be. Parents need an unhurried opportunity to talk over their experiences and feelings, and they need an understanding of the grief process so that they realize their feelings are normal."

Hospital Nurse: We seem to have so many adolescent mothers, and we can't spend the time we'd like during their short hospital stay. What about referring these mothers for a home visit?"

Community Nurse: "Yes, the community nurse can be very helpful to the adolescent who has newly become a mother. These young mothers are faced with immense reponsibilities and stress at a time of life which is already difficult. (See Chap. 21.) The adolescent's motherhood becomes a crises for her, for her family, and for the father of the baby.

Hospital Nurse: "What does the nurse do when she visits?"

Community Nurse: "The most important service the nurse can offer is a caring relationship. As she works with the family, she becomes aware of and does some assessment of family dynamics—coping mechanisms, roles, support systems, communication skills—and she strives to use this knowledge to strengthen the mother–daughter relationship. She works to find resources within the family and community to meet identified needs. And of course, she includes instruction about infants and satisfactory infant care, which is as important as for an older parent."

Hospital Nurse: "Well, thank you. I trust that we can work more closely to assure real continuity of care for our newborns and their parents!"

SUMMARY

This chapter discussed the importance of the first few weeks at home and the significance of the hospital nurse and community nurse in assuring continuity of care. Priorities for determining which mothers and infants most need a nursing visit at home were delineated. The functions of the visiting nurse and the way in which the nurse uses the nursing process were explored. We discussed assessment of the home and community, physical assessment of mother and infant, and assessment of readiness for parenthood. To better visualize the use of the nursing process and the role of the community nurse, a visit to a new family was described. Infant behaviors, feelings of new parents, parent–child bonding, the nurse's use of communication skills, and the integration of all aspects of nursing care were illustrated during this visit. Other aspects of maternal child nursing in the community were described by means of an interview.

study questions

1   Ideally, every new mother and infant should be visited at home by the nurse. When this is not possible, what priorities determine who is visited?
2   Describe at least five functions of the nurse in making a home visit to a new mother and infant.
3   What does the nurse look for when making a physical assessment of the mother? Of the newborn? Why are these appraisals so important?
4   Describe several typical infant behaviors that a new parent might expect in the first few weeks at home.
5   Describe some typical feelings a new parent might experience during the first few weeks at home.
6   Describe several behaviors observable in the parent that would suggest that a strong parent–child bond is developing. List several clues that would alert the nurse to a potential problem in bond development.
7   Identify the specific communication skills the nurse utilized in the visit. Why did she select these specific techniques?
8   Describe how the nurse utilized the nursing process in a home visit to a new mother and infant.
9   Identify the mother's "agenda" (areas of concern) in the visit described. Identify the nurse's agenda. Which topics do you feel take priority? Why?

references

1   J. Smiley, S. Eyres, and D. Roberts, "Maternal and Infant Health and Their Associated Factors in an Inner City Population," *American Journal of Public Health,* April 1972, p. 476.
2   N. Donaldson, "Fourth Trimester Follow-up," *Amercian Journal of Nursing,* **77** (7):1176, 1977.
3   J. Haight, "Steadying Parents as They Go—by Phone," *American Journal of Maternal Child Nursing,* **2** (5): 311–312, September/October, 1977.

bibliography

Allan, J.: "The Identification and Rx of 'Difficult' Babies," *The Canadian Nurse,* December, 1976, pp. 11–16.
Baird, S. F.: "Crisis Intervention Theory in Maternal–Infant Nursing," *Journal of Obstetric, Gynecol- ogic and Neonatal Nursing,* **5** (1):30, January/February, 1976.
Bishop, B.: "A Guide to Assessing Parenting Capabilities," *American Journal of Nursing,* **76**:1784, November, 1976.
Black, P.: "The Child at Risk—Interprofessional Cooperation," *Nursing Mirror,* April 21, 1977, pp. 56–61.
Bozian, W.: "Nursing Care of the Infant in the Community, Symposium on Care of Newborn," *Nursing Clinics of North America,* **6** (1):93, March 1971.
Brazelton, T.: *Infants and Mothers, Differences in Development,* Delacorte, New York, 1970.
Brown, M. S., and M. A. Murphy: *Ambulatory Pediatrics for Nurses,* McGraw-Hill, New York, 1975.
Bryan-Logan, B., and B. Dancy: "Unwed Pregnant Adolescents—Their Mother's Dilemma," *Nursing Clinics of North America,* **9** (1):5, March 1974.
Christensen, A.: "Coping with the Crisis of a Premature Birth—One Couple's Story," *American Journal of Maternal Child Nursing,* **2** (1):33, January/February, 1977.
Clark, A.: "Recognizing Discord Between Mother and Child and Changing It to Harmony," *American Journal of Maternal Child Nursing,* **1** (2):100, March/April, 1976.
———, and D. Alfonso: "Mother–Child Relationships," *American Journal of Maternal Child Nursing,* **1** (2):94, March/April, 1976.
Dubois, D.: "Indications of an Unhealthy Relationship Between Parent and Premature Infant," *Journal of Obstetric, Gynecologic and Neonatal Nursing,* **4** (3):21, May/June 1975.
Farrar, C. A.: "A Data Collection Procedure to Assess Behavioral Individuality in the Neonate," *Journal of Obstetric, Gynecologic and Neonatal Nursing,* **3** (3):15, May/June 1974.
Gruis, M.: "Beyond Maternity: Postpartum Concerns of Mothers," *American Journal of Maternal Child Nursing,* **2** (3):182, May/June 1977.
Harvey, K.: "The Empty Cradle: Caring Perceptively for the Relinquishing Mother," *American Journal of Maternal Child Nursing,* **2** (1):22, January/February, 1977.
Hobbs, D. F., and J. M. Wimbish: "Transition to Parenthood by Black Couples," *Journal of Marriage and the Family,* November, 1977, pp. 677–689.
Hurd, J. M.: "Assessing Maternal Attachment: First Step Toward the Prevention of Child Abuse," *Journal of Obstetric, Gynecologic and Neonatal Nursing,* **4** (4):25, July/August, 1975.
Hurwitz, A.: "Child Abuse: A Program for Intervention," *Nursing Outlook,* September, 1977, pp. 575–577.
Jones, W. L.: "The Emotional Needs of the New Family," *Nursing Mirror,* Oct. 23, 1975, pp. 49–52.
Kempe, C. H., and E. Helfer: *Helping the Battered Child and His Family,* Lippincott, Philadelphia, 1972.
Kennedy, J.: "The High-Risk Maternal–Infant Acquaint-

ance Process," *Nursing Clinics of North America,* **8** (3): 549, September, 1973.

Kleinberg, W.: "Counselling Mothers in the Hospital Postpartum Period: A Comparison of Techniques," *American Journal of Public Health,* **67** (7):672, July 1977.

Kowalski, K., and M. Osborn, "Helping Mothers of Stillborn Infants to Grieve," *American Journal of Maternal Child Nursing,* **2** (1):29, January/February, 1977.

Kreindler, S.: "Psychiatric Treatment for the Abusing Parent and The Abused Child," *Canadian Psychiatric Association Journal,* **21**:275, 1976.

Ludington-Hoe, S.: "Postpartum: Development of Maternicity," *American Journal of Nursing,* **77**:1171, July 1977.

Mercer, R.: "Postpartum Illness and Acquaintance-Attachment Process," *American Journal of Nursing,* **77**: 1174, July 1977.

Seiden, A.: "The Maternal Sense of Mastery in Primary Care Obstetrics," *Primary Care,* **3** (4):717, December, 1976.

Williams, C.: "Health Services in the Home," *Pediatrics,* **52** (6):773, December 1973.

Williams, J.: "Learning Needs of New Parents," *American Journal of Nursing,* **77**:1173, July 1977.

Wuerger, M. K.: "The Young Adult Stepping into Parenthood," *American Journal of Nursing,* **76** (8):1283, August 1976.

20
MATERNAL AND NEONATAL PHARMACOLOGIC FACTORS

MARTHA OLSEN SCHULT
ELIZABETH J. DICKASON

MATERNAL FACTORS

It is safe to say that the best drug to administer to a pregnant woman is no drug at all! While more and more drugs are being released into the pharmaceutical market daily, their effects on the growing fetus will become known only in retrospect. Americans consume exorbitant amounts of these drugs, especially sleeping medications, tranquilizers, amphetamines, antacids, laxatives, antibiotics, and vitamins. Pregnant women take drugs, both prescribed and unprescribed. The Collaborative Study of the National Institute for Neurologic Disease and Stroke found that among 50,000 women studied, 900 different drugs were taken during pregnancy.[1] Fofar and Nelson report that the number of drugs taken by pregnant women in one study averaged four to nine drugs per woman.[2] *Perinatal Press* reports that "middle to high socioeconomic gravid patients ingest between three to twenty-nine drugs (mean 10.3) during pregnancy."[3] They note that these drugs taken during pregnancy do not include cigarette smoking, alcoholic beverages, or anesthetic agents.

When taken according to prescribed amounts, most drugs are considered safe for the adult human body. However, some of the drugs considered safe to the adult body can have devastating effects on the unborn baby. The thalidomide tragedy of 1961–1962 is an example of such an effect; considered a "harmless" sleeping medication and taken by pregnant women, thalidomide caused thousands of babies to be born with phocomelia— the absence of limbs (Fig. 20-1).

Much research is being conducted to try to discover the effects of drugs on the fetus at various points in its development (see Fig. 20-2). A few effects of drugs on the fetus are known. For example, aspirin has the potential for causing gastrointestinal bleeding in the fetus. Large doses of phenobarbital can cause neonatal bleeding, and some vitamins taken in excess can harm the fetus. With the exception of a few drugs with high molecular weights, every drug ingested or inhaled by the pregnant woman crosses the placental

fig. 20-1 Phocomelia with absence of the upper extremities. (*From D. Bergsma (ed.), Birth Defects: Atlas and Compendium, The National Foundation—March of Dimes, White Plains, N.Y., with permission of the editor and contributor.*)

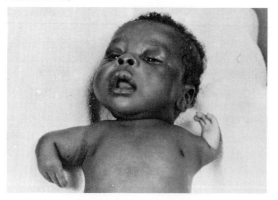

tissue in varying concentrations and has the potential for disturbing or altering the growth patterns of the fetus.

It is generally agreed that the period of *organogenesis* is the most critical period in the life of the fetus/embryo— the first 8 to 10 weeks of gestation when the major body organs are being formed. Any alterations in this delicately balanced act of nature could either change cell differentiation or affect cell growth. For this reason, all women who suspect that they might be pregnant should be warned against taking *any* medication at this time (including vitamins and minerals). Unfortunately, many women are not aware that they are pregnant until the second month of pregnancy. By that time, any harmful drug or disease organism may have already taken its toll on the fetus.

Every pregnant woman has the right to be told of the possible effects that a drug or drugs may have on her unborn baby. McCrory states, "Whenever a pregnant woman takes a drug, she should do it with educated awareness of the choice she is making between a therapeutic benefit to her and a toxicity risk to her unborn baby."[4] Most women would not deliberately take a drug that would harm a growing baby. But how are women to become informed? Nurses and doctors have a responsibility, along with the drug companies, to keep informed and to disseminate such knowledge to the public so that parents can become educated. Labels on drug bottles should warn the mother against taking certain drugs during pregnancy or lactation, and pregnant women should be told that too much caffeine in coffee or tea, as well as too many cigarettes, may affect the growth of the baby. This is information every woman needs to know.

In addition, the *benefit-to risk* ratio between the therapeutic effect of the agent and its possible effects on the fetus must be explained to a woman who, because of super-

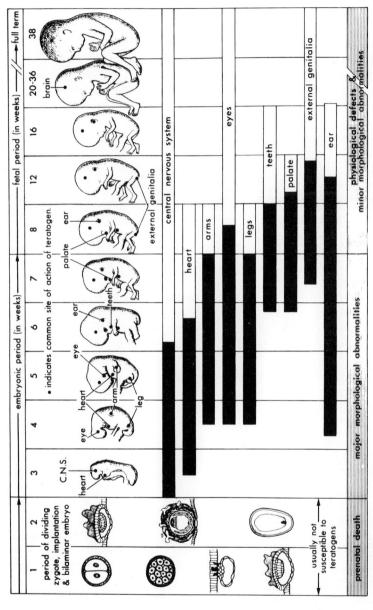

fig. 20-2 Schematic illustration of the sensitive or critical periods in human development. (Shaded areas denote highly sensitive periods.) *(From K. L. Moore, Before We Are Born: Basic Embryology and Birth Defects, Saunders, Philadelphia, 1975.)*

imposed problems, must receive medication. (Without clear understanding of the factors involved, it is always hard to make a choice, and lingering doubt can result in guilt or blame later on.) As the woman is informed and participates in the decision, she can gain understanding of the real dilemma that may result. (See Appendix 2, The Pregnant Patient's Bill of Rights.) Finally, when a drug must be given to a pregnant patient, the one with the least possible effects should be chosen (Table 20-1).

DRUGS USED IN PREGNANCY AND AFTER DELIVERY

antacids

During pregnancy the motility of the stomach is slowed, and early in pregnancy, gastric acidity is reduced. Therefore, an antacid is rarely necessary. Later, however, the cardiac sphincter becomes slightly relaxed, and the pressure of the enlarging uterus causes slight regurgitation of stomach acid through the cardiac sphincter into the esophagus. The acid reflux irritates the mucosa, causing a burning sensation. In addition to this discomfort of heartburn, increased movement of the diaphragm and the flaring rib cage may create a temporary hiatus hernia.

Nonpharmacologic remedies for these problems should be advised before drug therapy is begun. Such remedies include (1) drinking milk between meals, (2) eating small, frequent meals, (3) avoiding gas-producing and fatty foods, and (4) alternating dry and liquid meals.

Any antacid should be prescribed by the physician, and the patient should be advised against taking extra doses. Magnesium products have a laxative tendency, and aluminum and calcium have a constipating effect, but combinations of aluminum and magnesium seem to have few untoward effects and thus are the most commonly prescribed antacids. Large quantities of calcium carbonate can cause "milk-alkali syndrome" or acid rebound, inducing the stomach to secrete more acid. Schenkel and Vorherr report that large doses of magnesium trisilicate may damage fetal kidneys, and fetal neurologic and neuromuscular systems can be damaged by magnesium hydroxide.[5] Sodium bicarbonate should probably be avoided completely during pregnancy because of its high sodium content, its systemic absorption, and the gaseous carbon dioxide produced by it in the stomach. Whenever antacids are necessary, they should be used judiciously and avoided in the first trimester whenever possible.

antacids during labor During labor, many physicians will order that antacids be given immediately (stat) or q2h to neutralize stomach acidity. A dosage regimen of 15 mL of magnesium trisilicate q2h to raise the gastric pH to above 2.5 is recommended to reduce pulmonary complications should the patient vomit and aspirate during labor or delivery.

antiemetics

A common discomfort of pregnancy is the nausea and vomiting known as "morning sickness," which occurs in approximately 50 percent of all pregnant women. Before any drugs are prescribed for morning sickness, all other avenues of relief should be explored. If an antiemetic is needed, it should be used judiciously during the first 5 to 8 weeks of organogenesis.

Two of the several antiemetics prescribed for morning sickness are *Tigan* (capsules: 250 mg; suppository: 200 mg; ampuls: 200

table 20-1 Categories of drugs affecting the fetus and newborn

Teratogenic Effects

congenital defects	fetal death	reduced birth weights, or alter somatic growth	later: carcinogenic	mental retardation
Alcohol*	Chlorpropamide	Drugs of abuse	Hormones	Carbon monoxide
Anticonvulsants	Dicumarol	Alcohol*	Radiopaque dyes	Mercury
Cancer chemotherapeutic agents	Ergot	Smoking	Radioisotopes	Radiation
Corticosteroids	Lead, mercury	Corticosteroids	Radiation	Thioureas
Estrogens	Salicylates*	Ovulatory agents†	Chemotherapeutic agents†	Alcohol*
Progestins		Anticonvulsant agents		
Radiation, radioisotopes				
Lead, mercury				
Quinine*				
Tetracycline				
Thalidomide				
Hallucinogenic agents†				
Ovulatory agents†				

Dose-dependent Transitional Effects During Newborn Period

immediate adaptation	withdrawal effects	hematologic problems (hemorrhage, anemia, or thrombocytopenia)	thyroid function
Analgesics	Alcohol*	Alcohol	Radiopaque dye
General anesthetics	Amphetamines	Barbiturates	Radioisotopes
Local anesthetics	Anticonvulsant agents	Dicumarol	Iodine
Magnesium sulfate	Barbiturates	Dilantin	Thioureas
Valium, other tranquilizers	Glutethimide	Diuretics	
Oxytocin*	Heroin	Fat-soluble vitamin K	
(increased jaundice)	Propoxyphene	Quinine	
Hypotonic IV fluids plus	Psychotropic drugs	Promethazine	
Oxytocin		Salicylates	
Diuretics		Sulfonamides	
		Thioureas	

*In large amounts.
†Relationship still uncertain.
Source: Adapted from *Perinatal Press*, I(I)10, 1976.

mg/2 mL for intramuscular injection), and *Bendectin* (tablets: two at bedtime). Tigan is a well-tolerated antiemetic. Much research has been conducted on its effect on the developing embryo. Although there is no conclusive evidence that it is completely safe for the fetus, neither has it been proved harmful to mother or infant. The nurse should inform the patient that she may experience some drowsiness and ask her to report any allergic symptoms, such as a rash, to her physician.

Bendectin is a combination of Bentyl, Decapryn, and pyridoxine hydrochloride. Because the tablets are specially coated to produce a long-acting effect, when given at night they are beneficial the following morning, when spasms of nausea are most often experienced. Because of the antihistamine component of Bendectin, patients should be cautioned about drowsiness. Any adverse symptom such as diarrhea, rash, or excessive vomiting should be reported to the obstetrician. Bendectin is a researched drug and is primarily prescribed for nausea and vomiting of pregnancy.

antiemetics to avoid during pregnancy Buclizine, cyclizine, and meclizine are antihistamines not presently used in view of their teratogenic effects on animals. Compazine (prochlorperazine) is also not used during pregnancy because of the adverse reactions that can occur.

laxatives

Constipation is a common complaint during pregnancy. When counseling a pregnant woman regarding her dietary habits, the nurse should encourage her to include roughage in her meals, as well as ample fluids, in an effort to increase bulk and lubricate the bowel. This, along with exercise, usually will prevent constipation. Again, the advisability of avoiding

medications can be stressed to the pregnant woman.

Some of the commonly prescribed laxatives and stool softeners include:

Milk of magnesia: 30 mL (1 oz) orally at bedtime.

Colace: capsules (50- and 100-mg dioctyl sodium sulfosuccinate as a stool softener).

Peri-Colace: capsules (100 mg Colace, 30 mg Peristim, a mild stimulant laxative).

Psyllium hydrophilic mucilloid (Betajel, Metamucil, Mucilose): 1 rounded tsp (7 g) stirred into a glass of liquid, od, bid, or tid; a soft celloidal bulk which does not interfere with absorption of vitamins. Do not let mixture stand after mixing; drink immediately.

Senokap DSS: capsules (senna and dioctyl sodium sulfosuccinate).

Mineral oil should not be prescribed for the pregnant woman, as it interferes with the absorption of the fat-soluble vitamins A, D, E, and K. Harsh, gripping laxatives should also be avoided.

Constipation may be a problem in the postpartal patient. Slowed motility of the bowel during labor, tenderness of the birth tract, and the repaired episiotomy all contribute to the patient's inability to defecate or to her fear of pain upon defecation. Peri-Colace, Colace, and milk of magnesia are all effective laxatives for the postpartal mother.

nonnarcotic analgesics

Pain, other than an occasional discomfort, is abnormal during pregnancy, and its cause should be ascertained before any drug is dispensed. Analgesics should be used sparingly during pregnancy. It has been shown that aspirin, which had been commonly used, can cause problems in the neonate. Schenkel and Vorherr report that aspirin taken even 2 weeks prior to delivery has resulted in infants with a 10 percent higher risk of extra bleeding and the development of cephalhematoma, purpura, and a transient melena after birth.[6] Potential hazards of salicylates to developing infants include teratogenic effects on the central nervous sytem throughout pregnancy and upon the kidneys during the second to the fifth month, GI tract bleeding in utero, and salicylate poisoning of the newborn.

Para-aminophenol derivatives (acetonalid, acetaminophen, and phenacetin) also have the potential for causing teratogenic effects, particularly when taken in large doses and in combination with other drugs, as in headache mixtures.[7] In light of these findings, it is probably best for the infant if the mother refrains from taking *any* analgesics containing these substances during the first 8 weeks of her pregnancy and within 2 weeks of her EDD.

Postpartum patients do not have to take the same precautions because the neonate can no longer be affected by medication unless the baby is being breast-fed. Local anesthetic sprays, compresses, sitz baths, and/or ice packs are usually sufficient to alleviate the pain from the episiotomy site. In addition, Kegel exercises are also helpful for perineal discomfort.

The "after-birth" analgesics listed below will usually suffice to relieve *postpartum* discomfort. However, narcotic analgesics may be necessary to relieve more severe pain (such as the pain resulting from cesarean section).

Acetaminophen (Datril, Tylenol), 325 mg tablets, 1 to 3 tid or qid prn. Acetaminophen is a mild analgesic used for minor discomforts and postpartal pain. It is generally free from side effects when used according to directions. Since it contains no aspirin, it is suitable for use by those individuals who are sensitive to aspirin.

Propoxyphene hydrochloride (Darvon), 65-mg capsules, 1 qid prn and Darvon Compound 65 (propoxyphene hydrochloride, aspirin, phenacetin, and caffeine), capsules, 1 qid prn. Darvon is used for relief of mild to moderate pain in the postpartal patient. Gastrointestinal disturbances, dizziness, headache, and rashes may occur with its use. Do not administer Darvon compound to aspirin-sensitive individuals.

Acetylsalicylic acid (aspirin), 325 mg tablets, 2 qid prn. Aspirin is a mild analgesic used in postpartal patients for the relief of pain. It does not produce sedation or euphoria, nor does it disturb the memory. It can produce gastric irritation, and for this reason, it may be combined with a buffering agent in administration. Some of the side effects include sweating, skin eruptions, and disturbances of sight and hearing. It is often used in combination with other drugs, such as codeine, for synergistic action.

Percodan (oxycodone, aspirin, phenacetin and caffeine) 1 tablet q3-4h prn. Percodan provides relief from moderate and severe pain in the postpartal patient. Since its habit-forming potentiality is greater than that of its relative, codeine, it should be used discreetly. Nausea, vomiting, and constipation may occur with its use. Do not administer to aspirin-sensitive individuals.

sedatives, hypnotics

Restlessness and inability to sleep during the last trimester as a result of the large, protruding abdomen and other discomfort may warrant the use of hypnotics. As with other drugs, sedatives should not be given too close to delivery because of effects on the fetus/neonate (see Table 20-2). Some of the hypnotics used to induce sleep include the following:

Chloral hydrate (Noctec), 250 mg capsules, 1 to 2 capsules at bedtime. Noctec, one of the oldest hypnotics, provides restful sleep for pregnant patients. It has been used with benefit in alcoholics and in the elderly, as well as in children! Although it may be habit-forming, it is considered a mild hypnotic because patients can be aroused with little effort and seldom complain of a "big head" or hangover as an aftereffect.

Sodium secobarbital (Seconal), 100- to 200-mg capsules, may be given orally or rectally. Intramuscular and intravenous preparations are prepared in single-dose ampuls. Seconal is a quick-acting hypnotic or sedative. It produces degrees of drowsiness and depressed reflexes, according to the amount of barbiturate given. Large dosages may cause dangerous depression of the respiratory system.

Sodium pentobarbital, (Nembutal), 100- to 200-mg capsules may be given orally or rectally. It is a short-acting barbiturate and is used to induce sleep and relaxation. It acts as a depressant of the central nervous system of the body; consequently, overdosage can be detrimental.

Phenobarbital (Luminal), 30- to 100-mg tablets. This drug acts as a depressant of the central nervous system, producing a long-lasting and quieting effect on the individual. With reduced dosages given several times a day, it is possible to produce a sustained sedative or quieting effect on the nervous system. (See Chap. 23 for use in preeclampsia.) (All barbiturates may be habit-forming and also are likely to produce aftereffects ("hangover") if a sufficient time of rest has not ensued.)

Many mothers find it difficult to sleep the first night after delivery because of overtiredness from a long labor, excitement over childbearing, a strange bed, or the strange noises in the hospital. Because most mothers are in the hospital for only a few days, physicians may prescribe sedatives to ensure sufficient rest and relaxation. *Seconal, Nembutal, chloral hydrate,* or *phenobarbital* may be chosen to provide this desired effect in the postpartal mother.

When administering sedatives or hypnotics, nurses should see that external stimuli that interfere with rest and/or sleep are removed from the immediate area of the patient. These include loud talking, bright light or sunlight, offensive odors, and food odors that stimulate the olfactory and salivary glands. In the hospital setting, all barbiturates must be accounted for and signed for in the narcotic book.

Nurses must provide safety for the patient under sedation. Some patients may not need side rails, but others may; nurses should astutely exercise judgment concerning this question when administering sedatives or hypnotics.

As with all drugs, nurses should be alert to any adverse effects such as rash, diarrhea, GI disturbances, or respiratory depression. Hypnotics and sedatives can cause hyperactivity in some individuals instead of having a quieting effect and producing rest.

tranquilizers

In the 1950s, a whole new category of drugs called tranquilizers was introduced. Their ability to reduce anxiety and depression, without impairing mental ability and without being habit-forming, has aided tremendously in reducing the need for using habit-forming drugs such as the barbiturates. However, there has been mounting evidence that tranquilizers may adversely effect the fetus/neonate, and should not be prescribed lightly. Like other drugs, they should be avoided during the first trimester of pregnancy.

vitamins and minerals

One of the major contributing factors to illness during pregnancy is the lack of good nutrition prior to pregnancy as well as during pregnancy. One of the major teaching responsibilities of nurses is to help patients understand the necessity for good food habits and to guide them in choosing and preparing foods.

Helping the patient to understand how important proper nutrition is for her own health and particularly for the health and growth of her baby may require more than merely telling her she should eat properly every day. But even with encouragement, repetition of teaching, and help, many patients do not get their necessary daily vitamins and minerals and may need vitamin supplement therapy.

No vitamins or minerals should be taken without the direction of the physician. Without this precaution women who have been on fad diets may take "therapeutic" doses ten times more potent than prenatal doses. Special care should be taken to prevent ingestion of excessive amounts of fat-soluble vitamins A and D, which have been linked to fetal anomalies.

Some of the supplemental vitamins and minerals prescribed during pregnancy include the following:

Natabec Kapseals—multivitamin and mineral supplement with iron (ferrous sulfate) and calcium
Natabec R Kapseals—same as Natabec Kapseals plus folic acid
Natalins tablets—multivitamins and folic acid, iron and calcium
Ferrous sulfate,—200- and 300-mg enteric-coated tablets of iron
Ferrous gluconate (Fergon)—tablets, 300 mg iron

Vitron-C—ferrous fumarate, 200 mg, and ascorbic acid, 125 mg
Iron dextran injection (Imferon)—50 mg iron per milliliter.

iron Any patient receiving iron orally should be informed that dark greenish-black stools are to be expected. Some patients experience constipation or a laxative effect when taking iron. Although this is a side effect of iron, if the iron is begun on a low dose and gradually brought to the normal level, most women can adjust to it. Occasionally, the pregnant woman may have to discontinue the medication for several days and then restart (see Chap. 22 for a complete discussion of anemia). When liquid iron preparation is ordered, it should be given through a straw, well diluted to prevent staining of the teeth. Iron preparations should not be given with milk, as it prevents the absorption of iron. Iron preparations can also be administered before meals or between meals for maximum absorption.

Intramuscular iron is prescribed for the woman who does not respond to oral iron therapy. Improperly injected, iron dextran stains the subcutaneous tissue for 6 to 12 months. Deep intramuscular injection by the Z-track technique (with a needle that is long enough to reach muscle) is necessary to prevent staining. This is performed as follows:

1 Use a double-needle technique (one needle to draw up medication, another for injection).
2 Add 0.5 mL air to syringe after measuring dose. (Air provides a "plug" to seal off medication in muscle.)
3 Before injecting, twist skin away from site (always use the gluteus medius muscle).
4 After insertion, aspirate. (Iron is dark brown; therefore, increase in the volume in the syringe is the only indicator of the presence of blood.) Inject slowly.

5 Wait 10 s, remove needle, allow skin to return to normal location.
6 Do not massage the site.
7 Rotate sites to avoid tissue injury (never inject in deltoid or vastus lateralis muscles). (See Fig. 20-3.)

calcium The daily calcium requirement in pregnancy is 1200 mg. Since fetal bone formation requires extra calcium, every pregnant woman should drink at least 1 qt of milk per day. However, many pregnant women do not like milk or do not drink the required amount of milk. For this reason, physicians sometimes prescribe calcium during pregnancy as a nutritional supplement. Calcium is also prescribed for women who experience muscle spasms as a result of calcium-phosphorus imbalance. Milk intake is curtailed because milk contains phosphorus as well as calcium.

The following drugs contain calcium:

Natabec Kapseals—with calcium carbonate, 600 mg
Natalins—with calcium carbonate, 625 mg
Calcium gluconate—300 mg tablets
Calcium lactate—300- and 600-mg tablets

Calcium is also available in powdered form.

Other specific vitamins or minerals may be ordered by the physician according to the particular dietary deficiency or blood sample results.

DRUGS USED DURING LABOR AND DELIVERY

Although labor is a normal physiologic process for the healthy female, it does involve a degree of stress and discomfort, and for these reasons, certain tranquilizers and analgesics have proved useful. Because of the intimate

fig. 20-3 Z-track technique. (*a*) Skin layers. (*b*) Pull skin and top fatty layer to side. (*c*) Inject and wait 10 s. (*d*) Release skin when needle is withdrawn. (*e*) Do not massage.

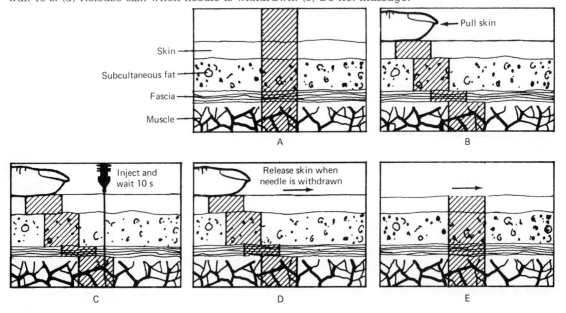

dependence of the fetus upon maternal circulation, whatever drug effect the mother experiences is also experienced by the infant. The placental barrier is not a barrier to most analgesics, sedatives, or anesthetics. Furthermore, the infant receives the maternal dosage, which usually will *equilibrate,* or become equalized on both sides of the placenta. If separated from the maternal processes of drug metabolism and excretion before the drug is totally excreted, the fetus will be born with an excessive dose of the particular drug in its system. Therefore, any substance which, by central action on the brain, relieves maternal pain and anxiety will also affect the fetus.

dose-time relationship

If drugs are to be used, the problems to be considered in every case are both the dose and the timing of the dose. Dosage affects the degree to which maternal responses are affected. Maternal CNS depression leads to respiratory depression of varying levels. If hypoxia results, the oxygen supply to the fetus is reduced. With large doses, maternal metabolic processes may be overwhelmed, and more free drug will then be available to pass to the fetus. For instance, fetal levels rise to 70 percent of maternal levels within 6 min of high intravenous meperidine dosage.[8] The intramuscular route demonstrates a slower uptake in the fetus and less placental transfer and may be the route of choice very early in labor. However, if small doses of such a drug are given intravenously and repeated once within 5 or 10 min, optimal effects will be achieved.[9]

Timing of the dose prior to delivery is hard to determine but important. The aim is to avoid birth during the peak period when drug effects are greatest. However, if birth occurs before a dose is transferred, or 3 to 4 h after

a dose, then the metabolic processes can control maternal levels reaching the fetus, or remove the drug from the fetal circulation.

Any infant born affected by analgesia and anesthesia must be observed in the nursery for delayed excretion of the drug. In addition, bonding must be especially supported during the recovery period.

The primary factors affecting the type of medication chosen during labor are determined by monitoring the fetal heart rate as a reflection of fetal condition and by the progress of labor as judged by the length, strength, and frequency of contractions and the descent of the fetus.

narcotic analgesics

Narcotics are used during labor to produce analgesic and hypnotic effects in the patient by means of central nervous system depression. The sensation of pain is alleviated or reduced but may not be completely obliterated.

Meperidine (Demerol) is most commonly used for women in labor to produce analgesia and relaxation. Aside from nausea in some patients, there are few maternal side effects provided that dosages are calculated to meet the needs and tolerance of each patient. A single intravenous dose may cause contractions to be felt less intensely for a period, but the work of the uterine muscle will continue, causing dilation and effacement of the cervix. Nurses should be alert to this factor and carefully note other signs of progress so that they are not surprised by a delivery when the patient suddenly appears to awake from the medication. When meperidine is used in conjunction with tranquilizers, the dose is usually halved because of the potentiated analgesic effect.

If meperidine is administered 1 to 2 h (IV) or 2 to 3 h (IM) before delivery, the high level in the maternal circulation may unduly depress the infant. This depressant effect is exaggerated in an immature preterm infant. Meperidine has been demonstrated to reduce significantly the cord blood oxygen level, and it therefore appears to contribute adversely to the normal biochemical asphyxia present at birth. Certainly, obvious signs of depression are seen in the nursery when a sleepy baby does not suck well for several days, when there is an excessive amount of mucus during the first 24 h of life, and when the infant does not respond with quick reflexes to neuromuscular tests. Recent research indicates that meperidine metabolites have a somewhat toxic effect on fetal nerve tissue; therefore, *high* doses, even if given early in labor, are not recommended. Brackbill and associates studied the long-term effects of obstetric medication on infant learning responses and have found subtle biochemical effects of meperidine metabolites, effects which persist in the newborn period. The long-term results of such biochemical effects are not yet known, however.[10]

A drug which is related to meperidine, *alphaprodine* (Nisentil) produces a rapid-acting analgesia with a short duration of 2 h when given intramuscularly, or 0.5 to 1 h when given intravenously. Its action lies somewhere between that of meperidine and that of morphine, with a greater potential for fetal respiratory depression. The last dose should be give more than 2 h before birth, and naloxone should be available.

Morphine sulfate is a most powerful central nervous system depressant. It has only rare use in obstetrics—e.g., to put to rest the overtaxed uterine muscle when hypertonic uterine dysfunction occurs. It is also used to control convulsions of eclamptic patients until appropriate treatment can be instituted.

Morphine crosses the placenta rapidly to depress the respiratory center of the fetus. If the drug has been used within 4 h of delivery,

apnea may be present at birth, and resuscitation will then be necessary. Other analgesics in current use are listed in Table 20-2.

narcotic antagonists

Narcotics used during labor, or present in the mother's circulation prior to delivery in cases of narcotic addiction, can cause *narcosis* in the newborn. Severely narcotized infants at birth are in respiratory difficulty and experience apnea and asphyxia. The interference with the respiratory center function results in biochemical asphyxia with hypoxia, hypercapnia, and a lower pH.

Naloxone hydrochloride (Narcan) is a narcotic antagonist which lacks the opiate or morphinelike qualities of the other narcotic antagonists, e.g., nalorphine hydrochloride (Nalline), especially. Because it has no side effects except nausea and vomiting in rare instances and produces no respiratory depression if given alone, naloxone has replaced nalorphine as the drug of choice to prevent narcosis in the infant. It acts to combat central nervous system depression and respiratory depression.

Naloxone can be administered intravenously, intramuscularly, or subcutaneously. When given intravenously, the drug usually acts within 1 or 2 min. If no response is evident, the dose may be repeated intravenously. If after two or three doses no response is evident, further investigation or other resuscitative actions are necessary. The dose is 0.01 mg/kg for the neonate. The mother may be given the drug prior to delivery in doses of 0.4 mg. Since the degree of placental transfer is unpredictable, resuscitative measures should be prepared for in the infant. If the mother is addicted to opiatelike drugs (heroin, methadone, etc.), acute narcotic withdrawal symptoms may occur in the infant; thus, such factors need to be known before administration. See Chap. 29 for a discussion of drug withdrawal in the infant.

antianxiety agents

Anxiety, along with anticipation, is part of the emotional state during labor. Tranquilizers have proved to be useful adjuncts during the labor process by alleviating the patient's anxiety without impairing her mental acumen. The most commonly used tranquilizers in labor are hydroxyzine, an antihistamine, and the phenothiazines, promazine (Sparine), promethazine (Phenergan), and propiomazine (Largon). All these agents potentiate the effects of a narcotic while relieving anxiety and apprehension and reducing nausea and vomiting. Both hydroxyzine and promethazine have strong antihistaminic effects, producing extra sedation as well as being very effective antiemetics (see Table 20-2).

Until the recent discovery that diazepam (Valium) had an adverse effect on newborn temperature control, the drug was commonly used during labor as an antianxiety agent. Now it is utilized only when timing would prevent passage across the placenta, i.e., on the delivery table. Studies have shown that within 12 min after intravenous administration, the level of diazepam was higher in cord blood than in maternal plasma. The drug accumulates in fetal brain, lungs, heart, and liver and, because it is highly protein-bound, is excreted very slowly in the newborn period. The time in which half of the drug is metabolized ranges between 21 to 45 h.[11] The remainder is not completely eliminated for up to 8 to 10 days in the infant. The younger the infant's gestational age, the more hazardous are the effects of diazepam; prolonged lethargy, hypotonia, hypoactivity, respiratory depression, and failure to suck have lasted up to 72 h after birth. If subjected to cold stress, the metabolic adjustments needed to restore temperature were poorly utilized by the young infant. In addition, even in a thermoneutral environment, a number of the infants studied had rectal temperatures of 35°C or below in the first 12 h.[12]

barbiturates

Barbiturates are rarely used to sedate the actively laboring patient because the adverse effects on the newborn are widely recognized. These effects include long-term depression of newborn responses and delayed maternal bonding with a sleepy, slowly responding infant. In addition, sucking is depressed, so that the early feeding experiences frustrate the mother.

Barbiturates have been useful as sedatives when given in small doses to the preeclamptic patient or to the hospitalized antepartum patient not in labor. Whenever enough time elapses for complete maternal metabolism and excretion of the drug, there is little carryover for the infant. However, when a drug such as phenobarbital has been used for extended periods in a preeclamptic or epileptic patient, doses of potentiating drugs must be reduced and the infant must be observed for possible withdrawal symptoms for 5 to 7 days after birth (see Chap. 29).

anticholinergics

Scopolamine, 0.2 to 0.6 mg (gr 1/320 to 1/100), IM or IV, is an anticholinergic commonly used as a preoperative medication to dry secretions of the oropharyngeal passages. In obstetrics, scopolamine has not been used primarily for this action but for a side effect of *amnesia*; when combined with a narcotic analgesic, the result is *twilight sleep*. The number (formerly great) of patients receiving twilight sleep has diminished in the last few years because of noted side effects.

Scopolamine lasts longer in the body than a narcotic and, as the analgesic effect diminishes, can cause excitation, delirium, and restlessness. Because of amnesia and lack of conscious control, patients may become difficult to manage; they must be kept under close observation and, in some cases, restrained. Many women are frightened by the stories they may have heard about "wild talking" under twilight sleep; others react with satisfaction to "not remembering a thing." As more public education about childbirth becomes available, most women prefer to be awake for their deliveries. Twilight sleep may be useful for a small number of extremely frightened patients.

Scopolamine raises fetal and maternal heart rates and smooths out the normal beat-to-beat variations as seen on the monitor record (Chap. 27); it thus can seriously mask fetal distress. Extreme thirst is the chief complaint of the mother. For these reasons, the use of this drug is decreasing.

ANESTHESIA

The word *anesthesia* indicates that the area affected will have no sensation. Anesthetics may provide local or regional numbness with loss of sensation to pain, or they may result in generalized muscle relaxation and loss of sensation because of varying degrees of central nervous system depression.

During labor, pain of uterine contractions and cervical dilatation is transmitted to the posterior roots of the eleventh and twelfth thoracic nerves. Pain of descent and expulsion of the fetus travels by way of the afferent fibers of the second, third, and fourth sacral nerves (see Fig. 20-4). At the same time, muscle innervation must continue uninterrupted. A balance must be sought between reducing pain effectively without obliterating nerve impulses to the muscles of the uterus.

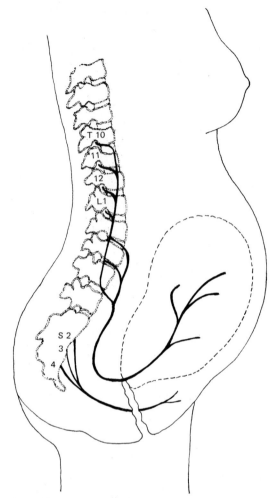

fig. 20-4 Pathways of pain in labor. (*Adapted from John Bonica, Mechanisms and Pathways of Pain in Labor, courtesy of Abbott Laboratories.*)

Local anesthetics have been used effectively after active labor has begun. Preparations such as lidocaine, mepivacaine, dubucaine and bupivacaine are *amides,* most of which are metabolized slowly and transfer fairly easily across the placental membrane. *Esters,* procaine, chloroprocaine, tetracaine, and cocaine are metabolized swiftly but are used less commonly now than is a newly developed ester, nesacaine. Although quite effective for the mother when utilized for local or regional anesthesia, local anesthetics may cause some problems in the infant, depending on the rate of transfer across the placenta. The major adverse effect in the fetus has been myocardial depression, resulting in bradycardia of varying degrees. After birth, depending again on dose-time intervals, the infant may demonstrate some differences in muscle tone and control; there may be greater irritability and decreased motor maturity.[13]

adverse effects

Primarily, local anesthetics cause varying degrees of vasodilatation with resultant hypotension. If absorbed in very large amounts, there can be central nervous system stimulation with excitement, apprehension, disorientation, tremors, and rarely, convulsions. Hypersensitivity may occur involving allergic dermatitis, asthmatic attack, or an anaphylactoid reaction. Because of this possibility, test doses are always used prior to full injection. Patients should be asked about prior experiences with local anesthesia as well.

local infiltration

A local anesthetic is injected into the tissues around the area to be anesthetized. *Local infiltration* provides a pain-free area for an episiotomy or repair of lacerations. A few minutes for absorption must be allowed before the procedure begins. Mild reactions include dizziness, palpitations, and headache. The mother may be apprehensive about episiotomy repair, as she will sense the tugging and pulling of the surrounding tissue and will expect to feel pain, an anxiety similar to that experienced during dental work. A simple explanation that she will have these sensations may help her to relax during suturing.

regional anesthesia

Anesthetics may be injected to block a group of nerves leading to a region of the body. Medication is injected into or around a nerve pathway or at the plexus of the nerve.

paracervical block The paracervical block anesthetizes the hypogastric plexus and ganglia and provides relief from the pain of cervical dilation, especially during the active phase of labor. The injection is made through the vagina at each side of the cervix; care is taken to aspirate before injecting because of the increased supply of blood vessels in the lower uterine area (Fig. 20-5a).

Anesthesia is effective for 1 to 2 h. Untoward effects are seen as fetal bradycardia, because of the rapid transfer of the drug across the placenta. Thus, careful monitoring of the FHT (fetal heart tone) is essential after paracervical block. Recovery to the normal rate should take place within 5 min. Should a fetus demonstrate persistent bradycardia—longer than 15 to 18 min—a cesarean section may be indicated for fetal distress. Because adverse effects are common (30 to 50 percent), this route is used infrequently.

pudendal block The pudendal block is an effective regional anesthetic for the second stage of labor and for the delivery. The pudendal nerve plexus lies just above and behind the ischial spine, and the nerve itself supplies sensation to the whole perineal area. A block done just before delivery is effective throughout the delivery and episiotomy repair (Fig. 20-5b).

Untoward effects are not seen in the infant. This safe method of anesthesia may not be completely effective for the mother if the injection is slightly out of place. A time period of 5 to 10 min after injecting the anesthetic is preferred to allow for complete numbing of the area. Recovery will take place within an hour.

table 20-2 Analgesics/sedatives/tranquilizers used during labor

narcotics

agent	dosage	effect begins/duration	maternal effects	fetal effects
Meperidine (Demerol, Pethidine)	30–100 mg IM. Doses of 25 mg IV, diluted in 5 mL normal saline. Dose reduced if given with tranquilizer.	10–20 min/2–3 h. 3–5 min/1.5–2 h. (SC administration not advised.) 70 to 90% relief of pain, and sedation.	Delays labor progress if dose excessive; may enhance labor for some. Nausea/vomiting, hypotension, some respiratory depression, urine retention.	Rapid placental transmission, possible CNS depression, respiratory depression. In newborn, large doses result in lowered oxygen saturation. Metabolites hinder adaptation to stimuli for more than 1 mo.
Alphaprodine (Nisentil)	40–50 mg SC. 15–20 mg IV.	10 min/2–3 h. 3 to 5 min/1.5–2 h. 70 to 90% relief of pain, and sedation.	Delays labor if given too early or with excessive dose. Enhances labor for some. Similar to meperidine in effect but shorter duration.	Rapid placental transmission, but since shorter duration of action in mother, if dose-time interval is observed, may not affect infant as much in newborn period. Studies incomplete.
Anileridine (Leritine)	30–40 mg SC. 20–40 mg IM. 15–20 mg IV.	15–30 min/4–5 h. 10–20 min/2.5–4 h. 3–5 min/2–3 h. Less sedation and sleep than meperidine.	Similar to meperidine but short duration of side effects: respiratory depression, hypotension. Some antiemetic and antitussive effects.	Depressant effects on fetus may be more severe than meperidine, in equigesic doses. Must have Narcan available.
Morphine	8–10 mg SC. 3–5 mg IV (diluted in 5 mL normal saline; give slowly over 2–3 min).	15–30 min/4–5 h. 3–5 min/1.5–2 h. Very effective relief of pain, plus sedation. Occasionally used for CNS sedation in severe preeclampsia.	Given in equigesic doses, morphine is no more depressing than other narcotics; time-dose interval before birth is critical, therefore SC route with high doses is not commonly used. Side effects of nausea/vomiting, slower respirations, hypotension; urinary retention may require intervention.	Rapid placental transmission, CNS depression in high doses. Respiratory depression counteracted by Narcan. Observe infant 2 to 3 h after delivery because action of Narcan may diminish before morphine effect is gone.

Drug	Dosage/Route	Action, Onset/Duration	Effects on labor	Effects on infant
Oxymorphone (Numorphan)	0.75–1.5 mg SC (postop only). 0.5–1.0 mg IM. 0.5–0.75 mg IV.	15–30 min/4–5 h. 10–20 min/2.5–4 h. 3–5 min/1.5–2 h. Pain relief and sedation.	Similar effects as morphine. Maternal respiratory depression may delay labor if given too early or in too large doses. Note that SC doses not recommended during active labor since duration is so long.	Similar to morphine effects.
barbiturates Used only in very early labor to provide sleep				
Secobarbital (Seconal)	50–200 mg PO.	20–30 min/4–5 h. Sleep and sedation, no analgesic or amnesic action. May enhance sensation of pain if given without analgesia during labor.	No effects on progress of labor but must be given so that drug is completely metabolized before time of birth. Depressive effect on respirations and circulatory system with higher doses.	If in infant's system, attention depressed for 2 to 4 days after birth. Enhances enzymes in microsomal portion of liver. Other drugs may be affected as well as bilirubin metabolism speeded.
Pentobarbital (Nembutal)	50–200 mg PO.	20–30 min/4–5 h. Sleep and sedation, no analgesic or amnesic action.	No effects on progress of labor. Drug must have time to be completely metabolized before time of birth.	If in infant's system, attention depressed for 2 to 4 days after birth. Enhances microsomal function of liver, thus metabolizing other drugs faster.
antianxiety agents				
Promethazine (Phenergan)	25–50 mg IM. 12.5–25 mg IV.	15–20 min/3–4 h. 3–5 min/2–3 h. Antihistaminic action adds extra sedation with narcotic. Potentiates narcotic; if given with narcotic, reduce dosage.	Stimulates respirations, decreases nausea/vomiting. Some disorientation, hypotension, tachycardia may occur. No effect on labor progress.	CNS depression, equilibrates with maternal level within 15 min (IV route). Transitional effects depend on level and time of dose.
Promazine (Sparine)	25–50 mg IM. 25 mg IV.	15–20 min/3–4 h. 3–5 min/2–3 h.	Effective in combination with narcotic. Labile hypotension may occur. Other effects as Phenergan.	CNS depression. Into fetal circulation by 4 min (IV route). Transitional effects depend on level and time of dose.

table 20-2 Analgesics/sedatives/tranquilizers used during labor (continued)

agent	dosage	effect begins/duration	maternal effects	fetal effects
Hydroxyzine HCl (Vistaril)	50–100 mg IM only.	15–20 min/3–4 h.	Reduces nausea, some sedation; potentiates narcotic, reduce dose by 50%.	CNS depression. In high doses, observe for infant sedation.
Propiomazine (Largon)	20–40 mg IM. 20–40 mg IV.	15–20 min/3–4 h. 3–5 min/2–3 h.	Avoid combination in syringe with other drugs. Same effects as above agents.	Minimal CNS depression.
Diazepam (Valium)	5–10 mg IM. 5–10 mg IV, by slow IV push. Well diluted in plain 5% dextrose in water to avoid injury to vein. Do not mix with other solutions.	10–15 min/5–6 h. Only given IM after delivery. 3–5 min/4–5 h. Only given just before delivery so does not cross to fetus. Sedation, hypnosis used as an induction agent for procedures other than delivery.	Not recommended in last few weeks of pregnancy or in first trimester (reports of cleft lip/palate). Low doses should have no maternal side effects; rarely, excitement, hallucinations, hypotension.	More than 30 mg within 15 h of delivery results in low Apgar, apnea. Higher doses concentrate in infant, affect thermoregulation, feeding up to 1 week. Since long half-life, effects persist. May interfere with bilirubin protein binding.

Source: Adapted from S. Anderson, "Labor and Delivery," in *McGraw-Hill Handbook of Clinical Nursing*, McGraw-Hill, New York, 1978, chap. 8.

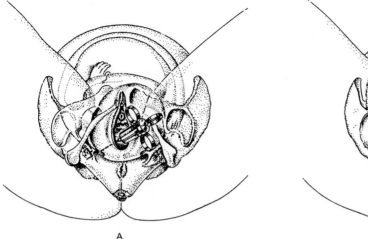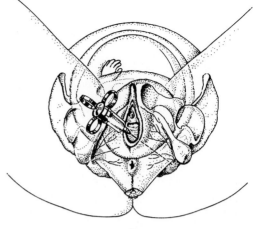

A   B

fig. 20-5 (a) Paracervical block. (b) Pudendal block. (*From Anesthesia in Obstetrics, Clinical Education Aid, No. 17, courtesy of Ross Laboratories.*)

peridural anesthesia Peridural anesthesia (outside the dura) is administered into the bony spinal canal without the needle penetrating through the dura into the spinal fluid itself. The local anesthetic surrounds the nerves as they exit from the spinal cord. Epidural and caudal routes are both peridural. Signs of effective anesthesia will be seen as the sensation diminishes in the uterus, cervix, and perineum. The lower extremities become tingly and flushed as vasodilation results. Motor control is weak but not absent in the legs unless the larger amounts needed for an operative delivery are injected.

Because of vasodilation, blood may pool in the extremities, causing maternal hypotension. The immediate treatment is to elevate both legs, in order to return blood to the central circulation. The patient is then turned on her side to reduce uterine pressure on the veins of the pelvic area. Intravenous fluids to maintain adequate blood volume and oxygen by mask to ensure fetal oxygenation are part of the available treatment for hypotension. Fetal bradycardia may result from the primary effect of the drug or as a result of maternal hypotension. Other effects may be dizziness, nausea, and a pounding heart.

CAUDAL BLOCK The injection is made through the opening at the lower end of the sacrum, the *sacral cornua*. The patient must be in a lateral Sims's position. After positioning and explanation, the anesthesiologist inserts a long needle into the caudal space. A test dose of anesthetic solution is injected, and the patient is observed for 5 min for changes in vital signs or any untoward response. The full dose is then administered slowly and the needle withdrawn. If a continuous caudal block is planned, a plastic catheter would be threaded through the needle and then taped in place after the needle is removed. The continuous method allows a smaller, more frequent dose to be administered throughout the active and advanced active phases and the second stage of labor.

A caudal block may be administered after the active phase of labor has begun. The anesthesia provides a complete lack of awareness of cervical and uterine discomfort. Depending upon dosage, the mother will not sense a full bladder nor know when to push during the second stage. The lack of sensation of bladder fullness may persist into the recovery period.

EPIDURAL BLOCK   The insertion site for an epidural block is through the lower lumbar area. The patient is positioned on her side, with her neck flexed and knees drawn up to the abdomen. The lower part of the back is prepared as for a spinal tap by cleansing with antiseptic solution. Local infiltration into the superficial tissues with anesthetic precedes the insertion of a needle into the epidural space. A small plastic catheter is then inserted through the needle and the needle withdrawn. Placement of the catheter allows higher or lower anesthesia. An epidural may thus be utilized for extensive anesthesia for cesarean section (Fig. 20-6).

Recovery care for the patient who has had an epidural block is similar to that for the patient who has had a caudal block. The patient is checked for all the signs of dimin-

ishing anesthesia, toe temperature, ability to maintain a normal blood pressure when sitting up or standing, and a return of complete sensation and an ability to control her legs.

The patient may sit or stand when control has returned to her extremities, but the nurse should watch for postural hypotension, fainting, and difficulty in voiding.

spinal and saddle block   The spinal and saddle block (low spinal) are closely related methods of anesthesia but differ in position of the patient, amount of medication, and area affected. The spinal is used for cesarean sections, as it blocks nerves of the lower part of the body to the level of the sixth or eighth thoracic nerve, just below the diaphragm. The patient is positioned on the side, asked to arch the lower part of her back and to flex her neck and knees. The nurse usually stands in front of the patient to help her hold her head and knees in this position. A spinal anesthetic is administered on the delivery table just prior to the operation (Fig. 20-7).

fig. 20-6   Caudal and epidural anesthesia and saddle block. (*From Clinical Education Aid No. 17, courtesy of Ross Laboratories.*)

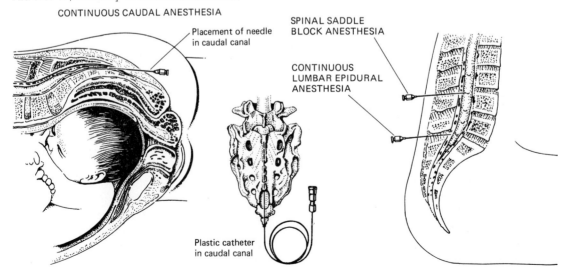

CONTINUOUS CAUDAL ANESTHESIA

Placement of needle in caudal canal

Plastic catheter in caudal canal

SPINAL SADDLE BLOCK ANESTHESIA

CONTINUOUS LUMBAR EPIDURAL ANESTHESIA

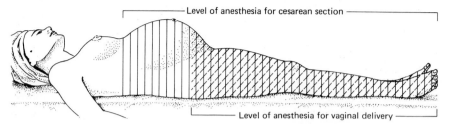

fig. 20-7 Level of anesthesia for vaginal delivery and cesarean section. (*From Clinical Education Aid No. 17, courtesy of Ross Laboratories.*)

SADDLE BLOCK   The saddle block is so named because the parts of the body that would come in contact with a saddle are the parts anesthetized. The saddle block can be administered after the patient has completed effacement and dilation of the cervix. The patient is positioned sitting on the side of the delivery table or bed. The nurse should place a stool so that the patient can support her feet, and arm support should also be provided for the patient while she rounds the lower part of her back for the injection. Since the patient is in the descent phase of labor, the position is most uncomfortable (Fig. 20-6).

After a small amount of anesthetic is administered, the patient is kept in a sitting position for about 1 min to allow for the anesthetic to diffuse downward in the spinal fluid. (The anesthetic has been mixed with a glucose solution so that it sinks to the base of the fluid around the cord.) The patient is then placed in a supine position with a slight lateral tilt, and with a pillow to flex the neck. In about 1 min the effects of the anesthetic become evident. It is during this period that careful observation of vital signs is especially important. Hypotension is a frequent side effect of either spinal or saddle block anesthesia, and vital signs should be observed throughout the delivery and into the recovery period (see Fig. 20-8).

Both methods of anesthesia puncture the dura and may result in a postpuncture headache. It is thought that this headache is caused by a disequilibrium of spinal fluid pressure as a result of seepage via the needle puncture site. With administration by a skilled person using a needle with the smallest possible gauge, and with careful nursing care during recovery, very few patients will experience this problem. The patient who has had a spinal anesthetic is kept flat in bed for up to 8 h; she then ambulates carefully, with the nurse watching for postural hypotension. Personnel on the postpartum unit should be aware of the presence of a patient who has had spinal anesthesia so that they do not inadvertently change her position before she has recovered.

general anesthesia

General anesthetics are given either by the intravenous route or by inhalation. In effective concentrations, they cause unconsciousness by depression of the central nervous system. General anesthesia continues to be one of the leading causes of maternal death because of complications such as vomiting and aspiration during anesthesia, and maternal hypotension. Preanesthetic preparation is often not possible for the mother in labor, so that vomiting can be a real danger. Digestion and stomach emptying slow naturally during labor, so that even if food and fluids were last taken several hours before admission, the mother may be a poor candidate. Patients who are to

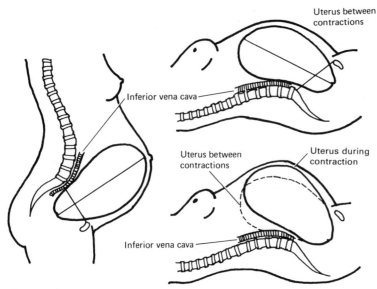

Uterus between contractions

Inferior vena cava

Uterus between contractions

Uterus during contraction

Inferior vena cava

fig. 20-8 Vena cava syndrome. The large uterus presses upon the vena cava as it lies beside the bony spine. When anesthesia relaxes the veins, the effect is aggravated. Turning the woman to her side relieves pressure, and blood pressure returns to normal. (*Adapted from John J. Bonica, Principles and Practice of Obstetric Analgesia and Anesthesia, Davis, Philadelphia, 1967, p. 32.*)

have general anesthesia must not be given foods or liquids by mouth during labor, and the last time that food was ingested must be carefully recorded for the information of the anesthesiologist. An antacid is routinely administered during labor to raise the gastric pH. Should vomiting and aspiration occur, the gastric acids would then not be as destructive to respiratory tissue.

Perhaps because of this danger, general anesthetics are rarely used today for normal deliveries; when used they are administered just before the actual delivery of the fetal head, and a rather light level of anesthesia is produced. Because whatever is injected or inhaled will pass quickly into the fetal circulation and depress the fetal respiratory center, anesthesia is induced rapidly, with the anesthetist keeping record of the length of time that the infant is subjected to the drug.

Of the available general anesthetics, nitrous oxide, methoxyflurane, and cyclopropane are most commonly used in obstetrics. Precautions against static in the area of inhalation anesthetics and oxygen are set up in each delivery area: conductive shoes; grounded metal fixtures and appliances; conductive rubber mattresses and pads on the table. Each person entering the delivery room wears conductive shoes or boots over shoes to reduce the possibility of static sparking.

recovery Recovery from general anesthetics is gradual and depends upon the depth of anesthesia. The patient should be protected from harm if confusion or restlessness occurs. Side rails are always to be in place. Hypotension is a possibility in recovery, and pain perception may be distorted. When the patient first requests pain medication, it should be given in half doses to prevent a possible hypotensive effect. Smooth-muscle activity may be affected, with slowed gastrointestinal motility, or some difficulty in voiding.

Vomiting and aspiration are always a danger, even during recovery. Although the patient has had no food or liquids by mouth and perhaps received an anticholinergic drug preoperatively to suppress secretions, suction equipment must always be available. The patient should be on her side or at least with her head turned to the side, so that aspiration will not occur if vomiting takes place.

DRUGS USED TO STIMULATE UTERINE CONTRACTIONS

oxytocics

Oxytocin injection (Pitocin and Syntocinon) (10 units/mL), acts on the smooth muscles of the uterus to stimulate contractions. From 3 to 10 units are diluted in 500 or 1000 mL. of Ringer's lactate or 5 percent dextrose in water. In order to have absolute control of the amount infused intravenously, a 5 percent dextrose-in-water intravenous solution should be started and the oxytocic added to a piggyback solution, i.e., the oxytocic is added to a second intravenous solution which is connected via a special insert to the first intravenous solution. The oxytocic solution is always controlled and titrated by the physician; the rate of administration is increased very slowly. As the uterine muscle begins to contract, the rate is adjusted according to the frequency, duration, and intensity of the contractions. As much as 40 drops/min may be given to stimulate beginning contractions; as time elapses the muscle will become more sensitive to the oxytocic solution and the rate

of administration must be slowed or the oxytocic discontinued as the status of labor warrants. (See Chap. 26 for nursing responsibility during induction.)

Constant monitoring of the fetus is very important. Contractions lasting more than 100 s, or more frequent than 2 min apart, will impair placental circulation and cause hypoxia in the fetus. These *hypertonic contractions* may cause the uterine muscle to tear, rupture, or become exhausted.

Ideally, infusion machinery such as the *Sage intravenous infusion pump,* the *Ivac peristaltic pump,* or the *Harvard pump* should be used to control the rate of infusion of intravenous solution and/or medication.

Postdelivery, involution normally does not require the use of drugs to be initiated nor to be sustained. If necessary, oxytocics are used to stimulate the uterine muscle, causing it to contract the open sinuses at the site of placental separation from the endometrium, to aid in preventing undue bleeding.

Oxytocin (Pitocin, Syntocinon). From 1 to 2 mL (10 to 20 units) is added to the IV solution left in the bottle after the time of delivery, and the rate of flow is increased to 20 to 40 drops/min, after the delivery of the placenta.

Ergonovine maleate (Ergotrate), 0.2 mg, orally, intramuscularly, or intravenously. Ergotrate causes the uterus to contract forcibly for a long period. An intravenous or intramuscular injection of ergotrate is given, therefore, *only when it is certain that the placenta is detached* and well into the process of explusion. Ergotrate may be given orally to sustain the uterine muscle in good contraction for the first 24 h after delivery, 0.2 mg is usually ordered every 4 h for six doses.

Ergotrate has been known to cause elevated blood pressure because of its vasoconstricting (smooth-muscle) effect. Therefore, the drug is *never* administered to patients with hypertension or preeclampsia.

Methylergonovine maleate (Methergine),

0.2 mg, orally, intramuscularly, or intravenously. Its action is similar to that of Ergotrate; it is contraindicated in patients with any sign of elevated blood pressure.

Injectable Ergotrate and Methergine should be refrigerated, since they deteriorate with age and exposure to heat and light.

prostaglandins

First identified in semen, prostaglandins (17 have been identified) have been subsequently found in many body tissues. Since they appear in higher than normal levels during labor and in amniotic fluid, their role in initiating or sustaining labor is being recognized and applied. Many therapeutic and adverse effects result from contraction of smooth muscle (especially PGF_2). Since these substances are so widely distributed, and their effects so numerous, they are still under study. Clinical use is limited to research centers (see Chap. 22).

DRUGS AND LACTATION

hormones to prevent lactation

The breasts have been prepared throughout pregnancy for the task of nourishing the newborn infant. When the placenta detaches from the wall of the uterus, there is an abrupt halt in the secretion of the placental hormones, particularly estrogen and progesterone. This seems to trigger the release of the lactogenic hormone, setting in motion the activities preparatory to milk production. However, many women want to feed their babies by bottle rather than by breast and wish to halt the lactation process. In order to do this, drugs may be prescribed, if necessary, and binders, ice packs, and/or analgesics may be helpful

to relieve her discomfort. Estrogen and progestational agents, as well as androgens, are capable of suppressing lactation, but estrogens are most frequently used, either alone or in combination with the other hormones. See Table 20-3 for a list of drugs that suppress lactation.

Before any agent to suppress lactation is given, several points must be checked:

1 Be sure the patient is *not* going to breast-feed.
2 Before any estrogenic product is given, check the patient for contraindications. Do not give if there is a history of reproductive tract cancer or hepatic, renal, or cardiac disease (including thrombophlebitis).
3 Hormones must be given as close to delivery as possible. Injections may be given just prior to placental separation. Oral agents should be given as early in the postpartum period as possible. Be sure the patient has reacted before giving her any oral medication.
4 If medication is to be continued at home, instruct the patient in the medication schedule.

drug excretion in breast milk

After decades of interest in bottle-feeding, the pendulum seems to be swinging in the other direction. A number of women are returning to breast-feeding, and physicians are recommending breast milk for its special qualities (see Chap. 16). The interest appears to parallel the growing concern in women to know what is happening in their bodies. Pregnant women especially want to know what affects their bodies during pregnancy, delivery, and recovery. Increasingly, they are asking questions about the safety of medication.

Nurses are challenged as they distribute medication and are questioned about the necessity of taking the drug and the effect on the infant. The nurse must have access to knowledge and resources on the subject to satisfy the patients' inquiries.

Drugs will transfer into breast milk in various amounts depending upon a number of factors. Especially important are the drugs' fat solubility, molecular weight, protein-binding capacity, and the pH and the fat content of the milk at that particular feeding.

Colostrum is low in fat content, and thus lipid-soluble drugs may be less concentrated there. Breast milk itself varies in fat content from 2 to 7 percent, depending on the time of day and whether the milk is the hind or fore milk. There is generally a higher concentration of fat in milk at midmorning and less in the early morning. Hind milk has a greater concentration af fat than the first part of the feeding, i.e., fore milk. Therefore, drugs with greater lipid solubility (such as barbiturates) would be found in greater concentration in hind milk.

Other factors which influence the passage of drugs include the concentration of the drug in maternal circulation in relation to the concentration in the breast milk; the higher concentration will move to the lower. Finally, the dosage level and the duration of drug intake will affect the amount of drug in milk.

If the mother is in poor health because of either liver or kidney dysfunction, drugs may not be metabolized or excreted normally, and the breast may become an organ of excretion, with excessive amounts entering the milk. Thus, breast-feeding is contraindicated in those cases.

If drugs must be prescribed for the breast-feeding mother, several guidelines may be employed to decrease ingestion by the infant. Have the mother take the medication just *after* a feeding. If the drug is given once a day, it may be prudent to take the drugs after an evening feeding and substitute a bottle for the next feeding. If medication can be delayed until the newborn is a few days older, when enzymatic functioning is better established, adverse effects may be reduced. Of course, the drug that has been shown to have the least side effects in the infant and mother should be employed. See Table 20-4 for a list of drugs which are best avoided during lactation or those that should be used with caution.

DRUGS AND THE NEWBORN INFANT

Fetology, the study of the fetus in its environment, is seeking, through extensive research, to determine the effects of nutrition, organisms, disease, chemicals, radiation, and other stresses on the development of the fetus. Amniocentesis, intrauterine treatment such as transfusion, and fetal monitoring are providing clues to the world of the fetus. *Teratology,* the study of the changes in a fetus resulting from environmental effects, is developing as a separate discipline.

Drugs may cause irreparable harm and fetal death, or may influence only one small part of the developing baby. Drug-induced defects in the infant are thought to be the cause of 2 to 3 percent of all congenital anomalies. The longer-lasting, more subtle effects some drugs may cause are not included in this figure. Some drugs may not change body structure but may be *fetotoxic,* causing metabolic changes, electrolyte imbalance, central nervous system or respiratory depression, and (in the case of narcotic addiction or alcoholism) withdrawal symptoms in the newborn.

The concept of a "placental barrier" that protects the fetus from maternal ingestants is

table 20-3 Drugs used to prevent lactation

drug	action	adverse reaction	dose	nursing implications
Chlorotrianisene (Tace, Tace 72)	Nonsteroid estrogen (synthetic); inhibits release of prolactin; prevents breast engorgement.	Occasional: skin rash, nausea, vomiting, edema. Rare: postpartum bleeding requiring treatment.	Tace: 12 mg PO qid for 7 d; 25–50 mg PO q6h for 6 doses, Tace 72: 72 mg PO bid for 2 d.	1. Give first dose just after delivery. 2. Do not give if any question of breast-feeding. 3. Do not give with history of reproductive tract cancer or hepatic, renal, or cardiac disease.
Dienstrol (DV, Restrol, Synestrol)	Same.	Same.	0.5–1.5 mg PO qd for 3 d, then 0.5 mg for 7 d	1. Same as above. 2. Protect from light. 3. Instruct patient on home schedule.
Diethystilbestrol (DES, Stilbestrol)	Same.	More severe and common—anorexia, nausea, vomiting, epigastric distress, diarrhea, dizziness, headache, thirst, anxiety, insomnia. In puerperium, may be associated with thromboembolic disorder.	PO or IM, only postpartum, 5 mg qd or tid to total dose of 30 mg	1. Same as Tace. 2. Do not give if patient has any history of thrombophlebitis.
Ethinyl estradiol (Diogyn-E, Estinyl, Esteed, Eticylol, Feminone)	Same as Tace.	Nausea, vomiting, headache, edema.	0.5–1 mg PO qd for 3 d, then 0.1 mg for 7 d	1. Same as Tace. 2. Remind patient of medication schedule at home.
Piperazine estrone sulfate (Ogen)	Steroid which inhibits prolactin and prevents breast engorgement.	Same as other estrogens.	3.75 mg PO q4h for first 20 h postpartum	Same as above.
Methallenestril (Vallestril)	Same as Tace.	Not as potent as other nonsteroid estrogens; therefore, fewer side effects.	20–40 mg PO qd for 5 d	Same as above.

combination drugs

Methyltestosterone esterified estrogens (Estratest)	Inhibits lactogenic hormone, suppressing lactation.	Minimal because of antagonism of hormones; breast tenderness or hirsutism may occur.	Methyltestosterone: 1.25 mg; esterified estrogens: 2.5 mg 1 tablet tid for 4 d, then 1 tablet qd for 10 d	1. Same as for other estrogens. 2. Remind patient of dosage schedule at home.
Testerone enanthate/estradiol valerate (Deladumone OB, Ditate-DS)	Same as Estratest; premixed in sesame oil for gradual release.	Virilization, incomplete suppression of engorgement. Rare: convulsions, jaundice, pain at injection site, and local dermatitis.	Testosterone: 360 mg; estradiol 16 mg: 2mL IM at onset of second stage or just after delivery.	1. Same as other estrogens. 2. Give via Z-track technique. 3. Store at room temperature. 4. Weight loss is slower after delivery.

other

Pitocin nasal spray	Relieves breast engorgement in non-nursing mothers; in nursing mothers, stimulates "letdown" reflex, thus promoting milk ejection by contracting myoepithelium of mammary glands.	None.	One spray delivers 1.7 units to nasal mucosa.	1. Use 2 to 3 min prior to nursing infant. 2. Intranasal spray most effective route. 3. Useful especially when breasts are so engorged that infant cannot grasp nipple.

Source: From E. J. Dickason, M. O. Schuit, and E. M. Morris, Maternal and Infant Drugs and Nursing Intervention, McGraw-Hill, New York, 1978.

table 20-4 Drugs to avoid in lactation

Analgesics
  Aspirin*
  Heroin†
  Methadone†
  Phenylbutazone*
Anticoagulants
  Bishydroxycoumarin*
  Ethyl biscoumacetate*
  Phenindione†
  Warfarin sodium*
Anticonvulsants
  Phenytoin*
  Primidone†
Antihistamines
  Chlorpheniramine maleate*
Anticholinergics
  Atropine sulfate*
Antihypertensives, diuretics
  Acetazolamide*
  Hexamethonium†
  Reserpine†
  Thiazides†
Anti-infectives
  Amantadine HCl†
  Aminoglycosides*
  Chloramphenicol*
  Erythromycin*
  Isoniazid†
  Mandelic acid†
  Metronidazole†
  Nalidixic acid†
  Novobiocin†
  Sulfonamides*
  Tetracyclines†

Cancer-chemotherapeutic agents†
  Best to discontinue breast-feeding if on chemotherapeutics
Hormones
  Corticosteroids†
  Estrogen, progestins, androgens†
Laxatives
  Aloe*
  Cascara†
  Danthron†
  Senna compounds*
Muscle relaxants
  Carisoprodol†
Oxytoxics
  Ergot preparations†
Psychotropics, psychotherapeutics
  Butyrophenones*
  Chlordiazepoxide*
  Diazepam*
  Imipramine*
  Lithium carbonate†
  Phenothiazines*
Sedatives, hypnotics
  Barbiturates†
  Bromides†
  Glutethimide*
  Meprobamate†
Thyroid and antithyroid preparations
  Carbimazole†
  Methimazone†
  Thiouracil†
  Thyroxine sodium†
Iodides
  ^{131}I (radioactive)†
Other
  Alcohol*
  Caffeine*
  Marijuana†
  Nicotine*
  Lead, mercury†

*Use with caution.
†Best avoided while breast-feeding.
Source: From E. J. Dickason, M. O. Schult, and E. M. Morris, *Maternal and Infant Drugs and Nursing Intervention,* McGraw-Hill, New York, 1978.

no longer valid. It must be assumed that whatever drug or chemical the mother takes the baby also receives and at approximately the *same dosage.* As long as the fetus is connected with its mother via the placental circulation, the drugs that are transferred to the fetus are returned to her circulation for breakdown and excretion. Metabolism and excretion of nontoxic drugs become a problem only when the child is born with the maternal dosage (or a high percentage of it) in its bloodstream. Its liver, kidney, and enzyme functioning will not be mature enough to handle the metabolism of such high drug levels. This immaturity of the metabolic and excretory functions may cause excessive levels of drugs and their metabolites to remain in the infant's body for many days after birth. Brackbill has stated, "Because of the improved technology in modern obstetrics and the proliferation of drugs, a major obstetric danger may now be medication itself."[14]

After being affected by labor analgesia and anesthesia, infants may have prolonged recovery periods. Sucking and feeding behavior may be slow, and extra mucus may be present, especially during the second period of reactivity. The mother finds it more difficult to feed her infant, who requires more stimulation to suck and falls asleep easily. This poor feeding behavior may disrupt the initial intimacy between mother and infant and have a cumulative and lasting effect on the development of the mother–child relationship.[15] The greater the environment demands on the infant, and the more complex the action required of the newborn to cope with these demands, the greater is the difference in quality of performance among infants in terms of their perinatal premedication history.[16]

With the concern over the large number of children in our society with learning disabilities and behavior disturbances, a great deal of attention is being focused on these studies of infant response to medication.

administration of medications

Drugs are administered to the newborn through intravenous, intramuscular, or oral routes, and by instillation. Medications may be instilled into the eyes or occasionally into the ears. With eye medications, care must be taken to place the medication in the conjunctival sac, *not* directly on the pupil. Silver nitrate, the most commonly used eye drug, illustrates this point (see Chap. 15).

Oral medications are administered with a plastic disposable dropper, a rubber-tipped dropper or are placed in a nipple so that the infant can suck the medication. Oral medications are usually given prior to the feeding while the infant is awake and eager to suck. Medication is not generally mixed with the formula unless it is administered by nasogastric or gavage tube, as the taste of the milk may be changed and the infant may refuse to finish the milk. Since such small doses are ordered, medication must be measured by a calibrated dropper or a tuberculin syringe. When medications are administered by dropper, place the dropper tip at the back of the tongue to stimulate the sucking reflex. Hold the baby in the usual feeding position to promote swallowing without aspiration (Fig. 20-9).

Intramuscular administration is usually into the *vastus lateralis,* the major muscle of the quadriceps femoris (Fig. 20-10). Gluteal muscles are not sufficiently developed to be used for injections. Injections into this area could impinge on the sciatic nerve, either directly or by the irritation and swelling resulting from the medication. Since nerve damage sometimes occurs, even when injections are carefully given in the vastus lateralis muscle, it is best to use the oral route whenever possible.

When giving intramuscular injections, the procedure is changed in minor ways from that used for adults. After checking the order and

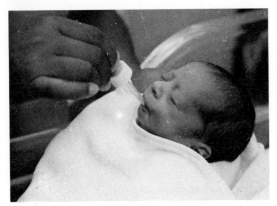

fig. 20-9 Feeding the infant with medication by dropper.

drug, determine the best way to measure the amount (usually a tuberculin syringe is used) and draw up the medication. Check the infant's arm band against the medication card. Paplate the area to determine the injection site (either midanterolateral or upper anterolateral is acceptable). Restrain the leg, and grasp the muscle tissue with one hand, inserting the needle with the other. Nurses need not *thrust* the needle into the muscle, since newborn skin is very tender and the needle readily inserted. Aspirate, and then inject very

fig. 20-10 Intramuscular injection sites for newborn and preterm infants. (*From E. J. Dickason and A. Ritz, Normal Premature Infant, McGraw-Hill, New York, 1970.*)

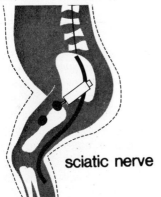

sciatic nerve

slowly. If injection is made too rapidly, the medication enters the surrounding tissue under pressure and causes more swelling and irritation than with slow injection. Each medication is then charted and the infant observed for the effect. Recently, the modified Z-track technique has been proposed for infants who are past the neonatal period.[17]

Intravenous administration may be ordered when the infant cannot retain fluids given orally, when high doses of antibiotics are needed, or when electrolyte or glucose imbalance is present.

A sick infant can become dehydrated very rapidly because of a rapid metabolic rate, immature kidneys that do not efficiently concentrate urine, and a large skin surface in comparison with body weight. The principles of intravenous therapy outlined in Chap. 30 for premature infants are readily applicable for full-term infants as well.

There is no standard dosage of drugs for the newborn, nor any rule for calculating dosages for premature or full-term newborn infants. Empirical evidence, suggestions from the drug companies, laboratory tests, and reports of adverse reactions of a particular drug are but guides for use in calculating dosages of drugs for the newborn. Drug response in the infant is often radically different from that in older children and adults. Factors affecting the response in the newborn are linked to the maturity of the body enzymes and the rate of absorption and route of excretion of the drug. It follows that the less mature the infant, the more difficulty there will be with drug dosage and response.

NURSING RESPONSIBILITIES

The expanding role of nurses should include both assessment and teaching aspects related to pharmacology in maternal and new-born care. As a result of understanding the implications of the wider definition of the teratogenic effects of drugs, nurses must include in their care plans both observation and assessment of drug effects on their patients and teach preventive care. The following steps can be taken to increase awareness and improve assessment and intervention.

1 Education about drugs should be included in antepartum and postpartum classes, as well as for every lactating woman.
2 Explain to each mother who must take a questionable drug the benefit-to-risk ratio for that drug.
3 Counsel all mothers about nonpharmacologic methods for alleviating minor discomforts of pregnancy and recovery.
4 Encourage women to take childbirth classes to help reduce medication levels during delivery, and then support the educated mother in her attempts to cope with labor and delivery.
5 During interview and assessment of the mother on admission to labor, include a record of any incidental nonprescription or prescription drugs taken prior to labor.
6 Inform nursery nurses of any transitional drugs that might affect newborn during recovery. Inform nursery nurses about timing and level of analgesia and anesthesia.
7 Increase ability to assess the newborn for normal behaviorial responses. Records must be more descriptive during the newborn period if long-term behavioral effects of drugs are to be evaluated.
    a Note iatrogenic factors affecting infant's responses.
    b Be alert for delayed excretion, cumulative effects, and altered physiologic states whenever noting drug effects in the newborn.
    c Note and record feeding ability. Check the mother's chart when her infant sucks poorly, falls asleep during feedings consistently, or will not interact with mother.
    d Make every effort to teach the mother how to feed and handle a sleepy baby and when to expect improvement.
    e Increase efforts to support the mother–infant bonding process when the infant is sick and receiving special care or when it is recovering from the effects of delayed excretion of drugs.
    f Support the breast-feeding woman, providing information to answer questions about drug effects on the infant.

When these steps are taken, it should be possible to provide informed nursing support to any woman during pregnancy or recovery and to discover subtle signs of medication influence on the infant.

study questions

1 Why is the first trimester of pregnancy so critical a period in terms of drug effect on the developing fetus?
2 Define the following terms: teratology, organogenesis, benefit-to-risk ratio.
3 What types of teratogenic effects can be caused by drugs? (See Table 20-1.)
4 How may drugs affect the infant during the transitional period?
5 Identify seven points important to the Z-track method of injection. For which types of medication should this technique be used?
6 Distinguish between the terms *anesthesia* and *analgesia*. Why is the time-dose relationship so important?
7 What precautions are always taken before administering a full dose of a local anesthetic?
8 Identify why naloxone has replaced other narcotic antagonists.
9 Before the nurse gives the patient any medication to suppress lactation, certain information about the patient must be checked. List three factors which must be assessed prior to administration.
10 If a drug must be taken during the breast-feeding period, what guidance can be given to the mother regarding reduction of drug effect in the infant?

11 Are there ways you might implement a "drug alert" in your setting while working with pregnant women or later with parents?

16 Brackbill et al., *American Journal of Obstetrics and Gynecology,* op. cit., p. 382.
17 Dickason et al., op. cit., p. 251.
18 Ibid., p. 20.

references

1 E. J. Dickason, M. O. Schult, and E. M. Morris, *Maternal and Infant Drugs and Nursing Intervention,* McGraw-Hill, New York 1978, pp. 1–2.
2 J. O. Fofar, and M. M. Nelson, "Epidemiology of Drugs Taken by Pregnant Women," *Clinical Pharmacology and Therapeutics,* **4:**632, July-August, 1973.
3 *Perinatal Press,* Ross Laboratories, 1976, vol. 1, no. 1, p. 10.
4 W. W. McCrory, Concluding Remarks, in "Symposium on Drugs and the Fetus," *Clinical Pharmacology and Therapeutics,* **14:**700, July-August 1973.
5 B. Schenkel and H. Vorherr, "Non-Prescription Drugs During Pregnancy: Potential Teratogenic and Toxic Risks Upon the Embryo and Fetus," *Journal of Reproductive Medicine,* **12**(1)27: January 1974.
6 Ibid., p. 40.
7 Ibid., p. 44.
8 S. M. Schinder and F. Moya, "Post Graduate Seminar of Anesthesiology," in S. M. Schinder (ed.), *The Anesthesiologist, Mother and Newborn,* Williams & Wilkins, Baltimore, 1974, p. 151.
9 J. S. McDonald, "Preanesthetic and Intrapartal Medications," *Clinical Obstetrics and Gynecology,* **20**(2):447, June 1977.
10 Y. Brackbill, J. Kane, R. L. Maniello, and D. Abramson, "Obstetric Meperidine Usage and Assessment of Neonatal Status," *Anesthesiology,* **40:**116, February 1974.
11 M. Mandelli et al., "Placental Transfer of Diazepam and Its Disposition in the Newborn," *Clinical Pharmacology and Therapeutics,* **17:**564, 1975.
12 J. E. Cree, J. Meyer, and D. M. Haeley: "Diazepam in Labor: Its Metabolism and Effect on the Clinical Condition and Thermogenesis of the Newborn," *British Medical Journal,* **4:**251, 1973.
13 K. Standley, A. B. Soule III, S. A. Copans, and N. S. Duchowney, "Local-Regional Anesthesia During Childbirth: Effect on Newborn Behaviors," *Science,* **186:**635, June 1974.
14 Y. Brackbill, J. Kane, R. L. Maniello, and D. Abramson, "Obstetrics Premedication and Infant Outcome," *American Journal of Obstetrics and Gynecology,* **118**(3):383, 1974.
15 G. Stechler, "Newborn Attention as Affected by Medication During Labor," *Science,* **144:**315, 1964.

bibliography

Anderson, G. G., and G. L. Schooley: "Comparisons of Uterine Contractions in Spontaneous and Oxytocin— or PGF2—Induced Labor" *Obstetrics and Gynecology,* **45:**284–286, March 1975.
Asperheim, M., and L. Eisenhower: *The Pharmacologic Basis of Patient Care,* 2d ed., Saunders, Philadelphia, 1973.
Babson, S. G., and R. C. Benson: *Management of the High-Risk Pregnancy and Intensive Care of the Neonate,* Mosby, St. Louis, 1971.
Baggish, M. S., and S. Hooper: "Aspiration as a Cause of Maternal Death," *Obstetrics and Gynecology,* **43**(2):327, 1974.
Bergerson, B. S., and A. Goth: *Pharmacology in Nursing,* 12th ed., Mosby, St. Louis, 1973.
Bonica, J. J.: "Obstetric Analgesia and Anesthesia: Recent Trends and Advances," *New York Journal of Medicine,* **70**(7):79, 1970.
Bowes, J., Jr., Y. Brackbill, E. Conway, et al.: "The Effects of Obstetrical Medication on the Fetus and Infant," Monograph of the Society of Research in Child Development, **35**(4):137, 1970.
Brackbill, Y.: "Psychophysical Measures of Pharmacological Toxicity in Infants," in P. L. Morselli (ed.), *Basic and Therapeutic Aspects of Perinatal Pharmacology,* Raven Press, New York, 1975.
Brent, R.L.: "Medicolegal Aspects of Teratology," Second Semmelweiss Seminar, New Jersey College of Medicine, September 1976.
Chez, R. A., and A. R. Fleischman: "Fetal Therapeutics—Challenges and Responsibilities," *Clinical Pharmacology and Therapeutics,* **14**(4)(pt. 2):754, 1975.
Dancis, J. (ed.): *Perinatal Pharmacology,* Raven Press, New York, 1974.
Eriksson, M., Charlotte S. Catz, and Sumner J. Yaffee: "Drugs and Pregnancy," *Clinical Obstetrics and Gynecology,* **16**(1):199, March 1973.
Goodman, L. S., and A. Gilman (eds.): *The Pharmacological Basis of Therapeutics,* 5th ed., MacMillan, New York, 1975, pp. 397–401.
Gottshalk, W. (ed.): "Anesthesia in Obstetrics," *Clinical Obstetrics and Gynecology,* **17**(2):139–287, June 1974.
Grad, R. K., and J. Woodside: "Obstetrical Analgesia and Anesthesia," *American Journal of Nursing,* **77:**241, February 1977.

Heinonen, O. P., and D. Slone, and S. Shapiro: *Birth Defects and Drugs in Pregnancy*, PSG Publishing, Littleton, Mass. 1977.

Klaus, M. H. and A. A. Fanaroff, *Care of the High-Risk Neonate*, Saunders, Philadelphia, 1973.

Matthews, A. E. B.: "Drugs in the First Stage of Labor," *Nursing Times*, **63:**648, 1967.

Meyer, M. B., B. S. Jones, and J. A. Tonascia: "Perinatal Events Associated with Maternal Smoking During Pregnancy," *American Journal of Epidemiology*, **103:**464, 1976.

Miller, A.: *Physicians' Desk Reference*, Medical Economics, Oradell, N. J., 1974–1977.

———: "The DES Controversy," *Contemporary OB/GYN*, **3**(1):81, 1974.

Nishamura, H., and T. Tahashi: *Clinical Aspects of the Teratogenicity of Drugs*, Experta Medica, American Elsevier, New York 1976.

Overbach, Arvin M.: "Drugs Used with Neonates and During Pregnancy," Parts I, II, III, *RN*, October, November, and December, 1974.

Pomerance, J. J., and S. J. Yaffee: "Maternal Medication and Its Effect on the Fetus," *Current Problems in Pediatrics*, **4:**1–60, 1973.

Sirrat, G. M.: "Prescribing Problems in the Second Half of Pregnancy and During Lactation," *Obstetric and Gynecological Survey*, **31:**1, 1976.

Thronburg, J. E. and K. E. Moore: "Pharmacologically Induced Modifications of Behavioral and Neurochemical Development," in B. L. Mirkin (ed.), *Perinatal Pharmacology and Therapeutics*, Academic Press, New York, 1976, chap 4, p. 331.

Wilson, James G.: "Present Status of Drugs as Teratogens in Man," *Teratology*, **7:**3–16, 1975.

———: *Environment and Birth Defects*, Academic Press, New York, 1977.

Yaffee, Sumner J.: "A Clinical Look at the Problem of Drugs in Pregnancy and Their Effect on the Fetus," *Canadian Medical Association Journal*, **112**(6):728, 1975.

Yerushalmy, J.: "The Effects of Smoking on Offspring," *Contemporary OB/GYN*, **1**(5):13, 1972.

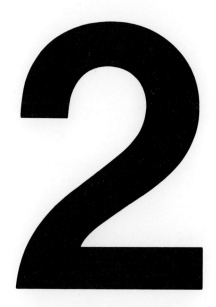

2
**THE HIGH-RISK
MOTHER
AND INFANT**

21

THE HIGH-RISK PREGNANCY: PSYCHOSOCIAL PROBLEMS

ELIZABETH J. DICKASON
CHRISTINE D. SOUTHALL

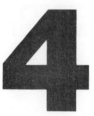

THE HIGH-RISK MOTHER

A high-risk pregnancy is one that does not progress according to the usual pattern. In severe problems, the term *reproductive wastage* aptly describes a pregnancy that is ended by death of the fetus or one that results in a disabled infant. On the other hand, a complicated pregnancy may result in a totally normal infant, while presenting a real stress to the mother's health and well-being.

Causes of difficulty during pregnancy include diseases existing prior to the pregnancy that impinge on the health of mother and fetus, complications caused by the pregnancy, and complications occurring during the delivery and newborn periods. In addition, psychosocial problems may greatly affect the health potential of mother and infant.

A high-risk pregnancy may result in the conception being lost by spontaneous abortion before the age of viability, i.e., 20 weeks. Although approximately 15 percent of all conceptions are lost in this way, many of the reasons for such abortions are unknown. The known maternal factors include poor nutrition, anemia, borderline fertility, and maternal chronic disease. In addition, about 30 percent of the aborted conceptions are lost because of poor implantation or because of a malformed, poorly developing embryo. After the age of viability, an abnormal outcome may result when pregnancies end in stillbirth or neonatal death or result in a compromised infant with less than an optimal chance for a healthy life.

If an infant is born before its development is completed, immaturity in every body system will handicap recovery. Immaturity and low birth weight are no longer synonymous, although about two-thirds of the low-birth-weight infants are also immature in development. One-third are fully developed but have poor fetal weight gain because of intrauterine stress or malnourishment. Whatever the case, if all low-birth-weight infants are included in a single group, they account for about 65 percent of all deaths in the first year of life, even though these infants make up only about 10 percent of all infants born.

The handicaps and long-term effects produced by intrauterine stress or malnourishment are being widely studied. If the infant is subjected to a reduced nutritional or oxygen supply, inevitable effects occur that prevent optimal development. Only in the last few decades have the results of reduced oxygen levels during the perinatal period been fully recognized.[1] The injury to the fetal brain may be severe (resulting in cerebral palsy or mental retardation) or less severe but just as significant (resulting in minimal brain dysfunction which may cause learning disabilities or disturbed behavior). Both retrospective and prospective studies are in progress to determine the full implications of perinatal asphyxia. For instance, in one study of a group of children who had suffered perinatal asphyxiation 16 years before, it was found that these children now had similar behavior patterns when compared with controls, but

that under stress they showed significantly more behavior disturbances.

It is clear that in dealing with the high-risk pregnancy we must be as concerned for the long-term outcome for the infant as we are for the immediate comfort and safety of the mother. For instance, medication to reduce the discomfort of labor is of immediate benefit to the laboring woman, but its ultimate value must be measured against the years of difficulty for the child should it become hypoxic and its functions depressed during the process of birth. Because of the many factors which we now know lead to future disability in children, a sense of responsibility for the future well-being of all children needs to permeate the thinking of those handling obstetric management and nursing support of the high-risk pregnancy.

MORBIDITY AND MORTALITY RATES

The term *morbidity* comes from the word *morbid*, meaning "abnormal," "pathologic," or "sick." The *morbidity rate* is the rate of occurrence of a particular disease, expressed in a ratio with a given nonsick population. *Mortality rate* is the number of deaths caused by a particular disease, expressed in a ratio with a given population. Such rates are compiled by the National Center for Health Statistics and are reported in monthly and yearly summaries. The accuracy of these statistics of course depends upon careful reporting from each health care institution. In addition, when one is reading such statistical statements, it is important to identify the given population in each instance.

infant mortality

The *infant mortality rates* include all deaths from the day of birth through the end of the eleventh month (the first birthday). From the brief listing in Table 21-1 it can be seen that most infants who die do so within the *neonatal period,* that period which extends from birth through the first 28 days of life. In this period, most of the deaths occur within the first 48 h of life. (To obtain the death rate for the period from 1 month through 11 months, subtract the neonatal from the infant mortality rate.)

The *perinatal death rate* includes all deaths from the period of viability (the beginning of the twentieth week in utero) through the first 28 days of life and is quoted as a ratio per 1000 births. In contrast, neonatal and infant death rates are quoted as a ratio per 1000 *live* births. Thus, in order to interpret the rates of death in a given year, one must know both the number of births and the number of live births for that year.

The main causes of infant mortality are listed in Table 21-2. It can be seen that there are some conditions that cannot be prevented. Supportive care and early diagnosis may contribute to a continued reduction in preventable conditions. It is encouraging to note that the mortality rate has fallen approximately 25 percent over the years 1968 to 1975. There has been a further reduction since 1975, primarily as a result of a reduction in deaths from RDS/HMD and of better monitoring during labor. Thus, deaths of immature infants and infants stressed by difficult labor have been prevented, in some cases. Prematurity still accounts for a large part of the total figure. Poverty, as reflected in the higher rates for nonwhite infants, continues to contribute to unnecessary mortality during the first year of life. Advances in perinatal care have been consistent and gratifying, and further reductions may occur when these two factors are affected by improved health care delivery.[2]

maternal mortality and morbidity

Maternal mortality refers to deaths of women while pregnant or within 90 days of the end of the pregnancy, no matter how the pregnancy was concluded. The overall United States maternal mortality rate is an average of all groups and is reported as per 100,000 live births.

When the average death rate is broken down into "white and nonwhite," an unacceptable discrepancy becomes apparent (see Table 21-3). The rate of death among nonwhite mothers in our society (three times higher than for white mothers) is a problem most directly attributable to the effects of poverty. This is underscored by the fact that the rates even out if women are divided along socioeconomic lines rather than along racial lines. The problem can be further illustrated by the regional statistics which show that areas of the country with higher mortality rates have more rural and urban poor mothers, both white and nonwhite.

Causes of death are currently listed as sepsis, toxemia, hemorrhage, abortion, ectopic pregnancy, and other complications. Table 21-4 gives the figures for 1975. In the last decade, deaths due to toxemia have dropped by 50 percent, whereas deaths due to sepsis have remained at approximately the same rate of occurrence. Increased under-

table 21-1 Infant and neonatal mortality rates*

	1950	1960	1970	1972	1977
Births	3,632,000	4,258,000	3,718,000	3,256,000	3,310,000
Infant death rate	29.2	26.0	19.8	18.5	14.1
Neonatal death rate	20.5	18.7	14.9	13.6	9.9

*Rates per 1000 live births.

table 21-2 Deaths under 1 year and infant mortality rates by color: United States, 1975 (for selected causes)

causes	classification*	number			rate†		
		total	white	nonwhite	total	white	nonwhite
All causes		50,525	36,173	14,352	1606.9	1417.4	2423.5
Early infancy							
Congenital anomalies	(740–759)	8528	7086	1496	272.9	277.7	252.6
Hyaline membrane disease/respiratory distress syndrome	(776.1–776.2)	7798	5896	1892	258.0	231.0	320.2
Asphyxia, anoxia, and other hypoxic conditions	(776.0, 766.3 776.4, 776.9)	4779	3258	1521	280.8	127.7	256.9
Immaturity, unqualified	(777)	4398	2843	1555	139.9	111.4	262.6
Complications of pregnancy	(762, 763, 769)	3372	2390	982	107.3	93.7	166.2
Difficult labor, with and without birth injury	(764–768)	2340	1749	591	74.5	68.5	99.8
Conditions of placenta and umbilical cord	(770–771)	1253	989	264	39.8	38.7	44.6
Later infancy							
Influenza and pneumonia	(470–474, 480–486)	2201	1410	791	70.0	55.3	133.6
Accidents	(E800–E949)	1337	927	410	42.5	36.3	69.2
Symptoms and ill-defined conditions	(780–796)	5121	3299	1822	162.9	129.3	307.7

Source: *Monthly Vital Statistics Report* **25**:11, Supplement, February 11, 1977, National Center for Health Statistics, Rockville, Md.
*From the eighth revision, *International Classification of Diseases*, Adapted 1965.
†Per 100,000 live births in a specific group. To obtain rate per 1000, move decimal two places to left. Infant mortality rate per 1000 is therefore 16.06 for Total, 14.17 for White, 24.23 for Nonwhite in 1975.

standing of how to diagnose and treat ectopic pregnancy and hemorrhage has reduced the deaths resulting from these causes by about 50 percent.[3] The advent of elective abortion has contributed to the decrease in deaths from illegal abortions with their resultant complications of sepsis, hemorrhage, and uterine perforation.

table 21-3 Maternal mortality rates*

	1950	1960	1970	1975
Overall rate	83.3	37.1	24.7	12.8
White	61.1	26.0	14.4	9.1
Nonwhite	221.6	97.9	55.9	29.0

Source: Division of Vital Statistics, National Center for Health Statistics, Rockville, Md.
*Rate per 100,000 live births.

SOCIOECONOMIC FACTORS AFFECTING HEALTHY PREGNANCY OUTCOME

Most studies come to the conclusion that the overall risk of a complicated pregnancy is influenced by the prior health and socioeconomic level of the mother. Despite the many advances of the last decade, many women in our country are at a disadvantage when it comes to preventive obstetric care. The location, expense, waiting, and travel time prevent poor women from seeking prenatal care, especially when they work during the day or have overwhelming family responsibilities. Medical practitioners and obstetricians are concentrated in the private care sectors, leaving a number of clinics only minimally staffed or partially staffed with foreign medical personnel who may have communication difficulties with patients.

We must recognize that poverty creates a cycle that is most difficult to break. Schneider states:

The socioeconomic factors making for high risk pregnancy reduce themselves in practice to one: poverty. In theory, a number of independent factors might be singled out, but in actuality, they manifest themselves as a vast Gordian knot of overcrowding, poor nutrition, fatigue, dirt, maternal stature, poor education, and the need to work even during a difficult pregnancy. . . .[4]

In urban areas where recent immigrants struggle with overwhelming adjustments, a visit to the clinic may be too frightening a process to undertake voluntarily. The woman waits until there is no alternative, because problems already exist. In rural areas, poverty, fear, and prejudice are as debilitating as they are in the city. Also, distances are more of a factor to consider in seeking care, for most poor women will not go for preventive care if the clinic is too far from their homes.

When we quote statistics showing nonwhite mothers with more than double the white mortality and morbidity rates, and a much higher infant mortality rate in our society, Schneider's statement should be burned into our minds: "The repeatedly noted higher risk among black women is not due to any genetic or racial factor but to the fact that so many of them are poor".[5] That statement can be applied to any group of poor women who show an increased rate of trouble during their pregnancies.

ADOLESCENT PREGNANCY

In 1975, 19 percent of all births were to teenagers, and in the last 8 years there has been an increase of 21 percent in births to girls 15 to 17 years of age. The rate of girls under 15 has not increased and continues to be about 0.5 percent of the females in that

table 21-4 Maternal deaths* and maternal mortality rates† for selected causes, by color: United States, 1975

cause of death	category numbers*	number of deaths total	white	all other	mortality rate† total	white	all other
Complications of pregnancy, childbirth and the puerperium	(630–778)	403	231	172	12.8	9.1	29.0
Ectopic pregnancy	(631)	50	19	31	1.6	0.7	5.2
Toxemias of pregnancy and the puerperium, except abortion with toxemia	(636–639)	77	45	32	2.4	1.8	5.4
Hemorrhage of pregnancy and childbirth	(632, 651–653)	48	28	20	1.5	1.1	3.4
Abortions	(640–645)	27	11	16	0.9	0.4	2.7
Abortions induced for legal indications	(640, 641)	10	4	6	0.3	0.2	1.0
Abortions induced for other reasons	(642)	4	1	3	0.1	0.0	0.5
Spontaneous abortions	(643)	3	1	2	0.1	0.0	0.3
Other and unspecified abortions	(644, 645)	10	5	5	0.3	0.2	0.8
Sepsis of childbirth and the puerperium	(670, 671, 673)	76	51	25	2.4	2.0	4.2
All other complications of pregnancy, childbirth and the puerperium	(630, 633–635, 654–662, 672, 674–678)	124	77	47	3.9	3.0	7.9
Delivery without mention of complication	(650)	1	—	1	0.0	—	0.2

Source: *Monthly Vital Statistics Report, Final Mortality Statistics, 1975*, The National Center for Health Statistics. **25**:11, Supplement, February 11, 1977.
*Maternal deaths are those assigned to complications of pregnancy, childbirth, and the puerperium; category numbers 630 to 678 of the Eighth Revision, *International Classification of Diseases*, Adapted, 1965.
†Rates are per 100,000 live births in specified group.

group. Recently there has been a notable decrease in pregnancies in the 18- to 19-year-old group, a decrease that reflects the general decline in births to older women (see Table 21-5).

Because the teenage girl is more likely to have a low-birth-weight, illegitimate baby and is more likely not to have finished her schooling or to have received adequate prenatal care,[6] her pregnancy is always regarded as a high-risk one. It is of concern that in today's society such a high rate of pregnancy should still occur in young girls when widespread information about sexuality and family planning is available.

If we view the adolescent age span as that from 11 to 19, developmental tasks during this period will divide adolescence into three groups, under 15 years, 15 to 17, and 18 to 19. Assuming that the level of maturity differs with experiences, exposure to challenges, and rate of body maturation, we will first consider the adolescent who might become pregnant between 11 and 14, the early adolecent.(See also Chap. 1.)

early adolescent pregnancy

Sexual involvement in early adolescence is naturally experimental, most often without much previous education or without assimilation of the education that has been received. Sometimes the young adolescent, beset by turbulent emotions, seeks love outside the family circle. In this case, she is often rebellious and is seldom directed toward parenthood but toward proving that she is lovable.[7] The father of the unborn child is often four or more years older or may be an adult.

For a variety of reasons, pregnancy may not be discovered in very young girls until the second and sometimes even the third trimester. The young girl's knowledge of menstruation and hormonal activity is limited; periods are often irregular for the first year or two, so that she herself may not suspect that she has become pregnant. Weight gain is natural during this period. Overweight girls often do not seem much larger until the fifth or sixth month of pregnancy. The girl may be frightened by

table 21-5 Birth rates* and live births for women 10–19 years of age: United States 1966–1975

age and race of mother	1966		1970		1975	
	live births	rate	live births	rate	live births	rate
10–14 years						
Total	8,128	0.9	11,752	1.2	12,642	1.3
White	2,666	0.3	4,320	0.5	5,073	0.6
All other	5,462	4.0	7,432	4.8	7,569	4.7
15–17 years						
Total	186,704	35.8	223,590	38.8	227,270	36.6
White	119,800	26.6	143,646	29.2	148,344	28.3
All other	66,904	92.9	79,944	95.2	78,926	82.0
18–19 years						
Total	434,722	121.2	421,118	114.7	354,968	85.7
White	345,312	109.6	319,962	101.5	261,785	74.4
All other	89,410	205.5	101,156	195.4	93,183	150.1

Source: *Monthly Vital Statistics Report*, 26(5): 9, Supplement, September 9, 1977.

*Rates are live births per 1000 women in a specified group.

the prospect of parental, teacher, or peer disapproval and may hide her symptoms by wearing a tight brassiere and girdle. Elaborate measures may be taken to conceal the pregnancy, and there are known cases of a girl's coming to term without parental knowledge of the pregnancy.

Once it becomes evident that the pregnancy is a fact, the girl and her mother are usually counseled. If the pregnancy has been discovered early enough, interruption is often recommended, for obvious reasons. The child is not mature enough to assume the role of parent, nor can she assume economic support of a child of her own. Medically, she is at risk for more complications than an older teenager. However, cultural, ethnic, religious, and socioeconomic constituents of the decision must be balanced against the girl's own attitudes and reactions. To force interruption may be more detrimental to her than to carry the infant to term. It is not a lightly reached conclusion and needs careful counseling and support from social worker, physician, psychiatrist, and nurse.[8]

If the girl goes on with the pregnancy, hospitals routinely provide concomitant psychiatric support in the child psychiatry department, or through social service. Some girls may be placed in foster care or in a home for girls with premarital pregnancies, especially if the parents are unable to be supportive during the pregnancy.[9]

The young adolescent experiences the pregnancy with detachment. For example, it is very difficult for her to be responsible in adjusting eating patterns. When the emphasis is on nutrition, the girl's mother needs to be brought into the conference for necessary health support. In fact, the mother will be needed at every step in health care during pregnancy, to ensure the keeping of appointments at the clinic and the carrying out of referrals.

Pregnancy may be viewed by the girl as a transient childhood disease, unpleasant, but soon over and "cured." During the last trimester, much support and preparation should be afforded for the process of labor and delivery. Growth of the girl is still in progress, so that cesarean section may have to be done in cases of a small pelvis. When this is the case, needless to say, the experience is even more unreal and similar to a disease for which surgery is necessary.

The medical approach to the delivery of young girls is made with very special humane, sympathetic care. To minimize the trauma during labor and delivery, medication will be used to keep the girl as comfortable as possible through the entire process. This is in keeping with the thought that future pregnancies will be experienced with less fear and fantasy and with more maturity if this one is not frightening.

mid-adolescent pregnancy

Older teenagers (15 to 17) are naturally viewed and counseled in a different light. Barring emotional immaturity, it is highly unusual that pregnancy within this age group is accidental because of ignorance. With more information available on family life, sex, and child-spacing methods, and with the growing availability of abortion services, the older adolescent may be fairly sophisticated about her options. Some of the reasons given by girls for not protecting themselves against pregnancy remain romantic—not wanting to plan ahead or to seem aggressive or to "spoil the mood." Rebellion and the desire to have a "baby of my own to love me" may lead desperately unhappy girls to seek pregnancy. Many documented studies attest to the unconscious wish for pregnancy.[10]

The nurse can expect to see this adolescent earlier in pregnancy, usually not for confirmation of the pregnancy but for medical care and counseling, either with the parent or with the father of the unborn child. As with the young adolescent, counseling, once the older girl reaches the clinic, is directed first toward assessing the family relationship and then toward attempting to reconcile any differences that may exist between parent and daughter on the plan of care.

late adolescent pregnancy

Girls in the 18- to 19-year-old group have had a chance to finish high school and to be employed. In 1970, reports showed that 77.5 percent were unmarried. For this group the illegitimacy rate decreased over the years 1966 to 1975 for white and nonwhite and the overall number of babies born was less. Thus, nearly one-third of all births to the 18- 19-year-old group were illegitimate. This trend may reflect the increased freedom of a single parent to keep her baby without a marriage to formalize parenthood. (It also reflects the increased use of family planning for married couples, resulting in a change in the ratio of babies born to married vs. single women).[11]

emancipated minors Hofmann states that the traditional definition of emancipated minors is "adolescents who are married, in the armed forces or who with parental consent are self-supporting or living away from home under such circumstances that (they) make most of (their) own decisions.[12]

There are, however, many cases of minors over 15 who have been treated by physicians without parental consent. An informed judgment must be made as to the adolescent's need, maturity, and life situation. Problems of consent apply to contraceptives, pregnancy testing, venereal disease treatment, and all other adolescent health services. As yet, not all states have realistic statutes reflecting adolescent needs for health care.*

In many urban areas, special facilities for adolescent health services are available for pregnancy and venereal disease (VD) testing. Some schools are using peer-group counseling by older prepared students to handle the common concerns of adolescents and to provide free referral for pregnancy and VD testing without parental consent. These school services, always backed up by medical personnel and clinics, are an attempt to teach teenagers, who are a high-risk group for VD and early pregnancy.[13]

continuing education Some schools have provided special programs for the pregnant teenager. These facilities are being phased out as public attitudes toward premarital pregnancy have become less stringent.[14] Girls are encouraged to stay in school. Finishing education is the practical solution to the situation, since if the girl keeps the child she will have to assume its economic support if the father of the child does not. In most programs it has been discovered that these girls benefit from personal attention and may bloom in confidence and ability to cope with their new situation. Therefore, even if education is provided in the same school, special supportive discussion groups and personal interest of a sympathetic counselor are important ways of assisting the girl to gain confidence.

Although there is increased awareness of the needs of the young teenage father of the child, specific programs have not generally been available to assist him through this crisis.

Depending on the ethnic makeup of the

*Information about laws in each state can be found in *Contraception, Family Planning and Voluntary Sterilization: Laws and Policies of the United States, Each State and Jurisdiction,* U.S. Department of Health, Education, and Welfare, January 1973.

school, the girl returning to school may have some difficulty with social pressures and adjustments. In black communities, the baby is usually assimilated into the family as another child, with the grandparents taking ultimate parental responsibility. The usual option in the white culture had been to require marriage or to give the child up for adoption. Adoption is traumatic for the mother, and teenage marriages have led to a much higher divorce rate, since both partners are immature. The recognition of these facts and the more permissive trend in society are making more options available. No matter what the situation, the emphasis with teenagers should be on the importance of finishing basic education and on becoming economically able to support a family. The task of becoming psychologically mature enough to assume the role of parent may not be achieved easily. Thus, the need for more widespread education for parenting is reemphasized each time a premarital teenage pregnancy occurs.

DRUG ADDICTION IN PREGNANCY

Drug addicts are the outcasts of our society. Recent trends reflect less sympathetic understanding than was accorded them in the past, largely because of the intensity with which public health agencies have worked to inform the population about addiction. Commonly existing feelings, both of medical personnel and of laymen, are that one who becomes addicted now does so by choice. In addition, there are feelings that already addicted persons are antisocial because of the existence of varied agencies with enough approaches to provide detoxification, regardless of the drug classification. It is still admitted, however, that widespread devastating socioeconomic conditions continue to ravish the poor, affecting ego strength and mental

hygiene. Such conditions may have a forceful impact on the individual who is ill prepared to cope with life. The alternatives, however, continue to remain philosophic.

Drugs used most commonly vary with locale, e.g., LSD has been more widespread on the West Coast, while 50 percent of heroin users in the United States are in New York.[15] Varying degrees of drug usage and habituation are common as well. Polydrug abuse (use of multiple controlled substances) is common in the drug-using pregnant woman. "Neonatal withdrawal has now been recognized following chronic maternal use of alcohol, amphetamines, barbiturates, codeine, diazepam (Valium), etchlorvynol (Placidyl), gluthethimide (Doriden), heroin, meperidine, morphine, pentazocine (Talwin), and propoxyphene hydrochloride (Darvon)."[16] Because heroin addiction is by far the most common drug problem in large innner-city hospital clinics, our discussion will focus on the female heroin addict who becomes pregnant.

To begin with, pregnancy and the birth of the baby may represent to the female drug addict the last claim to a worthwhile purpose. The pregnancy can represent a new lease on life—another beginning. Sometimes it means a release of old guilt feelings. Often, at the time, the woman makes a sincerely felt resolution to reform and be different.

The woman may or may not be aware that heroin addiction has contributed to irregularities in her menstrual cycle. Thus, pregnancy may be several months advanced before she realizes that she is pregnant. She may conceal the fact then, for her own ego gratification and to prevent being forced into a decision, or she may come at once to the clinic for confirmation to ensure the health of the baby.

prenatal care

On first visits to the clinic, most addicts are defensive and paranoic. They expect that the initial counseling will include pressure and suggestions to interrupt the pregnancy. They have usually been involved with prostitution, for themselves and often for their male counterparts; and often they have been jailed for shoplifting and other misdemeanors. Statistics show that the majority of drug-addicted women have had two to four pregnancies.[17] Thus some women may have children placed in foster care, or, as they perceive it, "taken away from them." In abortive attempts to reclaim other children or to gain credentials in an effort to reestablish in some measure their claim to be responsible, they may have gone into institutions for treatment.

In spite of all the expressed and unexpressed goals of a drug addict, general traits of the addicted personality need to be kept in mind. Some of the more common characteristics are that they will attempt to be manipulative by trying to please the counselor, while seldom being truthful. They may falsify the amount of daily drug intake because a large amount reinforces a feeling of being "bad." They may make unsolicited promises, that they are in the process of becoming involved in rehabilitation or are already involved.

The nurse must have an understanding approach regardless of personal feelings, keeping in mind the addictive profile. This means adopting a firm, consistent, direct manner in seeking information for medical purposes and in counseling for the possible prevention of deterioration during the pregnancy.

If the nurse sees the patient early, it can be assumed that the mother has made the choice to come of her own accord for the sake of the baby. Because the mother usually feels a sense of worthlessness and uselessness, the pregnancy then represents her one act of decency, a way to feel human again. Nonsympathetic personnel who may not be acquainted with the psychology of the addicted female might be inclined to force their solutions on her through manipulative, threatening persuasion. Such an approach would eradicate any cooperation the patient might give and would most likely result in complete loss of rapport or possibly in loss of contact with the woman until the time of delivery.

On the other hand, counseling toward traditional health maintenance is a waste of time with the addict in early pregnancy. She is likely to continue in her same destructive patterns until late in pregnancy. Recognizing this, the nurse should not become frustrated in attempts to counsel or place restrictions on her regarding nutrition, hygiene, and rest.

Usually toward the end of the second trimester, the nurse counselor has the best chance of helping the expectant mother safeguard the outcome of the baby because the woman begins to worry about the infant's health. It is at this point that the counselor can encourage the mother to adhere to some of the most important aspects of prenatal care.

Nutrition is critical. In every possible way the nurse can encourage the mother to increase her protein intake. For example, sweets probably constitute the major part of her usual diet. To be useful and realistic, diet substitutions should be in keeping with what she *will* eat. Vitamins, folic acid, and iron will be prescribed and should be stressed as supplements necessary for the baby's health.

Personal hygiene and sexual habits are serious considerations for counseling. Prostitution often continues to term, so that it is not unusual for the patient to contract venereal disease very late in pregnancy after routine screening.

The addict's irregular life pattern with regard to rest, food, and hygiene contributes to the detrimental environment experienced by the growing fetus. Medical complications in patients who do not seek care or follow prenatal care guidelines include problems related to drug dependency. Infections, especially venereal disease and hepatitis, and thrombophlebitis and iron-deficiency anemia may occur. Obstetric complications include preterm labor with low-birth-weight babies, preeclampsia, and precipitate labor.[18] However, when a woman participates in prenatal care and in a rehabilitation program, the incidence of complications drops sharply.

detoxification or maintenance

Withdrawal of the client without some kind of drug therapy is contraindicated during pregnancy because of the possible dangers to the fetus. For instance, smooth-muscle spasms affect the circulation through the placenta. In severe cases of maternal withdrawal, the fetus may die. Thus, detoxification is often delayed until after delivery to minimize fetal risks.[19]

Detoxification of heroin addicts is now accomplished almost universally in the United States with methadone. It is not recommended in either the first or third trimesters, and if given in the second trimester, it should be at a very slow rate, using low-dose methadone.[20]

To remain drug-free after this period, a woman must be in a strongly supportive program. The alternative is to place her on a methadone maintenance program. The use of methadone in this way must be recognized as simply a substitute addiction. The benefits are those of control of dosage, regular dosage, and continued supervision and counseling in the center. These benefits accrue, of course, only if the client is cooperative.

delivery and infant response

Toward the latter part of pregnancy, the client will be concerned about the infant's response. The nurse needs to give her as much infor-mation as possible about the drug's effect on the infant. She should know that the baby will be passively addicted and that the degree of difficulty the infant will have will depend upon the extent of her habit. She can be reassured, however, that in the absence of psychologic dependency, medical treatment of the baby usually alleviates withdrawal symptoms. The baby's recovery may be affected by its poor intrauterine environment, most commonly causing *intrauterine growth retardation,* a complex result of many factors—among them poor nutritional supply and intrauterine stress.

Deliveries are often premature (30 to 40 percent). Prematurity coupled with withdrawal symptoms will doubly handicap the infant, and mortality rates are high (5 to 10 percent).

Stone states that in the study from Metropolitan City Hospital in 1969, 80 percent of the drug-addicted mothers admitted to, or gave evidence of, drug use on the day of admission to labor.[21] Because of inability to determine how much drug a mother has in her system, regional anesthetics are commonly used.

Finally, remembering that this patient usually has not attended the clinic regularly or participated in classes in preparation for childbirth, the nurse must be especially alert and watchful for untoward responses during labor.

postpartum care

Following delivery, the patient's first concern is usually to satisfy her need for drugs. If the patient is not on a methadone regimen or receiving tranquilizers, she will make attempts to acquire drugs from the outside through visitors to avoid withdrawal symptoms (nausea, tremors, sweating, abdominal pain, cramps, and yawning) which may appear in 2 or 3 h after delivery.

The nurse must be alert to the possibility of stealing from other patients, must notice the length of time the patient spends in the bathroom, and must not leave medication rooms or carts unguarded. Some way must be planned for unobtrusive surveillance of visitors to drug-addicted patients when they are not separated from other patients. Withdrawal is not attempted without drug therapy because of the complex changes in the woman's body during this recovery period.

Fears of separation from the baby may be intensified following delivery because in most instances, the infant is placed in an intensive care unit for observation and treatment. (Care of the infant is discussed in Chap. 29.)

The social worker has usually been involved in discussing placement of the baby in foster care until the mother is either completely drug-free or involved in an approved program for rehabilitation. Guidelines for approved programs are set up by the bureau of child welfare in most cities or states when policies are regulated by a governmental agency.

Care of the addicted pregnant patient is one of the most difficult aspects of maternal and infant nursing. The outcome is often negative and sad. Nurses in this area find themselves wanting to become more and more involved in prevention of drug addiction. Certainly the high infant morbidity and mortality rates and the tragedy in the mother's life appear to justify aggressive programs to this end.

other addictions

Drug abuse of alcohol and excessive smoking remain current public health concerns. Education about the adverse effects of these substances is being made more widely available. Effects are discussed in Chap. 20 and 27.

HIGH-RISK PREGNANCY PROTOCOL

Most institutions have developed a protocol for medical management of the high-risk pregnancy. Such a protocol includes identifying the risk factors and rating them on a scale similar to the one in Table 21-6. Planning the steps in careful management of the pregnancy follows such identification of problems. Of chief concern is the decision of when to terminate the pregnancy. To achieve the best assessment of the infant's condition, tests such as those described in Chap. 27 are planned toward the end of the pregnancy. Technical supportive care appears easier to achieve than does support for psychosocial problems, and further work needs to be done to identify the ways the woman can be assisted to reduce the stresses of poverty, premarital pregnancy, or drug abuse. Table 21-7 summarizes the major problems in high-risk pregnancies which will be discussed in detail in the chapters to follow.

study questions

1 List three preexisting problems underlying a high-risk pregnancy, with a high incidence in your area.
2 Define morbidity rate.
3 Identify the populations for perinatal, infant, and neonatal mortality rates and that for the maternal mortality rate.
4 Which causes of infant mortality are not preventable? Study Table 21-2 and identify those causes of death which might be prevented by better education and more available health care.
5 Are there factors in your geographic area that lead to a difference in health care for poor women?
6 Identify at least six reasons why poor women may receive less complete health care.
7 Briefly differentiate between the expected responses to premarital pregnancy in the young, the mid, and the late teenage years. List factors contributing to the increase in total numbers of births in mid-teenage girls. Why do you think that total births to young teenagers have not increased so much?

table 21·6 Antepartum fetal risk score

baseline data		obstetrical history	
Age 12–16	2	Abortion	
Age 35+	1	Stillbirth	
40+	2	Neonatal death	
Para 0	1	Surviving premature	
6+	2	Antepartum hemorrhage	
Interval over 2 years	1	Toxemia	
Obesity over 200 lb	1	Difficult mid-forceps	
Diabetes, B,C,D,	2	Cesarean section	
F	3	Major congenital anomalies	
Chronic renal disease	1	Baby over 10 lb	
with decreased function	3		
with increased BUN	3	one	1
Hypertension (preexisting)		two or more of above	2
$\frac{140+}{90+}$	1	Rh-immunized mother	
		+ homozygous father	2
$\frac{160+}{110+}$	2	+ erythroblastosis	3

Score (circle one)   0   1   2   3

present pregnancy			
Bleeding before 20 wk		Toxemia I (mild)	1
Alone	1	Toxemia II (severe)	3
With pain	2	Eclampsia	3
Bleeding after 20 wk		Hydramnios	3
Ceased	1	Multiple pregnancy	2
Continued	2	Abnormal GTT	1
With pain	3	Decreasing insulin	
With hypotension	3	requirement	3
Spontaneous premature		Maternal acidosis	3
rupture of membranes	1	Maternal pyrexia	1
Latent period over 24 h	2	Pyrexia + FHR 160+	2
Anemia below 10 g	1	Rh negative	
below 8 g	2	with rising titer	2
No prenatal care	2	Liley zone 3	3
Less than 3 visits	1		

Score (circle one)   0   1   2   3

gestational age			
28 weeks or under	4	37 weeks or under	1
32 weeks or under	3	42 weeks or more	1
35 weeks or under	2	43 weeks or more	2

Score (circle one)   0   1   2   3   4

Total Score   0   1   2   3   4   5   6   7   8   9   10

Source: Originally published in *Canadian Medical Journal* **101:**57–66, October 18, 1969. Used by permission.

table 21-7 High-risk pregnancy

problems	how pregnancy is complicated	how supportive care is changed
1. **Adolescent pregnancy** Age: 10–14 Age: 15–17	1. Increased risk of anemia, poor nutrition. 2. Psychosocial problems, poor adaptation, ambivalence, etc. 3. Increased incidence of preeclampsia, preterm delivery. 4. Increased anxiety about labor, parenting.	Continuity of care should be provided for. Classes in pregnancy, labor, child care more intense, thorough. Provide for follow-up in postdelivery period. Need of ego strengthening; support by family, peer acceptance may be missing. Intervention by social worker always needed, occasionally psychiatrist.
2. **Elderly primigravida,** 35+ or 40+	1. Increased risk of obesity, other underlying health problems. 2. Increased risk of psychosocial problems, anxiety, ambivalence. 3. Higher incidence of preeclampsia, hypertension. 4. Increased risk of congenital defects (Down's syndrome, 1:100 risk)	Increased need for support, nutritional counseling. More difficulty expected during pregnancy and labor. Provide information on adult level, gain cooperation. Assessment of underlying diseases. Follow through in postpartum period for parenting support. May need and request genetic counseling and diagnostic amniocentesis.
3. **Anemia** (iron deficiency) Below 10 g Below 8 g	1. Fatigue, poor iron reserves. 2. Reduced oxygen-carrying capacity. 3. Increased risk of infection postdelivery. 4. Reduction of hemoglobin below 11.0 g and hematocrit below 31–33%	Nutritional counseling is a high priority. Iron PO or IM may be ordered. Blood transfusion in severe cases. Observe carefully postdelivery.
4. **Bleeding** a. Prior to twentieth completed week of gestation (1) *Spontaneous abortion:* incidence, 1:15 (a) *Threatened*	1. Usually indicates problem with morphogenesis, placental or hormonal function, or an ectopic implantation. (a) Low hormonal levels, poor development of embryo/fetus/placenta. Maternal chronic disease.	Observation, bed rest, pad count. Above, plus supportive fluids, blood replacement, if necessary. Watchful waiting, and a D and C if abortion proceeds to completion, but bleeding continues.

table 21-7 High-risk pregnancy *(continued)*

problems	how pregnancy is complicated	how supportive care is changed
(b) *Inevitable* Early: 8–10 weeks Late: 13 weeks and after	(b) Defective embryo or placental inadequacy (50–60%), unknown causes (20–30%) (which may include environmental agents), and maternal disease (15%) (Assali)	Recognize that there will be increased anxiety and grieving afterwards, if pregnancy was desired.
(c) *Missed* abortion	(c) Unknown causes, death of embryo without passage out of uterus for 8 or more weeks.	
(d) *Habitual* abortion	(d) Repeated spontaneous abortion, occurring the third or more times. Often due to incompetent cervix, low fertility.	
(2) *Ectopic pregnancy* Incidence between 1:2000 and 1:800; depends on socioeconomic level (higher incidence in poverty).	Due to tubal pathology. Obstruction in passage, low fertility.	A number of diagnostic procedures—culdocentesis, culdoscopy—may precede surgical removal of pregnancy.
b. Bleeding after 20 weeks (1) *Placenta previa* (a) Complete (total) (b) Partial (incomplete) (c) Low-lying (marginal) (Total incidence, 1:100–150)	1. Painless spotting, then moderate bleeding usually indicates placenta previa. If it continues, anemia in mother and hypoxia in fetus will be a problem. Blood will coagulate. 2. Early delivery after assessing fetal risk vs. maternal risk. 3. Postpartum hemorrhage more possible because of larger placental site in lower uterine segment.	Serial hemoglobin, hematocrit for mother plus observation, bed rest, pad count, supportive fluids, and blood replacement. Estriols, ultrasound, BPD to estimate fetal age and condition. Watchful waiting. Cesarean section when any placenta covers undilated internal os. Judgment used when placenta is low-lying or marginally near dilated cervix. Extra intervention needed for grieving, anxious family. Extra observation of involution.
c. Bleeding at time of labor (1) *Premature separation of placenta* (placental abruptio) (a) Complete: incidence, 1:500 (b) Partial: incidence, 1:85–139 (i) Concealed (hidden bleeding) (ii) Marginal (open bleeding)	1. Bleeding beginning during or just before labor usually indicates some degree of placental separation. 2. Usually accompanied by fetal distress and hypotension and/or severe pain (if concealed bleeding). Symptoms may be subacute or abrupt. 3. Fetal mortality depends on degree of	Continuous monitoring and support of maternal blood pressure, observation of contractions, condition. Assessment of fetal jeopardy. With emergency cesarean section, or vaginal delivery if partial abruption occurs late in labor. Observe for hypofibrinogenemia; blood will be unclotted.

	abruption. Maternal mortality depends on availability of emergency treatment.	

5. **Hemoglobinopathies**

a. Folate deficiency anemia: incidence, 50:100 of all women show some signs of deficiency before pregnancy ends.	1. Macrocytic anemia may occur. 2. May underline conditions such as abruptio placenta, spontaneous abortion, or preeclampsia.	Replacement with folate supplements, accompanying iron supplements. More frequent blood tests. Teach diet with adequate folic acid sources.
b. Thalassemia (1) Major (Cooley's anemia) (2) Minor (heterozygous)	1. Autosomally transmitted disease; hemoglobin has altered globin production because of defect in alpha or beta chain. 2. Patients with major disease rarely become pregnant; those with minor have minimal anemia until under stressors such as pregnancy.	Screen populations from Mediterranean and Southeast Asia countries. Supportive care if anemia worsens; blood transfusions.
c. Sickle cell (1) Trait (S-A): incidence 8–10:100 of U.S. black population (2) Disease (S-S): incidence, 0.3–1.2:1000 in U.S. black population	1. Autosomally transmitted disease. Hemoglobin has poor solubility for oxygen at low oxygen tensions, crystallizes into sickle shape; sludging of cells and hemolysis; hypoxia to vital organs. 2. 25–50:100 pregnancies with sickle-cell disease terminate in abortion, stillbirth, or neonatal death. 3. Increased incidence of complications; preeclampsia, infection, premature labor, sickling crises. 4. Urinary infection, hematuria more common with sickle trait women.	Treatment of infections and prevention of stressors critical. High folic-acid-bearing foods, iron supplements. Folic acid (1–2 mg) often prescribed, qd. Exchange transfusion in pregnancy when crises occur. Screen more frequently for bacteriuria.
d. Hemoglobin C (1) Trait (C-A): incidence, 2:100 in U.S. black population (2) Disease (S-C) linked with sickle cell	1. Homozygous state tolerated well with only mild anemia, but pregnancy may precipitate severe crises, with maternal mortality 7:100; fetal death 35:100.	Best possible supportive care if homozygous woman becomes pregnant. Genetic counseling; advise to avoid pregnancy.
e. Erythrocyte enzyme deficiency (1) Glucose 6-phosphate dehydrogenase (G-6-P-D) (2) Pyruvate kinase (PK)	1. May cause chronic hemolytic process or be triggered into severe hemolytic crises by stress of certain drugs or metabolic stresses such as infection, pregnancy.	Screening of all patients with family history suggesting enzyme deficiency. Teach patient to avoid stressors which precipitate hemolytic crises.

table 21-7 High-risk pregnancy (continued)

problems	how pregnancy is complicated	how supportive care is changed
6. **Polyhydramnios (hydramnios)**	1. Aggravates all pressure symptoms, severe supine hypotension, pressure on renal vessels. 2. Infant is small, often with associated GI or GU anomalies. Preterm labor is common.	Possibly repeated amniocenteses and removal of amniotic fluid. Extra support for anxiety. Expect a compromised infant.
7. **Cardiac disease** Incidence, 1.7%, but becoming increasingly rare, since rheumatic fever is treated in childhood. Congenital defects and hypertensive heart disease incidence rising.	1. Stress of hypervolemia of pregnancy reaches peak at 34 weeks, lasting until delivery. 2. Depending on functional classification, superimposed pregnancy may increase risk of fatigue, cardiac arrhythmias, anemia, and dyspnea; rarely, congestive heart failure. 3. Postdelivery, sudden increase in blood volume just after placental delivery may precipitate crisis. Recovery is slower. Ambulation depends on cardiac function. 4. Thrombophlebitis more common, with danger of emboli. 5. Stillbirth rate and low-birth-weight incidence is doubled over healthy pregnancies.	More frequent medical supervision. Low-salt diet, diuretics may be continued. Special care that anemia and infections do not occur. May be on prophylactic iron and antibiotics. Hospitalization at thirty-fourth week to check cardiac function. Promote bed rest in side-lying position for best kidney function. Both mother and fetus must be monitored during delivery. Delivery effected without heavy medication. Vaginal delivery unless obstetric complications demand cesarean section. Postdelivery: tight abdominal binder applied to maintain pressure on deep abdominal veins. Elastic stockings. IV fluids monitored carefully. Assess cardiac function before encouraging activity.
8. **Multiple pregnancy** Incidence: varied since ovulatory agents in use.	1. Aggravates all pressure symptoms, causing orthopnea, varicose veins, hemorrhoids, constipation, vena cava syndrome. 2. Anemia, nutritional inadequacy possible. Fetal growth retardation, or disproportional growth of one fetus may occur. 3. Preeclampsia, third trimester bleeding from low-lying placenta. Difficulty in labor/delivery and preterm labor all more common. 4. Postdelivery uterine atonia, hemorrhage, and delayed involution more common.	Bed rest in side-lying position for last 6 weeks of pregnancy to promote renal function. Extra care for other discomforts. Correction of anemia, high protein intake important. Additional iron, folic acid. Complicated delivery needs advanced planning, notification of support personnel. Postdelivery: extra support in bonding, teaching to cope with more than one baby.

9. **Hypertensive states of pregnancy** a. Preexisting hypertension: (present before pregnancy or occurring before twentieth week)	1. Renal function may be compromised already. Diuretics, antihypertensives may be required. 2. Increased blood volume may increase edema, headaches. 3. Higher risk of superimposed preeclampsia, abruptio placenta. Placental function compromised. Increased incidence of IUGR, small-for-date, chronically distressed infants.	Low-salt, high-protein diet required. Medication will be adjusted to those safe during pregnancy. More frequent monitoring of bp and symptoms related to hypertension. More frequent studies of placental function. Bed rest in side-lying position near end of pregnancy. Hospitalization may be necessary.

b. *Preeclampsia* (hypertension occurring after twentieth week, plus edema, proteinuria) Incidence, 6 to 7:100
  (1) *Mild:* bp under 140/90 but may have risen 30/15 over baseline, some edema
  (2) *Moderate:* bp between 140/90 and 160/110, edema, albuminuria
  (3) *Severe:* bp 160/110 and above, severe edema, oliguria, albuminuria.
	1. After twentieth week, adds physical, mental stress to pregnancy.
	2. Increased risk of stillbirth, abruptio placenta, chronic fetal distress, IUGR.
	3. Increased risk of eclampsia, with hazard of hypoxia to mother and fetus
	4. Renal function affected by deposit of fibrin in glomeruli. Sodium and water retention becomes extreme. Oliguria, proteinuria severe.
	5. Eye grounds show retinal arteriolar spasm: papilledema, hemorrhages; result is visual disturbances. Epigastric pain and amnesia are late cues to impending convulsions (*eclampsia*).
		Careful instructions about warning signs of worsening symptoms. Preventive care is a high priority. High-protein diet, fluids, moderate salt intake, bed rest in side-lying position for mild preeclampsia.
		Moderate preeclampsia: medications may be ordered—sedative, antihypertensive, magnesium sulfate, and rarely, a trial of diuretics.
		Hospitalization for any condition more than mild symptoms. Early delivery when OCT positive, estriols falling, and rising bp uncontrolled by interventions.

10. **Rh-negative mother with a rising antibody titer**	1. No risk to mother. 2. Repeated amniocentesis required to measure bilirubin density, OD∆ 450, in amniotic fluid. 3. Fetus may become either hyperbilirubinemic or extremely anemic. 4. Infant may need exchange transfusion; rarely, intrauterine transfusion.	Antibody titers done at regular intervals. Oxygen may be given during labor. Preterm induction may be done to deliver baby in order to do exchange transfusion. No RhoGam can be given to mother.
11. **Diabetes** (a) Class A Total incidence, 1:100–200 pregnancies	1. Higher incidence of preeclampsia, fetal anomalies, hydramnios, infection. 2. Hyperglycemia affects fetus, causing pancreatic hypertrophy, Class A infant often large for gestational age, with higher risk of RDS, hypoglycemia in neonatal period.	Intensive instruction and supervision diet; insulin and urine testing. More frequent visits to be regulated. May need hospitalization for adjustment of insulin dosage, serial FBS, postprandial sugars. Serial biparietal diameter, L/S ratio estriols, OCT.

table 21-7 High-risk pregnancy (continued)

problems	how pregnancy is complicated	how supportive care is changed
(b) Insulin-dependent diabetics (Class B-D)	3. Insulin imbalance with hypoglycemia, hyperglycemia, or acidemia has adverse effect of fetus. Placental dysfunction common, and Class C, D infants are small for gestational age. Preterm delivery may occur or be planned to rescue compromised infant.	Postdelivery regulation important before discharge. Extra support for anxiety about fetal outcome or if infant is born with anomalies.
12. **Renal disease** Incidence: varied	1. Multiple underlying problems will affect pregnancy by changing renal excretory ability: chronic glomerulonephritis, nephrotic syndrome, solitary kidney, polycystic kidney, and severe diabetic renal changes. 2. Proteinuria may be massive; hypertension, edema, vomiting, and accompanying discomforts of nausea, headache, palpitations, visual disturbances may cause the diagnosis to be confused with severe preeclampsia.	1. Risk is mainly to fetus unless mother goes into renal failure. Spontaneous abortion, preterm labor, and intrauterine death are possible. 2. High-protein, low-salt diet; antihypertensives; and sometimes diuretics and cardiac glycosides. 3. Bed rest in side-lying position is important. 4. Urinary infections are treated vigorously.
13. **Preterm labor** a. With intact membranes	1. Regular contractions and beginning effacement and dilation of cervix prior to 37 weeks' gestation. 2. Termination of pregnancy before fetal growth is complete; preterm infant his higher risk of RDS, hypoglycemia, infection, mental retardation.	Inhibition of preterm labor attempted, alcohol IV. vasodilan, bed rest.
b. Ruptured membranes less than 12 h Total incidence of preterm labor resulting in premature infants, 15:100		Premature rupture of membranes changes waiting for labor, since infection may ensue. Careful induction is necessary without analgesics or anesthetics if infant is preterm. Exception if infant is under 33 weeks. Careful waiting to gain maturity.
c. Ruptured membranes with more than 24 h, with maternal pyrexia.	3. Labor must be induced before ascending infection begins. After 24 h, infection always possible. Aspiration syndrome and pneumonia common in infant, and postdelivery endometritis in mother.	Bethamethesone given to mother if infant is less than 32 weeks to induce maturation of surfactant production in lungs. Prophylactic antibiotics often begun. Careful fetal monitoring, and gentle delivery. Involvement of neonatal personnel in immediate care in delivery room and transitional period.

8 What does *polydrug abuse* mean? Study the adverse effects of chronic high use of the less commonly recognized drugs of abuse: ethchlorvynol, glutethimide, pentazocine, and propoxyphene.

9 List the major problems in providing consistent prenatal supervision for a drug-abusing woman.

10 Discover, for your area, the way a baby is cared for if the mother refuses detoxification or a regular program of maintenance. Talk with the social worker.

11 After studying the chapters on high-risk pregnancy and delivery, return to Table 21-7 and review the ways nursing care is changed by the presence of these risk factors.

references

1 Y. Brackbill, J. Kane, R. L. Manniello, and D. Abramson, "Obstetric Premedication and Infant Outcome," *American Journal of Obstetrics and Gynecology* , **118**(3):377, 1974.

2 R. L. Manniello and P. M. Farrell, "Analysis of United States Neonatal Mortality from 1968 to 1974 with Specific Reference to Changing Trends in Major Casualties," *American Journal of Obstetrics and Gynecology*, **129**(6):667, November 15, 1977.

3 K. R. Niswander and M. Gordon, *The Women and Their Pregnancies*, The Collaborative Perinatal Study of the National Institute of Neurological Diseases and Stroke, W. B. Saunders, Philadelphia, 1972.

4 J. Schneider, "The High-Risk Pregnancy," *Hospital Practice*, October, 1971, p. 133.

5 Ibid., p. 135.

6 "Teenage Childbearing: United States, 1966–1975," *Monthly Vital Statistics Report*, National Center for Health Statistics, **26**(5):1, Supplement, September 1977.

7 F. L. Curtis, "The Pregnant Adolescent," *Nursing '74*, March, 1974, p. 77.

8 American Academy of Pediatrics, "Teenage Pregnancy and the Problem of Abortion," Report of the Committee on Youth, *Pediatrics*, **49**:303, 1972.

9 National Council of Illegitimacy, *Directory of Maternity Homes and Residential Facilities for Unmarried Mothers*, New York, 1966.

10 L. B. Johnson, "Problems with Contraception in Adolescents," *Clinical Pediatrics*, **10**:316, 1971.

11 "Teenage Childbearing: United States, 1966–1975," op. cit., p. 7.

12 A. D. Hofmann and H. F. Pipel, "The Legal Rights of Minors," *Pediatric Clinics of North America*, **20**(4): 989, 1973.

13 S. L. Hammar, "The Approach to the Adolescent Patient," *Pediatric Clinics of North America*, **20**(4): 1973.

14 A. Foltz, L. V. Kleeman, and V. Jekel, "Pregnancy

and Special Education: Who Stays in School?" *American Journal of Public Health*, **62**:1612, 1972.

15 American College of Obstetrics and Gynecology, "Addictive Drugs and Pregnancy," Technical Bulletin 21, April, 1973, p. 1.

16 S. R. Kandall, "Transitional Effects of Drugs in the Newborn," in E. J. Dickason et al.,*Maternal and Infant Drugs: Nursing Intervention*, McGraw-Hill, New York, 1978, p. 271.

17 American College, op. cit., p. 3.

18 Ibid., p. 4.

19 J. F. Connaughton, et al., "Perinatal Addiction: Outcome and Management," *American Journal of Obstetrics and Gynecology*, **129**(6):685, November 15, 1977.

20 Ibid., p. 685.

21 M. L. Stone et al., "Narcotic Addiction in Pregnancy," *American Journal of Obstetrics and Gynecology*, **109**(5):717, 1971.

bibliography

Boulette, T. R.: "Parenting: Special Needs of Low-Income Spanish-surnamed Families," *Pediatric Annals*, **6**(9):95, September 1977.

Chabot, M. J., J. Garfinkel, and M. W. Pratt: "Urbanization and Differentials in White and Nonwhite Infant Mortality," *Pediatrics*, **56**(5):777, November 1975.

Crane, J. P., J. P. Sauvage, and F. Arras: A High-risk Pregnancy Protocol," *American Journal of Obstetrics and Gynecology*, **125**(2):227, May 15, 1976.

Curtis, F. L.: "The Pregnant Adolescent," *Nursing '74*, March 1974, p. 77.

——:*11 Million Teenagers: What Can Be Done About the Epidemic of Adolescent Pregnancies in the United States*, The Alan Guttmacher Institute, New York, 1976.

Finnegan, L. P., and B. A. MacNew: "Care of the Addicted Infant," *American Journal of Nursing*, **74**(4): 685, 1974.

Kramer, J. P.: "The Adolescent Addict: The Progression of Youth Throughout the Drug Culture," *Clinical Pediatrics*, **49**:303, 1972.

Krepick, D. S., and B. L. Lang: "Heroin Addiction: A Treatable Disease," *Nursing Clinics of North America*, **8**(1):41, 1973.

McKenzie, R. G.: "A Practical Approach to the Drug-using Adolescent and Young Adult," *Pediatric Clinics of North America*, **20**(4):1035, 1973.

Raugh, J. L., L. B. Johnson, and R. L. Burket: "The Reproductive Adolescent," *Pediatric Clinics of North America*, **20**(4):1021, 1973.

Wright, N. M.: "Family Planning and Infant Mortality Decline in the United States," *American Journal of Epidemiology*, **101**(3):182, 1975.

22
HEMATOLOGIC PROBLEMS AND HEMORRHAGE

ELIZABETH J. DICKASON

BLOOD LOSS ANEMIA

Anemia, by far the most common hematologic problem of pregnancy, may be considered in one of three general categories:

1 Blood loss from the vascular system (hemorrhage)
2 Inadequate production of erythrocytes (hypoproliferative or maturational anemia)
3 Premature destruction of erythrocytes (hemolytic anemia)

With all factors considered together, hemorrhage is the chief cause of maternal morbidity and mortality. In a number of instances, bleeding can be prevented by early diagnosis, by providing improved diets and prenatal care, and by careful supervision of all aspects of delivery and postpartum care. There are, however, certain unpredictable causes of bleeding, which must then be treated as quickly and precisely as possible to prevent further morbidity or mortality.

basis of hemorrhage during pregnancy

In pregnancy, the blood supply to the uterus increases enormously to provide for placental circulation. The myometrium is supplied mainly from the uterine and ovarian arteries, and as these arteries enter the uterine muscle, they coil and loop to allow for the stretching of the growing uterus. (Fig. 22-1). Their pathways into the myometrium at every level of the uterus, from cervix to fundus, allow the uterine muscle to act as an elastic web to control blood flow—constricting vessels which pass through it as the uterus contracts, allowing normal flow as the uterus relaxes.

The normal characteristic action of the uterine muscle is to contract and relax in a rhythmic pattern; early in pregnancy, mild irregular contractions can be observed. Later in pregnancy these increase enough in frequency and intensity to be confused with true labor. As true labor begins, these rhythmic contractions are essential to the blood flow and muscle relaxation that maintain adequate oxygenation of the fetus, of the placenta, and of the myometrium itself.

For hemostasis of any bleeding originating in the vessels of the uterus, the myometrium must function as the primary vasoconstricting agent. This unusual action of the uterus in regulating blood flow relates to three basic obstetric problems, the first two of which will be considered in this chapter:

1 Hemostasis in cases such as ectopic pregnancy where the placental blood supply is not under the control of uterine contracture
2 Pre- and postpartal hemorrhage when the causes relate to uterine dysfunction
3 Hypertonic contractions that reduce blood to the placenta and thus oxygen to the fetus during labor (Chap. 27)

fig. 22-1 Blood supply to the uterus.

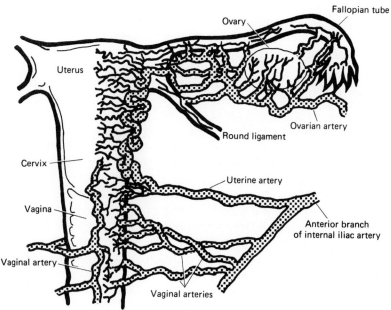

Any tearing or separation of the placenta will precipitate bleeding through the arterial openings into the placental bed. After delivery of the placenta, relaxation or interference with normal contracture of the myometrium allows a rapid flow of blood into the uterine cavity. The volume of blood that can be lost from the uterus is a reflection of the abundant supply (500 mL/min, at term, flows through the placental area). Thus, bleeding from the placental site can be so severe as to imbalance the supply of oxygen and nutrients to both mother and fetus alike.

hypovolemic shock   Hemorrhage which suddenly reduces blood volume causes symptoms of *hypovolemia*. Rapid loss of blood of the equivalent of more than 1 percent of body weight or more than 10 percent of blood volume causes *hypovolemic shock*. [One milliliter of blood is considered equivalent to 1 g of body weight. Therefore, in a woman weighing 50 kg (110 lb) or 50,000 g, 1 percent of body weight equals approximately 500 mL.[1]]

The state of shock is a result of inadequate tissue perfusion, leading to deprivation of all nutrients to vital tissues, especially glucose and oxygen, and to a buildup of waste products in these tissues.

Although a variety of body responses occurs as a result of hypovolemia, intricate processes for hemostasis and reflex vasoconstriction also begin (Fig. 22-2). To support the body's own efforts to restore volume, intervention to repair the cause of bleeding must take place immediately. Treatment follows three main avenues:

Replacement of fluid to restore adequate blood volume
Repair or removal of the causes of bleeding
Support of the patient during the process of treatment

The main medical and nursing support and observations that are carried out during hypovolemic shock in obstetrics are outlined in Table 22-1.

ECTOPIC PREGNANCY

Ectopic implantation always leads to bleeding within the first trimester. An embryo and placenta located outside the normal implantation area cannot grow for more than 10 or 12 weeks without showing the classic signs of pressure and bleeding. The rate of occurrence varies from group to group and appears to be especially influenced by low health and economic levels. For instance, an extremely high rate occurred in Saigon: a rate of 1 in 40 pregnancies, which probably reflected the wartime conditions and lack of care there. The rate in inner-city areas of the United States is from 1 in 80 to 1 in 120, whereas in areas of higher income levels the rate may be as low as 1 in 500 or 1 in 800. Thus an average figure for the United States of 1 in 200 pregnancies is somewhat misleading.[2]

Cell growth will proceed at the same phenomenal rate of speed whether the blastocyst implants in the fallopian tube, ovary, cervix, interstitial area of the fundus, or peritoneal cavity (Fig. 22-3). The rapidly developing embryo with its placental tissue will usually begin showing specific pressure effects by 10 weeks' gestation without excessive bleeding. Wherever the trophoblast cells burrow into the implantation site, the effect is the same. Placental implantation stimulates an increase in blood supply, forms maternal pools of blood (lacunae), and produces a spongy vascular area which will bleed profusely should it somehow later become detached from its site.

Breen found in his survey of 654 patients

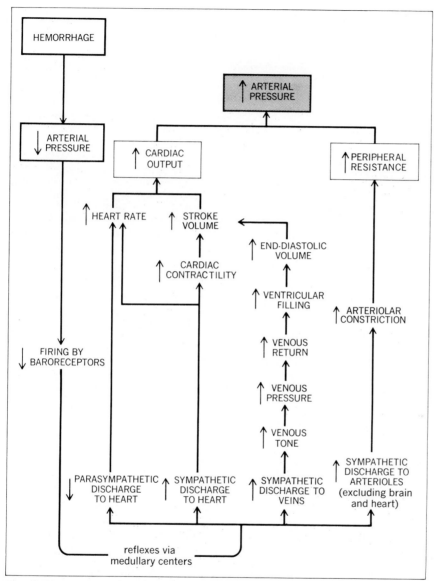

fig. 22-2 Reflex mechanisms to raise blood pressure after blood loss. (From A. J. Vander, D. Sherman, and D. Luciano, Human Physiology, McGraw-Hill, New York, 1970.)

with ectopic pregnancy that 97.7 percent were in the tube.[3] This number corresponds to the incidence in other studies. The other 2.3 percent were distributed, as shown in Fig. 22-3, at interstitial, cornual, cervical, ovarian, and abdominal sites, and are so rare that discussion here will center on tubal implantation.

table 22-1 Hypovolemic shock

physiologic changes	patient symptoms	interventions
cardiac/circulatory status *Deceased* venous pressure, cardiac output, pulse pressure, arterial pressure	Feels weak, dizzy; may feel rapid heartbeat	Record vital signs; if necessary, take apical pulse. Monitor CVP; if severe hypotension persists, line should be inserted by doctor. Support blood volume with plasma expanders, whole blood, Ringer's lactate.
Peripheral vasoconstriction To protect vital organs; adrenal medulla stimulated to produce catecholamines, adding to vasoconstriction	Feels cold, peripheral tissues are pale, nails blanch slowly; feels restless, anxious, fearful	Keep patient warm, check skin color, turgor, mucous membrane moisture, temperature. Reassure patient, stay with her. Record expressed statements, observations.
respiratory status Tachypnea Respiratory center stimulated by hypoxia	Complains of "air hunger," shortness of breath	Note rate, rhythm, depth of respirations. Administer oxygen by mask (do not use Trendelenburg position during pregnancy; instead, place patient in side-lying position).
gastrointestinal status Fluid shift from interstitial tissues and intestinal tract to vascular compartment (takes several hours to shift).	Sensation of thirst increases	Drop in hematocrit observed after shift. Draw blood for serial hemoglobin/hematocrit determinations. Keep NPO if returning to OR or delivery room for correction of bleeding.
Decreased parasympathetic activity + reduced GI motility, secretions	Nausea may occur	
renal status Conservation of fluids and salts stimulated by vasoconstriction of renal arterioles (needs 70 mmHg pressure to effectively filtrate blood)	May have no sensation of need to void	Observe closely for oliguria (lower limit of normal 30 mL/h). Record hourly output and specific gravity, from Foley catheter.

tubal pregnancy

Since the tube is 8 to 14 cm in length and 0.5 to 1 cm in diameter, its size cannot support an embryo for long. Normally, the inner mucosal lining of the tube goes through cyclic changes similar to the changes in the endometrium, without the shedding of cells and blood that make up the menstrual flow. Cilia are present to sweep the ovum along the tube;

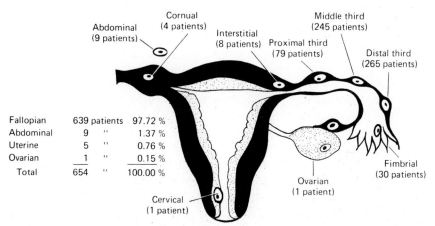

Fallopian	639 patients	97.72 %
Abdominal	9 ''	1.37 %
Uterine	5 ''	0.76 %
Ovarian	1 ''	0.15 %
Total	654 ''	100.00 %

Cornual (4 patients)
Abdominal (9 patients)
Interstitial (8 patients)
Middle third (245 patients)
Proximal third (79 patients)
Distal third (265 patients)
Fimbrial (30 patients)
Ovarian (1 patient)
Cervical (1 patient)

fig. 22-3   Ectopic pregnancy: implantation sites. (*From J. L. Breen, "A 21 Year Survey of 654 Ectopic Pregnancies," American Journal of Obstetrics and Gynecology,* **106:***1004, 1970.*)

they are assisted by rhythmic contractions that produce the effect of a slow current moving toward the uterus. The fluids produced by the tube appear to be essential for the support of the ovum as it is transported.

causes   Although the exact reasons for many tubal implantations can not be discovered, delayed movement down the tube appears to be the major cause. The most common hindrances to movement of the zygote are inflammatory changes and scar tissue, usually the result of infection. *Salpingitis* (tubal infection) may be a sequel to endometritis after surgery, childbirth, or abortion, or may be caused by venereal disease. Scar tissue or adhesions may also be a sequel to abdominal surgery, e.g., for appendicitis, ovarian cyst, or cesarean section.

The health or function of the fallopian tube may be affected by lowered progesterone or estrogen levels and by endometriosis, both factors in infertility problems. Occasionally, an ovum may migrate from one ovary to the opposite fallopian tube. This unusual trip has been diagnosed when surgery is done to remove the tubal pregnancy, only to find the corpus luteum located in the opposite ovary.[4] The delay caused by the time for migration of this ovum to the opposite fallopian tube caused implantation to occur in that tube.

When tubal or any type of ectopic pregnancy is confirmed, the treatment is usually surgical removal of the conception. By the time the pregnancy has developed 10 or 12 weeks, the damage to the tubal tissue is so extensive that it usually cannot be left in place. As an exception to this, if the diagnosis is made early enough, the physician may be able to remove the gestation and repair the tube so that it maintains its function. The procedure is called a *tuboplasty*.[5] The surgery may be of an emergency nature, within an hour of admission, or may be delayed if the diagnosis is difficult to make. In any case, the danger of hemorrhage is the primary concern.

recurrence   Since the pathologic condition that caused the tubal implantation is usually bilateral, the woman has a much greater chance of a second tubal pregnancy or of subsequent sterility.

diagnosis   When an ectopic pregnancy is suspected, a careful history of symptoms is taken (Table 22-2). The common indications are amenorrhea, with varying degrees of spotting or heavier bleeding, anemia, syncope, general pregnancy symptoms, and abdominal pain beginning approximately 10 to 12 weeks after the last menstrual period.

To confirm the diagnosis, the physician may, after a vaginal examination, perform a *culdocentesis*, or aspiration of fluid from the cul-de-sac of Douglas (Fig. 22-5). The procedure is done with the patient in a lithotomy position and does not require anesthesia. A needle is inserted into the wall of the vagina just behind the cervix. In cases of slow leaking from an enlarging placental site in the tube, dark unclotted blood can be aspirated from the cul-de-sac where it has collected.

If a culdocentesis is inconclusive, and the diagnosis is still to be determined, a *culdoscopy* may be the physician's next choice. A small probe with a fiberoptic light is inserted into the cul-de-sac for direct visualization of the tubes. Other physicians prefer a *laparoscopy*, i.e., insertion of a similar probe through the abdominal wall for visualization of the tubes. Both procedures require preparation of the patient, consent, and at least local anesthesia.

These procedures may be carried out on an emergency basis or may be delayed until diagnosis is first sought by nonsurgical means, such as ultrasound evaluation or the culdocentesis. If an emergency *laparotomy* is decided upon to remove the products of conception from the tube, the usual preoperative orders are as follows:

1   Give nothing by mouth.
2   Put Foley catheter in place for straight drainage.
3   Type and cross-match for 2 to 4 units of blood.
4   Determine hemoglobin and hematocrit levels.
5   Perform abdominal shave (or perineal shave, depending on hospital policy).
6   Have intravenous equipment in place, with large-bore intracatheter.
7   Premedicate only after consent is obtained.

supporting care   Care is based on the main problem of preventing life-threatening hemorrhage. The patient is maintained on complete bed rest while the diagnosis is confirmed by tests. Sedation may be administered if the patient is not bleeding acutely. The amount of vaginal bleeding is recorded at specific intervals.

Vital signs are recorded frequently. It is important to note that unless there is accompanying infection, the temperature is usually normal. Of course, when extensive bleeding has occurred, the patient will show signs of hypovolemic shock. Preparations are made for each treatment and for surgery.

recovery period   The recovery period should theoretically follow that of a tubal ligation. However, since most patients have lost a considerable amount of blood and have had the trauma of losing the pregnancy under these conditions, the recovery period may be more complex. These patients are liable to postoperative abdominal distension and to infection because of prior anemia and trauma; a few have postoperative depression. Supportive, anticipatory nursing care can help to reduce complications for the patient.

CYSTIC DEGENERATION OF THE CHORION

The hydatidiform mole, a molar pregnancy, is a rare but potentially dangerous change in the normal placenta. The rate of occurrence in the United States is about 1 in 2000 pregnancies. The chorionic syncytium grows erratically, forming fluid-filled vesicles that are

table 22-2 Symptoms noted with tubal implantation

symptoms	comments
Various types and degrees of bleeding:	
Painless, periodic vaginal spotting may resemble a light menstrual period	Patient may not notify doctor
	Bleeding may be caused by breakdown of decidual tissue after death of embryo in tube
Hidden bleeding into peritoneum ("a slow leak") causes symptoms of lower abdominal pressure (dark unclotted blood collects in cul-de-sac)	Caused by slow separation of placenta
Sudden massive bleeding associated with rupture of the tubal site causes mother to go into hypovolemic shock	Bleeding is usually preceded by pain
Anemia:	
Fatigue; pale mucous membranes (out of proportion to observed blood loss)	Hemoglobin/hematocrit levels fall slowly, especially with hidden slow bleeding
Abdominal pain of various types:	
Feeling of fullness in lower part of abdomen or backache and mild abdominal aching	3 to 5 weeks after missing the first period, symptoms begin, gradually increasing in intensity
May be referred pain and occur at time of usual menstrual period	(See Fig. 22-4 for sites of referred pain)
May be exquisite pain on vaginal examination when cervix is moved	Vaginal examination often brings first clue to what is wrong
Intense "tearing" pain may occur at time of rupture of tube	May still masquerade as appendicitis
Syncope:	
Light-headedness and fainting have been observed in 35 to 50% of ectopic pregnancies. Termed the "bathroom sign," as fainting often occurs while straining to defecate	Response to feeling of fullness and pressure in rectal area
	Cause: pressure of growing embryo or collection of blood in cul-de-sac, pressure on nerves of the perineal area
Early symptoms of pregnancy:	
There will be breast tenderness, nausea, and for about 50% a positive pregnancy test, uterus enlarged to about an 8-week size	As long as corpus luteum is functioning, effects of pregnancy hormones will be experienced

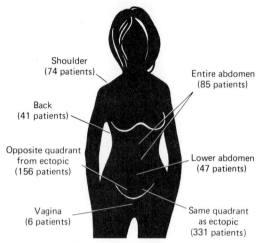

fig. 22-4 Ectopic pregnancy: sites of referred pain. (*From J. L. Breen, "A 21 Year Survey of 654 Ectopic Pregnancies," American Journal of Obstetrics and Gynecology,* **106:***1004, 1970.*)

fig. 22-5 Cul-de-sac of Douglas: behind cervix, in front of rectum.

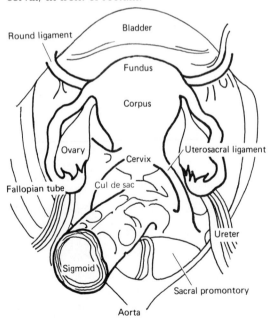

best described as grapelike clusters. (Fig. 22-6). The growth of these vesicles causes the uterus to enlarge much more rapidly than in a normal pregnancy. Strangely, there may also be accompanying hypertensive symptoms similar to those of preeclampsia, but occurring much earlier. Abnormally increasing uterine size and hypertension are accompanied by uterine bleeding, beginning as spotting and progressing slowly to a more serious amount.

Striking changes in laboratory findings indicate a hydatid change in the placenta. The levels of human chorionic gonadotropin (HCG) rise rapidly, since the excessive growth takes place in the chorion. Other laboratory findings in the presence of molar pregnancy are lower estriol levels, lower pregnanediol levels, and lower 17-ketosteroid levels than in a normal pregnancy of the same gestational age.[6]

supportive care

The treatment is to empty the uterus of all tissue by careful dilation and curettage, or if the pregnancy is too far advanced, by hysterotomy. After treatment, frequent urine tests are made to check on levels of HCG. Levels should have fallen to the normal nonpregnant rate by the end of 2 months after treatment.

malignant changes

This follow-up is important because, in a few *very rare* instances, molar pregnancy progresses to one of two malignant changes: to locally *invasive mole,* sometimes called *chorioadenoma destructens,* or to *choriocarcinoma.* Choriocarcinoma is the most malignant form; without treatment, it is invariably fatal. Treatment consists of intravenous therapy with antimetabolite drugs such as methotrexate and actinomycin-D. Early treatment at the first

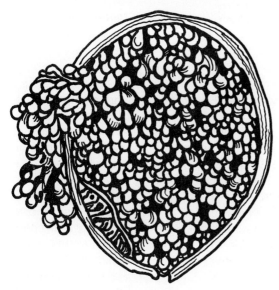

fig. 22-6 Hydatidiform mole. Grapelike clusters fill the uterine cavity.

sign of a rising HCG level has led to a cure rate as high as 98 percent.[6]

There is a possibility that the changes will be undiscovered if the woman spontaneously aborts the gestation early and completely. In one study 40 percent of the tissue from spontaneous abortion showed some degeneration of the chorion.[7] In another study 70 percent of the actual cases of choriocarcinoma were in patients who had had spontaneous abortions.[8] In these cases, symptoms causing the woman to seek medical attention would stem from already existing metastatic disease.

ABORTION

An abortion is a termination of pregnancy before the fetus is able to survive. An *early* abortion takes place before the sixteenth week of gestation; a *late* abortion occurs during and after the sixteenth week. To be classed as the product of an abortion or as *previable,* the fetus must weigh less than 500g and have

a crown to rump length of less than 16.5 cm.[9] Should the fetus weigh more than 500 g and be born without any signs of life, it is registered as an immature (viable) fetus and a *stillbirth.* If there are any signs of life, such as respiratory or muscle movements or heartbeat, the birth should be listed as liveborn fetus, and as a *neonatal death* if it does not survive.

The age of viability has now been set at the beginning of the twentieth week of gestation, even though few of the 20- to 27-week-old infants are able to survive with modern techniques of neonatal intensive care. These infants between 500 and 1000 g have a small but significant chance of survival and thus are counted as potentially viable infants.

The word *abortion* can be defined as stopping short of the full growth, or not completing the pregnancy. The word is always modified by an adjective to be specific. Terms describing types of abortion may be classified into two groups:

Spontaneous (*involuntary*)	*Induced* (*voluntary*)
Threatened	Legal
Inevitable	Therapeutic
Complete	Elective
Incomplete	Illegal
Habitual	Criminal
Missed or retained	Self-induced

spontaneous abortion

Seventy-five percent of all spontaneous abortions take place between 8 and 12 weeks of gestation. In fact, many women have experienced early abortions without realizing that they were actually pregnant. Spotting at the first period, then extra bleeding and cramping at the next, may be the only indications of the pregnancy loss; even by 8 weeks the embryo is so small that a woman may pass all the tissue easily. Since an estimated 15 percent of all gestations end in spontaneous abortion, almost every gravida will have experienced an involuntary loss of a pregnancy at some time in her reproductive period.

causes Causes of spontaneous abortion have been classified by Assali as embryonic and fetal causes (50 to 60 percent), maternal causes (15 percent), and a combination or unknown (20 to 30 percent).[10]

Embryonic or fetal causes include chromosomal and germ plasm defects and placental abnormalities. What is termed a "blighted ovum" is abnormal development or implantation that is inconsistent with growth. Since most of the early abortions show embryonic defects, women who have lost such a pregnancy may find comfort in the fact that early abortion may be a protection against an abnormal fetus.

Maternal causes tend to initiate late abortions. These include various infections (Chap. 25), poor nutrition, and, rarely, trauma. Rh incompatibility may be so severe as to prevent the pregnancy from continuing past the first trimester. Systemic diseases that are not well controlled may cause abortion; examples of these are diabetes, sickle-cell anemia, or hypertensive cardiovascular disease. Endocrine imbalance may cause low sex steroid levels which prevent maintenance of the pregnancy without replacement therapy by hormones. Thyroid imbalance, if poorly controlled, often leads to abortion.

threatened abortion The warning signals of a threatened abortion are those of varying degrees of bleeding, cramping, and abdominal aching. On vaginal examination the physician finds no cervical dilation in process. The lack of dilation distinguishes a threatened abortion from an inevitable abortion. A closed cervix allows hope that treatment with bed rest, sedation, abstinence from coitus, and therapy with uterine relaxants or hormones may avert the progression to an inevitable abortion.

SUPPORTIVE CARE   Since the cause is rarely known early enough to use preventive therapy, treatment is symptomatic. Bed rest and sedation may calm the patient. If tests for progesterone and human chorionic gonadotropin reveal low levels, replacement with progesterone may be started. Sometimes thyroid supplements help to maintain a pregnancy. If an abortion is threatening because of psychogenic causes, calm listening and counseling may be helpful. In every case, intercourse will be contraindicated until the pregnancy seems to be well established.

inevitable abortion Since no therapy really works after true dilation begins, the term *inevitable* is used to describe the inability of therapy to reverse the process of cervical dilation or to save the fetus.

COMPLETE ABORTION   The cervix dilates to 4 to 5 cm, and all parts of the placenta and embryo are passed out of the uterus. The recovery period is one of normal involution. Many women do not receive medical care but go through the complete abortion at home.

INCOMPLETE ABORTION   After cervical dilation, bleeding, and cramping, fragments of the embryo and placenta are passed. The retained portions of the placenta cause excessive bleeding. In this case the woman must be admitted for evacuation of the uterine contents.

Incomplete abortion may be due to a poorly performed criminal abortion and may be accompanied by injury to the cervix or uterine wall and infection as well. Careful questioning may elicit an admission from the woman that she sought illegal termination of pregnancy.

In a New York City hospital, admissions for incomplete abortions were reduced by 50 percent the year after the liberalized abortion law was passed.[11]

habitual abortion A woman who has lost three or more consecutive pregnancies is called a habitual aborter. The cause may be maternal infertility, chronic disease, or blood group incompatibility. The chief cause is cervical insufficiency, due to prior birth trauma or induced abortion trauma to the cervix, or to intrinsic anatomic problems. The process follows a specific pattern: the cervix begins dilating after 16 weeks, the membranes bulge out of the external os, and the uterus begins the contractions which will lead to delivery of a tiny fetus.

Unless insufficiency, or *cervical incompetence,* is diagnosed and treated, the mother may lose a series of pregnancies between 16 and 26 weeks in gestation. The treatment is to use a *cerclage* procedure, or the placement of a nonabsorbable suture around the cervix to hold it closed. The procedure may be done before conception; if it is done after conception, special precautions must be taken to maintain the pregnancy after the cervical manipulation. Postoperatively, the patient is placed in Trendelenburg position for 48 h to relieve the pressure of the fetus on the cervix. Sedation and complete bed rest for 48 h are usually ordered. Special checking will be done for vaginal bleeding, contractions, and the fetal heartbeat. Of course, before delivery is possible, this suture must be removed.

missed abortion After a pregnancy has been noted, there may in a few cases be a regression of symptoms—or lack of progression—leading the examiner to suspect a missed abortion. In the previable period, the retention of a conceptus 4 or more weeks after intrauterine death is called a *missed abortion* or a *retained abortion.* The placental function may continue for some time after fetal death, thus causing confusing pregnancy screening tests. However, it is the nature of things that fetal growth and activity follow a rapidly changing schedule. Absence of the usual weekly changes is a strong indication of fetal death.

Once a missed abortion is recognized, the physician will plan to empty the uterus with suction, or with dilation and curettage, using oxytocin infusion to control bleeding. Late abortion will be treated with oxytocin infusion to soften the cervix. Should this be ineffective, an intraamniotic injection of saline solution may be attempted. Prostaglandin F_2-alpha (dinoprost) is currently approved for intraamniotic instillation for late abortion.

stillbirth Death after the age of viability is termed an intrauterine fetal death (IUFD). After the delivery, such a death in utero is called a *stillbirth.* Signs and symptoms of an IUFD follow those of a missed abortion, with the additional changes that are appropriate to the length of time in weeks that the pregnancy had lasted. There are a diminishing of amniotic fluid, a regression of the breast changes, and a reversal of the other physiologic changes of pregnancy. Fetal movements have been felt since 18 weeks and should reach a maximum in the last trimester, decreasing slightly the few weeks before delivery. The mother who has become accustomed to feeling every movement and frequent change of position of the child will state that she feels "empty" when fetal death occurs.[12]

Tests for fetal life are the same as those for pregnancy. Especially useful are estriol levels and fetal electrocardiograms. An x-ray view of the fetus some time after fetal death shows overlapping of the skull bones and a generally flaccid posture. If radiopaque dye were introduced into the amniotic fluid, the absence of swallowing (see Chap. 27) would indicate fetal death.

induced abortion

The changing laws regarding voluntary abortion reflect the social turmoil of the society. The Supreme Court ruling of January 1973 removed all restrictions on an elective abortion in the first 12 weeks of gestation. The decision was made on the grounds of protecting the woman's right to privacy, leaving the abortion decision to her and her physician. The decision called for clear state restrictions on abortion between 13 and 29 weeks of gestation and asked state prohibition of abortion after 30 weeks.

Today, the risk of dying from an abortion is less than that of dying from complications of pregnancy. However, every week that a pregnancy progresses, the risk increases. Gestational age appears to be the most important factor in mortality risk. The risk of induced abortion causing death is nine times greater at 11 to 12 weeks than if performed earlier than 9 weeks. At 16 to 20 weeks, the risk is 49 times higher than with early abortion. During the period 1972–1974 the overall abortion risk was 3.9 per 100,000 procedures, a figure still considerably below the 14.9 per 100,000 live births for pregnancy/delivery risks.[14] The conclusion is clear: if a woman wishes to have an induced abortion, she should seek it early, before the ninth week.

As a result of the elective abortion rate (one out of four pregnancies each year), the rate of *criminal* abortion has dropped markedly, and with it the high maternal morbidity from hemorrhage, infection, and trauma. Such illegal abortions caused untold psychologic and physical damage to women desperate enough to seek a termination of pregnancy.

In one New York City hospital, during 1970–1972 as a result of the increase in elective abortions, the incidence of out-of-wedlock births dropped 11.8 percent, mortality rate was 28 percent lower, and illegal and septic abortions had almost disappeared.[13]

The legal status of abortion on demand is under challenge by Right-to Life groups and others opposed to the Supreme Court ruling. The reader is referred to Berry (see Bibliography) for a more complete discussion of various religious approaches to the issue. It is important for nurses to develop an understanding of their own attitudes toward the idea of pregnancy termination so that they can effectively approach a person seeking abortion without carrying the emotional "baggage" of unclear feelings. The confusion which results from ambivalent feelings or incompletely understood ideas will only interfere with a therapeutic approach to such patients.

Burchell has identified five possible positions on abortion and effectively discusses professional questions, attitudes, and approaches to the controversy.[15] He notes that legal changes do not usually affect deeply held attitudes.

1   The first position allows no indication for abortion. Carried to its extreme, an ectopic pregnancy could not be removed, nor could a patient with pelvic cancer be treated until the baby was born.
2   The second position holds that no direct abortion is accepted, but if necessary, an indirect abortion secondary to a life-saving procedure may be performed. It appears that most people against elective abortion hold this position.
3   The third position allows medical indications to govern whether an abortion is necessary. This position was that which promoted therapeutic abortions. However, the indications became so vague that restrictions were almost negligible if the patient could afford to get different medical opinions. The physician became the one who governed the choice of instituting an abortion.
4   The fourth position, the one sanctioned by the Supreme Court, allows direct abortion based on the judgment of the physician

and the patient. The reasons may be social, economic, or medical, but it is a fairly joint decision. The physician, however, may refuse to perform the procedure.

5 The fifth position allows the patient to be the only deciding factor, i.e., abortion on request, based on the woman's judgment alone. This last position has no restrictions, and although she may be counseled otherwise, the woman has the responsibility of the final decision.

Most people are agreed that abortion should not be used as a method of contraception. Therefore, our efforts as professional nurses involved in health education can go toward helping a woman to prevent future conception when pregnancy is so unwelcome as to cause her to seek to terminate one that has already begun. Nurses who have gained a degree of empathy with a woman going through the turmoil of unwanted pregnancy can begin to comprehend the aspects of her choice. Making a decision when one is in the center of the choice is far different from making it when one is merely observing or debating issues intellectually.

That the choice of abortion constitutes a life crisis situation is clearly stated by Mace:[16]

One thing is clear: you must do something, or rather you must decide what to do. Pregnancies do sometimes end of their own accord, but you can't count on that. You need a policy, a plan, and you need it without delay. Every day that passes, the developing life within you grows bigger, more active, more mature. Nine months seems a long time, but it can pass very quickly.

Pregnancy itself is a crisis event for a woman; when it is an unwelcome event the crisis is intensified. Nurses are called upon to use every skill in supporting the mother through the period of the abortion and recovery.

methods of pregnancy termination

DILATION AND SUCTION EVACUATION Suction evacuation of uterine contents is the method of choice for an early termination of pregnancy between 6 and 10 weeks (Fig. 22-7). The cervix must be dilated wide enough to allow the passage of instruments. Dilatation is the most difficult part of the procedure for it must proceed slowly and may be met with considerable resistance, expecially in a nullipara. To overcome this problem many physicians are turning to the use of *Laminaria,* a form of seaweed that is hygroscopic (i.e., it swells when wet). Small laminaria sticks can be placed into the cervical os and left in place overnight. Their slow increase in size does painlessly what the physician would have to do under anesthesia. The next day the patient returns for suction curettage with a cervical dilatation of 2 to 3 cm. Laminaria are widely used in Japan and only recently have been tried in this country.

DILATION AND SHARP CURETTAGE A D and C may be done toward the end of the first trimester. Instead of a suction device, a spoon-shaped instrument is used to scrape the lining out of the uterus. Dilatation of the cervix is done as in a suction evacuation.

Either suction or sharp curettage can be done under paracervical anesthesia on an outpatient basis when the duration of gestation is less than 11 weeks. Abortion under general anesthesia should be done with admission to the hospital when any question arises about gestational age or when any medical problems are present. Whichever method is chosen, several precautions are necessary.

1 A complete history should be taken and a complete physical examination made.
2 Ample time should be given for counseling in order for the patient to be clear in her own mind about the decisions. (See references by Keller and Shainess.)

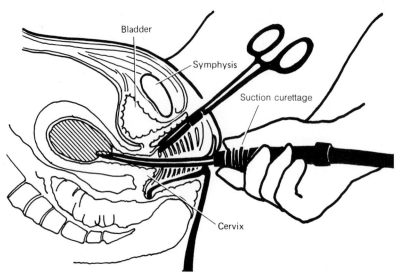

Bladder

Symphysis

Suction curettage

Cervix

fig. 22-7 Suction abortion.

3 The statement of the patient's consent should be clearly explained to and understood by her before she signs it.

4 Blood tests must be made. A complete blood count is done, and a tube for type and cross-match should be held in case a transfusion becomes necessary. All prospective patients should be screened for the Rh-negative factor.

5 The patient is instructed to come for her appointment having fasted, i.e., with an empty stomach.

6 She is to be accompanied by a friend who can go home with her after the operation is over.

Adverse Effects Infection, hemorrhage, and cervical injury are the major adverse effects. Occasionally the uterine wall is perforated during the procedure. Retained fragments of the placenta may lead to delayed bleeding.

After the procedure, the patient rests until able to go home. Instructions are as follows: Report any untoward symptoms of bleeding in excess (soaking pad, passing clots), fever, or pain. Do not use tampons or douche or have sexual intercourse until 2 weeks have

passed and the physician has checked recovery. If the patient is unreliable about contraception, some physicians will insert an IUD just after an abortion procedure (with consent, of course).

The prevailing mood for a woman who has chosen to terminate a pregnancy is one of relief. There still may follow a period of grieving, and the counselor can prepare the woman for such an event. The importance of good counseling cannot be overemphasized; it is critical to the complete success of the elective abortion process.

HYPERTONIC SALINE INSTILLATION After gestational age has been determined as *over 14 weeks* (to allow for sufficient amniotic fluid), a saline induction can be used to terminate pregnancy or to begin labor when there has been an intrauterine fetal death (see Fig. 22-8).

The preparation for the procedure is the same as for a D and C. The patient voids just before the procedure. The abdomen is washed with antiseptic solution and draped. The procedure follows that of amniocentesis (see Chap. 27), but the needle is placed in the miduterus. Local anesthetic is used to anesthetize the skin and area of descent of the needle. A 4- to 5-in needle is used to enter the amniotic fluid; free flow of fluid indicates correct placement. A Teflon catheter is inserted through the needle. Amniotic fluid is aspirated and replaced with 20 percent saline solution to a total of 200 mL. At the end of the instillation, 1 million units of aqueous penicillin is instilled and the catheter withdrawn. *Adverse Effects* A flushed face, thirst, headache, tachycardia, and numbness and tingling in the extremities indicate inadvertent injection into the vascular system. *Hypernatremia* results and must be treated at once with a rapid infusion of 5 percent dextrose and water, plus oral water intake.

Pain in the abdomen indicates incorrect injection into the peritoneum. In some cases, membranes rupture during the procedure and some the hypertonic saline solution leaks out through the fallopian tubes into the abdominal cavity.

Bladder injection is indicated by a *burning sensation* and urgency. The bladder must be irrigated at once with physiologic saline solution to dilute the hypertonic fluid and prevent sloughing of the bladder mucosa. *Fever* may occur as a result of chorioamnionitis, but patients appear to respond effectively to antibiotic therapy. Finally, *hemorrhage* from retained placenta occurs at a rate of about 1:100.

All these are reasons why a saline induction should never be treated as a minor procedure. Staff should be prepared for any eventuality, and clear instructions should be given to the patient to report any untoward symptoms. Most patients are discharged after the procedure with instructions to return when labor begins.

Labor will ensue within an average of 1 to 3 days (for about 80 percent of women). Other women deliver earlier or have delayed abor-

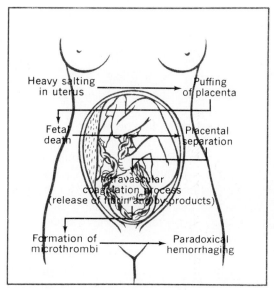

fig. 22-8 Saline abortion: how it seems to happen. (*From Marius N. Trinique, Medical World News.*)

tions. Usually the cervix dilates rapidly once the process begins, and many women pass the products of conception at home. Thus, patients need a great deal of support and teaching.

Some services use a tape recording, to which the patient listens during the procedure, and in addition provide her with written instructions. An important point to emphasize to the patient is that she will go through a labor process, albeit shortened, and will experience uterine contractions and discomfort. When labor takes place in the hospital, the nurse is the one who monitors the patient's condition and supports her during the process. All the points of postdelivery care are valid for postabortion patients.

PROSTAGLANDIN INSTILLATION Dinoprost tromethamine (prostaglandin F_2-alpha) is used as a method of inducing contractions in the second trimester. Several routes have been investigated; the intrauterine instillation pro-

vides the best results with the least side effects. One or two milliliters of amniotic fluid is removed by amniocentesis, and 40 mg of dinoprost tromethamine is injected slowly, after a test dose is given. If there is no response to the first instillation, 10 to 20 mg may be repeated after 6 h. Cervical dilatation and abortion should follow within 8 to 20 h.[17]
Adverse Effects Side effects vary in intensity depending upon the route of administration. Should the prostaglandin be absorbed systemically, nausea, vomiting, and diarrhea are common (50 percent). Fever, dizziness, headache, and hypertension may also occur. Rarely, bronchospasm, cardiac arrythmias, chest pain, hiccups, and hyperventilation have been seen. Should the medication be injected intravascularly, a hypotensive episode of 15 to 30 min duration is precipitated. Since prostaglandins are very quickly metabolized, the shock period is self-limiting, as are the other reactions. Nevertheless, immediate care must be available and all personnel prepared to treat shock. The most difficult problem associated with this method is bleeding, which may result from cervical or lower uterine laceration or from retention of portions of the placenta. Exploration of the uterus and cervix under anesthesia must be done as soon as the diagnosis is made.

In spite of these problems, prostaglandin instillation is probably a faster, safer method of second-trimester induction of labor. It is becoming the method of choice in many settings.

HYSTEROTOMY, HYSTERECTOMY Sometimes, termination of pregnancy is performed later in the second trimester by means of a *hysterotomy* (incision into the uterus) or a *hysterectomy* (removal of the uterus). The risks are high and are usually related to uterine pathology. Most often, one of these procedures must be done when another method of abortion has failed or complications have occurred. Rarely are either of these methods chosen as the initial procedure.

PLACENTA PREVIA

On occasion the blastocyst implants in the lower uterine segment. Because the decidua there is less nourishing and the blood supply less adequate, the placenta will spread out over a larger surface and may cover the internal os, *completely, partially, or marginally* (Fig. 22-9). Placenta previa occurs in about 0.5 to 1 percent of all pregnancies and is more common in older gravidas and in those with a multiple pregnancy.

Because low implantation does not favor fetal growth, many of these pregnancies are lost by spontaneous abortion in the first trimester. If the pregnancy is sustained, warning hemorrhages usually do not then occur until the second half of pregnancy. Bleeding is due to the slowly effacing cervix *pulling away* from the overlying placenta. Hemorrhage may be so severe as to necessitate interruption of the pregnancy to save the life of the mother, with the result of an immature or nonviable infant.

The mother who has been looking forward to this baby will suffer grief at its loss as acutely as the mother who loses her baby at term. Support during the critical decision to terminate the pregnancy is important, because the mother may blame herself for being the cause of the bleeding. She can be reassured that the low-lying placenta is an accident of implantation and is unpredictable, unavoidable, and not usually repeatable.

diagnosis

The only observable sign of placenta previa is the evidence of degrees of *painless* bleeding; the woman may notice persistent spotting, or she may wake to find a large amount

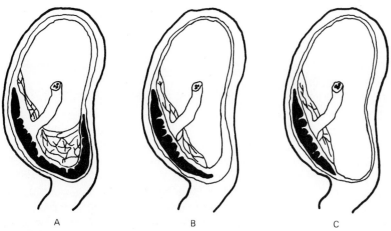

fig. 22-9 Types of placenta previa: (a) total, (b) partial, and (c) low implantation.

of blood in her bed. Thus, *any* bleeding in pregnancy must be reported to the physician at once. On examination the physician is careful not to manipulate the cervix as that might cause further bleeding. However, a gentle speculum examination is necessary to rule out other causes: cervical polyps, infection, cervical erosion, or capillary fragility with blood vessel disruption after sexual intercourse.

Soft-tissue x-rays may help to locate the placenta when it is preventing engagement of the fetal head. Ultrasonography is also a useful diagnostic tool for locating the site of the placenta.

supportive care

Bed rest until bleeding stops has allowed many pregnancies to mature a few more weeks. Each day in the uterus gives the fetus a better chance of survival. To encourage bed rest, the physician may order sedation (see Chap. 26 for premature labor therapy). Nursing care is planned around keeping the mother quietly in bed, and observing the amount of bleeding. If the bleeding is serious,

vital signs are taken more frequently than every 4 h. Since unsuccessful tries may raise unnecessary anxiety in the mother, it is preferable to use an amplified fetoscope to obtain the fetal heart rate.

Daily laboratory tests will be ordered to keep track of hemoglobin and hematocrit levels. Blood type and cross-match are determined in order to have at least 2 pt of blood available at all times. Except for the initial gentle speculum examination, vaginal examinations usually are not done, since any manipulation of the cervix may cause an increase in bleeding. The one exception is the "double setup," in which the patient is examined in the delivery room only after preparations have been made for an immediate vaginal delivery or an emergency cesarean section, should excessive bleeding be precipitated by the examination itself.

Vaginal delivery is possible only when the placenta is marginal or low-lying and the fetal head is well engaged. In this case, the fetal head acts as a ball valve, or tamponade pressing on the edge of the placenta, thus preventing further bleeding during the process of descent.

postpartum care

The placenta site will be larger than usual and *friable,* or easily torn. When the placenta has been located in the lower uterine segment, which is thinner and passive during labor, there may have been small tears during delivery that may result in considerably more bleeding during the immediate recovery period. Therefore, any woman who shows signs of placenta previa is watched very carefully for excessive bleeding after delivery.

PREMATURE SEPARATION OF THE PLACENTA

In 2 percent of all pregnancies, some degree of placental separation occurs before delivery. Another term used to describe placental separation is *abruptio placentae,* a term that reflects the suddenness of the occurrence. The severity of separation has been classified by grades:[18]

Grade 0	No clinical symptoms but examination of placenta after delivery shows from one cotyledon to one-third separation of placenta
Grade 1	External hemorrhage only Mild uterine contraction More than one-third of placenta, less than two-thirds
Grade 2	External and internal hemorrhage Uterine contraction, "uterus de bois" (woodlike) Up to two-thirds separation of placenta
Grade 3	Internal hemorrhage Severe separation and uterine contraction Maternal shock and clotting defect Intrauterine death

Although the causative factors are not clear in every case, 40 to 50 percent of all premature separations are accompanied by maternal hypertension. A multipara has a higher risk of premature separation, as will a woman with folic acid deficiency. Also, abruptio placentae is more likely to occur in a woman who has already experienced one such episode. The mechanism of separation is thought to be associated with vascular changes causing a reduction of blood flow to the uterus. If this reduction is severe enough, vessel necrosis and placental infarcts may occur. As an *infarct,* or area of dead tissue, enlarges, it splits away from the decidua, and hemorrhage from the site begins (Fig. 22-10).

diagnosis

Premature separation usually produces symptoms suddenly, just before or during labor, although the underlying process may have gone on for some time prior to labor. Continuing abdominal pain accompanied by severe bleeding and a change in the character of the uterine contractions are signs that can be easily noted. However, variations in severity of symptoms and grades of separation cause some confusion with placenta previa.

With concealed bleeding, or *internal hemorrhage,* the uterus will become rigid and very painful. If touched by the attendant the patient will complain of exquisite uterine tenderness, an unusual sign during labor. The cause of this rigid, hard contracture of the muscle is

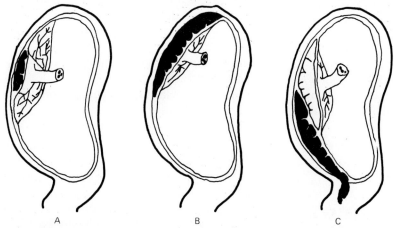

fig. 22-10 Types of abruptio placentae: (a) partial separation (concealed bleeding), (b) complete separation (concealed bleeding, and (c) partial separation (apparent hemorrhage).

that blood has been trapped between the decidua and the placenta. The maternal arterial pressure forces more blood into the space, further separating the placenta and disturbing any clots that may have formed; thus the blood may be forced by mounting pressure to *extravasate* into the uterine muscle, forming what looks like a big bruise, leaving the muscle painful, swollen, and unable to relax. The description of the uterus as woodlike, "uterus de bois," is an accurate one for grades 2 and 3.

External, or visible, bleeding occurring with placental separation indicates that the *edge* of the placenta has broken away, allowing the blood to leave the uterus without building up the intense internal pressure that causes so much pain. With grades 0 and 1, the contractions may become erratic but the intense pain of concealed bleeding may be absent.

Fetal survival depends on the ability of the remaining intact placenta to provide oxygen exchange. Fetal death is certain with grade 3 and may occur with grade 2.

supportive care

Treatment depends primarily on the severity of symptoms and the stage of labor when they occur. The only way to stop the bleeding is for the obstetrician to effect delivery and remove the placenta so that the uterus can contract enough to clamp off arteries leading to the placental site. In case of an extremely bruised uterus with extensive extravasation, uterine contraction may be impossible and a hysterectomy may be required to stop bleeding.

When a great deal of bleeding has occurred, blood coagulaton defects cause difficulty in hemostasis. Thus in every delivery accompanied by moderate to severe premature separation, tests for fibrinogen levels and clotting time will be made.

outcome

Maternal mortality is less than 1 percent when treatment is available, yet fetal mortality from fetal anoxia and immaturity remains at about 40 to 50 percent. Those women who experience abrupt separation when they are some distance from a hospital are usually the ones who succumb to the effects of rapid, uncontrollable bleeding. As a result, statistics from rural areas of the United States may show a higher mortality rate than those from urban areas, where medical care is usually more readily available.

EARLY HEMORRHAGE AFTER DELIVERY

After the placenta has separated, the placental site is a raw wound having numerous arteriole and venule openings that spill out blood if no hemostasis takes place. Normally, strong myometrial contractions pinch off the blood supply, and blood clots form. If the uterus stays firmly contracted, all is well, and blood loss is minimal. If for some reason it relaxes, the blood flow begins again, pushing out the newly formed clots.

During immediate recovery, oxytocin given intravenously or intramuscularly will actively support normal uterine contracture. When oxytocin is not available or is not given, the infant can be put to breast so that its sucking action can stimulate pitocin release from the posterior pituitary.

uterine atony

Uterine *atony* is the main cause of early postpartum hemorrhage (i.e., in the first 24 h). Frequent checking on the degree of uterine contraction is an important part of nursing care. The likelihood of uterine atony is increased if the newly delivered woman had:

1 A long, exhausting labor
2 Uterine dystocia
3 A traumatic delivery
4 An overdistended uterus, polyhydramnios, twins, etc.
5 Prior bleeding from abruptio placentae, with extravasation
6 Placenta previa with a large placenta site in the lower uterine segment
7 Fibroids preventing symmetric contraction of the uterus
8 A generally poor condition when she came to delivery, with anemia, preeclampsia, or extreme fatigue

A completely preventable cause of bleeding is that due to overdistension of the bladder. The distended bladder, attached to the tissues of the uterus, pulls it up and pushes it to the right or left of midline, thus preventing contracture. Without the mother herself being aware of bladder distension (see Chap. 12 for reasons), extensive bleeding may occur. If the fundus is to the side and above the umbilicus during early recovery, it will contain many clots. After massage, very firm pressure on the fundus will then expel the clots out into the vagina and then into the bedpan. The amount must be measured, with an estimation of the amount of urine mixed with the blood. Of course, prior emptying of the bladder before massage will allow the uterus to contract properly. In many cases pain, tension, and anxiety will inhibit voiding. After all techniques to assist the patient have been tried, catheterization may be needed before hemostasis can be obtained.

lacerations

Oxytocin cannot stop bleeding if there are undetected lacerations of the uterine wall, cervix, vaginal wall, or perineum. Lacerations (Chap. 26) are the second most common cause of early bleeding and will show signs of a steady trickle of arterial blood. The mother may show signs of shock without much observable bleeding if the lacerations are deep within the birth passage or in the uterus. The immediate treatment is to return her to the delivery room to repair the laceration, all the while working to restore blood volume.

retained placental fragments

The third major cause of bleeding after delivery is retention of fragments of the placenta or tissues of the amniotic sac. Good obstetric care includes checking the placenta to see that it has been delivered intact.

If the bleeding is caused by placental fragments, the patient is returned to the delivery table. With light anesthesia, the obstetrician curettes the uterus with a gloved wrapped in a sterile gauze sponge, or uses gentle exploration of the uterus with instruments.

hematoma

A hematoma, or bleeding into the tissues, produces symptoms of swelling, exquisite pain at the site, and often shock symptoms out of proportion to the loss of blood that is evident. Hidden bleeding into the broad ligament, rectal or vaginal wall, or the labia may be the cause of these acute symptoms. Immediate treatment involves a return to the delivery room for examination, clamping, and suturing of the bleeding site. The collected blood in the tissues may be removed as much as possible to reduce the painful pressure.

Severe pain is *always* unusual after a normal delivery. Nonnarcotic analgesics are usually adequate for postdelivery discomfort. Therefore, a patient complaining of severe pain should always be examined at once for the condition of the perineal area, the bladder, and the uterus.

manual compression If bleeding continues and all factors have been explored, oxytocics have been given, and fluids and blood are being replaced intravenously, the uterus will be compressed manually by the physician. Before or after internal manual compression, *external compression* can be applied by the nurse by grasping the fundus of the uterus firmly with the palm of one hand and pushing down just above the symphysis pubis with the other palm, so that the uterus is compressed between the palms. Massaging the fundus will cause reflex contracture of the muscle, but too much stimulus, too long, will eventually cause exhaustion of the muscle. When bleeding still does not stop, the uterus may be packed to provide a tamponade. The last resort, a lifesaving measure in severe uterine hemorrhage, is for the obstetrician to do a hysterectomy or to tie off the main arteries leading to the uterus.

LATE POSTPARTUM HEMORRHAGE

One or two weeks after delivery, fresh bleeding is usually the result of retained placental fragments or infection. Rarely, a fibroid tumor of the uterus will delay involution and may cause some extra bleeding. When infection of the endometrium, *endometritis,* is present, *subinvolution,* or poor reduction of the placental site, occurs. This leads to a recurrence of bleeding when the patient is home after having apparently been progressing normally before discharge. Any patient with delayed hemorrhage will be readmitted to the hospital for curettage, oxytocin infusion, blood transfusion, and antibiotic therapy if infection is present.

ANEMIA RESULTING FROM INADEQUATE ERYTHROCYTE PRODUCTION*

Inadequate blood production to maintain a normal hemoglobin level may result from a variety of causes, including lack of "blood-cell building blocks," e.g., iron, folic, acid, vitamin B_{12}; lack of hormonal stimulus for erythrocyte production; or damage to the bone marrow structure or to the hematopoietic (blood-producing) stem cells in the marrow.

iron deficiency anemia

Iron deficiency is the most common cause of anemia in both pregnant and nonpregnant women (90 percent). If hemoglobin levels fall below 11.0 g and if the hematocrit value is below 31 to 33 percent in the second half of pregnancy, iron lack is suspected. Iron deficiency is more common in women than in men. The total store of iron is less in women, and the physiologic requirement in females is greater because of blood loss during menstruation or delivery and the iron needs of the fetus during pregnancy and lactation (see Fig. 22-11).

The daily requirement of iron in a physiologic steady state averages 1 to 2 mg. The additional requirement of about 400 mg iron for pregnancy itself and 150 mg for the placenta would require nearly two more milligrams in additional *daily* iron absorption for the mother to remain in iron balance. For the pregnant woman, this usually necessitates iron supplementation, since this amount is not available for absorption from usual dietary sources.

The marrow will respond to iron lack by

* The author wishes to acknowledge the contribution of Evert A. Bruckner, M.D., to this section.

"economizing," with a resultant moderate decrease in the number of erythrocytes it produces and the development of mild anemia. As the iron deficiency state becomes more severe, additional "economizing" includes the production of smaller erythrocytes (microcytes) and later the production of pale erythrocytes with a lower concentration of hemoglobin in each one (hypochromic cells).

folate deficiency anemia

DNA (deoxyribonucleic acid) is a key part of cell nuclei and chromosomes and is basic to cellular life. Folic acid and vitamin B_{12} are necessary for the synthesis of nucleic acid, and thus for the synthesis of DNA. The more cell division and growth, the greater the amount of DNA required and thus the greater is the requirement for folic acid and vitamin B_{12}. The fetus has the capacity of selectively absorbing folate and vitamin B_{12} (as well as other factors necessary for its development, including iron) and will absorb these substances at the expense of the mother. Thus, if the available supply of these substances is inadequate for the needs of both the mother and the fetus, the available amount will go primarily to the fetus.

The folate stores in human beings are relatively small and are fairly readily depleted by either increased utilization or decreased intake. A deficiency may result from poor intake, poor absorption from the intestine, liver damage, or frequent pregnancies, which may not allow adequate time for replenishing the body folate stores. Other causes include certain anticonvulsant drugs and tapeworm infestation of the intestine. In many tropical areas, multiple causes of anemia will often include malaria as well.

Body stores of vitamin B_{12} are somewhat larger than those of folic acid and its sources from the diet are more varied; therefore, de-

INPUT   OUTPUT

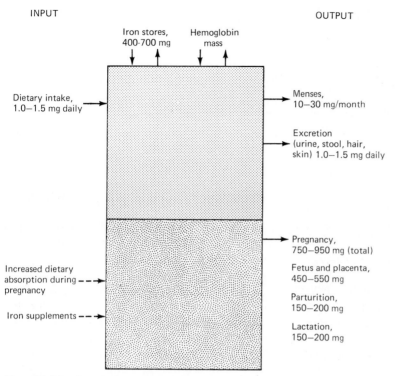

fig. 22-11 Iron balance in women.

pletion is considerably less common. Lack of folate or vitamin B_{12} results in failure of blood cells to divide and mature properly. The cell nucleus matures more slowly than the cytoplasm, and thus the growth patterns of these two cell components become out of phase with each other. Bone marrow that shows these changes typical of deficiency of either folate or vitamin B_{12} is described as *megaloblastic.*

In addition to exhibiting slower maturation in the presence of folate deficiency, the erythrocyte precursors typically may skip one of the several mitotic divisions which they would ordinarily make and thus may remain larger than normal at the end of the cycle. These erythrocytes are called *macrocytes.*

Daily folate requirements are 50 to 100 μg/day before pregnancy. Folate deficiency dur-

ing pregnancy is largely preventable by folate supplements of 100 to 300 μg/day.[18] Approximately 50 percent of pregnant women show some evidence of deficiency before the end of gestation unless supplementation is prescribed.

thalassemia

A third type of hypoproliferative anemia exists which has a distinctively different mechanism and effect. Thalassemia is characterized by a *hypochromic microcytic* anemia, usually associated with an abnormality of erythrocyte shape. Thalassemia shares with iron deficiency the characteristic of inadequate hemoglobin production. However, at this point a key difference emerges: in iron deficiency the inadequate hemoglobin production is a result of decreased *heme* synthesis, whereas, in thalassemia, anemia results from inadequate *globin* production plus an excessive breakdown of the defective erythrocytes which are produced. Thalassemia is thus both a hypoproliferative anemia and a hemolytic state.

Thalassemia is genetically determined and may occur in either the homozygous or heterozygous state. In homozygous thalassemia (also called *thalassemia major,* Mediterranean anemia, or Cooley's anemia), the anemia is severe and very little normal adult hemoglobin is present. This severe hemolytic anemia is associated with an enlarged spleen, decreased resistance to infection, and other complications. These patients usually do not live beyond adolescence, and pregnancy is rarely encountered in girls with thalassemia major. If it occurs, there is striking anemia and severe congestive heart failure.

The heterozygous form of the disease is called *thalassemia minor.* In general it is not nearly as serious, and there is a wide variation in the symptoms that are experienced. Some patients have very minimal anemia; in others there may be frequent episodes of rapidly worsening anemia, produced by various types of stresses, including pregnancy. Further complications arise when thalassemia coexists with other hemoglobinopathies such as hemoglobin S (i.e., sickle thalassemia).

The thalassemia syndromes primarily affect populations originating in countries bordering the Mediterranean Sea and in Southeast Asia, but are not strictly limited to these geographic boundaries.

HEMOLYTIC ANEMIA

Hemolytic anemia results from the premature or excessive destruction of erythrocytes, associated with an inability of the bone marrow to replace these cells rapidly enough to maintain a normal hemoglobin and hematocrit level. This group of anemias may be categorized as *intrinsic,* in which an inherent defect in the erythrocyte is the basis for premature cell destruction, or *extrinsic,* in which factors outside the erythrocyte are primarily responsible for hemolysis.

Although there are many potential causes of anemia, we shall focus on two groups of *intrinsic* erythrocyte defects which account for the great majority of cases of hemolytic anemia: those with abnormal hemoglobin structures and/or production (hemoglobinopathies), and those in which an enzyme deficiency results in an alteration of erythrocyte metabolism (enzymopathies).

The hemoglobinopathies consist of those disorders in which the percentage (95 percent) of adult hemoglobin (hemoglobin A) in the red cell is decreased. This can result either from an inability to produce adequate globin to form hemoglobin A, as in thalassemia, or from a condition in which the hemoglobin A has been replaced by an abnormal hemoglobin, as in sickle-cell disease.

A few comments about the structure of hemoglobin may facilitate an understanding of some of the causes of anemia associated with the hemoglobinopathies. The hemoglobin molecule is made up of an iron-containing component called *heme* and, for the most part, two pairs of polypeptide chains called *alpha* (α) and *beta* (β). Table 22-3 indicates the percentage of other hemoglobin chains found in normal adults. These chains are attached to heme group, which in turn has the property of reversibly combining with oxygen. The polypeptide chains are made up of 574 amino acids joined in linkage. If a single amino acid is substituted in either of these chains, an abnormal hemoglobin will result. Such substitutions may occur on either the alpha or beta chain. More than 100 abnormal hemoglobins have been discovered thus far, but the most common and clinically most

table 22-3 Structure of adult hemoglobin

type	ratio	structure
Hemoglobin A (adult)	95%	2 alpha, 2 beta chains (α_2, β_2)
Hemoglobin A_2	2 to 3%	2 alpha, 2 delta chains (α_2, δ_2)
Hemoglobin F (fetal)	1 to 2%	2 alpha, 2 gamma chains (α_2, γ_2)

important is hemoglobin S, or sickle hemoglobin, which is produced by the substitution of the amino acid *valine* for *glutamic acid* in the beta chain of the molecule.

hemoglobin S—sickle-cell disease

Sickle-cell disease is transmitted equally by males and females. The heterozygous form (designated S-A) is called sickle-cell trait; the homozygous form (designated S-S) is called sickle-cell disease. In sickle-cell disease, most of the hemoglobin in the affected individuals is hemoglobin S, with the remainder usually being hemoglobin F, a fetal form of hemoglobin.

The deoxygenated form of hemoglobin S has approximately one-fortieth the solubility of hemoglobin A. At the lower range of oxygen tensions, it crystallizes out of solution and assumes a characteristic crescent, or "sickle" shape. A resultant increase in the viscosity or thickness of the blood results in a "sludging effect" on the blood and a decrease in the blood flow in the very small blood vessels of the tissues, particularly in the spleen, bones, kidneys, lungs, and gastrointestinal tract. Sickle-cell crises may result from these cells, forming "log jams" in small vessels. Ischemia and infarction are responsible for painful crises and the systemic problems of this disease.

sickle-cell trait

Sickle-cell trait is a relatively benign condition, and there is little evidence indicative of any serious complications of pregnancy associated with sickle hemoglobin trait. Urinary tract infections are present with increased frequency in pregnant patients with sickle-cell trait, and hematuria is also relatively common.

incidence The incidence of sickle-cell anemia in the black population of the United States is about 0.2 percent. The sickle-cell trait is present in 8 to 10 percent of the American black population. In tropical Africa the incidence of this gene is considerably higher overall, with considerable variation from one population group to another, with some having an incidence as high as 45 percent.

Sickle-cell disease follows a geographic distribution related to the high incidence of malaria, for it somehow offers protection against malaria. Therefore, persons with S-A and S-S can usually trace their roots to tropical Africa and Asia, with a few from Mediterranian countries.

Large-scale screening programs to detect unrecognized hemoglobinopathies, particularly hemoglobin S, have been advocated, and numerous projects for this purpose are now operative. These studies understandably have generated much discussion pro and con, with a number of difficult questions having been raised concerning the implications of these data. For example, to what extent might the theoretic or practical value of knowing that one is heterozygous—or homozygous—for hemoglobin S be offset by possible social penalties of various kinds (e.g., relating to employment, obtaining medical and other

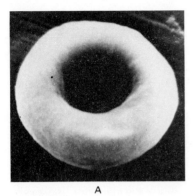
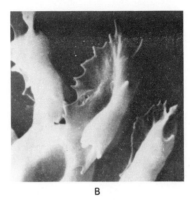
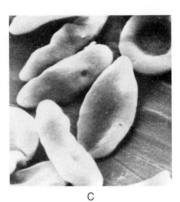

A   B   C

fig. 22-12   Process of sickling and unsickling of red cells. (a) Stereoscan electron micrograph of a normally oxygenated red cell showing classic biconcave disk with central cavity and slight surface irregularity. (b) When deoxygenated, cells take on the typical holly-leaf sickle shape. If reoxygenated, the cells unsickle. The process may go on to an irreversible state (c). (c) In the oxygenated state, irreversibly sickled cells have a characteristic oval or cigar shape with a smooth membrane. If deoxygenated and then reoxygenated again, cells return to this shape. (From "Sickling Damages Red-cell Membrane," Medical World News, Jan. 26, 1973; courtesy of Drs. Lessin, Jensen, and Klug.)

types of insurance, etc.)? These are difficult questions and will require searching and imaginative interdisciplinary study and action, combined with a broad-spectrum approach to education of the public-at-large regarding these issues.

sickling crisis   Crises of sickle-cell disease are of two general types, which frequently coexist. In a *painful crisis*, pain in the back, abdomen, or long bones is frequent, but virtually all the organ systems may be involved in one way or another. Pulmonary infarction, hematuria, and cerebrovascular accidents also may occur. Bone crises have repeatedly been reported as complications of late pregnancy and the puerperium. In a *hemolytic crisis*, anemia typically develops with great rapidity, which, when superimposed on the already existent moderately severe anemia which is characteristic of sickle-cell disease in the stable state, may result in additional complications such as congestive heart failure, angina, and myocardial infarction. Fever and jaundice are commonly present during hemolytic crises.

supportive care   The management and treatment of the pregnant patient with sickle-cell disease is difficult. Infections, particularly recurrent urinary tract infections, are common and are treated with appropriate antibiotics. Folate deficiency, common in sickle-cell patients, may become much more severe in pregnancy, and the administration of oral folic acid supplements, 1 to 2 mg daily, is helpful. Sickle crises are treated with adequate hydration and analgesia. If anemia becomes severe, blood transfusion is routine. Exchange transfusions are used prophylactically in the third trimester as the possibility of a crisis mounts. These consist of removing a quantity of blood from the patient and replacing it with normal (i.e., non-hemoglobin S) blood, thereby increasing the proportion of non-hemoglobin S blood and decreasing the concentration of the hemoglobin S cells, which are predisposed to clumping and hemolysis.

Extreme care must be taken not to diminish oxygen tension by anesthesia or analgesia during labor; oxygen by mask is often provided. The risk of crisis and development of anemia can continue into the postpartum period.

morbidity and mortality Both a high fetal wastage and increased perinatal maternal mortality occur in patients with sickle-cell anemia. Complications are frequent and varied, including an increased incidence of toxemia, infectious complications, increased severity of anemia, painful crises in the bones, and premature labor. Up to one-fourth to one-half of all known pregnancies in women with sickle-cell anemia terminate in neonatal death, abortion, or stillbirth, compared with a fetal wastage of about 15 percent in black patients without sickle-cell disease.[18]

hemoglobin c

Hemoglobin C is a relatively common abnormal hemoglobin having an incidence second only to hemoglobin S in the black American population. Approximately 2 percent of American blacks carry the gene of hemoglobin C, which is approximately one-fourth the incidence of hemoglobin S. Hemoglobin S and hemoglobin C may coexist, with resultant hemoglobin S-C disease. Hemoglobin C disease (S-C disease) is relatively well tolerated, with only mild to moderate anemia. However, during pregnancy and the puerperium, both morbidity and mortality are increased and pregnancy in a woman with hemoglobin S-C disease is nearly as hazardous as in a woman with sickle-cell disease. Maternal mortality averages about 7 percent, with fetal wastage being considerably higher, averaging about 35 percent.[19-21] Because of the frequency and potential seriousness of complications, as well as increased danger of maternal death,

avoidance of pregnancy is to be encouraged; contraception or sterilization should be considered. On the basis of these facts a case can be made for an early therapeutic abortion in the event of pregnancy. Strong differences of opinion related to both philosophic and moral presuppositions as well as to the manner in which the available data are interpreted, exist regarding these issues.

genetic counseling In order that they may understand the risks entailed and associated potential problems in any offspring, genetic counseling is of considerable importance to patients with hemoglobinopathies. If the identities of any hemoglobinopathies present in the prospective parents are known, a prediction of probability of occurrence of the entity in question in offspring can be made. For example if one parent is homozygous (e.g., has sickle-cell disease) and the other is heterozygous (e.g., has sickle-cell trait), *half* their children may be expected to have the disease and the other half the trait. If both parents are homozygotes, all their children would also be expected to inherit the disease. Data of this type may be of great assistance to prospective parents in understanding possible risks to any offspring they may have. (See Chap. 28.)

erythrocyte enzyme deficiencies (enzymopathies)

Another form of genetically inherited hemolytic anemia is that caused by abnormalities in erythrocyte metabolism resulting in defective energy production within the cell and a subsequent shortening of the erythrocyte lifespan. Enzyme deficiencies are the most common example. A large number of erythrocyte enzyme deficiencies have been discovered; glucose 6-phosphate dehydrogenase (G-6-

PD) is the most frequently found. Pyruvate kinase (PK) deficiency is less common but is not rare. Both these enzyme defects may either cause a chronic hemolytic process or trigger an acute hemolytic reaction. Various types of stress may trigger such a hemolytic reaction, including oxidative drugs (in the case of G-6-PD) and various other metabolic stresses (infection, fever, pregnancy). Many variants of G-6-PD are known, and the distribution of their deficiency varies widely among different population groups. One common variant is found in approximately 11 percent of American black males, but is much less frequent in black females. Another variant is found in about 50 percent of certain Jewish populations.[22] A G-6-PD screening test is indicated in those cases where a hemolytic process is suspected, or where the family history suggests an enzyme deficiency. It is important to identify this enzyme deficiency in order to try to avoid the precipitation of an acute hemolytic crisis by the introduction of medications or other chemicals which may trigger it.

DISEASES OF THE LEUKOCYTIC CELL SERIES

nonneoplastic proliferative states

Proliferative disorders of the leukocytic cell series may be either of malignant or nonmalignant type. Examples of nonmalignant or self-limited processes include infectious mononucleosis, lymphadenopathy due to various infections (measles, toxoplasmosis, streptococcal infections, etc), and allergic reactions. The complications related to these processes are caused by the primary process

itself, and the proliferative changes in the bone marrow and lymph nodes are merely reflections of this primary process. These changes in the blood, nodes, and bone marrow have no known direct detrimental effect on pregnancy.

leukemia and lymphomas

Examples of a malignant form of neoplastic proliferation of the white cell series include leukemia in its various forms and various types of lymphoma. Leukemia is infrequently encountered in pregnancy. Since chronic myelogenous leukemia has its greatest incidence between the ages of 35 and 50 years, i.e., during later reproductive years, it would be expected to be the most common type of chronic leukemia to accompany pregnancy.

Currently available data would suggest that the course of chronic leukemia is not significantly changed by pregnancy. Fetal wastage is considerably increased because of stillbirth and prematurity, but, on the basis of limited data available, maternal mortality does not appear to be markedly increased. Transmission of leukemia from mother to child during pregnancy is not a significant risk.

hodgkin's disease Pregnancy is an uncommon occurrence in Hodgkin's disease, even though the incidence of this disease is relatively high in the reproductive age group. The available data do not provide convincing support for the common view that pregnancy, per se, has a deleterious direct effect on the course of Hodgkin's disease. However, pregnancy may alter the approach to therapy in a given case, and thus indirectly alter the course of the disease. A history of treated Hodgkin's disease is not in itself a strong basis for terminating pregnancy. Circumstances in which this may be considered or advised include (1) a history of previous radiation to the pelvis, with the associated possibility of fetal abnormality due to radiation effect on the ovaries, (2) the occurrence of pregnancy during the course of an ongoing chemotherapeutic program, or (3) the occurrence of pregnancy in the presence of active or progressive clinical disease.

In the event of recurrence of Hodgkin's disease in sites distant from the uterus, if radiation therapy is deemed the therapy of choice it can be carried out despite pregnancy. Available data provides no evidence of increased fetal wastage in association with radiation therapy to distant sites.

PROBLEMS OF THE COAGULATION SYSTEM

Coagulation of the blood is a complex phenomenon involving many interrelated factors which are of varying importance in their role in the overall process. The coagulation system exhibits a somewhat precarious balance between excessive coagulation (and thrombosis) and deficient or defective clotting (and hemorrhage). When we speak of "the coagulation system" or "the hemostatic mechanism" it is important to bear in mind that the phenomenon referred to involves *both* the factors that participate in the clotting of blood and those that are involved in the breakdown or lysis of the blood clot. These factors include clotting substances in plasma and tissue fluids, blood platelets, and the function of the blood vessel wall. During pregnancy, increased synthesis of most clotting factors occurs on an average of 1.8 times the nonpregnant level. If there is a question about blood coagulability, screening tests are done: bleeding time, clotting time, and prothrombin time (factors II, V, VII, X) and partial thromboplastin time (all factors except VII and XIII).[23]

thromboplastin

One of the key factors in initiating the coagulation sequence which results in a blood clot is thromboplastin. When this material is introduced into the circulation the coagulation system is activated. Thromboplastin is present in most types of body tissue to some degree, but certain tissues contain a relatively high concentration of this substance. Damaged tissues may release thromboplastin into the circulation. For example, abruptio placenta or a retained dead fetus may activate the coagulation sequence by this mechanism. Abruptio placenta is probably the commonest cause of coagulation defect in pregnancy. Shock, gram-negative sepsis, and surgery are examples of other circumstances which may predispose to derangement of the blood clotting mechanism and result in thrombosis or hemorrhage. Of specific importance in obstetrics is the fact that amniotic fluid also contains a significant concentration of thromboplastin. If the thromboplastin is introduced into the circulation in amniotic fluid embolism, it may likewise trigger clinically inappropriate coagulation.

the role of thrombin One step in the coagulation process is the generation of thrombin from its precursor substance prothrombin, in the presence of certain other necessary clotting factors. Thrombin is an extremely active substance which catalyzes several other reactions related to the clotting-bleeding process. It activates other clotting factors (factors V, VII, and XII), exerts a direct effect on platelets, and splits the molecule of fibrinogen, which is one of the clotting factor proteins produced by the liver. The effect of thrombin on the platelets causes them to clump together, and they are subsequently removed from the circulation by the reticuloendothelial system. Thrombocytopenia (platelet count of less than 100×10^9/L) may develop as a result of this increased platelet aggregation and destruction, and a "vicious cycle" may be established, with increased utilization of clotting factors (including fibrinogen), decrease in platelet supply, further activation of the coagulation system, and increased thrombin generation, which causes further platelet clumping and their removal from the circulation, and the cycle is thus perpetuated.

disseminated intravascular coagulopathy (DIC)

Disseminated intravascular coagulopathy is uncommon in the pregnant or parturient woman, but it is perhaps the best known of the coagulation problems. It well illustrates the interaction of multiple factors active in the coagulation process, and will therefore be considered here in more detail than its frequency of occurrence would otherwise indicate. DIC is that condition in which the coagulation sequence is activated in a clinically inappropriate manner, with a resultant series of events which may result in either hemorrhage or thrombosis (or both), but thrombosis occurs more uncommonly. Other terms which are sometimes used to describe various aspects of this clinical entity include *consumptive coagulopathy* and *defibrination syndrome*.

Hemorrhage is usually generalized, with symptoms of petechiae, ecchymosis, and purpura. Bleeding into the GI tract and urine also occurs. Early signs may be oozing at the venipuncture site or bruising on the arm after a blood pressure cuff has been used.

management of dic Although DIC of a clinically significant degree is uncommon, self-limiting episodes of increased activity of the coagulation system (including fibrinolysis,

that part of the coagulation system which relates to the dissolving or breakdown of the blood clot) may occur following certain types of surgery. These episodes usually clear up spontaneously within a few hours, with little or no clinical expression, and do not initiate the "vicious cycle" mentioned above.[24]

In those situations in which the pathologic state is transient or can be effectively dealt with (e.g., abruptio placenta or removal of a dead retained fetus), treatment for the DIC may not be indicated or required. If, however, a serious bleeding/clotting process results from a condition that cannot be corrected, response to treatment is frequently poor. Administration of platelet transfusions, or cryoprecipitate (factor VII and fibrinogen) may be ordered. Supportive measures such as fluids to maintain fluid and electrolyte balance, blood cells in cases of hemorrhage, and oxygen are necessary.

platelet disorders

Pregnancy is not a proved etiologic factor in disorders of platelet function or production. It may uncommonly be an intermediary factor in the development of thrombocytopenia due to folate deficiency. A preexisting folate deficiency may be worsened in a pregnant woman because of the folate demands of the developing fetus. Thrombocytopenia may result from the severe folate deficiency thus produced. Pregnant women are subject to the same risks, but not to increased risks of development of an idiosyncratic response to medications, sepsis, or excessive alcohol intake. Of serious concern in pregnancy is the development of so-called idiopathic (immune) thrombocytopenic purpura (ITP), an immunologic disorder in which a circulating humoral IgG, immunoglobin, accelerates the destruction of platelets because of changes in the platelet surface. Signs show as petechiae and purpura on skin and mucous membranes when the platelet count is lower than 20 to 30 × 10^9/L.[25]

Children born to mothers with ITP frequently have thrombocytopenia because of placental transfer of antibodies, but it usually clears up spontaneously. Fetal mortality is somewhat higher than normal, however.

management Corticosteroids and sometimes a splenectomy are utilized to control platelet destruction. Platelet transfusions are of no benefit.

SUMMARY

Hematologic problems in pregnancy are usually a reflection of (1) continued or increased expression of a hematologic problem which was present prior to pregnancy, such as a hemoglobinopathy or enzymopathy, (2) increased stresses or metabolic requirements directly associated with the pregnancy, such as anemia resulting from iron or folate deficiency or hemorrhage, or (3) changes in the blood-clotting mechanism, such as the development of disseminated intravascular coagulation as a result of the introduction of thromboplastin into the bloodstream in certain pathologic conditions.

It is important to pinpoint as precisely as possible, and as early in the pregnancy as possible, the presence or potential development of hematologic problems so that appropriate corrective or preventive measures may be taken.

study questions

1 Identify the three general problems causing anemia during pregnancy.
2 What structural factors make bleeding in pregnancy a likely possibility? How is bleeding corrected?
3 Ms. Jones, 21, in her eleventh week of pregnancy, is diagnosed as having a right ectopic tubal pregnancy. Identify the probable symptoms she has and describe the diagnostic tests which must be done before treatment begins.
4 What questions would you include in her admission history?
5 How is a molar pregnancy diagnosed? Why is follow-up care so important?
6 Describe the differences between each type of abortion.
7 Think about which position you take regarding elective abortion. How are you able to respond to a person who adopts a different position?
8 How would you explain the value of an early decision regarding elective abortion as compared with a procedure performed after 12 weeks?
9 Compare placenta previa and premature separation of the placenta as to (a) method of diagnosis, (b) treatment, (c) supportive care, and (d) fetal outcome.
10 Which causes of postpartum bleeding can the nurse prevent? What are the important interventions?
11 Compare the effects of folate and iron deficiency. Identify foods high in these factors which can be included in a patient's diet.
12 Hemolytic anemia is inherited as an autosomal recessive trait. After you have studied Chap. 28, plot inheritance for sickle-cell anemia if the father is a carrier of the trait and the mother has sickle-cell anemia.
13 If the mother becomes pregnant when her sickle-cell anemia is under control, what special management is required to achieve a healthy pregnancy and delivery? (See reference by C. C. Ruff.)
14 Identify the situations in which DIC might occur. What signs and symptoms should alert the nurse to the presence of a coagulation disorder?
15 Thrombocytopenia may occur rarely in mother or baby. What signs or tests might indicate this condition? Define the term.

references

1 R. C. Benson, *Handbook of Obstetrics and Gynecology*, 4th ed., Lange, Los Altos, Calif., 1971, p. 182.
2 T. F. Halpin, "Ectopic Pregnancy," *American Journal of Obstetrics and Gynecology*, **106**(2):234, 1970.
3 J. L. Breen, "A 21 Year Survey of 654 Ectopic Pregnancies," *American Journal of Obstetrics and Gynecology*, **106**(7):1017, 1970.
4 Halpin, op. cit., p. 236.
5 W. B. Stromme, "Conservative Surgery for Ectopic Pregnancy," *Obstetrics and Gynecology*, **41**(2):215, 1973.

6 C. B. Hammond and R. T. Parker, "Diagnosis and Treatment of Trophoblastic Disease," *Obstetrics and Gynecology,* **35**(1):134, 1970.

7 Ibid., p. 138.

8 N. S. Assali and C. R. Brinkman, *The Pathophysiology of Gestation: Maternal Disorders,* Academic Press, New York, 1972, vol. 1, p. 194.

9 K. R. Niswander and M. Gordon, *The Women and Their Pregnancies,* The Collaborative Perinatal Study of the National Institute of Neurological Diseases and Stroke, Saunders, Philadelphia, 1972, p. 92.

10 Assali and Brinkman, op. cit., p. 192.

11 J. J. Rovinsky, "The Impact of a Permissive Abortion Statute on Community Health Care," *Obstetrics and Gynecology,* **41**(5):781, 1973.

12 J. M. Johnson, "Stillbirth—A Personal Experience." American Journal of Nursing, **72**(9):1595, 1972.

13 Rovinsky, op. cit., p. 787.

14 W. Cates, D. A. Grimes, J. C. Smith, and C. W. Tyler, "Legal Abortion Mortality in the U.S.: Epidemiologic Surveillance, 1972–74," *Journal of American Medical Association,* **237**:452, 1977.

15 R. C. Burchell, "Professional Perspectives on Abortion," *Journal of Obstetric, Gynecologic, and Neonatal Nursing,* **3**(6):25, 1974.

16 D. R. Mace, *Abortion: The Agonizing Decision,* Abingdon, New York, 1972, pp. 13–14.

17 *AMA Drug Evaluations,* 3d ed., Publishing Sciences Group, Littleton, Mass., 1977, p. 625.

18 Assali and Brinkman, op. cit., p. 223.

19 W. R. Bell, "Hematologic Abnormalities in Pregnancy," *Pediatric Clinics of North America* **24**(3): 170, August 1977.

20 R. P. Perkins, "Inherited Disorders of Hemoglobin Synthesis and Pregnancy," *American Journal of Obstetrics and Gynecology,* **111**:120, 1971.

21 E. O. Horger III, "Hemoglobin C Disease During Pregnancy," *Obstetrics and Gynecology,* **39**:873, 1972.

22 M. G. Freeman and G. J. Ruth, "S-S Disease and C-C Disease; Obstetric Considerations and Treatment," *Clinical Obstetrics and Gynecology,* **12**:134, 1969.

23 W. W. Williams, W. Beutler, A. Ersley, and W. Rundeles (eds)., *Hematology,* McGraw-Hill, New York, 1972, p. 392.

24 M. M. Conklin, "DIC in the Pregnant Patient," *Journal of Obstetric, Gynecologic, and Neonatal Nursing,* **3**(3):29, 1974.

25 G. J. Kliener and W. M. Greston, "Current Concepts of Defibrination in the Pregnant Woman," *Journal of Reproductive Medicine,* **17**(6):309, December 1976.

bibliography

Berry, S. L.: "Abortion," in J. Clauson (ed.), *Maternity Nursing Today,* McGraw-Hill, New York, 1977.

Hall, Robert E.: *A Doctor's Guide to Having an Abortion,* Signet, New York, 1971.

Hammond, B., L. G. Borchet, L. Tyrey, W. T. Creasman, and R. T. Parker: "Treatment of Metastatic Trophoblastic Disease: Good and Poor Prognosis," *American Journal of Obstetrics and Gynecology,* **115**(4):451, 1973.

Hematologic Disorders in Pregnancy, vol. 2, *Clinics in Haematology,* Saunders, Philadelphia, 1973.

Keller, C., and P. Copland: "Counseling the Abortion Patient Is More than Talk," *American Journal of Nursing,* **82**:102–106, 1972.

Lebfeldt, H.: "The Psychology of Contraceptive Failure," *Medical Aspects of Human Sexuality,* May 1971.

Lewis, J. L., Jr.: "High Risk Pregnancy: Hydatidiform Mole and Choriocarcinoma," *Journal of Reproductive Medicine,* **7**(2):57, 1971.

McFarlane, J.: "Sickle-Cell Disorders," *American Journal of Nursing,* **77**:1948, December 1977.

Nelson, B. H., and J. E. Huston: "Placenta Previa: A Possible Solution to the Associated High Fetal Mortality Rate," *Journal of Reproductive Medicine,* **7**(4):188, 1971.

Neubardt, S. and H. Schulman: *Techniques of Abortion,* Little, Brown, Boston, 1972.

Palomaki, J. F.: "Abortion Techniques: What Are Their Risks and Complications?" *Contemporary OB/GYN* **9**:73, January 1977.

Pritchard, J. A., R. Mason, M. Corley, and S. Pritchard: "The Genesis of Severe Placental Abruption," *American Journal of Obstetrics and Gynecology,* **108**:22, 1970.

Quinlivan, W. L. G., and J. A. Brock: "Blood Volume Changes and Blood Loss Associated with Labor," *American Journal of Obstetrics and Gynecology,* **106**:843–849, 1970.

Ruff, C. C.: "Childbearing in Sickle-Cell Anemia: A Nursing Approach," *Journal of Obstetric Gynecologic and Neonatal Nursing,* **6**(3):23, May/June 1977.

Scott, J. R.: "Vaginal Bleeding in the Mid-trimester of Pregnancy," *American Journal of Obstetrics and Gynecology,* **113**(3):329, 1972.

Shainess, N.: "Abortion, Social, Psychiatric and Psychoanalytic Perspectives," *New York State Journal of Medicine,* **68**:23, 1968 (Reprint C 34).

Tanner, M. L., C. B. Stamler, E. Klein, and B. Lee: "Attitudes of Personnel: Determinants of or Deterrents to Good Patient Care," *Clinical Obstetrics and Gynecology,* **14**:4, 1971.

23

CARDIOVASCULAR AND RESPIRATORY PROBLEMS DURING PREGNANCY

ELIZABETH J. DICKASON

Cardiovascular changes during pregnancy are quite distinct and would be considered a disease state in a nonpregnant adult. Each of the adjustments that take place has a purpose, and each affects the symptoms experienced by the woman as well as affecting the healthy outcome of the pregnancy. Understanding cardiovascular problems in pregnancy requires a knowledge of these normal changes.

NORMAL CARDIOVASCULAR CHANGES

The circulatory system can be thought of as a closed system made up of long elastic tubes of varying diameters which are already full of fluid. Pressure must be applied at one end to move the fluid through the system. The amount of pressure, measured as blood pressure, and the rate of flow depend on many factors. Figure 23-1 identifies these factors.

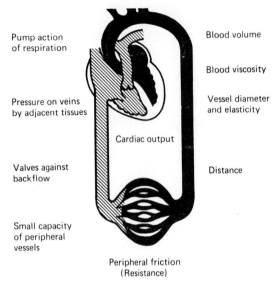

Pump action
of respiration

Blood volume

Blood viscosity

Pressure on veins
by adjacent tissues

Vessel diameter
and elasticity

Cardiac output

Valves against
backflow

Distance

Small capacity
of peripheral
vessels

Peripheral friction
(Resistance)

fig. 23-1 Factors influencing circulation. (*From E. L. Coodley, "Anatomy of Circulation"; reproduced with permission of the copyright owner, Consultant, The Journal of Medical Consultation.*)

cardiac output

Cardiac output (the volume of blood the left ventricle pumps into the aorta per minute) and *stroke volume* (the amount of blood sent into the aorta with each systole) can both be measured and are used to determine how effectively the heart is working. During pregnancy an increase of about 30 percent in cardiac output appears as early as the tenth week. Nonpregnant women average an output of 4.5 L/min. The change of 1.5 L/min raises the volume to a total of 6 L/min in the last two trimesters of pregnancy.

The nonpregnant heart rate averages 70 beats per minute. An overall increase of about 15 beats per minute helps to accomplish the extra work and push through this extra volume, until after delivery when the rate slowly returns to normal.

blood volume

Blood pressure will usually rise in cases of *hypervolemia,* or increased blood volume, and always will drop in cases of *hypovolemia.* In pregnancy, however, the blood volume rises 30 to 40 percent (1500 to 1800 mL over the normal nonpregnant average of 4000 mL). This large increase in volume does not seem to cause a basic elevation of blood pressure because most of the fluid is accommodated in the growing placenta, uterus, body tissues, and breasts. In later pregnancy, about 500 mL/min travels through the placenta. The placenta now acts as an arteriovenous shunt, actually causing a *decrease* in blood pressure during the first two trimesters of pregnancy.

Blood volume increases early in pregnancy and then is maintained at about the same peak level until just before delivery, when there is a slight decrease. After delivery there is a sudden rise in blood volume as 300 mL of blood is suddenly forced into the circulation with the removal of the placenta.[1] The blood pressure may rise 10 to 20 mmHg during the immediate recovery period, and then will decrease slowly until the blood volume returns to normal by 4 to 6 weeks postpartum.

An increase of 1200 to 1500 mL of *plasma* makes up most of the increase in blood volume. The *hematocrit* level, or the ratio of red blood cells to plasma, may drop from the normal ratio of 35 to 45 percent to about 30 to 35 percent because the volume of red cells increases only by about 250 to 400 mL. This results in a state of *hemodilution.* The oxygen-carrying capacity of the hemoglobin is unchanged, and the physiologic change is considered normal.

blood viscosity

The viscosity of blood affects the flow rate, the resistance to flow, and the pressure needed to pump the blood from the heart. Blood is about five times more viscous than water. Obviously, the thicker, more viscous fluid flows more slowly, and more pressure is needed to move it. When there is a state of dehydration with reduction in plasma volume and a rise in hematocrit, or *hemoconcentration,* the blood becomes even more viscous. If there is fluid retention in the vascular system, with a slight reduction in hematocrit, the blood becomes less viscous.

quality of vessels

The flow rate varies with the lumen of the tube: in a wider tube the blood will flow faster, in a narrower one it will flow more slowly. Any disease of the vessels, such as arteriosclerosis, affects the diameter of the lumen and the elasticity of the vessels. Mechanisms of vasoconstriction and vasodilation affect the lumen of the vessels and thus the flow rate and blood pressure.

Some capillaries in the circulatory system are so small that red blood cells go through in single file, even squeezing through by changing shape. Flow slows down in these small capillaries to about 1 mm/s, quite a change from the speed of flow in the large superior vena cava of 200 mm/s, and in the aorta, of 300 to 500 mm/s! The average round trip takes 25 s.[2] Circulation time is usually measured from arm to tongue, using a liquid injected intravenously which causes a burning sensation when it reaches the tongue. The nonpregnant rate is 15 to 16 s; during pregnancy the rate averages 12 to 14 s.

distance of flow

Blood pressure is affected by the distance the blood has to travel; pressure is highest in the large arteries and lowest in the vena cava. One estimate is that the adult system covers

70,000 miles through all the capillary beds of the body.[2] Figure 23-2 shows the relationship between the rate of flow and blood pressure. Age makes a difference: blood pressure rises as the infant matures to adulthood and the heart must pump through a longer circuit.

peripheral resistance

Peripheral resistance, or the forces causing friction as fluid and cells pass through the vessels, is a major factor in the amount of pressure needed to move fluid through the circulatory system.

> Total peripheral resistance . . . the measure of the totality of all the factors which affect the blood flow: effective viscosity of blood, the lengths of the vessels, their cross sectional areas as determined by intrinsic tone, vasomotor nerve impulses, presence of constrictor or dilator substances and extravascular pressures provided by tissue tensions.[3]

body water

Tissue tension increases as *total body water* rises all during pregnancy to 20 percent

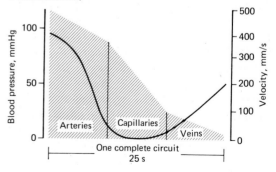

fig. 23-2 Blood pressure and velocity. (*From E. L. Coodley, "Anatomy of Circulation"; reproduced with permission of the copyright owner, Consultant, The Journal of Medical Consultation.*)

above normal, accounting for some of the weight gain and mild dependent edema of pregnancy. In the postpartal period, diuresis occurs in the second through fifth days, ridding the body of most of this excess water (Fig. 23-3).

direction of flow

The direction of flow of fluid affects the pressure needed to move it. Human beings have adjusted to standing upright, but as a result, blood must flow against the force of gravity through the venous system for 4 to 5 ft. Any pressure or process which hinders this flow will cause pooling, or *stasis* of fluid in the lower portions of the body. In many cases fluid moves into the interstitial spaces as pressure rises in the venules. Body position, posture, constriction of circulation, lack of muscle movement, or pressure of the growing uterus on the muscular veins of the pelvis may hinder fluid flow.

supine hypotension syndrome

An example of obstructed venous return is the supine hypotension syndrome, or the *vena*

fig. 23-3 Distribution of increased cardiac output in pregnancy. (*From F. E. Hytten, and I. Leitch, The Physiology of Human Pregnancy, Blackwell, Oxford, 1971.*)

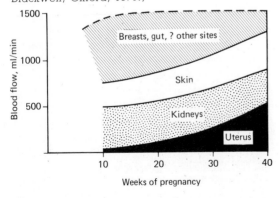

cava syndrome. The large uterus pressing on the inferior vena cava and the iliac and femoral arteries as the woman lies supine causes a pooling of venous blood in the legs. The result is an elevated pressure in the femoral vessels, with reduced volume and pressure of blood returning to the right atrium. The result is a falling blood pressure and stroke volume, profuse diaphoresis, and pallor; if the woman is in labor, fetal bradycardia may be recorded. A woman near term, lying supine 3 to 7 min, could experience the effect. Most women will, as a reflex, turn to one side unless they are heavily sedated in labor. A clearly documented syndrome such as supine hypotension must be recognized by the nurse at the bedside as she monitors vital signs (see Chap. 27). Basic treatment is to turn the patient to a side-lying position. In addition, near term, women should be encouraged to assume a side-lying position for sleep and rest.

The vena cava syndrome seems to occur more commonly in the woman with an extra large uterus, as in multiple pregnancy or polyhydramnios. It occurs more often in primigravidas with firm abdominal muscles and taut uterine muscles. Any type of interference with vascular return will predispose the mother to uterine pressure on the vena cava. Severe varicosities, where blood pools in veins in larger than normal amounts, will aggravate the condition. During regional anesthesia, loss of neural control affecting venous dilation in the lower extremities may cause the same symptoms.[4]

HYPERTENSIVE PROBLEMS

Approximately 23 million Americans are hypertensive, but most of them are not currently under treatment.[5] Because a woman may see a physician for the first time when she becomes pregnant, it is important to screen for benign essential hypertension (BEH), renal disease causing hypertension, or pregnancy-induced hypertension (preeclampsia).

Diagnosis may be difficult. Many women have been treated for pregnancy-induced hypertension only to discover that hypertension persists into the period beyond pregnancy. In other cases, preexisting hypertension has been masked by the normal reduction in pressures in the first half of pregnancy. It is important to identify clues to symptoms, as untreated disease will cause cardiovascular damage and may cause fetal morbidity or mortality.

Certain women develop, toward the end of their pregnancies, an increased vascular sensitivity to angiotensin II, a substance which is a powerful vasoconstrictor and a stimulator of the mineralocorticoid, aldosterone. Aldosterone, in turn, increases reabsorption of sodium and water in the distal renal tubule. Renin, the precursor of angiotensin II, is produced mainly in the kidney in response to a lowered blood volume or pressure and is an essential part of the homeostatic mechanism to maintain blood pressure. This renin-angiotensin-aldosterone negative feedback system is the current key to understanding hypertensive

responses of all kinds. Disturbances in any part of the system will affect blood pressure control.[6,7]

Increased vascular sensitivity to angiotensin II has been demonstrated at least 6 weeks prior to the development of clinical signs of hypertension in pregnant women,[8] and tests have been developed which have a high degree of accuracy in predicting those women who are likely to develop an elevation in pressure as pregnancy progresses (see Table 23-1).

This type of hypertension has an insidious onset. In the early phase, there is sodium retention and edema, with an increased plasma volume. If uncorrected, a late phase develops, characterized by sodium retention, vasoconstriction with hypertension, albuminuria, and hemoconcentration. Without effective treatment, the woman may progress to a state of coma and convulsions as a result of vasoconstrictive ischemia of brain tissue (the state of eclampsia). Accompanying symptoms are visual disturbances resulting from arteriospasm of retinal vessels, oliguria or anuria from vasoconstriction of renal vessels, and albuminuria from injury to the glomeruli by fibrin deposits originating from placental lesions.

table 23-1 Supine pressor test (the roll-over test) (*testing begins at 28 weeks*)

	position	
	left lateral recumbent	**supine**
Blood pressure schedule	1. Take q5 min until two identical diastolic readings are obtained. 2. Then turn to supine position.	3. Take bp at once. 4. Then again at 5 min.

Positive test = rise in diastolic reading (step 4 above) of at least 20 mmHg.[8] Two or more positive tests are associated with a 46% incidence of pregnancy-induced hypertension. When mean arterial pressure of 85 mmHg occurs, incidence rises to 88%.[9]

pregnancy-induced hypertension

From the Greek word *eklampnis,* meaning "shining forth" or "sudden development," comes the word *eclampsia,* which describes the state of convulsions or coma. The word *preeclampsia* is used to describe the earlier phases of a complex process of the disturbed adjustment to pregnancy before convulsions occur.

The classic symptoms of preeclampsia are edema, hypertension, and albuminuria. Reliance on only a single symptom will be misleading, however, since renal disease may also result in such symptoms, as may severe essential hypertension.

Women most likely to develop preeclampsia during pregnancy are those who already have hypertension or diabetes, those who have complications of pregnancy such as multiple pregnancy, hydramnios and hydatidiform mole, and those primigravidas at either end of the age range—very young or elderly. The association of preeclampsia with poverty, protein malnutrition, and primiparity is recognized but not fully explained.

Currently, preeclampsia has a wide range of incidence, depending upon the population reported. However, the incidence has dropped markedly in the last 20 years—again for no clear reason, except that when recognized early and treated symptomatically, preeclampsia can be controlled before the severe preeclampsia and/or the eclamptic state is entered.

hypertension   Hypertension is defined as a lasting elevation of blood pressure to 140/90 or above, or a change of 30 systolic points and 15 diastolic above a normal baseline reading. Thus, a woman who normally has a blood pressure of 100/70 would be affected by hypertension if her pressure changed to 130/85.

All blood pressure is relative to the individual's physiologic state and is affected by many factors. The diastolic pressure is more significant than the systolic and should be recorded at the change of sound (Korotkoff's phase 4), since, in pregnancy, the vascular hyperkinetic state may cause a sound to be heard at zero cuff pressure. There tends to be great inaccuracy in taking indirect blood pressure readings. Some improvement is made by having the patient's arm relaxed and well positioned and by using a well-fitting cuff. Stress, excitement, and activity which might cause transient elevation must be reduced by rest before an accurate blood pressure reading can be recorded.

The observation has been made that during the first 28 weeks of pregnancy, both the systolic and diastolic pressures are slightly decreased from normal nonpregnant averages.[10,11] For instance, if the blood pressure is 120/80 at 4 weeks, it will drop to approximately 114/65–70 by the second trimester. As the third trimester progresses, increased peripheral resistance and fluid retention cause a slight rise in blood pressure even in normal pregnancies. The nurse must get from the chart the baseline prepregnant or first-trimester reading in order to recognize any pathologic significance in a third-trimester elevation.

edema   Seventy-five percent of pregnant women normally experience edema in the lower extremities, especially toward evening. This edema is called *dependent edema,* since its development is caused by elevated femoral venous pressure, mechanical obstruction produced by the enlarging uterus, and the effects of gravity when the woman is in the upright position. Changing to a horizontal position by resting in bed relieves the collection of fluid in the interstitial spaces and causes diuresis to occur.

In hypertensive states, edema is associated

not only with mechanical factors but also with salt retention. Fluid may move into the intracellular spaces and may be seen "above the waist" or in face, hands, and abdomen and is unrelated to body position. This kind of edema, is *generalized* body edema. Weight gain may indicate early edema and is the earliest observed sign during the antepartum period. Ten pounds of excess water is stored before pitting edema can be demonstrated in the lower legs.

Sodium conservation is a normal physiologic change in pregnancy. During pregnancy, the glomerular filtration rate in each kidney increases 50 percent, from about 500 mL/min to 750mL/min. If sodium were not reabsorbed by the kidney, the woman would soon be suffering from hyponatremia. For many years, retained sodium was considered the major cause of preeclampsia, and women were put on rigid low-sodium diets. Now it is thought that this regimen is hazardous to the mother, and dietary salt intake is only modified or not restricted at all.[12] In fact, a low-salt diet stimulates renin output, while a high-salt diet and bed rest inhibit renin production.[13]

albuminuria   The serious pathologic sign in hypertensive states is *albuminuria,* or proteinuria. Protein is normally screened out by the glomeruli but is passed into the urine in cases of renal disease or moderate to severe hypertensive disease. When proteinuria occurs in pregnancy-induced hypertension, it is a sign of a rapidly worsening condition.

The degree of proteinuria is determined by a 24-h collection of urine. A level of 100 mg or more per 100 mL, or 5 g or more in 24 h, is considered abnormal. When using test tapes on single urine specimens, a reading of 3+ or 4+ is considered a serious amount. Since extra cervical secretions are common in pregnancy, the protein tests may be distorted unless the nurse obtains a clean-voided midstream urine specimen from the patient.

effects on fetoplacental function
Widespread vasospasm affects the kidney, the placental circulation, arterial and venous flow, peripheral resistance, and eye grounds. The results are seen most clearly in the fundus of the eye, where constriction of the retinal arteriolar lumen is one of the earliest signs of preeclampsia. In later phases of preeclampsia, retinal edema may result from ischemia (lack of blood supply) because of this vasoconstriction. The visual disturbances experienced in the severe phase of preeclampsia may come from these changes.

Vasospasm appears to be part of the reason for the rising blood pressure; forcing the same amount of fluid through a smaller arteriolar lumen causes the heart to work harder and with greater pressure. Vasospasm also appears to injure the placenta, causing typical changes seen only in preeclampsia: small, degenerative *infarcts* in the placenta. These injuries may release thromboplastin, which in turn triggers a slow intravascular coagulation process with glomerular fibrin deposits.[14] Clearance of dehydroepiandrosterone-sulfate (DHEA-S), initially greater in women who later develop hypertension, decreases 3 to 4 weeks prior to the appearance of clinical symptoms of hypertension. Such a decrease reflects reduced placental function. It is thought that this may be caused by the areas of ischemia or that there may be a gradually developing immunologic host-rejection of placental trophoblastic tissue. Whatever the theory, there are these characteristic lesions of placental tissue which diminish placental function.[15]

Finally, the degenerating placenta may fail to nourish the fetus adequately or may be subject to premature separation. Premature separation of the placenta occurs in 5 to 6 percent of the cases of hypertension in pregnancy. Some infants of preeclamptic mothers suffer from the effects of placental insufficiency and are growth-retarded or "small-for-dates" babies. It has been noted that once full signs of preeclampsia are present the fetus usually fails to grow in size; thus the decision is made to induce labor or deliver by cesarean section as soon as symptoms are controlled.

prenatal care Good prenatal care provides screening tests to detect early signs of developing hypertensive problems. Each visit includes measurement of weight, a urine test for glucose and protein, a blood pressure reading, and a quick check for edema. The roll-over test should be done at 28 and 34 weeks[16] (Table 23-1).

Every patient should be taught the warning signals of rapid weight gain (more than 2 lb a week in the last trimester), scanty concentrated urine, visual disturbances, headache, and edema in face, hands, or extremities upon arising from sleep.

The patient should understand the importance of following rest, diet, and fluid instructions. The nurse should telephone any patient who skips her appointment, and a home visit should be made if a patient does not return to clinic after showing signs of preeclampsia.

If the condition is diagnosed early, and treated by bed rest, adequate diet, and an increased fluid intake, the progression will most often be arrested in the mild phase. In rare instances, however, severe preeclampsia may develop without the usual warning signals. Sometimes a woman who has not had prenatal supervision enters the eclamptic state at home. She has had symptoms but has not reported them or sought care. For example:

A 16-year-old, obese girl kept her pregnancy a secret from her parents. She was admitted to the emergency room in a convulsive state. Her parents thought she had become an epileptic. The baby was delivered soon after admission, precipitously, stillborn, and of about 32 weeks' gestation.

Blood pressure on admission while patient was in postseizure coma was 160/100. There was no prenatal care.

supportive care The patient will be hospitalized if any symptoms of moderate preeclampsia occur. Nursing care is based on the therapy of providing rest in the side-lying position as the most effective way to reduce blood pressure and promote diuresis. An explanation of the therapy of bed rest can help the patient to understand and cooperate:

You are in bed here for two reasons—your heart is pumping blood at a high pressure and you have gained a lot of weight, mainly water in the tissues. Your treatment is to stay resting in bed on your side and to drink up to 3 qt of water a day. Staying in bed puts your body in a relaxed horizontal position, so that the heart doesn't have to push blood uphill against gravity. Resting helps to lower your blood pressure. When you lie on your back the uterus may press on some of the veins connected to the kidneys, so you must remember to lie on either side. The side-lying position allows free circulation to your kidneys, to that more urine is made. The more you void, the less water stays in your tissues—so you lose weight.

The patient may get up at intervals, and walking is encouraged, rather than sitting. On such a regimen, many patients will improve markedly and can be discharged to be followed by weekly visits.

laboratory tests Very few tests are specific, but the following are done as screening tests or to check on the progress of preeclampsia.

Excretion in the urine of vanillylmandelic acid (VMA), a metabolite of the catecholamines epinephrine and norepinephrine, is measured as a screening test to see whether excessive amounts of these adrenal hormones are being excreted. Excessive excretion occurs, for instance, in the presence of an adrenal tumor. These hormones have a marked effect on blood pressure.[17] *DHEA-S,* dehydroepiandrosterone, clearance is evaluated toward the end of the second trimester for high-risk patients. A decrease is present in many women who later develop preeclampsia.

Estriols in the blood and urine tell something about the fetal state. If estriol levels are falling below the normal pattern (Fig. 27-9), the fetus may be in danger of intrauterine death.

Blood uric acid shows higher levels in severe preeclampsia. Levels of 5 mg/100 mL or more are significant. Uric acid levels will not be elevated in patients with preexisting hypertension.

tests for fetal maturity   If there is no resolution of symptoms and labor must be induced, tests for fetal status are carried out (see Chap. 27).

pharmacologic therapy

anticonvulsants

MAGNESIUM   The magnesium ion provides neuromuscular blockade at the myoneural junction, reducing acetylcholine release. It also causes peripheral vasodilation and reduces smooth muscle tone, although the effect on blood pressure level is small. Magnesium sulfate has been used as a means of reducing uterine contractions of preterm labor (see Chap. 26) while improving uterine blood flow. Its primary use is to prevent convulsions in cases of severe preeclampsia. It does not cause CNS sedation but reduces muscle function and, in high doses, results in hypotonia, loss of deep tendon reflexes, respiratory failure, and cardiac arrest. Therefore, regulation of Mg^{2+} levels must be exact and is best

achieved by monitoring serum levels. Dosage is planned to maintain a level between 4 to 6 meq/L. Normal levels are 1.8 meq/L. Daily serum levels may be drawn before the dose is ordered. In addition, three standard observations are used at regular intervals.[18]

1   Determination of the presence of knee-jerk response. Reflexes are lost if levels rise above 7 to 10 meq/L.
2   Respiratory rate must remain above 12 to 14 breaths per minute.
3   Urine output should be above 30 mL/h. The magnesium ion is excreted by the kidney; oliguria would lead to a cumulative effect.

Specific antidotes to overdose are calcium gluconate (20 percent IV), neostigmine, and tylenetetrazol (Metrazol).[19]

The infant may be born with elevated Mg^{2+} levels and should be observed for hypotonia and respiratory depression. Fortunately, the ion is excreted fairly rapidly.

The drug is administered to the woman as a 20 percent solution either by intravenous drip or intravenous push (no faster than 1 g/min). IM injection (50% solution) may be given into the gluteus medius, but this is quite painful. Some physicians order 1 mL of 1 percent procaine to be added to the solution if the patient has no allergies. The drug must be administered by Z-track injection, using a long enough needle to place solution well into the body of the muscle. Subcutaneous injection results in swelling, pain, and sometimes, abscesses.

DIAZEPAM (VALIUM)   Intravenously administered diazepam is utilized as an anticonvulsant with excellent results. Its major drawbacks are the effects on fetus and neonate (see Chap. 20). It reduces beat-to-beat variability of the heart rate, thus masking fetal distress, and in the neonatal period, seriously affects temperature control. Therefore, diazepam is used mainly in severe, life-threatening cases where the fetus is already in severe jeopardy. It is almost always given intravenously.

PHENOBARBITAL Phenobarbital (30 to 60 mg PO tid or q6h) is given to every preeclamptic patient during the early phases of the syndrome. It is an effective sedative and in higher doses, given intravenously or intramuscularly, controls and prevents convulsions by means of CNS depression.

antihypertensives

HYDRALAZINE Opinions differ on use of antihypertensives for treatment of preeclampsia. The usual approach is to delay their introduction unless the diastolic pressure rises above 100 mmHg. Hydralazine (Apresoline) may then be started, first by intravenous push or intravenous infusion, titrated to blood pressure response. Action is on peripheral arterioles to reduce tone and thus decrease peripheral resistance. Side effects in the mother include tachycardia, flushing, palpitations, and headache, but reducing the flow of the intravenous solution will diminish these symptoms. There appears to be no adverse effect on the fetus.

DIAZOXIDE In hypertensive emergencies, diazoxide is being used more frequently. It exerts action directly on arteriolar smooth muscle. Side effects are similar to hydralazine: tachycardia, flushing, headache, nausea, and vomiting. Retention of sodium and water and hyperglycemia are additional problems. Both drugs cause postural hypotension. Supportive care must take these common side effects into consideration. Diabetic patients may have extra problems with insulin control. Diuretics such as furosemide may be ordered to counteract the effects of sodium retention.

As soon as possible, the patient is placed on a less potent antihypertensive.

The drug must be given as a *bolus*, by rapid intravenous injection over a period of 5 to 10 s. The dose is 300 mg, or 5 mg/kg and the aim is to reduce diastolic pressure to 90 mmHg.

Extravasation can cause severe pain and phlebitis, so it is important to have a well-running intravenous and intracatheter already in place. Care must be taken to monitor blood pressure frequently, and effects will be noted within 5 min, lasting about 6 to 8 h. Some patients will metabolize this drug more rapidly than others, so duration is not predictable.

METHYLDOPA A patient with chronic hypertension may come to pregnancy already controlled on an antihypertensive. During pregnancy, drugs such as propranolol or reserpine are used less often than methyldopa (Aldomet). Methyldopa does not adversely affect uteroplacental blood flow and acts to reduce plasma renin levels. Minimal side effects include sedation, sodium retention, constipation, and a change in the direct Coombs' test to positive, for about 20 percent of patients.

diuretics

THIAZIDES The use of thiazide diuretics is a standard method of treating preexisting hypertension. Concern about their use in pregnancy has developed because of their action in reducing plasma volume and promoting sodium loss. They are effective for these reasons, however, in addition to causing reduced peripheral vascular resistance. Since it would be possible to cause electrolyte imbalance in both mother and fetus, and since adverse effects have been noted in the immediate newborn period, thiazides are no longer prescribed for the normal dependent edema of pregnancy but are reserved for chonic hypertension unaffected by other medication. The decision to medicate with any of these drugs depends on the type of hypertension, a matter difficult to determine during pregnancy. Shortly after delivery, further regulation should take place if blood pressures remain high.

MANNITOL   In severe preeclampsia, when vasoconstriction affects renal function, the use of mannitol, an osmotic diuretic, can be helpful. Mannitol is given intravenously, and because of its hyperosmolality, it causes an increase in blood volume. Excreted totally by the kidney, it takes water with it, thus increasing urine volume. Mannitol may only be used, therefore, if it is determined that kidney function is adequate. Otherwise, the increased blood volume might precipitate congestive heart failure.

FUROSEMIDE   Furosemide (Lasix) may be added to the therapeutic regimen in hypertensive crises to move fluid quickly out of extracellular and vascular spaces. The drug has a short duration of action and is best given intravenously at first, in doses of 20 to 40 mg. Combined with hydralazine, for instance, furosemide is very effective in reducing diastolic pressures in severely hypertensive patients.

severe preeclampsia-eclampsia

If, in spite of treatment, the trend in blood pressure continues to rise, the patient may enter the phase of severe preeclampsia. Equipment must be made readily available and convulsion precautions started (see Table 23-2).

Convulsions are preceded by periods of amnesia, although the patient appears awake and rational. The chief complaint will be severe frontal headache, *unrelieved by an-*

table 23-2   Preeclampsia precautions

Padded side rails on bed
Padded tongue blade (Fig. 23-5) and an airway at bedside
Tracheostomy set at bedside
Oxygen available by mask
Suction equipment at bedside
Foley catheter (urinary output recorded every 1 to 4 h as ordered)
Nothing by mouth or clear fluids as ordered
Fluids intravenously, using intravenous catheter, well secured
Darkened, quiet room
Vital signs checked every 1 to 4 h as ordered; fetal heart tone (FHT) every 4 h
Close nursing observation

algesics. The patient may complain of visual disturbances, ringing in the ears, or girdling epigastric pain, caused by edema of the liver capsule. Convulsions may occur during sleep and, contrary to some types of seizures, are not specifically triggered by light or noise (Fig. 23-4). A dark, quiet room is set up to reduce stimuli to the patient's edematous, irritated brain and to encourage rest. Levels of consciousness should be checked at intervals because the patient can slip into coma without a convulsion. A rising blood pressure, decreasing urinary output, and increasing amounts of albumin in the urine, are alarming signs of rapid progress of the illness (see Table 23-3).

Care during the convulsion is limited to protecting the patient and providing adequate oxygenation (Fig. 23-5). Oxygen is given by mask. If there is a rapid series of convulsions, a tracheostomy may be needed to provide a clear airway. Anoxia of the mother will affect the infant, but no labor will be induced until the convulsions are controlled for at least 24 h. "Immediate delivery of a convulsing patient doubles her chances of dying."[20] In some instances labor begins during a convulsive period. In these cases labor usually progresses rapidly to a precipitate delivery in

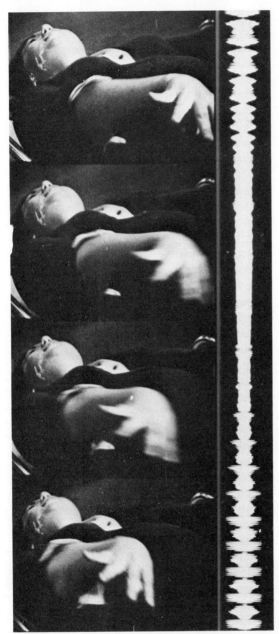

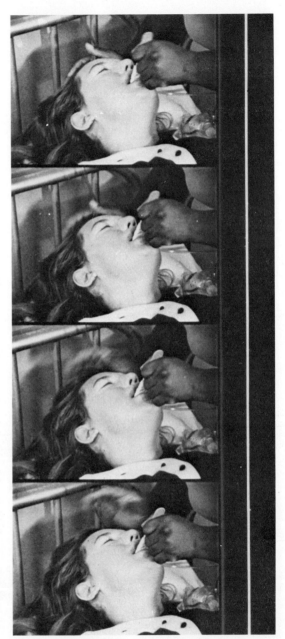

fig. 23-4   The first phase of a convulsion is tonic, rigid muscle contraction. (*From "Modern Obstetrics: Preeclampsia-Eclampsia"; courtesy of Ortho Pharmaceutical Corporation.*)

fig. 23-5   A padded tongue blade is placed to the side of the mouth between the molars. (*From "Modern Obstetrics: Preeclampsia-Eclampsia"; courtesy of Ortho Pharmaceutical Corporation.*)

table 23-3   Signs and symptoms of preeclampsia-eclampsia

mild	moderate	severe preeclampsia-eclampsia
Weight gain—edema		
More than 1–2 lb/wk	More than 1–2 lb/wk	Excessive weight gain; usually face puffy, rings hard to get off, etc.
No visible edema	Some edema above waist in abdomen, fingers, face, and extremities	
Hypertension		
30/15 rise over baseline reading	Diastolic, 90 or above; 140/90 or above	Systolic, 160 or above; diastolic, 110 or above; with preexisting hypertension—may be very high
Feels some lethargy, fatigue	Complains of headaches, lethargy, fatigue	Complains of frontal headache, lasting, unrelieved by analgesics. Cerebral and visual disturbances, ringing in ears, fainting episodes
		Grand mal convulsion may occur in sleep
Check status by roll-over test		May experience amnesia up to 48 h before convulsion.
		Patient appears alert and functions normally unless heavily sedated
		Epigastric girding pain, result of edema/hemorrhage in liver capsule
Urine—quality/quantity		
No proteinuria or just a trace	+1, +2 proteinuria	Proteinuria +3, +4, 5 g or more in 24-h specimen
Not much change	Scanty concentrated urine, DHEA-S reduced clearance	Oliguria—1000 mL or less in 24 h, progressing to severe oliguria; sometimes anuria—400 mL or less in 24 h
Blood changes		
Some increase in plasma volume	Blood estriols may be reduced, reflecting impaired placental-fetal function	Hematocrit elevated because of hemoconcentration; plasma volume lowered; platelets lowered
		Uric acid above 5 mg/100 mL
Fundal changes		
Some retinal arteriolar spasm	More extensive spasm can be seen	Edema—papilledema, ischemia of retina
Infant		
If delivered at this time, usually no problem	Usually no major problems if delivered at this phase	Infants may be malnourished or "small-for-dates" babies because of placental changes
		Precipitate delivery may occur; infant anoxic, stillborn. Premature separation may occur

bed, often with an abruptio placentae and excessive bleeding.

The seriousness of eclampsia is borne out by the statistics: the maternal death rate has been as high as 10 to 15 percent. Death results from uncontrolled convulsions, precipitate delivery, bleeding, and in some cases DIC.[21]

Recovery from eclampsia may be very rapid, with the blood pressure returning to moderate levels within 48 h of delivery. However, the danger of convulsions is not over for any preeclamptic or eclamptic patient until 3 or 4 days after delivery. Even without radical changes in blood pressure, convulsions have been known to occur on the delivery table and in the postpartum period. The patient with hypertension is in danger until her pressure is safely near her normal nonpregnant levels. (See Table 23-4 for summary of treatment for preeclampsia-eclampsia.)

chronic hypertension

The second group of hypertensive patients in pregnancy are those who have preexisting chronic hypertension from various causes. Elevation of blood pressure is always a secondary symptom of a primary disease in the body; many diseases cause hypertension. If pregnancy is superimposed on chronic hypertension the patient's symptoms may be aggravated. Close medical attention is needed throughout the gestational period. Severely hypertensive women may be warned not to become pregnant or may be advised to have a therapeutic abortion.

Because of the slight *decrease* in blood pressure during the first two trimesters, there may be an improvement in the symptoms, only to have a return to hypertension in the third trimester. Table 23-5 outlines the symptoms and severity of hypertension that was present before pregnancy.

The *cause* of hypertension is treated where

possible. There is a high fetal mortality rate in pregnancies with moderately severe hypertension, as well as a much higher risk of the woman's developing preeclampsia. Very often infants are growth-retarded and placentas are smaller than usual. Patients with moderate to severe hypertension are treated as cardiac patients are, with as much bed rest as possible, a controlled diet, and hospitalization during the last trimester.

hypertension with superimposed preeclampsia

About 25 percent of hypertensive pregnant women develop preeclampsia in some form. Of these, those with moderate to severe hypertension existing before pregnancy are in the most danger (refer to Table 23-5). Note the pathologic bodily changes which can be aggravated by the effects of superimposed preeclampsia. The disease develops earlier in pregnancy and moves to a crisis more rapidly than in normotensive women. Severe renal failure, an increased incidence of abruptio placentae, and more stillbirths are found in this group of women. Finally, preeclampsia tends to recur with each subsequent pregnancy when the woman is already hypertensive.

The signs of preeclampsia in these women are a rise in diastolic blood pressure of 15 mmHg over the usual reading, and any of the classic symptoms of headache, fatigue, edema, oliguria, and proteinuria. Hospitalization is the only safe way to care for this class of hypertensive patients.

transient hypertension in pregnancy

Transient hypertension occurring *only* in pregnancy parallels *preclinical* or *gestational diabetes* in its prognosis. It has been predicted

table 23-4 Treatment for preeclampsia-eclampsia

mild	moderate	severe preeclamp-sia-eclampsia
Home care Rest in bed as much as possible. Stay home—no shopping, tiring activities, etc.	*Hospitalize* Bed rest in side-lying position, with bathroom privileges	*Hospitalize* Strict bed rest, padded side rails, tongue blade at bedside, close observation. Check levels of consciousness
Diet Moderate salt intake; high protein; limit carbohydrates if overweight; fluids	Fluids, high protein, moderate salt intake	Clear fluids or IV fluids only
Intake and output Record not necessary	Careful output record	Measured intake and output; balance intake against output q4h. Hourly output from Foley catheter
Vital signs Roll-over test	q4h while awake; FHT bid	May be more often than q4h, depending on medication and condition Oxygen by mask prn, tracheostomy set at bedside. Suction at bedside
Medical supervision See doctor 1–2 times a week	Daily Ophthalmoscope exam	Prn Ophthalmoscope exam
Tests Urine for protein DHEA-S clearance Estriols	Urine for protein (24 h)/estriols Blood uric acid Vanillylmandelic acid(VMA) Serum electrolytes Creatinine Blood uric acid	Same as for moderate preeclampsia Hematocrit, platelets
Medication None, or low dose phenobarbital, 30 mg, tid	Phenobarbital, 30–60 mg, q6h Diuretic: short trial to see effect(?)	Phenobarbital, 30–60 mg, q6h Depending on condition: Magnesium sulfate IV, IM, Diazepam IV

table 23-5 Classification of severity of hypertension in gravid women

| | by diastolic blood pressure | |
	first and second trimesters	third trimester
Mild	80	90
Moderate	100	110
Severe	120	130

| | by other clinical criteria | | |
	cardiac	fundoscopy*	renal
Mild	Normal cardiac size. Normal electrocardiogram	Normal/minimal (KW I)	Normal renal function 30–50% increment in pregnancy
Moderate	Cardiac enlargement may be evident. ECG evidence of left ventricular hypertrophy. Few symptoms	Spastic or sclerotic changes (KW I, II)	Renal function decreased to approximately that of normal nonpregnant women, i.e., 500 mL/min. Filtration fraction may be increased
Severe	Cardiac enlargement usually evident. ECG evidence of hypertrophy and ischemia. Some symptoms (i.e., headache, palpitations)	Above and occasional hemorrhages and exudates (KW III)	Decreased renal function Increased filtration fraction
Accelerated and malignant	Above symptoms of cardiac failure, ischemic pains, and/or encephalopathy	Frank hemorrhages and exudates, papilledema (KW IV, malignant phase)	Rapidly decreasing renal function, hematuria, proteinuria

Source: Reproduced by permission from Philip J. Feitleson and Marshall D. Lindheimer, "Management and Hypertensive Gravidas," *Journal of Reproductive Medicine,* **8**(3):1972.
*KW = Keith Wagener classification.

that women who develop hypertension without preeclampsia in pregnancy will develop essential hypertension later in life.[10,11] Blood pressure returns to normal soon after delivery. There are no other untoward symptoms. Once the diagnosis of transient hypertension is made, treatment is symptomatic: adequate rest in bed in a side-lying position, and an adequate, controlled diet. No salt restriction is made, nor are diuretics given.

VARICOSE VEINS

Varicose veins in the lower extremities occur fairly often in pregnancy. Precipitating factors may be some inherent weakness in the wall of the superficial veins, aggravated by obstructed venous return, hypervolemia of pregnancy, obesity, poor muscle tone, and lack of exercise. With care, varicose veins can be minimized and chronic problems prevented.

During pregnancy, treatment is conservative and aimed at reducing any venous obstruction by rest in bed and elevation of the legs several times a day. Ace bandages or firm elastic stockings simulate good muscle tone and prevent stasis of blood in the lower legs. An increase in the amount of mild exercise will help, as will weight reduction.

To prevent obstructed venous return, instruct the patient to:

Avoid tight constricting clothing

Elevate legs when sitting

Exercise moderately; walk 1 or 2 miles daily

Lie down on her side several times a day to rest

Sleep using a side-lying position in later pregnancy

Use elastic stockings or ace bandages if varicosities exist

Varicosities may also occur in the vulvar, vaginal, inguinal, and rectal veins. Each site is affected by the normal pressure factors during pregnancy. Vulvar varicosities, especially, complicate delivery because they may tear and bleed excessively. During pregnancy, a foam pressure pad held in place over a sanitary pad by a perineal belt may be used to reduce discomfort in the vulva.

hemorrhoids

Rectal varicose veins are called hemorrhoids. From 20 to 50 percent of all pregnant women have some problem with hemorrhoids, beginning early in the first trimester. Hemorrhoids are aggravated by constipation, sitting for long periods, and obstruction of venous flow by the uterus. These rectal varicose veins are painful, itchy, and odorous, as some liquid leaks from the rectum in severe cases. Good perineal hygiene is essential for the pregnant woman with hemorrhoids. Treatment is symptomatic, and the varicosities tend to subside in the postpartal period.

The following are recommended for *treatment of hemorrhoids:*

Medication:
  Stool softeners
  Glycerin suppositories
  Topical anesthetic spray or ointment
  Sitz baths
  Witch hazel soaks to anus
  Ice bag to perineum

Diet:
  High bulk, nonconstipating, with increased fluid intake

THROMBOPHLEBITIS

superficial vein thrombophlebitis

Thrombophlebitis is clot formation in the venous system with accompanying moderate to severe inflammation, causing pain, swelling over the site, and some generalized fever. *Superficial vein* thrombophlebitis in the saphenous veins occurs more commonly than deep femoral vein phlebitis, and occurs more often when the woman has preexisting varicose veins. Because the clot tends to be fixed, there is little danger of an *embolus* traveling up to the heart or lungs with superficial thrombophlebitis. With treatment, the symptoms usually subside within 2 weeks.

Women at risk of having this condition should be taught that the early signs of thrombophlebitis are swelling and aching in the legs; they should be reminded to use prophylaxis, i.e., bed rest, elevation of legs, ace bandages or elastic stockings. The highest incidence occurs in the first 4 days of the postpartal period. Early ambulation has reduced the incidence markedly because the muscle activity of walking increases circulation and thus reduces venous stasis. Women discharged early may develop the symptoms at home, and with their attention on the infant, may ignore their own condition until it is full blown. Basic treatment for superficial thrombophlebitis is:

Complete bed rest with *elevation of both legs,* to shunt blood to deep veins and reduce edema

Heat (dry or moist) to assist in improving circulation

Analgesics to manage the pain of swelling and inflammation

Elastic stockings to reduce swelling when condition has improved and patient is out of bed again

In a comprehensive 19-year study by Aaro at the Mayo Clinic, thrombophlebitis of some type occurred in 457 out of 32,337 deliveries, or an incidence of 1.4 percent.[22] The majority of these were superficial vein thrombophlebitis and occurred during the postpartum period (85 percent). Observations made during the study indicated that superficial vein involvement almost always occurred in women who had experienced former episodes or who had varicose veins, whereas deep vein involvement was linked with delivery trauma, bleeding, infection, and operative delivery.

deep vein thrombophlebitis

When a thrombus forms in the deep veins of the leg, the term *phlegmasia alba dolens* has been used to describe the edematous, pale, painful leg. Reflex arteriolar spasm causes severe pain and turns the skin a cyanotic color. There is a deep aching along the line of the vein, plus chills, high fever, and usually an absent popliteal pulse. The onset varies— a few cases begin during the antepartum period, most of them begin within 72 h of birth, with some beginning as late as 22 days after delivery.

Basic treatment parallels that of superficial vein thrombophlebitis, plus use of antibiotics and anticoagulant medication. Heparin, given subcutaneously, is most often used antepartally, as the large molecule does not easily pass the placenta to affect the baby in the uterus. Heparin is quickly metabolized and removed from the system, so that, if necessary, it may be used until a few hours before

delivery. When labor begins, heparin is discontinued and vitamin K given to the mother. Later, if necessary, it will be administered to the infant.

septic pelvic thrombophlebitis

When infection of the endometrium or parametrium follows a traumatic or infected delivery, phlebitis of the femoral, ovarian, uterine, or iliofemoral veins may follow. Signs are tachycardia, chills, spiking fever, and a boggy, very tender uterus. This type of phlebitis is extremely serious, because small emboli and infected particles can easily break off and drift through the venous system to the heart and lungs. Treatment focuses on the infection, as it is usually very severe (see Chap. 25).

PULMONARY EMBOLISM

The first signs of pulmonary problems are a sharp sticking pain in the chest, shortness of breath, and, in some cases, hemoptysis, or coughing up blood-tinged mucus. Small warning emboli may be thrown off in deep septic phlebitis. The disease may progress very rapidly, with infected particles causing widespread infection or abscesses in the lungs.

In *very rare* instances, a large clot will break off from the deep femoral vein thrombus, travel to the heart, and then to the pulmonary artery, causing sudden death. Signs of such an accident are sudden severe dyspnea and extreme cyanosis.

Pulmonary embolism was the third leading cause of death in reports from New York City in 1967 to 1969.[23] Recently, in England and Wales, pulmonary embolism was second only to abortion as the cause of maternal death. Seventy percent of these deaths occurred in the puerperium.

When the patient who is beginning to be active after delivery experiences dyspnea, diaphoresis, or chest pain, the first thought should be of embolism. The patient should be put to bed immediately, a chest x-ray made, sedation and oxygen administered, and anticoagulants given.

AMNIOTIC FLUID EMBOLISM

In high-risk delivery where there may have been tumultuous, hypertonic labor and/or abruptio placentae, amniotic fluid may be drawn up into the venous circulation. Acting as an embolus, the fluid enters the arterioles of the lungs. Since the fluid contains meconium, vernix, lanugo, and fetal cells, these substances will act as foreign bodies in the system. There ensues what appears to be anaphylactic shock, with collapse, hypotension, and uterine hemorrhage. DIC occurs regularly as one additional complication of this syndrome. Uterine atony also occurs, leading to excessive bleeding. These symptoms are more likely to occur when there has been intrauterine fetal death, a condition which often precipitates DIC.

Mortality is over 80 percent, accounting for 4 to 6 percent of all maternal deaths,[24] or 1 death in 20,000 to 30,000 deliveries. In an otherwise healthy woman, the cardinal signs of sudden infusion of amniotic fluid into the circulatory system are as follows:

1 Respiratory distress
2 Cyanosis
3 Cardiovascular collapse
4 Hemorrhage
5 Coma

Initial signs are chilling, shivering, diaphoresis, anxiety, coughing, vomiting, and convulsions. The initial symptoms come on during late labor, delivery, or cesarean section. Rarely, they may occur in the immediate recovery period. With cardiopulmonary resuscitation, some women can survive the crisis.[25]

Right-sided heart failure with pulmonary edema will complicate recovery. Resolution of the debris of lanugo, vernix, meconium, and epithelial cells found in amniotic fluid may take time. Hydrocortisone in large doses may be used initially, as well as digitalization, rotating tourniquets, and aminophylline for pulmonary edema. Measures to control bleeding include packing the uterus, manual compression, and cautious use of blood transfusion or fibrinogen.

HEART DISEASE IN PREGNANCY

When heart function has been affected by heart disease, pregnancy may be complicated for the woman and her infant. The three major types of heart disease seen in pregnancy are rheumatic heart disease (RHD), congenital heart anomalies, and heart changes resulting from severe hypertension.

incidence

The incidence of rheumatic heart disease, though decreasing because rheumatic fever is being treated more successfully, is still 60 to 80 percent of all pregnant patients with cardiac disease. The number of fertile women with congenital heart disease has increased because of better survival to adulthood as a result of improved care in childhood. Multiparas with hypertension predating pregnancy may have damaged hearts, but newer methods of detecting hypertension and treating it effectively will, it is hoped, reduce heart damage from this cause.

The Combined Maternal Infant Study found an incidence of about 1.7 percent, or 622 cases, of cardiac disease out of 38,823 pregnancies.[26] There was a doubled stillbirth rate and a doubled low-birth-weight incidence among infants of these women.

classification

The Functional Classification of Heart Disease classifies women with heart disease in groups according to symptoms of dyspnea, palpitations, pain, or cyanosis on different levels of exertion.[27]

Class I	No symptoms on exertion
Class II	Symptoms on ordinary exertion
Class III	Symptoms on limited activity
Class IV	Symptoms at rest

Eighty percent of women with heart problems are in classes I and II and go through pregnancy with minimal trouble. Mothers in classes III and IV are treated as having very high-risk pregnancies and are guarded carefully; extended bed rest and hospitalization during pregnancy are required. The more severe the heart ailment, the higher the incidence of maternal complications and fetal death. In fact, for some women in classes III and IV, therapeutic abortion may be recommended.

signs and symptoms

In the examination of a pregnant woman, the doctor will look for signs of heart disease:

Cardiac enlargement seen on chest x-ray
Heart murmur either on diastole or systole
Changes in normal heart *rhythm* or *rate*
Symptoms of *dyspnea, orthopnea,* or *anginal pain*

Congestive heart failure is the big problem to be avoided in cardiac disease. Failure may be precipitated by the normal cardiovascular changes in pregnancy as they stress the weakened heart. Signs of failure are cough, increased dyspnea on exertion, a feeling of being smothered, hemoptysis, tachycardia, and increasing edema.

supportive care

Treatment of the cardiac patient will be carefully regulated according to her functional ability and diagnosis. Basic problems to avoid in pregnancy are anemia, infection, overweight, fatigue, and emotional stress. The visiting nurse in home visits can determine how the patient is carrying out her diet, rest, and medication orders, Ideally, the mother needs a full-time home aide in order to avoid fatigue, but realistically, many of the women in poorer sections of the country have to manage with heavy social and economic burdens. When high-risk obstetric clinics are alert to social and economic needs of the mothers, some assistance can be arranged. Ideally, too, the pregnant cardiac patient is admitted to the hospital 2 weeks early for evaluation of cardiac and fetal status. Worry about home problems may aggravate her condition; the staff must be alert to this aspect of cardiac care.

As long as the mother's condition is good and tests show that the fetal state is positive, labor may begin naturally. Induction or cesarean section is used only when fetal problems are present. The question of the safety of vaginal delivery as against cesarean section is decided on the basis of obstetric factors. The cardiac strain is much the same in vaginal and abdominal delivery, similar to that of moderate exercise.[28] Thus, women in classes I and II functionally can go through labor and delivery without great difficulty, whereas those in classes III and IV show increasingly severe symptoms of cardiac strain.

During labor the patient's condition should be continuously monitored to detect signs of strain. She should be in a semi-Fowler's position and have oxygen by mask available at the bedside. It has been noted that for the cardiac patient, *fear, pain,* and *excitement* are more harmful in terms of elevated pulse, respirations, and blood pressure than is the work of labor. Women who have had childbirth classes are helped by relaxation techniques and an understanding of the labor process. Nurses should work to aid the mother during labor and delivery with her relaxation techniques.

Normal amounts of analgesia are used (with the exception of scopolamine, because of the tachycardia and agitation this drug can precipitate). Epidural anesthesia is ideal for late first stage and second stage, as the stress of bearing down with contractions is eliminated. Hypnosis has been used in a few instances for labor and delivery and seems to be an ideal method. Low-outlet forceps are used to speed the second stage.

postdelivery care

Just after delivery, the mother is at risk of having cardiac failure and shock. With the sudden drop in intraabdominal pressure, blood quickly pools in the large abdominal vessels. This, plus the sudden elevation in blood volume as the reservoir of the placenta is eliminated, may imbalance the precarious adjustment of her cardiac function.

Special precautions must be taken to see that the mother does not receive intravenous fluids too rapidly. Oxygen is given by mask as occasion demands, vital signs are taken frequently, and a firm abdominal binder is applied to supply pressure on the deep ab-

dominal veins during the postpartum adjustment period.

In the postpartum period, the need for bed rest is countered by the need for early ambulation to prevent thrombophlebitis in these especially susceptible patients. There are no clear-cut rules for activity[29] except that patients in classes II, III, and IV will be kept in bed until cardiac function has stabilized.

Patients in classes I and II may breast-feed their infants if they wish. Postpartum care at home parallels antepartum care and includes activity based on tolerance, assistance in the home, and careful medical control of symptoms.

RESPIRATORY PROBLEMS AFFECTING PREGNANCY

Respiratory tract allergic responses of hay fever or asthma are only minimally affected by pregnancy. Any improvement may be the result of a higher circulating level of adrenal steroidal hormones and higher levels of histaminase.

Asthma has an incidence of slightly over 1 per cent in pregnant women.[30] Hay fever and other forms of respiratory allergy are more common but have less problematic effects on fetal development. The normal nasal congestion of pregnancy (see Chap. 4) may be aggravated by allergic rhinitis.

asthma

Pregnancy itself may either improve or complicate asthma. Improvement comes in the first two trimesters unless psychological stress over the pregnancy is present. More frequent attacks may occur in the third trimester, perhaps aggravated by edema of preeclampsia, weight gain, and pressure of the uterus on the diaphragm. Any respiratory infection should be treated vigorously, and allergens should be avoided as much as possible.

adverse effects Two basic problems are precipitated by severe asthmatic attacks. The first result from the stress of hypoxia on the fetus. The fetal mortality is higher than in nonasthmatic population when women have severe asthma attacks or, worse, status asthmaticus. In addition, the number of children with an abnormal 1-year neurologic examination is higher.[30] The other problem is the suspected teratogenicity of steroids when used in the first trimester. Clearly teratogenic in laboratory animals, corticosteroids may or may not cause cleft palate deformities in the human fetus. This effect does not persist beyond the period of organogenesis, however.

supportive care Any of the control drugs may be used in their customary doses, with the exception of corticosteroids in the first trimester. The woman is maintained on her usual regimen while taking care to avoid stress, allergenic insult, upper respiratory infections, and fatigue.

Regional anesthetics are chosen for delivery, and oxygen is administered as necessary. Patients receiving steroid therapy must be carefully managed throughout labor and into recovery, with dosages adjusted from time to time.

Desensitization by intradermal injection of minute doses of suspected allergens is carried out by some physicians during pregnancy; others believe it best to defer desensitization until the pregnancy is over.

CASE STUDY
Apr. 12
A 16-year-old, white primigravida at first visit to the prenatal clinic has a blood pressure of 130/80; pulse, 88; respirations, 18. Height, 5 ft 7 in. Weight, 168 lb. Estimated gestational age—32 weeks.

Counseled, sent home on a restricted-carbohydrate, high-protein, moderate-salt diet. Instructed to rest in bed several times a day and to return in 2 weeks. Instructed to call doctor for any signs of edema, headache, dizziness, visual disturbances. Parents appear to be supportive.

Apr. 26
Kept appointment, complained of headache. Bp, 144/98; weight, 181 lb. 1+ pitting edema. Admitted to antepartum unit.
Orders: Modified bed rest, side-lying position
Record of liquid intake and urinary output
Preeclampsia check; bp, q4h while awake; FHT, bid; weight, qd.
Regular diet, force fluids
Urinalysis, qd for sugar, albumin, and specific gravity.
Urine test for VMA, SMA 12, estriols
Blood for uric acid. CBC, hematocrit
Medications: Hygroton, 50 mg PO qd × 2
Phenobarbital, 60 mg PO q6h

Apr. 28
Bed rest and diuretic have caused 8-lb weight loss. 36 h after admission, 1 A.M., labor began. Patient very anxious about labor. Bp, 180/100. Seen by resident, who on basis of diastolic reading, ordered:
Magnesium sulfate, 2 g IV and 8 g IM stat.
7:30 A.M. At 7:30 A.M. in good labor; bp, 140/100; temperature, 36.7°C; pulse, 110; respirations, 24
8:30 A.M. FHT, 140. Membranes ruptured at 8:30, FHT to 180 for 20 min. Patient very wild and restless; Demerol, 50 mg, and Phenergan, 25 mg, administered

9:00 A.M.   Blood pressure dropped from 140/100 to 120/90 to 100/80; turned to side, quieted; pressure rose slowly to 140/114; FHT steady at 144

12:00 P.M. Delivered by low forceps with pudendal anesthetic, a 5 lb 3 oz, healthy baby, Apgar score 8–9

1:00 P.M.   BP, 160/110
1:30 P.M.   BP, 140/90

Returned to ward. Orders: Continue pree-clampsia check, record intake and output, administer phenobarbital, 60 mg tid.

May 2

The patient had an uneventful recovery and was discharged on the sixth postpartum day, with a blood pressure of 124/75; weight, 155 lb. Plans to bottle-feed baby.

study questions

1   If a 20-year-old woman entered prenatal care at 8 weeks of pregnancy with a blood pressure of 124/76, what would you anticipate her normal reading should be at 18 weeks? Why would there be a change?

2   What changes in pulse rate would be present?

3   Define hemodilution of pregnancy and compare normal lab reports with those indicating iron deficiency anemia.

4   Give at least three reasons why the side-lying position for rest is so helpful during pregnancy.

5   List the conditions most likely to aggravate vena caval compression during pregnancy.

6   Differentiate between mild pregnancy-induced hypertension and severe chronic preexisting hypertension, as to (a) onset and incidence, (b) symptoms, (c) pharmacologic treatment, and (d) fetal outcome.

7   Plan care for the teenager in the above case study. What nursing interventions were needed?

8   How does pregnancy complicate the symptoms of varicose veins? What relief measures can you advise?

9   Plan to teach a patient with varicose veins how to be alert, in the postpartum period, for signs of deep vein thrombophlebitis.

10 Who is more likely to experience pulmonary embolism? Compare these risk factors with the risk factors for amniotic fluid embolism.

11 Identify signs and symptoms of cardiac stress for a class I and a class III patient. Compare the expected progress of their pregnancies and deliveries.

12 What two adverse effects might be caused by severe asthma during pregnancy?

references

1   R. C. Benson, *Handbook of Obstetrics and Gynecology,* 4th ed., Lange, Los Altos, Calif., 1971, p. 198.

2. E. L. Coodley, "Anatomy of Circulation," *Consultant,* May 1972, p. 103.

3   J. J. Rovinsky, "Blood Volume and the Hemodynamics of Pregnancy," in E. E. Phillip (ed.), *Scientific Foundations of Obstetrics and Gynecology,* Davis, Philadelphia, 1970, Chap. 6, pp. 335, 336.

4   N. S. Assali and C. R. Brinkman, *Pathophysiology of Gestation: Maternal Disorders,* Academic Press, New York, 1972, vol. 1.

5. V. Vertes, "Aids in the Diagnosis of Hypertension," *Angiology,* (**10**) 545, 1977.

6   F. Finnerty, "Hypertension in Pregnancy," *Angiology,* (**10**) 535, 1977.

7   L. C. Chesley, "The Renin-Angiotensin System in Pregnancy," *Journal of Reproductive Medicine,* **15**(5):173, November 1975.

8   N. F. Gant and G. L. Daley, "A Study of Angiotensin II, Pressor Response Throughout Primigravida Pregnancy," *Journal of Clinical Investigation,* **52**:2682, 1973.

9   J. P. Phelan, "Enhanced Prediction of Pregnancy-induced Hypertension by Combining Supine Pressor Test with Mean Arterial Pressure of Middle Trimester," *American Journal of Obstetrics and Gynecology,* **124**(4):394, Oct. 15, 1977.

10 I. MacGillivray, "Blood Pressure in Pregnancy," in E. E. Phillip (ed.), *Scientific Foundations of Obstetrics and Gynecology,* Davis, Philadelphia, 1970, chap. 2, p. 293.

11 P. J. Feitleson and M. D. Lindheimer, "Management of the Hypertensive Gravida," *Journal of Reproductive Medicine,* **8**(3):106, 1972.

12 E. N. Ehrlich and M. D. Lindheimer, "Sodium Metabolism, Aldosterone, and the Hypertensive Disorders of Pregnancy," *Journal of Reproductive Medicine,* **8**(3):106, 1972.

13 Vertes, op. cit., p. 546.

14 N. M. Simon and F. A. Krumlovsky, "The Pathophys-

iology of Hypertension in Pregnancy," *Journal of Reproductive Medicine,* **8**(3):102, 1972.

15 J. Willems, "The Etiology of Preelampsia: A Hypothesis." *Obstetrics and Gynecology,* **50**(4):495, October 1977.

16 T. M. Peck, "A Simple Test for Predicting Pregnancy-induced Hypertension," *Obstetrics and Gynecology,* **50**(5):615, November, 1977.

17 R. M. French, *The Nurse's Guide to Diagnostic Procedures,* 2d ed., McGraw-Hill, New York, 1967, p. 35.

18 J. R. Woods and C. R. Brinkman. "The Treatment of Gestational Hypertension," *Journal of Reproductive Medicine,* **15**(5):195, November 1975.

19 P. Butts, "Magnesium Sulfate in the Treatment of Toxemia," *American Journal of Nursing,* **97**(8):1294, August 1977.

20 D. Haynes, *Medical Complications During Pregnancy,* McGraw-Hill, New York, 1969, p. 161.

21 L. T. Hibbard, "Maternal Mortality Due to Acute Toxemia," *Obstetrics and Gynecology,* **42**(2):263, 1973.

22 L. A. Aaro and J. L. Jeurgens, "Thrombophlebitis Associated with Pregnancy," *American Journal of Obstetrics and Gynecology,* **109**(8):1128, 1971.

23 J. J. Rovinsky, "Correlated Seminar on Thromboembolic Disease in Pregnancy," ACOG meeting, New York, 1970.

24 L. D. Courtney, "Amniotic Fluid Embolism," *Obstetrical and Gynecological Survey,* **29**(3):169, 1974.

25 R. Resnick et al., "Amniotic Fluid Embolism with Survival," *Obstetrics and Gynecology,* **47**(3):295, March 1976.

26 K. R. Niswander and M. Gordon (eds.), "The Women and Their Pregnancies," *The Collaborative Perinatal Study of the National Institute of Neurological Diseases and Stroke,* Saunders, Philadelphia, 1972, p. 226.

27 Ibid., p. 227.

28 W. Niswonger and C. F. Langmade, "Cardiovascular Changes in Vaginal Deliveries and Cesarian Section," *American Journal of Obstetrics and Gynecology,* **107**(3):337, 1970.

29 Benson, op. cit., p. 304.

30 E. A. Leontic, "Respiratory Disease in Pregnancy," *Pediatric Clinics of North America,* **24**(3):122, August 1977.

bibliography

Anderson, W. A., and G. M. Harbert: "Conservative Management of Preeclamptic and Eclamptic Patients: A Re-evaluation," *American Journal of Obstetrics and Gynecology,* **129**(3):260, October 1977.

Christianson, R., and E. W. Page: "Diuretic Drugs and Pregnancy," *Obstetrics and Gynecology,* **48**(6):647, December 1976.

Dickason, E. J., M. O. Schult, and E. M. Morris: *Maternal and Infant Drugs and Nursing Intervention,* McGraw-Hill, New York, 1978, Chaps. 5, 6.

Flowers, C. E.: "Magnesium Sulfate Obstetrics," *American Journal of Obstetrics and Gynecology,* **96**:763–776, 1965.

Hauth, J. C., F. G. Cunningham, and P. J. Whalley: "Management of Pregnancy-induced Hypertension in the Nullipara," *Obstetrics and Gynecology,* **48**(3):253, September 1976.

Hytten, F. E., and I. Leitch: *The Physiology of Human Pregnancy,* Blackwell, Oxford, 1971.

Kelly, J. V.: "Drugs Used in the Management of Toxemia of Pregancy," *Clinical Obstetrics and Gynecology,* **20**(2): 395, June 1977.

24

METABOLIC PROBLEMS DURING PREGNANCY

HILDA KOEHLER

VOMITING

Nausea in early pregnancy may progress in some instances to cause serious metabolic imbalance. When constant and excessive vomiting continues to the sixteenth week of pregnancy, resulting in 5 percent or more loss of body weight, it is termed *hyperemesis gravidarum*. If it continues without treatment, ketosis, ketonuria, neurologic disturbances, liver damage, retinal hemorrhage, renal damage, and finally death result. Before 1941, this condition was a prominent cause of maternal mortality; however, modern understanding of fluid and electrolyte balance has eliminated hyperemesis as a cause of maternal death.[1] Incidence varies with different times and different places. The only constant factor is that a previous history of hyperemesis gravidarum or unsuccessful pregnancy is associated with an increased frequency of hyperemesis in subsequent pregnancies.

Although no one knows the cause of hyperemesis gravidarum, the following have been offered as contributing reasons:

1 High levels of chorionic gonadotropin (HCG)
2 Decreased secretion of free hydrochloric acid simultaneously with reduced gastric motility
3 Psychologic intensification of physiologic factors

The peak of vomiting, coinciding with the peak level of chorionic gonadotropin in the blood, is at the tenth week (see Fig. 4-4). Because of the higher levels of HCG in those conditions, pernicious vomiting is more common when there is a multiple pregnancy or hydatidiform mole. Since gastric secretion and motility are decreased and the stomach is displaced upward and to the left early, this seems a reasonable factor in causing vomiting.

Conflicts surrounding the prospect of motherhood—such as fear of the responsibilities, worry about the threat to body image posed by the changing figure, dread of losing independence, or difficulty in thinking of oneself as a mother rather than a daughter—may provide the type of stress that produces vomiting as a reaction.

diagnosis

Since the woman is unable to retain anything ingested, she may lose an enormous amount of weight, to the point of emaciation. Resulting dehydration may lead to hemoconcentration; calorie depletion will result in ketosis. Existence of acetoacetic acid and acetone in the blood and urine confirms the diagnosis.

supportive care

Hospitalization for correction of electrolyte balance and dehydration with intravenous infusions, until oral intake can be resumed, is usually necessary. Vitamin supplements (particularly the B complex group, because of its action on the nervous system and because the B vitamins are needed for the metabolism of carbohydrates) are frequently added to the intravenous infusions. Sedation in injectable or suppository form is usually ordered; the most common drugs are phenobarbital and/or prochlorperazine. Psychologic counseling is instituted, either formally, by a psychiatrist or social worker, or more informally by the attending physician and nurses. Once oral feedings are possible, the patient is allowed to progress at her own pace from clear liquids to a regular diet, preferably with frequent small meals.

When the woman begins to gain weight, she is well on the way to recovery. Patients discharged before weight gain is resumed have a high readmission rate.

The sympathetic but deliberately firm care given by nursing staff contributes immensely to the recuperation of patients with hyperemesis. By maintaining a calm, compassionate atmosphere, projecting confidence in the certain effectiveness of treatment, and accepting vomiting episodes matter-of-factly, the nurse will truly provide reassurance. Previously there was a tendency to isolate the patient and prohibit or limit visitors; this is currently considered punitive and unscientific. The woman should be served only foods that are palatable to her. Hot foods must be hot and cold foods cold; lukewarm foods are intolerable to some.

prognosis

Complete recovery can be expected. For the fetus, there is little evidence that hyperemesis, per se, causes any increased risk of deformity or congenital malformation.[2]

A rare but possible complication from the severe, persistent vomiting of hyperemesis is aspiration of gastric juice, leading to pulmonary edema, which can result in death.

prevention

Leppert suggests that if young people receive education promoting healthy attitudes toward adult sexual roles, with emphasis on prevention of disturbed relationships—mother-daughter, parent-child—the incidence of hyperemesis will decrease.[3] Meanwhile, the obstetric health team must become more skillful and consistent in providing family-centered care which supports couples in assuming their new parenthood roles.

OBESITY

Approximately 60 million Americans are overweight.[4] There are always a number of pregnant women who are obese and whose bodies are thereby taxed by two simultaneous stresses. The following facts about the overweight pregnant patient illustrate the handicap under which pregnancy occurs:

1 Chronic hypertension is more common.
2 Babies tend to be larger—8 lb or more.
3 Latent diabetes may become overt during pregnancy.
4 Uterine dysfunction is more common, because of:
   a The oversized fetus
   b Compromised pelvic capacity
5 Perinatal mortality is four times greater than for women of normal size.[5]

Present practice discourages weight loss during pregnancy. Even the obese woman should gain at least 20 lb for best infant outcome.

THYROID DISORDERS

Iodine uptake and thyroxine secretion are controlled in the body by the thyroid-stimulating hormone. Iodine trapped in the thyroid gland is essential for the synthesis of thyroid hormone; if the synthesis into the hormone does not take place, a goiter will develop. Large amounts of iodine can be used to inhibit the hypertrophied thyroid gland by inhibiting the release of the thyroid-stimulating hormone from the pituitary.

hyperthyroidism (Graves' disease)

Hyperthyroidism occurs in about 2:1000 pregnancies.[6] It is related to increased frequency of premature delivery, postpartum hemorrhage, and possibly preeclampsia, but it does not cause abortions or fetal anomalies.[7] Pregnancy itself contains some of the ingredients of mild hyperthyroidism: the thyroid gland enlarges, women tend to be bothered by heat, their pulse is faster, they are more moody, and, of course, they have no menses.

Overtreatment of the mother with hyperthyroid drugs may result in fetal hypothyroidism and deficient development, especially of the central nervous system.[8] Radioactive iodine is not used because it would pass freely across the placenta, concentrating in and causing damage to the baby's thyroid and gonads.[9]

supportive care In severe cases, the internal medicine specialist and the obstetrician collaborate in caring for the hyperthyroid gravida. Drugs are prescribed to suppress the activity of the thyroid (Prophylthiouracil, with or without thyroxine), so as to improve the mother's condition without compromising that of the fetus. In the second trimester, a subtotal thyroidectomy may be performed, if indicated, by an experienced surgeon.

The factors determining how much and what kind of intervention the patient needs include the following: (1) the severity and specific manifestations of the hyperthyroidism, (2) the medical or surgical therapy prescribed, (3) the living conditions of the woman, and (4) her capabilities.[10]

The combination of hyperthyroidism and pregnancy leads to increased need for food intake and, fortunately, to increased hunger. Guidance as to the appropriateness of food choice for a well-balanced intake, with suggestions for snacks and extra fluid intake to compensate for increased perspiration, urination, and metabolism, is a real contribution by the nurse-counselor. Some of these women are afflicted with diarrhea; discovering with the patient what foods particularly cause diarrhea for her (frequently highly seasoned and fibrous foods speed peristalsis) can be helpful. Also important are suggestions about how to make her environment conducive to rest, as well as exploring possible diversions for absorbing excess energy (reading, crafts, visiting quietly) without becoming overtired.

Regarding medication, the following points are helpful in teaching these patients:

1   Remember that the hyperthyroid patient may be quite anxious, so go slowly with instruction, repeat when necessary, and have her repeat for verification of understanding. Write as well as personalize instructions.
2   Teach names and dosages of drugs, and specify exact hours for taking each.
3   Be sure the woman knows she must continue medication as long as the physician considers it necessary. She will soon feel better but must not stop her medication.[11]

The thyroid patient's increased susceptibility to infection is further reason for her to report immediately any signs of infection: fever, sore throat, rash, or "swollen glands."

prognosis   The mother will recover completely. The baby's thyroid function should be monitored carefully so that if it has been suppressed the baby can receive prompt treatment.

The only thyroid disease unique to pregnancy is hyperthyroidism accompanying hydatidiform mole, which is due to placental secretion of thyroid stimulator. Removing the mole effects the cure.[12]

hypothyroidism (myxedema)

Conception and hypothyroidism are usually incompatible.[13] A hypothyroid woman under treatment may become pregnant. Early diagnosis is mandatory, because abortion, premature delivery, preeclampsia, and congenital anomalies (most notably cretinism and/or mental retardation) are common. Since the baby's thyroid develops independently of the mother's, however, a normal infant may be born to a hypothyroid mother. Nonetheless, since thyroid disease has a familial tendency, there is a slightly greater expectation of thyroid disturbance in the fetus if the mother is hypothyroid.[14]

supportive care   A drug such as sodium L-thyroxine is prescribed in gradually increasing doses until symptoms disappear.

Like her nonpregnant counterpart, the hypothyroid gravida needs assistance in coping with her symptoms and achieving a euthyroid state. Since most are intolerant of cold, creativity and innovation are often needed to encourage planning to maintain body warmth. Poor appetite may compromise good nutrition, and these women will probably need help finding ways to nourish themselves and their unborn babies properly. Pregnant women tend to have dry skin, and the hypothyroid woman has extremely dry, flaky skin and so should be encouraged to use soap sparingly and to use cream or oil generously. Constipation can be a severe problem; stressing the need for adequate fluids and recommending increased roughage should correct or prevent difficulty. Sometimes stool softeners or laxatives are necessary. The importance of taking her thyroid preparation every day must be emphasized; the woman should feel better within 2 days to 2 weeks. And, of course, the need for continued medical supervision can never be overstressed.[15]

prognosis The mother's condition will be stabilized by the thyroid hormone. (In untreated patients, a characteristic exquisite sensitivity to anesthetic agents can be a hazard to the mother.[16]) The infant can be expected to be normal when the mother receives proper treatment; however, with delayed or insufficient treatment permanent mental or physical retardation is likely.

DIABETES

Diabetes mellitus, from the Greek *diabetes,* meaning "siphon," and the Latin *mellitus,* "honey-sweet," is the inability to metabolize glucose properly. The current definition states that diabetes is a chronic, hereditary disease characterized by hyperglycemia and glycosuria; the basic defect is an absolute or relative lack of insulin, which leads to abnormalities of metabolism, not only of carbohydrates but also of proteins and fats.[17]

It is inherited through recessive genes, with 75 percent of the population free of diabetes, 20 percent not diabetic but able to transmit the gene, and 5 percent who are diabetic, although not necessarily symptomatic, and who can and do transfer the disease to offspring.[18] It is not race-related. In women, symptoms of diabetes occur more frequently during menopause or in their fifties.

Before the discovery of insulin in 1921, diabetic women rarely became pregnant. Infertility and sterility were probably related to loss of ovarian function secondary to malfunction of the anterior pituitary gland, and severe dietary restriction to control the diabetes reduced the nutritional elements nec-

essary for reproduction.[19] Of the diabetics achieving pregnancy, 25 percent died; and 60 percent of the babies died.[20] Currently the incidence of diabetes is 1:100 to 200 pregnancies. Since the gravid state frequently unmasks unsymptomatic (latent) diabetes, many cases of diabetes are discovered for the first time during pregnancy.

Diabetes is manifested by an increased amount of glucose in the blood and subsequently in the urine. Abnormality is dependent upon actual or relative deficiency of insulin, resulting from functional disturbance of the islets of Langerhans in the pancreas. Insulin acts in the following ways:

1 It stimulates the cellular uptake of glucose, which is then oxidized in muscle and adipose tissue, and it regulates the rate at which this occurs.
2 It promotes the conversion of glucose to glycogen for storage in the liver, but it inhibits the conversion of glycogen to glucose
3 It promotes both the conversion of fatty acids into storable fats and the synthesis of protein within the tissues, while inhibiting their conversion into glucose.

When glucose is not metabolized, it accumulates in the blood. Since the cells cannot use this form of carbohydrate for energy, they metabolize fat instead; thus the person loses weight. The kidneys attempt to excrete the excess glucose, and the liver is unable to store glycogen properly.

The following are *signs and symptoms of diabetes:*

Polyuria (excess urination)
Polydipsia (excess thirst/fluid intake)
Polyphagia (excess hunger/food intake)
Neuritis (there may be pain in fingers and toes)
Skin disturbances, e.g., pruritus and slow healing

Weight loss
Weakness, fatigue, drowsiness
Visual disturbances

Because of the metabolism of fats, the liver produces an oversupply of ketone bodies; these combine with sodium, tending to make the blood more acid. If untreated, polyuria causes dehydration, with loss of valuable water-soluble minerals. Shifts of electrolytes from cells to body fluids result in the following:

Hemoconcentration and dehydration (elevated hematocrit)
Loss of base and chlorides, reduction of carbon dioxide—combining power, and thus, a shift of pH to the acid side
Fall in blood pressure, circulatory collapse
Labored breathing (Kussmaul respirations)
Depressed renal activity, retention of nonprotein nitrogen
Subnormal temperature

Sugar in the urine during pregnancy may occur from three main causes: lactose (milk sugar), transient glycosuria (benign), or diabetes. Investigation is needed to determine the cause.

The following conditions should *prompt suspicion of diabetes:*

A family history of diabetes, particularly in parent(s) or twin
History of large babies (weight above 9 lb)
History of increasing birth weights with each child
Unexplained perinatal mortality
Unexplained congenital anomalies
Maternal obesity
Glycosuria during current pregnancy
History of delayed wound healing
Hydramnios
History of repeated abortions
History of repeated infections

Priscilla White's classification for diabetes during pregnancy has been the most specific and is the most commonly used. It is outlined below:

Class A: Slightly abnormal glucose tolerance test; dietary control sufficient; no insulin required
Class B: Onset after age twenty; duration less than 10 years; no vascular disease
Class C: Onset between ages ten and twenty; duration 10 to 19 years; minimal or no vascular disease (retinal arteriosclerosis or calcification of leg vessels only)
Class D: Onset before ten; duration more than 20 years; vascular disease demonstrated by retinitis, transitory albuminuria, or transitory hypertension
Class E: Calcification of pelvic arteries evident on x-ray
Class F: Kidney involvement
Class R: Diabetes with pathologic changes of the retina, including preretinal hemorrhages and evidence of new blood vessels or scars.

Classification may change during the course of pregnancy and may be different in subsequent pregnancies (see Table 24-1).

supportive care

Close collaboration among internist, obstetrician, and pediatrician is mandatory in the care of the pregnant diabetic and her fetus during pregnancy and through the puerperium and neonatal period. Ideally, both the woman and her physician should agree that she is in good control as she plans to become pregnant, and since she will need extra care, both she and her partner should understand the cost of pregnancy in both money and time spent in the hospital and away from home.[21]

table 24-1 Interaction of diabetes and pregnancy

diabetes changes pregnancy	pregnancy changes diabetes
Oversized babies (metabolic acceleration: true skeletal growth, fat, water retention)	Subclinical (latent) diabetes may become clinical (overt, gestational) diabetes
Fetal death after 36 weeks likely (because of acidosis or placental dysfunction)	Renal glucose threshold is increased: a. Glucose tolerance test is changed b. 2-h postprandial level is elevated
Fetal anomalies more common (3% are lethal)	Glucose tolerance is changed:
Infertility and spontaneous abortion rate higher	a. Elevated needs for insulin, but sometimes b. Lowered needs for insulin if fetal pancreas functions to provide mother's need
Higher incidence of hypertension	Status of diabetes changes because of differing metabolic needs throughout pregnancy
Higher incidence of preeclampsia (one-third to one-half of patients are affected)	Metabolic complications (hyperemesis, nausea) difficult to treat
Placenta ages more rapidly	Work of labor depletes glycogen stores; ketosis may result
Abruptio placentae more common; hemorrhage more common	Anabolic activity changes to catabolic activity after delivery, upsetting diet and insulin needs
Premature labor more common	High estrogen levels may affect glucose tolerance of liver
Hydramnios 10 times more common in the diabetic	
Higher incidence of infection	

A thorough history is basic. When a known diabetic suspects that she is pregnant, she is most wise to get immediate medical attention, to minimize the chances of risk. Oral hypoglycemics should not be used during pregnancy because of adverse effects on fetal differentiation and development,[22] however, it is not unusual for a diabetic to present herself to the obstetrician already 8 to 10 weeks pregnant, having maintained herself on oral agents!

Management of diabetes and pregnancy aims at careful evaluation and classification of the condition of the diabetic woman before or early in pregnancy, meticulous and constant supervision and intervention throughout pregnancy, labor, and the puerperium, early termination of pregnancy, and careful pediatric care of the newborn. Prevention of acidosis, toxemia, infections, and intrauterine death are ongoing goals. Usually the obstetrician and internist take turns seeing the patient every 2 weeks until the twenty-eighth week; then she will be seen weekly or more often, depending on her intelligence and cooperation and the severity of the disease (Table 24-1).

To determine dietary and insulin management, the following tests are made at frequent intervals during pregnancy: fasting blood sugar level (70 to 120 mg/100 mL is the normal range in most facilities); 2-h postprandial blood sugar level; urinalyses for glucose, ketone bodies, and albumin; and blood urea nitrogen. Periodic eye examinations by an ophthalmologist are recommended; cardiovascular and renal function tests may be needed.

dietary management*

The aim of dietary management for the pregnant diabetic woman is to stabilize her blood glucose level. The carbohydrate, protein, and

* Written by Beatrice Lau Kee.

fat content of her food intake should be relatively constant from day to day, since these nutrients contribute to blood sugar levels.

There are two methods of dietary management for the diabetic patient. The liberal dietary management is known as the "free diet." The more conservative method is the measured calorie-restricted diet using the diabetic exchange system, developed by the American Dietetic Association, the American Diabetic Association, and U.S. Public Health Service.

The patient on the free diet is taught to eat an adequate diet and to avoid sugar and concentrated sweets. It is based on a more tolerant view toward glycosuria. The patient does not measure the amount of food she eats but is taught to eat foods in the basic four food groups. During pregnancy, she should eat foods as outlined in Chap. 6.

If meticulous dietary management is desired, the physician will prescribe a calorie-restricted diet for the patient, giving the desired level of carbohydrate, protein, and fat. The diabetic exchange system is based on the grouping of foods according to their similarity in carbohydrate, protein, as well as in fat content (see Table 24-2). Foods that do not need to be measured are coffee, tea, clear broth, bouillon, lemon, unsweetened gelatin, vinegar, spices, and seasonings. Foods which are not allowed are sugar, syrups, and other concentrated sweets.

An example of a diabetic diet suitable for a woman in her second and third trimesters is the 2200-kcal diet containing 230 g carbohydrates, 95 g protein, and 100 g fat. If insulin is used, the daily meal plan should include an evening or afternoon snack. This diet allows the following daily food plan:

FOOD EXCHANGE	PORTIONS
Milk, skim	4 cups
Vegetable	3 exchanges
Fruit	3 exchanges
Bread	9 exchanges
Meat	6 exchanges
Fat	16 exchanges

See Table 24-3 for some diabetic meal plans.

insulin requirements

Insulin requirements vary considerably. Some diabetic gravidas need none; unpredictable variations call for constant surveillance. In general, insulin requirements become greater, peaking at about the seventh month. Ordinarily satisfactory regulation can be attained by administering one of the long-acting preparations. Complications, notably hyperemesis gravidarum, infections, gastrointestinal upset, toxemia, or the stress of labor, require a shift to regular insulin to secure more accurate regulation[23] (Table 24-4).

table 24-2 Diabetic exchanges

exchange	portion size	carbohydrate, g	protein, g	fat, g	kcal
Milk, skim	8 oz	12	8		80
Vegetables	½ cup	5	2		28
Fruit	Varies	10			40
Bread	1 slice or varies	15	2		
Meat, low fat	1 oz or varies		7	3	53
Meat, medium fat	Omit ½ fat exchange				
Meat, high fat	Omit 1 fat exchange				
Fat	1 tsp			5	45

table 24-3 Typical diabetic diet during pregnancy

meal plan	sample menu
Breakfast	
1 fruit exchange	½ cup orange juice
1 meat exchange	1 egg (omit ½ fat exchange)
2 bread exchanges	½ cup bran flakes
	1 slice bread
4 fat exchanges	2 slices crisp bacon
	1½ tsp margarine
1 milk exchange	1 cup skim milk
Lunch	
2 meat exchanges	2 oz tuna fish
2 bread exchanges	2 slices bread
1 vegetable exchange	celery
4 fat exchanges	3 tsp mayonnaise
	5 small olives
1 bread exchange	2 graham crackers
1 fruit exchange	1 small apple
1 milk exchange	1 cup skim milk
Dinner	
3 meat exchanges	3 oz meat loaf (omit 3 fat exchanges)
2 bread exchanges	1 slice bread
	1 small baked potato
2 vegetable exchanges	½ cup green beans
	½ cup squash
4 fat exchanges	1 tsp margarine
1 fruit exchange	½ cup fruit cocktail
1 milk exchange	1 cup skim milk
Snack	
1 milk exchange	1 cup whole milk (omit 2 fat exchanges)
2 bread exchanges	1 English muffin
4 fat exchanges	2 tsp margarine

Additional information about diabetic diets may be obtained from:

The American Diabetes Association
1 East 45 Street
New York, New York 10017
or
The American Dietetic Association
620 North Michigan Avenue
Chicago, Illinois 60611

The local health department is another resource for patients who are put on diabetic diets by their physicians.

other problems

During the first trimester nausea and vomiting may lead to acidosis and must be treated after examination rather than over the telephone. During the second trimester, infec-tions, especially of the urinary tract, are most likely to be a problem. Pyelonephritis must be prevented. In the third trimester, signs of sugar intolerance and toxemia are potential hazards.

Deciding on the best time for delivery of

table 24-4 Characteristics of various types of insulin

type	indications	peak action, no. of hours after administration	duration, h
Regular	Emergencies Acidosis Acute and chronic infections Surgery, delivery Very young children Supplement to other insulins	1	5–7
Protamine zinc	If more than 30 units insulin required daily	14–20	36
NPH	If more than 30 units insulin required daily	10–16	24–28
Lente	If more than 30 units insulin required daily	10–16	24–28
Semilente	To speed action	4–6	12–16
Ultralente	To prolong action	18–20	36+

the baby is considered the biggest challenge; hospitalization at about 35 weeks as an aid in making this determination is the usual practice. Regardless of what the test for fetal maturity may show, early delivery is required when preeclampsia, repeated ketoacidosis, marked hydramnios, advancing retinopathy, preexisting renal disease with hypertension, or albuminuria occur. Delivery may be as early as 33½ to 34 weeks, as the hazard of intrauterine death is much greater than risk of neonatal death.[24] The following tests are performed: determination of size and age of the baby by palpation; x-ray for presence of distal femoral epiphysis and/or edematous fetus (halo sign); sonogram; urinary estriol determination (Fig. 24-1); and/or amniocentesis for determination of creatinine and pulmonary lipid levels. Most medical centers follow these tests with an oxytocin challenge test (OCT) to determine feasibility and safety for allowing this mother and baby to labor. (See Chap. 27 for description of OCT.) Because a diabetic fetus tends to be large, the possibility of maternal dystocia is greater, the placenta ages more rapidly, and the infant tends to

have a higher mortality rate if left until term, most obstetricians consider the thirty-seventh week optimum delivery time. Seventy percent will have a cesarean section.[25]

special problems of the infant of a diabetic mother (IDM)

The fetus developing within an abnormal intrauterine environment is subject to a number of risks. Infants of diabetics have a higher incidence of congenital anomalies and a higher perinatal mortality. The quality of metabolic control during the pregnancy is most important. Investigators have found mothers who had acetonuria fairly often had offspring with lower IQs than control infants.[26] Most infants are large for gestational age unless the mother has relatively severe diabetes with additional complications; then the infants can be undersized. There is an increased incidence of intrauterine death, a risk which rises sharply after 36 weeks (see Fig. 24-2).

After birth, there is increased risk of respi-

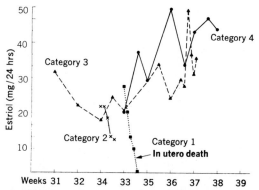

fig. 24-1 Patterns of urinary estriol excretion in four categories of diabetic patients. *Category 1:* fetal death occurred when estriol remained below 4 mg for 24 h. *Category 2:* mother needed an early cesarean section when estriol level fell rapidly; infant survived. *Category 3:* section scheduled for thirty-seventh week; infant survived. *Category 4:* labor ended pregnancy naturally, with infant survival. (*From John W. Greene, "Assessing Maternal Estriol Excretion," Contemporary OB/GYN, **2**(3):63, 1973. Estriol levels reflect laboratory techniques used by Dr. Greene.*)

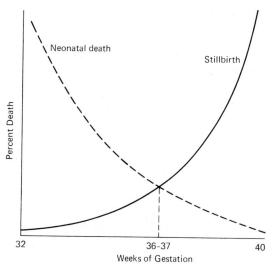

fig. 24-2 Hypothetical dilemma of high-risk pregnancy. The risk of neonatal death diminishes as term approaches, but the risk of intrauterine death sharply rises after 36 weeks in diabetic pregnancies. (*From J. L. Duhring, "Diabetes in Pregnancy, How to Diagnose and Treat it," Contemporary OB/GYN, **9**(2):119, 1977.*)

ratory difficulty either with hyaline membrane disease or with tachypnea having rates of 100 to 140 breaths per minute.[27] Since extra insulin has been produced to handle maternal elevated levels, most IDM have responded to the growth-promoting effects of insulin. The pancreas produces extra insulin in the immediate newborn period, and the infant experiences severe hypoglycemia (see Chap. 28). Often there is hypokalemia and hypomagnesemia as well. Temperature control is unstable, although the infant appears red, as though too warm, and, with fat puffy cheeks, looks older and more mature. Every IDM is cared for in an intensive care nursery through the transition period. With excellent care during the prenatal period and during labor and recovery, there should be a 90 percent survival rate.

education for the pregnant diabetic

With the rest of the health team, the nurse helps the expectant diabetic mother to understand the complications that might arise, the manifestations of her disease, its treatment, and its prognosis.[28] The following areas are worth exploring with the newly pregnant diabetic:

1 The age and circumstances under which the diagnosis of diabetes was made
2 How she perceived the course of her diabetes (particularly if she is a teenager)
3 Her attitude toward previous pregnancies, including her birth experiences
4 Her attitude toward health care, her family, and childbearing[29]

Information from this exploration will provide the basis for effective nursing intervention, especially as the need increases for tedious tests, careful dietary and insulin control, and even periods of hospitalization.

The care plan agreed on by the diabetic gravida and the nurse (and the rest of the health team) should consider the following factors, as identified by Garber:[30]

1 The importance of early prenatal care in pregnancy and of keeping all appointments.
2 The role of the diet, both for good nutrition and for diabetic control. Keeping a diet diary is a helpful practice, as this can be used as a tool for reviewing or learning meal planning, calorie counting, and food values.
3 How to test urine for sugar and acetone. The recommended method is as follows:
   a Empty bladder completely (the "long specimen")
   b Void again and collect specimen 30 min later (the "short specimen")
   c Test "short specimen"
   d Repeat daily before meals and at bedtime unless otherwise instructed
   e Use clean container for collecting specimen
   It is good practice to keep a daily record of urine tests, insulin, and unusual activities. The professionals can use the record to evaluate trends in the patient's condition, and the diabetic can use it as a tool for her education. (Toward the end of pregnancy, it may be necessary to use a urine-testing method specific for glucose, as some methods do not differentiate between lactose and glucose.)
4 Ability to recognize the signs and symptoms of hypoglycemia and hyperglycemia (see Table 24-5).
5 Alertness to report any infections of illness to the physician.

6 Importance of care of teeth, skin, feet, personal hygiene.
   a General skin care
      (1) Bathe daily with good perineal hygiene; dry well
      (2) Avoid tight clothing
      (3) Avoid skin exposure to temperature extremes (hot-water bottles, heating pads, frostbite)
      (4) Use extreme caution to avoid cuts, bruises
      (5) Use lotion, cream, oil for dry skin
      (6) Brush teeth and gums at least twice daily, preferably also after meals; use dental floss carefully
   b Foot care
      (1) Wash and dry feet well daily
      (2) Inspect feet carefully, using mirror if necessary
      (3) Use well-fitting shoes, stockings faithfully—no bare feet
         (a) Clean stockings daily; no repair work that create seams
      (4) Cut toenails straight across; get professional advice for difficult nails, corns, calluses, and bunions
7 Need for exercise and rest.
   a Be sure colleagues/friends know of diabetes
   b Do not vary meal patterns or skip meals
   c Wear identification as a diabetic; carry fast-acting carbohydrate
   d Adjust diet according to physical activity; if a marked increase in activity is expected, consult physician regarding insulin and diet (overfatigue decreases carbohydrate tolerance).
8 Administration of insulin, if needed. (The nurse must know the information in Table 24-4 in order to anticipate insulin reaction.)

table 24-5 Signs and symptoms of diabetic coma and insulin shock

	diabetic coma (hyperglycemia)	insulin shock (hypoglycemia)
Signs:		
Onset	Slow	Rapid
Skin	Dry	Sweating
Reflexes	Normal or absent	Positive Babinski's reflex
Eyeballs	Soft	Normal
Color	Florid face	Pallor
Urine	Sugar	Negative for sugar
Breath	Acetone odor	Normal
Breathing	Kussmaul (deep, labored)	Shallow
Pulse	Rapid	Normal
Symptoms:	Thirst	Inward nervousness
	Nausea/vomiting	Hunger
	Headache	Weakness
	Abdominal pain	Paresthesia
	Dim vision	Blurred vision
	Dyspnea	Stupor, convulsions
	Constipation	Psychopathic behavior

    a Familiarity with type or types of insulin to be used

    b Protocol for sites of injection, rotation of sites, and skin inspection

    c Technique for preparing materials, and injection skill

9 If 24-h urine specimen is needed for estriol determination, learn collection method

10 Referral to other health personnel (visiting nurse, Diabetes Association, homemaker, dietician, other physicians) as indicated.

When the woman goes into labor, all the technology and increased attention to assure safety for mother and infant can make for a very mechanized experience unless the team is sensitive to the personal and psychological needs of this human female.[31]

After delivery, diabetes is most difficult to control. Wide and sudden changes in blood sugar level occur because of endocrine and metabolic disruption associated with the termination of pregnancy, slight postpartum infection, change of blood glucose to lactose for breast milk, and perhaps the withdrawal of the availability of fetal insulin. After the second day, placental lactogen is gone and the nursing staff must be alert to the possibility of insulin shock.

prognosis

Maternal mortality of less than 2:1000 is expected with adequate modern therapy. Eye and kidney disorders are usually increased during gestation.[32] After delivery, it is important to reinvestigate women with an abnormal glucose tolerance to determine if glucose intolerance returns to normal. The test is best repeated 6 weeks after delivery. Some studies indicate that the appearance of symptomatic diabetes is no higher in those who have had gestational diabetes than in the general population.[33] The baby's prognosis depends on the severity of the diabetes, complications (either medical or obstetric), and prematurity, as well as on method of delivery (vaginal delivery is preferred). Infant mortality rate is currently between 10 and 15 percent, and anomalies occur in about 5 percent of cases.[34]

KIDNEY DISEASE

From early in pregnancy through the puerperium the renal collecting structures become dilated to produce the so-called physiologic hydronephrosis of pregancy.[35] Hormone activity accounts for ureteral hypomotility and ureteral muscle changes, resulting in a greater volume of urine staying in the pelvis and ureters. Later in gestation, either the supine or the upright position can cause partial ureteral obstruction,[36] since the enlarged uterus may entrap the ureters at the pelvic brim (Fig. 24-3). During pregnancy, many changes affect the excretion of salt, water, and total fluid balance maintained by the kidney. Normally 6 to 8L water is retained, both within and outside the cells.[37] Various hormones concerned with electrolyte filtration (aldosterone, renin substrate, progesterone, and estrogen) increase, modifying the kidney's ability to excrete, especially its ability to excrete sodium (Fig. 24-4).

Ideally, the woman with a known renal disorder should consult her physician before attempting to conceive.[38] Among the background renal conditions that may be complicated by pregnancy are chronic glomerulonephritis, nephrotic syndrome, solitary kidney, polycystic kidney, and, of course, class F diabetes.[39] Significant proteinuria will invariably accompany these conditions, leading the physician to investigate. Normally the blood pressure falls during pregnancy. The *absence* of the normal fall in blood pressure and serum urea may be the earliest sign of a developing renal problem.[40]

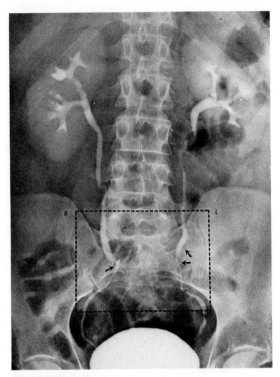

fig. 24-3 Intravenous pyelogram demonstrates ureteral dilation of pregnancy. *Note:* Right ureter is sharply cut off at pelvic brim (single arrow). (*By permission of Dr. Marshall Lindheimer and Dr. Adrian Katz, "Managing the Patient with Renal Disease," Contemporary OB/GYN, 3(1):49, 1974. Photo courtesy of Dr. Peter Dure-Smith.*)

chronic glomerulonephritis

Ranging in severity from tolerable impairment of kidney function to severe disability, chronic glomerulonephritis used to be incompatible with pregnancy but now is considered manageable in a cooperative patient. Usually a sequel to a severe systemic disease, most notably streptococcal glomerulophritis, chronic glomerulonephritis results in proteinuria and/or persistent urinary sediment. In

Renal Hemodynamics in Pregnancy

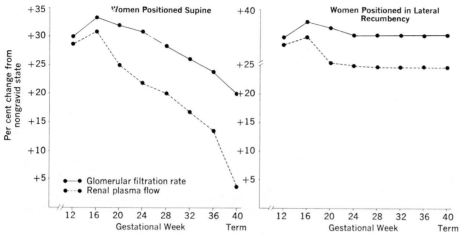

fig. 24-4 Renal hemodynamics in pregnancy. Differences in glomerular filtration rate and renal plasma flow in supine and lateral positions. Increases occur early in pregnancy and are sustained to term if women maintain lateral recumbency position. (*By permission of Dr. Marshall Lindheimer and Dr. Adrian Katz, "Managing the Patient with Renal Disease," Contemporary OB/GYN* **3**(1):49, 1974.)

pregnancy it produces palpitation, visual disturbances, headache, fatigue, dizziness, nausea, vomiting, edema, hypertension, and eventually some degree of cardiovascular disease and renal insufficiency.[41] Anemia is usually severe enough to require transfusion.[42]

supportive care Care is based on laboratory and clinical findings, which must be closely monitored. Generally therapy includes a high-protein diet, sodium restriction, administration of antihypertensive agents, and, with cardiac insufficiency, digitalis and perhaps diuretics. Preeclampsia necessitates hospitalization. Azotemia (nitrogen in the blood), hyperkalemia (high potassium content in the blood), and continuing blood pressure rise indicate the need to interrupt the pregnancy.

prognosis The mother's condition is basically unchanged following pregnancy. The primary risk is to the fetus, although without

hypertension or renal failure 90 percent fetal salvage can be expected.[43] Even with the best of management, however, there is a risk of spontaneous abortion, premature labor, or intrauterine death. Induction of labor must not be delayed beyond the end of the thirty-seventh week, and the neonate should be placed under intensive care immediately.[44]

nephrotic syndrome

If the nephrotic syndrome appears during pregnancy, the findings may be thought to indicate preeclampsia: edema, massive protein in the urine, low blood protein, and lipemia, with or without hypertension. Renal biopsy is required for definitive diagnosis.[45] Usually the kidney functions sufficently to allow the pregnancy to continue; interruption is indicated in the presence of severe malfunction, hypertension, or uremia. Thromboembolism (caused by elevated fibrinogen or depressed antithrombin level) and infection as a consequence of low gamma globulin level must also be anticipated.[46]

treatment Nephrotic syndrome is treated according to symptoms and the other conditions accompanying it. Bed rest in the lateral recumbent position, high-protein/restricted-sodium diet, and diuretics are commonly ordered. Steroids are contraindicated during the first 2 months of gestation. Infections must be vigorously treated.[47]

prognosis Depending on the cause, recovery may take place or the disease may progress to renal failure and death; pregnancy itself seems to have no serious effect on the course of the disease.[48]

solitary kidney

Usually when a person has only one kidney it enlarges to compensate for the extra demands put upon it; pregnancy does not seem to cause any special problems. The duration of the solitary-kidney condition, the present ability of that kidney to function, and the cause of the condition must all be taken into account.

supportive care Monthly urine cultures are the minimum for scrupulous monitoring against infection. Provided that no infection or hypertension intervenes, pregnancy progresses to term.

prognosis Excellent in the absence of the above complications.

In all patients with known renal disorder, frequent evaluations are necessary. If renal function deteriorates at any stage of gestation, reversible causes—such as urinary tract infection, subtle dehydration, and electrolyte imbalance—should be sought. Failure to find

such a cause is grounds for recommending termination of the pregnancy.[49]

Nursing actions and teaching are concerned with enabling the woman to cope with the various changes in her activities necessitated by her condition. She may need assistance in determining the best way for her to plan her diet around increased protein and decreased sodium requirements. All the drugs she may be given (e.g., digitalis, diuretics, antihypertensives, steroids, antibiotics) require interpretation and teaching whether she is going to take them at home or be given them as an inpatient. She will need instruction or review in the collection of urine specimens. If she is on bed rest, she will need to explore her emotional response to this order and discover activities that can keep her from total boredom. And, of course, if the baby is less than completely normal, the nurse can provide support and information, as well as providing help during the grieving process.

study questions

1 Define and describe possible causes of hyperemesis gravidarum. What is the primary danger if this condition goes unchecked?
2 What possible difficulties face the obese pregnant woman?
3 Write an initial nursing care plan for a hyperthyroid gravida being followed on an outpatient basis who has been well controlled with her medication(s).
4 What history would indicate that the patient might have diabetes?
5 Write a nursing care plan for a class C diabetic admitted to the hospital at 35 weeks for evaluation of her pregnancy.
6 What are the differentiating signs and symptoms of diabetic coma and insulin shock?
7 How does pregnancy affect the kidneys normally?
8 What are the two main handicaps under which the diabetic infant is born? What special observations must be carried out in the first days after birth?

references

1 R. C. Corlett, Jr., "Hyperemesis Gravidarum and Pancreatitis," *Contemporary OB/GYN* **9**(5):28, 1977.

2 G. N. Burrow, *Medical Complications During Pregnancy,* Saunders, Philadelphia, 1975, p. 29.

3 P. Leppert, "Hyperemesis Gravidarum: A Discussion of a Symptom Complex with a Connecting Bridge to Anorexia Nervosa," *Journal of Nurse-Midwifery,* **17**(4):20, 1973.

4 D. Lindner, "The Nurse's Role in a Bariatric Clinic," *RN* **37**(2):28, 1974,

5 N. J. Eastman and L. M. Hellman, *Williams' Obstetrics,* 14th ed., Meredith Press, New York, 1971, p. 799.

6 A. B. Gerbie, "Endocrine Diseases Complicated by Pregnancy," in D. M. Haynes (ed.), *Medical Complications during Pregnancy,* McGraw-Hill, New York, 1969, chap. 6, p. 352.

7 S. G. Babson and R. C. Benson, *Management of High Risk Pregnancy and Intensive Care of the Neonate,* Mosby, St. Louis, 1971, p. 51.

8 Ibid, p. 51.

9 M. B. Dratman, "Managing Hyperthyroidism in Pregnancy," *OB/GYN Observer,* May 1971, p. 6.

10 J. C. Hallal, "Hyperthyrodism," *American Journal of Nursing* **77**(3):421, 1977.

11 Ibid., p. 424.

12 J. Hershman, "Some Births Normal Despite Enlarged Thyroid in Gravida," *OB/GYN News,* **8**(23):44, 1973.

13 Dratman, op. cit., p. 6.

14 Ibid

15 J. C. Hallal, "Hypothyroidism," *American Journal of Nursing,* **77**(3):429, 1977.

16 Gerbie, op. cit., p. 356.

17 A. Marble et al. (eds.), *Joslin's Diabetes Mellitus,* 11th ed., Lea & Febiger, Philadelphia, 1971, chap. 1.

18 S. Berger, "Medical Management of the Diabetic," *Hospital Topics,* **49**(12):64, 1971.

19 Eastman and Hellman, op. cit., p. 791.

20 A. Gerbie, "Obstetrical Management of the Diabetic," *Hospital Topics,* **49**(12):64, 1971.

21 B. B. G. Christman, "Pre-Pregnancy Education Is Recommended for Diabetic Women," *OB/GYN NEWS,* **11**(16):14, 1976.

22 Berger, op. cit., p. 62.

23 Gerbie, "Endocrine Diseases Complicated by Pregnancy," p. 344.

24 J. W. Greene, Jr., "Diabetes Mellitus in Pregnancy," *Obstetrics and Gynecology,* **46**(6):724, 1975.

25 Green, op. cit., p. 725.

26 Kandall. S., "Problems with Drugs During Newborn Transition," in E. J. Dickason, *Maternal and Infant Drugs and Nursing Intervention,* McGraw-Hill, New York, 1978, chap. 8, p. 266.

27 Gerbie, "Obstetrical Management of the Diabetic," p. 64.

28 E. Laugharne and F. Duncan, "Gestational Diabetes: When Teaching is Important," *The Canadian Nurse,* **59**(3):34, 1973.

29 M. S. Cranley and S. A. Frazier, "Preventive Intensive Care of the Diabetic Mother and Her Fetus," *Nursing Clinics of North America,* **8**(3):493, 1973.

30 R. Garber, "The Use of a Standardized Teaching Program in Diabetes Education," *Nursing Clinics of North America,* **12**(3):377, 1977.

31 Cranley, op. cit., p. 497.

32 Babson and Benson, op. cit., p. 77.

33 D. A. D. Montgomery and J. M. G. Harly, "Endocrine Disorders," *Clinics in Obstetrics and Gynecology,* **4**(2):365, 1977.

34 Babson and Benson, op. cit., p. 78.

35 J. B. Nettles, "Renal Complications of Pregnancy," in Douglas M. Haynes (ed.), *Medical Complications During Pregnancy,* Meredith Press, New York, 1969, p. 444.

36 M. D. Lindheimer and A. I. Katz, "Managing the Patient with Renal Disease," *Contemporary OB/GYN,* **3**(1):49, 1974.

37 Ibid., p. 50.

38 R. Ramón de Alvàrez, "The Kidney in Pregnancy," *Hospital Practice,* May 1973, p. 133.

39 Ibid

40 M. G. McGeown, "Renal Disorders and Renal Failure," *Clinics in Obstetrics and Gynecology,* **4**(2):319, 1977.

41 de Alvàrez, op. cit., p. 133.

42 Nettles, op. cit., p. 504.

43 Ibid

44 de Alvàrez, op. cit., p. 134.

45 Ibid.

46 Ibid., p. 135

47 Ibid

48 Nettles, op. cit., p. 550.

49 Lindheimer and Katz, op. cit., p. 55.

bibliography

Bear, R. A.: "Pregnancy in Patients with Renal Disease," *Obstetrics and Gynecology,* **48**(1):13, July 1976.

Beller, F. K. et al.: "Renal Disease in Pregnancy," *American Journal of Obstetrics and Gynecology,* **125**(4): 845, Dec. 1, 1976.

Burrow, G. N.: "The Thyroid in Pregnancy," *Medical Clinics of North America,* **59**:1089, 1975.

Burt, R. L.: "How to Reduce the Hazards of Diabetes in Pregnancy," *Consultant,* June 1972, p. 37.

Carrington, E. R.: "Diabetes in Pregnancy," *Clinical Obstetrics and Gynecology,* **14**(1):28, 1973.

Cortlett, R. C., Jr.: "Hyperemesis Gravidarum and Pancreatitis," *Contemporary OB/GYN,* **9**(5):25, 1977.

Cranley, M. S. and S. A. Frazier: "Preventive Intensive Care of the Diabetic Mother and Her Fetus," *Nursing Clinics of North America,* **8**(3):489, 1973.

Duhring, J. L.: "Diabetes in Pregnancy: How to Diagnose and Treat It," *Contemporary OB/GYN,* **9**(2): 117, 1977.

Eastman, N. J. and L. M. Hellman: In *Williams' Obstetrics,* 14th ed., Meredith Press, New York, chaps. 27, 29, 1971.

Emslander, R. F. et al.: "Hyperthyroidism in Pregnancy," *Medical Clinics of North America,* **58**:835, 1974.

Gabbe, S. G. et al.: "Maternal Mortality in Diabetes Mellitus," *Obstetrics and Gynecology,* **48**(5):549, 1976.

Garnet, J. D.: "Pregnancy in Women with Diabetes," *American Journal of Nursing,* **69**(9):1900, 1969.

Garofano, C.: "Deliver Facts to Help Diabetics Plan Parenthood," *Nursing '77,* **7**(4):13, 1977.

Goluboff, L. G. et al.: "Hyperthyroidism Associated with Pregnancy," *Obstetrics and Gynecology,* **44**(1):107, July 1974.

Gottesman, R. L., and S. Refetoff: "Diagnosis and Management of Thyroid Diseases in Pregnancy," *Journal of Reproductive Medicine,* **11**(1):19, 1973.

Greene, J. W., Jr.: "Diabetes Mellitus in Pregnancy," *Obstetrics and Gynecology,* **46**(6):724, 1975.

Gugliucci, C. L. et al.: "Intensive Care of the Pregnancy Diabetic," *American Journal of Obstetrics and Gynecology,* **125**(4):435, June 15, 1976.

Guthrie, D. W. and R. A. Guthrie: "The Infant of the Diabetic Mother," *American Journal of Nursing,* **74**(11): 2008, 1974.

Haynes, D. M. (ed.): *Medical Complications During Pregnancy,* McGraw-Hill, New York, 1969, chaps. 6, 9.

Hazlett, B., and D. Gare: "The Pregnant Diabetic," *Modern Medicine,* **27**(12):37, 1971.

Kinch, R. A.: "Management of the Diabetic Pregnancy," *Journal of Reproductive Medicine,* **7**(2):40, 1971.

King, B. et al.: "Problem-Oriented Diabetic Day Care," *The Canadian Nurse,* October 1974, p. 19.

Kucera, J.: "Rate and Type of Congenital Anomalies Among Offspring of Diabetic Women," *Journal of Reproductive Medicine,* **7**(2):61, 1971.

Laugharne, E., and F. Duncan: "Gestational Diabetes: When Teaching Is Important," *The Canadian Nurse,* **69**(3): 34, 1973.

Leeper, R. D.: *Laboratory Tests in Diagnoses of Thyroid Disease,* vol. 1, no. 1, Upjohn, Kalamazoo, 1972.

Lindheimer, M. D., and A. Katz: "Pregnancy and the Kidney," *Journal of Reproductive Medicine,* **11**(1):14, 1973.

Man, E. B. and S. A. Serunian: "Development or Retardation of Seven Year Old Progeny of Hypothyrinemic Women. Part IX." *American Journal of Obstetrics and Gynecology,* **125**(8):949, 1976.

——— et al.: "Thyroid Function in Human Pregnancy," *American Journal of Obstetrics and Gynecology,* **111**(7): 905, 1971.

McConnell, E. A.: "Meeting the Special Needs of Diabetics Facing Surgery," *Nursing '76,* **6**(6):30, 1976.

Mestman, J. H. et al.: "Hyperthyroidism and Pregnancy." *Archives of Internal Medicine,* **134**:434, 1974.

O'Sullivan, J. B. et al.: "Treatment of Verified Prediabetics in Pregnancy," *Journal of Reproductive Medicine,* **7**(2):21, 1971.

———: "Screening Criteria for the High-Risk Gestational Diabetic Patient," *American Journal of Obstetrics and Gynecology,* **114**(7):895, 1972.

———: "Gestational Diabetes and Perinatal Mortality Rate," *American Journal of Obstetrics and Gynecology,* **116**(7):901, 1973.

———: "Medical Treatment of Gestational Diabetes," *Obstetrics and Gynecology,* **43**(6):817, June 1974.

Porter, A. L.: "Student Participation in Diabetic Patient Education," *Nursing Clinics of North America,* **12**(3):407, 1977.

Prout, T. E.: "Thyroid Disease in Pregnancy," *American Journal of Obstetrics and Gynecology,* **122**(3):669, 1975.

Roberts, M. F. et al.: "Association Between Maternal Diabetes and Respiratory Distress Syndrome in the Newborn," *New England Journal of Medicine,* **294**:357, 1976.

Schneeberg, N. G.: "Thyroid Therapy: First Do No Harm," *Consultant,* September 1971, p. 89.

Souma, J. A. et al.: "Comparison of Thyroid Function in Every Trimester of Pregnancy," *American Journal of Obstetrics and Gynecology,* **114**(7):905, 1972.

Tsai, A. et al.: "Diabetes and Pregnancy," *Journal of Reproductive Medicine,* **11**(1):23, 1972.

Tunbridge, W. M. G., and Hall, R.: "Thyroid Function in Pregnancy," *Clinics in Obstetrics and Gynecology,* **2**:381, 1975.

White, P.: "Pregnancy and Diabetes. Medical Aspects," *Medical Clinics of North America,* **49**:1015, 1965.

———: "What It Means to Be Female and Diabetic, Parts I, II, and III," *Diabetes Forecast,* January/February 1976.

25

INFECTIOUS DISEASES DURING PREGNANCY AND THE PUERPERIUM

HERBERT S. HEINEMAN

During pregnancy, the types of infection acquired and their method of acquisition are essentially the same as during the nonpregnant state. Etiologically, therefore, infection during pregnancy is mere coincidence. The need to consider this coincidence arises in part from the alterations in physiology which may modify the woman's response to infection, but even in this respect, as far as the mother is concerned, such modifications are only quantitative. Of much greater concern is the fetus, for whom maternal infection may have farreaching, possibly fatal, consequences.

Puerperal infections, on the other hand, are strictly complications of childbirth. In the true sense of the term, they may be regarded as wound infections. As such, they are significant, sometimes fatal, for the mother but of no consequence to the infant.

When infection occurs during pregnancy, questions naturally arise about the safety of both mother and child. It is reassuring to know, therefore, that the majority of infections may be treated in the usual manner without harm to either. Little thought needs to be given, for example, to the common respiratory and intestinal infections which most women may experience at least some time during a 9-month pregnancy. In some cases, such minor upsets lead to excessive disability when added to the burden of pregnancy. It is difficult to determine, however, whether the physiologic or metabolic alterations of pregnancy have anything to do with this phenomenon or whether fatigue, muscle strain, and health consciousness merely lower the threshold for symptoms. From a practical point of view, since infected cuts, colds, and intestinal upsets are virtually unavoidable in any case, it is in the best interest of the pregnant woman to permit normal human contact and activities.

Life-threatening infections, such as meningitis, pneumonia, or septicemia, may result in abortion or stillbirth. In these cases, however, damage to the fetus is merely an extension of the extreme metabolic or circulatory insult suffered by the mother; in the less severe cases, the pregnancy may proceed normally to term following control of the infection.

This chapter is concerned chiefly with those infections that bear a unique relationship to pregnancy. The relationship may take one of two forms: (1) the pregnant woman is particularly susceptible to the infection, copes with it less well, or more readily suffers complications than her nonpregnant counterpart; (2) development of the fetus, or the pregnancy itself, is threatened out of proportion to the severity of the maternal illness. In the management of infections, furthermore, consideration must be given to the effect of antimicrobial drugs on the fetus.

INFECTIONS RELATED TO INCREASED SUSCEPTIBILITY DURING PREGNANCY

infections and heart disease

The mere presence of heart disease does not prevent successful pregnancy. The limiting factor is the ability of the damaged heart to cope with the added circulatory demands of the last trimester. Three infections present particular hazards in terms of heart failure: streptococcal pharyngitis, bacterial endocarditis, and influenza.

streptococcal pharyngitis Streptococcal sore throat must be prevented in patients with rheumatic heart disease, for it may be followed by a recurrence of rheumatic fever, with possible heart failure or additional damage to compromised valves. Fortunately, prevention is available in the form of penicillin or other antibacterial agents; their effectiveness is limited only by the regularity with which they are taken. Monthly injections of long-acting benzathine penicillin G (Bicillin) counteract the problem of forgetfulness; many physicians prefer this regimen over any other.

bacterial endocarditis Bacterial endocarditis occurs in patients with rheumatic and many forms of congenital heart disease in which the inner lining (endocardium), including the heart valves, is already damaged either by previous inflammation (rheumatic fever) or by misdirected blood flow (congenital abnormalities). Bacterial infection occurring on these scarred surfaces, especially the valves, may inflict enough damage to cause acute heart failure. Severe kidney damage, cerebral embolism due to fragments of bacterial growths, and other complications may occur, necessitating termination of the pregnancy. Bacteria that cause this infection frequently enter the bloodstream from the gums, especially if the periodontal tissues are diseased. Antibiotic prophylaxis (usually penicillin) is therefore recommended at the time of dental treatments. Similar considerations apply to instrumentation of the urinary tract, such as cystoscopy.

influenza   For the great majority of people, influenza is, at worst, temporarily incapacitating, with eventual complete recovery. For the person with heart disease, however, even when the influenza is so slight as to cause only minimal restriction of activity, it poses a real danger of progression to pneumonia; this viral pneumonia is much more serious, with a considerably higher mortality, than the common bacterial (pneumococcal) pneumonias, partly because no effective treatment is available. The combination of pregnancy and heart disease predisposes a woman more to this complication than does either factor alone. A woman thus predisposed should be protected by immunization as early as possible in the influenza season. Influenza immunization, which involves the injection of killed virus, is harmless to the fetus and can therefore be safely performed during pregnancy.

other infections

poliomyelitis   Poliomyelitis is, fortunately, more of historic than of current interest, although it is by no means extinct in the United States. One of the interesting observations in past outbreaks was the susceptibility of pregnant women to the severest paralytic form. Susceptibility probably resulted both from the pregnant state and from the more intimate exposure of these women to young children, who frequently were carriers of the virus. The

only protection is immunization, which should be completed in early childhood but can be accomplished at any age and even during pregnancy if exposure seems unavoidable, as in an epidemic.

tuberculosis   Pulmonary tuberculosis may relapse during pregnancy or following delivery, leading to the reopening of healed cavities and the shedding of tubercle bacilli (*Mycobacterium tuberculosis*) in the sputum. Extrapulmonary foci may also be reactivated. In addition to deterioration in the mother's health, consideration must be given to the danger in which the newborn infant is placed. Infection in utero is very rare in this form of tuberculosis, so that the infant is normal at birth. However, the infant is also highly vulnerable to infection by airborne bacteria, and if the mother is coughing up tuberculosis-positive sputum close to the newborn's face, infection of the neonate can be anticipated.

Good prenatal care should, therefore, include a tuberculin skin test early in pregnancy. If positive, it should be followed by a chest x-ray and such additional studies as are clinically indicated. If active tuberculosis is diagnosed at this time, it can usually be brought under control with appropriate therapy before term, so that the mother can care for her infant in the normal manner. If the infection is not controlled, drastic measures are necessary to protect the infant, including total separation from the mother until the danger of transmission no longer exists.

urinary infection   Even in nonpregnant women, the urinary tract is host to more bacterial infections than any other organ system. Most commonly, infection takes the form of *asymptomatic bacteriuria* or cystitis, the latter characterized by burning and the frequent urge to void. Acute pyelonephritis, which is accompanied by shaking chills, high fever, other constitutional symptoms, and pain and tenderness in the area of the kidneys, is the most severe but fortunately quite uncommon form of urinary infection. Pregnancy and the puerperium, however, are associated with an increased incidence of acute pyelonephritis. The altered physiology and anatomic relationships in the abdomen of the pregnant woman probably help account for this fact, but the actual mechanisms are not fully understood. For practical purposes, it has been found that many potential pyelonephritis victims can be identified early in pregnancy by examination of their urine. The syndrome *asymptomatic bacteriuria in pregnancy* has assumed great importance among obstetricians, since one-quarter to one-third of women affected, if not treated, have been found to develop overt symptoms. Fortunately, this development can be largely prevented by antibiotic treatment during the asymptomatic phase. Culture of the urine (which must be properly collected, under professional supervision, in order to prevent contamination) is, therefore, one of the important components of good prenatal care.

In the majority of women with no history of prior urinary infection, the responsible organism is *Escherichia coli,* which is susceptible to most broad-spectrum antibiotics. If there has been previous infection with antibiotic therapy, less common and more resistant organisms, such as *Klebsiella, Proteus,* and enterococci, may be found. Therapy must then be more carefully selected and the chances for success are diminished.

Women discovered at any stage of pregnancy to be bacteriuric should be followed throughout pregnancy and during the postpartum period for possible recurrence. Although sterilization of urine is usually easy, this does not guarantee permanent cure.

vaginitis Of the various kinds of vaginitis, that caused by *Candida* (*Monilia*) *albicans* is most characteristically linked to pregnancy. It is a benign but uncomfortable fungal infection of the vaginal mucous membrane characterized by intense itching, redness, and frequently a creamy discharge. Although it occurs commonly without apparent predisposing cause, pregnancy (and the pseudopregnant state induced by oral contraceptives) is associated with a higher incidence and greater resistance to treatment. Symptoms respond fairly readily to topical therapy—e.g., use of vaginal tablets containing nystatin—but relapse is common; definitive cure usually follows the end of pregnancy.

Vaginitis caused by *Trichomonas vaginalis* is also common during pregnancy. However, pregnancy is not etiologically related to this infection and provides no obstacle to successful therapy. Metronidazole has been the treatment of choice for many years, and no serious effects on mother or fetus have been linked to it. However, carcinogenic effects have been noted in mice, and some caution in its use is probably justified.

INFECTIONS IN PREGNANCY THAT AFFECT THE FETUS

The chief characteristic of the group of infections that affect the fetus during pregnancy is their severity in the fetus—often leading to death or irreversible developmental defects—compared with their benign manifestations in the mother. Their essential features are summarized in Table 25-1.

cytomegalovirus infection (cytomegalic inclusion disease)

Cytomegalovirus is one of a group of viruses that are capable of traversing the placenta

table 25-1 Maternal infections posing a threat to the fetus

infection	ease of recognition in mother*	critical months of pregnancy	most common manifestations in newborn†	prevention of fetal infection	therapy
Cytomegalovirus	vs	Unknown	Microcephaly; cerebral calcification; jaundice	None available	None available
Gonorrhea	(C)B	9	Ophthalmitis; septicemia	Antepartum treatment of mother	Antibiotics
Hepatitis‡	CS	Unknown	Hepatitis	None available	None available
Herpes simplex	Cvs	9	Disseminated infection	Cesarean section§	Chemotherapy¶
Listeriosis		8–9	Septicemia; meningitis	Antepartum treatment of mother	Antibiotics
Malaria	CMs	Unknown	Fever; nonspecific signs	Antepartum treatment of mother	Chemotherapy
Mumps‡	CvS	Unknown	Endocardial fibroelastosis	Immunization of mother before pregnancy	None available
Rubella	CvS	1–3	Cardiac defects; cataracts; deafness	Immunization of mother before pregnancy	None available
Smallpox; vaccination	Cvs	Unknown	Disseminated infection	Vaccinia immune globulin	None available
Syphilis	(C)S	5–9	Bone and tooth deformities; progressive nervous system damage	Antepartum treatment of mother	Antibiotics
Toxoplasmosis	(C)S	4–6**	Microcephaly; cerebral calcification; chorioretinitis	Unknown	None available††
Tuberculosis	CB	Postpartum	Tuberculous pneumonia; meningitis; disseminated infection	Antepartum treatment of mother; separation from mother after birth	Chemotherapy

*C, clinical; B, bacteriologic; V, virologic; S, serologic; M, microscopic. Small letters indicate that tests are specialized and not routinely available. Parentheses indicate that typical features are more often absent than present.

†Only characteristic manifestations are listed; many others may be present.

‡Relationship not firmly established.

§Value not definitely established.

¶Iododeoxyuridine and cytarabine; insufficient data available for evaluation.

**Best available information.

††Irreversible damage present at birth.

and infecting the fetus in utero. The severe congenital malformations first drew attention to this agent because infection acquired after birth is rarely serious and cannot be recognized without special laboratory studies.

Most commonly, acquired cytomegalovirus infection is a rather mild febrile illness in childhood, unaccompanied by specific physical findings even though the virus is disseminated throughout the body. In the great majority of affected children, the illness runs its course without diagnosis. If, however, hematologic tests are performed, *lymphocytosis* with many atypical cells may be found, leading to a mistaken diagnosis of infectious mononucleosis (see also "Toxoplasmosis," below). Antibodies are formed, which prevent dissemination of the virus should subsequent reexposure occur.

A woman who has escaped infection during childhood may acquire the virus for the first time during pregnancy. She will then undergo a characteristically mild illness, recovering without any damage to herself but with possible extreme damage to, or even lethal effects on, the fetus.

The most vulnerable organ in the young fetus is the brain, which may remain underdeveloped, leading to microcephaly and mental retardation. Jaundice, enlargement of the liver and spleen, purpura, hernias, and other complications may occur. Furthermore, serologic surveys suggest that this infection may be responsible for some cases of subnormal intelligence and partial hearing loss, representing congenital damage to the nervous system that is not recognized at birth.

The magnitude of the problem is illustrated by the fact that as many as 1 percent of newborns have been found to excrete virus and therefore to be infected. Even though the great majority of these escape damage, the unfortunate minority is considerable in absolute numbers.

No preventive measures are available, either in the form of a vaccine or in early treatment of the mother. Since acquired infection is so difficult to recognize, elimination of this source of congenital anomalies appears to be a formidable task at present. It would be reasonable and feasible to investigate all febrile illnesses during pregnancy at least with a blood count. If atypical lymphocytosis is found, further studies for cytomegalovirus infection would be indicated.

gonorrhea

Although birth defects resulting from fetal maldevelpoment have not been reported, maternal infection with *Neisseria gonorrhoeae* may endanger the fetus in two ways. *Ophthalmia neonatorum,* or conjunctivitis of the newborn, is believed to result from inoculation of one or both eyes during passage through an infected birth canal. Improperly treated, the infection may result in corneal perforation, destruction of the eye, and blindness. The universal use of topical prophylaxis (generally silver nitrate drops or antibiotic ointments) in the eyes of infants born in American hospitals has reduced the incidence of this infection. Care must be exercised however, to ensure that the material is actually delivered to the conjunctiva.

More recently, evidence has been presented that gonococcal infection may occur in utero during maternal septicemia; the infant may then be born with neonatal sepsis or pneumonitis.

At least three obstacles prevent total control of neonatal gonococcal infection. The first is the sheer number of women infected, which is constantly increasing. Second is the lack of acquired immunity following infection, making it possible to become infected repeatedly. Third, more than 80 percent of women with active gonorrhea have no symptoms and therefore do not attract attention to the possibility of this diagnosis.

Proper handling of this problem requires routine culture of the cervix during the last month of pregnancy. Because of the intensified care of pregnant women at this time, obtaining a cervical culture should be an easy matter, but the obstetrician must be aware of the special growth requirements of gonococci and use appropriate culture technique. (Public health departments cooperate very willingly in this endeavor.) Treatment can then be instituted, usually with penicillin, and danger to the newborn can be minimized.

hepatitis

Because of the occasional occurrence of hepatitis in the newborn infant, a possible relationship has been sought with infectious hepatitis in the mother. The relationship, however, awaits final proof. With the recent discovery of hepatitis-associated antigen (Australia antigen), it has been possible to use laboratory techniques to look for transplacental transfer of a possible etiologic agent in hepatitis; this research has suggested that at least hepatitis B can be transmitted across the placenta. For other forms of hepatitis, the evidence is less convincing.

herpes simplex

Two strains of herpes simplex virus commonly infect human beings. The genital strain (type 2) causes *herpes progenitalis,* a recurrent vesicular eruption of the genitalia that can be venereally transmitted. In its typical form, it is fairly easily recognized by the clinician. Using special laboratory diagnostic techniques, however, it has been determined that the infection occurs also in atypical and even asymptomatic forms; just how often is unknown, but it may safely be assumed that, like gonorrhea, genital herpes is much more common than would be suspected on the basis of symptoms alone. Congenital malformations have not been reported, but it is suspected by some that spontaneous abortion may occur with excessive frequency if the mother contracts genital herpes in the first half of pregnancy.

The best known threat to the fetus occurs as a result of maternal herpes active at the time of delivery. The infant may be infected at birth, and the virus spreads throughout his body to produce a frequently fatal disease characterized by necrotizing lesions in lungs, liver, brain, and other organs, and a vesicular skin eruption (resembling chickenpox).

In the belief that infection is acquired during passage through the birth canal, some obstetricians advocate cesarean section if active herpetic infection can be diagnosed at term. However, the additional possibility of in utero infection via the placenta has not yet been excluded, and prevention of neonatal herpes by abdominal delivery has not been conclusively proved.

listeriosis

Listeriosis occurs in several forms. An adult occasionally develops a severe disease associated with septicemia or meningitis. More often, however, infection is mild and escapes identification. Infection in this form, manifested as a cold, fever, or malaise days to weeks before term in the pregnant woman, may transmit the bacterium, *Listeria monocytogenes,* to the fetus. Depending on the stage of pregnancy and the severity of the infection, the result may be abortion, stillbirth, or neonatal sepsis. The last of these is best known. An older term, *granulomatosis infantiseptica,* describes the tissue pathology in newborn infants dying of listeria sepsis. Meningitis may also occur in newborns. If promptly recognized, these infections can be treated successfully with penicillin or other antibiotics.

malaria

Malaria, a parasitic infection, is quite uncommon in American women, although intercontinental travel sometimes leads to exposure in endemic areas. A less obvious danger confronts the mainline drug user who shares a needle with others, for she may acquire malaria by direct transmission from an asymptomatic carrier. Infection thus acquired seldom poses great danger to the mother in the absence of other debilitating conditions because the species of malarial parasites usually involved (*Plasmodium malariae* and *P. vivax*) cause relatively benign infection; the diagnosis may not be suspected, however, because the woman has never visited an endemic area.

In many cases, mothers who have borne malarious infants have had no symptoms at all during pregnancy but have been long-term carriers, thus further obscuring the diagnosis. Fever, irritability, and other nonspecific signs may then appear, often without any clue to the true diagnosis because the periodic fever pattern typical of adult infection may not be present in the infant. The diagnosis of malaria is worth considering in any infant with fever of unknown origin if the mother has ever been in an endemic area or has taken illicit drugs intravenously.

mumps

The majority of women are immune to mumps by the time they reach maturity, either through natural infection or through immunization. A substantial minority, however, escape both and may have their first exposure when a young child (commonly preschool age) transmits the infection to a pregnant woman. It has been proposed, on the basis of a small group of children studied, that endocardial fibroelastosis, a serious congenital cardiac condition in which the inner lining of the heart is thickened and stiffened, is the result of intrauterine mumps virus infection. This correlation is not proved, however, and mumps is not considered sufficient cause for interrupting pregnancy. On the other hand, the Advisory Committee on Immunization Practices of the U.S. Public Health Service does not recommend immunization with live mumps vaccine during pregnancy. Pending further knowledge of possible consequences, no routine preventive measures are taken against mumps in pregnancy. The best safeguard, as with rubella (see below), is to ensure immunity before conception.

mycoplasma

The mycoplasmas are a group of microorganisms resembling bacteria but lacking their characteristic shape and cell wall. The best known is *Mycoplasma pneumoniae,* the cause of what was formerly called "primary atypical pneumonia." Other species, *Mycoplasma hominis* and *Ureaplasma urealyticum* (formerly called "T-strain"), are frequent inhabitants of the female genital tract. Their full pathogenic potential has not yet been elucidated. It has been suggested that they may be responsible for some cases of spontaneous abortion, stillbirth, prematurity, and low birth weight, and that the risk of these complications may be reduced by treatment during pregnancy with a tetracycline, to which the organisms are susceptible. However, tetracyclines are very undesirable antibiotics in the pregnant woman, and in the absence of more definitive indication, their use for mycoplasma prophylaxis is contraindicated. No fetal maldevelopments have been attributed to mycoplasmas.

rubella

German measles, or rubella, has achieved notoriety as the prototype of *teratogenic* infections (i.e., infections causing embryonic developmental defects) (Table 25-2). Infection acquired after birth is almost universally benign, but rubella, unlike a number of other maternal infections dangerous to the fetus (such as cytomegalovirus infection, listeriosis, and toxoplasmosis), produces a characteristic syndrome of rash and swollen lymphs glands which readily attracts attention. It is this property that first led to recognition of the association between rubella and congenital deafness, cataracts, and heart disease. The more recent development of serologic tests has made it possible to confirm the diagnosis or rule it out in cases of other illness with similar clinical findings. Equally important, a woman can be tested before or during pregnancy for susceptibility to rubella. A positive test (titer greater than 1:10) indicates immunity and the virtual absence of any danger to the fetus from this infection. A negative test (titer less than 1:10), on the other hand, if discovered during the childbearing age but in the nonpregnant state, is a strong indication for immunization. Early in pregnancy, immunization cannot be carried out for fear of infecting the fetus with the live vaccine; women discovered at this stage to be nonimmune must be observed for symptoms and, in such circumstances, retested for developing antibody titers, which would prove that rubella had occurred and that the fetus had been exposed to the virus in utero.

The management of pregnancy complicated by rubella depends on a number of factors. Underlying the choice of alternatives is the central fact that there is no known way to protect the fetus once infection of the mother has occurred, nor, indeed, any way to reduce the chance of infection in a susceptible woman if she has been exposed. (Gamma globulin has been shown to be worthless for this purpose.) Thus the decision involves (1) determining whether maternal infection has occurred, which can be done reliably in each case by serologic tests; (2)

table 25-2 Probability of rubella-associated congenital abnormality according to time of maternal infection*

gestational month	congenital abnormality,%†
1	50–60
2	25–35
3	7–15
4	5
5–9	‡

*Based on various reports.
†Percentages of live births; additional losses through spontaneous abortion not included.
‡No significant risk due to rubella.

determining whether the fetus has been damaged, which cannot be done on an individual basis but requires an estimate of probability. The estimate is based on the stage of pregnancy at which infection occurs. Table 25-2 shows current estimates of the frequency of fetal maldevelopment related to the time of infection. The high probability of severe congenital defects following first- and second-month infection has led to consideration of therapeutic abortion for these mothers. Purely medical judgment has to be tempered by appropriate legal, moral, and religious considerations that vary from case to case. Universal immunization of girls before puberty holds the best hope for future control of congenital rubella. A woman who is discovered while pregnant to be nonimmune, and who shows no serologic evidence of infection during pregnancy, should be immunized as soon as practical after delivery to avoid future difficulties.

smallpox

Smallpox no longer occurs in the United States and deserves only passing mention. However, *vaccination* is an important consideration, because the live virus (vaccinia) used has been known to cross the placenta and lead to disseminated infection in the fetus, which may then be stillborn. Since this infection has been all but eradicated, even vaccination is no longer performed except in unusual circumstances. If a pregnant woman is thought to have been exposed or vaccination is considered for any reason, public health authorities should be consulted before any action is taken. The only indications for vaccination now are travel to endemic areas and work in some special laboratories. Since vaccination is contraindicated in pregnancy, a pregnant woman without immunity must weigh very carefully her risk of exposure before undertaking either of these activities.

syphilis

The causative organism of syphilis, *Treponema pallidum,* can cross the placenta and infect the fetus, with disastrous results. Congenital syphilis can range in severity from stillbirth, at one extreme, to a positive serologic test unaccompanied by clinical findings, at the other. Between these extremes are various forms of damage. Some, such as skeletal and dental malformations, may be evident in infancy or early childhood, while others, such as general paresis (dementia), may not develop until adolescence. Special conditions are required for placental passage to occur: (1) Treponemes must be circulating in the bloodstream, which is characteristic of primary and secondary syphilis but rarely occurs more than 2 to 4 years after maternal infection first took place. (2) The pregnancy must be beyond the fifth month, because up to that time the placenta affords an effective barrier. The latter feature permits prevention of congenital syphilis by treatment of infected mothers during the first half of pregnancy, usually with penicillin. Identification of such women is achieved by a simple serologic test, which is routinely performed in any good prenatal care program.

Although therapy for syphilis is well standardized, its effect is not immediately apparent. Only a steady diminution in titer of antibodies, or their total disappearance, can be accepted as evidence of cure, and this takes many months to determine. In addition, if the maternal titer is sufficiently high, placental transfer of antibody will occur and the infant will be born *seropositive.* Providing the mother has received standard treatment during pregnancy, the infant should not be treated unless his titer persists unchanged for 3 months or actually increases; a positive serologic test resulting from transplacental passage of maternal antibodies reverts to negative in 3 to 6 months. Conversely, an infant born seronegative to a seropositive mother should be retested in 3 months; infection could have occurred shortly before birth, with antibodies first becoming detectable several weeks later.

toxoplasmosis

Toxoplasma gondii is a protozoan parasite of mammals. The usual source of acquisition by human beings has not been identified, although incompletely cooked meat and contamination by cat feces have occasionally been implicated. Regardless of how it is acquired, human infection is much more common than realized, as evidenced by serologic tests. These tests, although well standardized and not difficult to do, are seldom performed unless an infant with characteristic abnormalities is born or, in the case of older children and adults, a characteristic retinal lesion is discovered. Only in these two instances is the infection readily suspected by the clinician. In fact, toxoplasmosis is usually clinically unrecognizable, being manifested as pneumonia, skin rash, myocarditis, meningoencephalitis, or, most commonly of all, fever and lymphadenopathy resembling infectious mononucleosis. Atypical lymphocytosis may further confuse the diagnosis (see also "Cytomegalovirus Infection," above), but the specific heterophil antibody test is negative. Most infections undoubtedly go undiagnosed, and if one occurs during pregnancy, especially in the second trimester, the protozoon may reach the fetus and cause a syndrome characterized by destructive inflammation of the retina (chorioretinitis), maldevelopement of the brain (microcephaly or hydrocephalus), and cerebral calcifications; other organs, particularly liver and spleen, may be involved also. It is suspected, furthermore, that some infections that escape detection at birth may be responsible for subsequent neurologic or mental deficits.

Much remains to be learned regarding prevention of congenital toxoplasmosis. For one thing, since maternal toxoplasmosis is not readily diagnosed by the clinician (unlike, for example, rubella), the statistical probability of fetal infection can only be estimated; the risk is thought to be about one in three. Second, although treatment for acute toxoplasmosis is available, the main drug used (pyrimethamine) itself may be *teratogenic* and is therefore not appropriate for use in pregnancy; thus, the treatment may be more dangerous than the disease. No vaccine is available.

A third consideration is the tendency of this infection to recur after periods of dormancy. This makes it possible for a mother to infect infants of subsequent pregnancies; fortunately, such cases appear to be rare.

tuberculosis

The chief danger to the infant from tuberculosis occurs after birth. Infection in utero or at the time of delivery is not an important consideration.

ANTIMICROBIAL DRUGS IN PREGNANCY

All antimicrobial agents have the potential for entering fetal tissues via the placenta. Whether the fetus suffers ill effects depends both on the drug and on the stage of pregnancy at which it is given.

Practically all that is known about adverse effects has been learned in retrospect, i.e., through the study of damaged infants whose mothers received drugs that were not known to be harmful during pregnancy. The safety of other drugs has been established in the same haphazard way. Unfortunately, this is the only way. While fully informed volunteers are routinely used to determine the safety of new drugs in their own bodies, it is quite a different matter for a mother to volunteer her unborn child to show that a new drug does not produce a crippling congenital defect. Information derived from animal experiments (which are always conducted before human volunteers are subjected to new drugs) have limited relevance to human beings, because the experimental dosages often are not comparable to those used in human therapy and because there are unpredictable species differences in pharmacology. New drugs are therefore marketed with the warning that safety during pregnancy has not been established. When the life of a pregnant woman depends on the use of a new drug, a calculated risk is justified, and from accumulated experiences of this sort effects on the fetus eventually become known.

Following is a summary of relevant information about current antimicrobial agents.

1   Amantidine (prophylactic for type A influenza). Found to be embryo-toxic and teratogenic in rats. Not considered safe for pregnancy.

2 Aminoglycosides (streptomycin, kanamycin, gentamicin). Chief side effect is ototoxicity. Prolonged use in pregnancy has resulted in impaired hearing in the infant.

3 Cephalosporins. Safety is not strictly established. So far, they have not been incriminated in congenital abnormalities.

4 Chloramphenicol. Beyond the well-publicized myelotoxic effects, there is no known danger unique to the pregnant state or the intrauterine fetus. However, the metabolic process for detoxifying the drug is not fully developed in the newborn, who may retain excessive blood levels and develop the so-called gray syndrome (cyanosis and circulatory collapse).

5 Clindamycin and Lincomycin. In a rare prospective study involving some 300 pregnant women, the safety of lincomycin for both mother and fetus appears to be established. The newer derivative, clindamycin, has not been similarly tested.

6 Erythromycin. Safety is not strictly established, but years of use have not revealed any problems related to pregnancy.

7 Ethambutol. Safety not strictly established, but no pregnancy-related problems have been reported.

8 Isoniazid. Safety is not strictly established, but years of use have not revealed any problems related to pregnancy.

9 Methenamine compounds (methenamine mandelate, hippurate). Safety is not strictly established, but years of use have not revealed any problems related to pregnancy.

10 Metronidazole. Used for many years without any reported serious adverse reaction. Current status uncertain because of carcinogenic effects in mice.

11 Nalidixic acid. This drug is considered safe during the second and third trimesters. Caution is advised in the first trimester because of insufficient controlled data.

12 Nitrofurantoin. Safety is not strictly established, but years of use have not revealed any problems related to pregnancy.

13 Para-aminosalicylic acid. Safety is not strictly established, but years of use have not revealed any problems related to pregnancy.

14 Penicillins. Penicillin G and penicillin V are considered safe. For the newer, semisynthetic penicillins, safety is not established, but their popularity and extensive use promise to yield sufficient information for practical purposes. So far, they have not been incriminated in congenital abnormalities.

15 Polymyxins (polymyxin B, colistimethate). Safety is not established.

16 Rifampin. Safety not strictly established, but no pregnancy-related problems have been reported.

17 Sulfonamides. These drugs are considered safe for mother and intrauterine fetus. The newborn, however, is unable to handle sulfonamides and may become jaundiced (see also "Chloramphenicol," above). It is wise not to give the drug so close to delivery that the baby might be born before the mother has completely excreted it; long-acting sulfonamides should be avoided altogether.

18 Tetracyclines. These drugs are unsafe for both mother and fetus. Pregnant women have developed fatal fatty degeneration of the liver and pancreas, usually when treated with very high doses. Dysplasia of the teeth occurs in the child because of the affinity of tetracyclines for calcifying tissues; although not apparent until months after birth, these deformities can be traced back to pregnancy.

IMMUNIZATION DURING PREGNANCY

Because of the variety of agents used to produce immunity to infection, their effects on the fetus must be considered individually. Table 25-3 shows the most commonly used immunizing substances and their relative safety during pregnancy.

The only questions concern live virus vaccines. Theoretically, none can be considered safe because they all cause maternal infection and viremia, with unpredictable effects on the fetus. Their use is a matter of individual judgment regarding the danger of the unmodified disease to the mother.

MATERNAL INFECTIONS DURING THE PUERPERIUM

Labor is a traumatic event. Wounds are regularly inflicted on the uterus, cervix, and vagina. The urethra may be contused, and the anus may be lacerated. It is surprising that infection occurs as infrequently as it does, although it is well known that excessive trauma or hemorrhage during labor increases susceptibility.

bacteriology

A variety of bacteria may be isolated in puerperal infections. Some are frequently associated with distinct syndromes, so that the clinical picture may suggest the bacterial cause. However, the overlap is too great to justify choice of antimicrobial therapy on this basis alone. Laboratory diagnosis is essential, because the antimicrobial susceptibilities of the different bacteria are quite unpre-

table 25-3 Safety of immunization during pregnancy*

immunizing agent	use in pregnancy
Toxoids	
Diphtheria	Safe
Tetanus	Safe
Killed viruses	
Influenza	Safe
Poliomyelitis (Salk)	Safe
Rabies	Safe
Live, attenuated viruses	
Measles	Not recommended†
Mumps	Not recommended†
Poliomyelitis (Sabin)	Not recommended†
Rubella	Unsafe
Vaccinia (for smallpox)	Unsafe‡
Yellow fever	Not recommended†
Killed bacteria§	
Cholera	Safe
Plague	Safe
Typhoid	Safe
Gamma globulin¶	
Human	Safe
Equine	Safe

*Based on recommendations of the Public Health Service Advisory Committee on Immunization Practices, 1972.

†Based on theoretic grounds. No solid information available.

‡In emergency (proved exposure), may be used together with vaccinia immune globulin.

§All these agents are used only under special circumstances.

¶Used mostly in emergencies following exposure. Provides only temporary protection against severer forms of hepatitis, measles, rabies, and vaccinia. May also suppress rubella in mother, but without protection to the fetus.

dictable. Since the nurse frequently assists in, and may actually be responsible for, obtaining culture material, it is important that he or she understand the bases of meaningful microbiologic diagnosis. The most important principle is that the information obtained from a clinical specimen can be useful only in so far as the specimen, *at the time of examination in the laboratory,* reflects conditions in the patient. The following guidelines should be remembered:

1   Skin and mucous membranes are *always* colonized by bacteria. A wound culture must therefore be taken from *deep* within the wound—if possible, after sterilizing the surface.

2   A Gram stain helps in interpretation of culture data, frequently gives additional information, and can be reported within minutes of submission to the laboratory. A smear should therefore be made at the bedside when culturing a wound and submitted for staining along with the culture specimen; a telephone report may be very helpful.

3   A culture specimen consists of *live* material. It changes constantly, in that some bacteria may proliferate, proportions may change, contaminants may assume predominance, and some pathogenic species may die out completely within a short time. Unless the specimen is processed soon after it leaves the patient, the results may not reflect the true state of affairs. In other words, it should be rushed to the laboratory. (One reason for preferring a bedside smear over one made in the laboratory is that further delay has no effect on a dried smear.)

4   Anaerobic bacteria are frequently implicated in pelvic infections. Their tolerance of oxygen is sometimes so poor that sealed specimen tubes with prereduced atmospheres have been specially prepared and are commercially available for use in anaerobic infections. Whether or not such methods are used, liaison with the microbiology laboratory is important if anaerobic organisms are to be recovered.

5   Blood cultures are important sources of information in puerperal fevers. The proper time to culture the blood is the moment someone suspects that bacteremia may be present. The oft-repeated recommendation to culture the blood when the temperature is rising (which may require waiting for it to fall first) is based on fallacious reasoning. During septic fever, temperature fluctuations are determined by the hypothalamus, not by the intermittent entry of bacteria into the blood. Two blood cultures from different veins 1 h apart, regardless of the temperature during that hour, are sufficient; thereafter, empiric antibiotic therapy may be started if the clinical condition does not permit waiting for culture and sensitivity results.

clinical syndromes

amnionitis   Amnionitis results from excessive delay in delivery after rupture of the fetal membranes. Once the "seal is broken," access of bacteria from the vagina is uninhibited, and prompt emptying of the uterus is essential in preventing infection. If delivery is delayed beyond 24 h, the danger is increased to as much as 15 to 20 percent. The infection may disseminate in the mother via the placenta, but the chief victim is the fetus, who aspirates the infected fluid and may show signs of sepsis with or without meningitis shortly after birth. The most commonly implicated bacteria in neonatal sepsis are *Escherichia coli* and group B streptococcus. Respiratory distress is a common presenting sign, and its differential diagnosis should always include neonatal sepsis, especially in premature infants.

urinary infection   Danger of overt acute pyelonephritis in bacteriuric women continues throughout pregnancy (see Chap. 24) into the early postpartum period. An added danger is the introduction of bacteria into the bladder by catheterization. While this procedure may occasionally be necessary, it should be done with the utmost care and avoided altogether if possible during labor or immediately following delivery, because the danger of infection may be as high as 20 percent as compared to 2 percent in healthy, nonpregnant women. Very likely, trauma to the urethra and bladder during delivery increases their susceptibility to bacterial invasion.

puerperal fever Obstetricians are not alarmed at low-grade fever [up to 38°C (100.4°F)] on the first postpartum day, ascribing it to absorption of pyrogen from damaged tissues or unknown self-limiting factors. Needless to say, fever of this type may occasionally persist longer than one day. For practical purposes, however, higher, or more prolonged fever is usually taken as a sign of infection. In the past, infections arising during this period have been collectively termed "childbed fever" or "puerperal fever." Advances in understanding of anatomic and microbiologic varieties of postpartum infections have rendered these terms obsolete, and a satisfactory diagnosis nowadays must include a reference to anatomic location as well as to bacteriologic agent. Depending on these factors, a number of different infections can be recognized.

episiotomy wound infection Infection of the episiotomy wound involves the skin and underlying soft tissue of the posterior portion of the vulva. Staphylococci or enteric gram-negative bacilli are commonly involved. The process tends to localize but may lead to disruption of the wound. Local drainage is usually curative, with antibiotics playing an auxiliary role.

The nurse must include observation of the suture line in the daily assessment and identify for the patient the symptoms that she should report, i.e., pain, warmth, swelling, purulent drainage.

pelvic cellulitis (parametritis) In pelvic cellulitis the loose connective tissue supporting the internal genitalia, including the broad ligament of the uterus, are invaded by extension from the cervix or, less commonly, the uterus. Although not usually serious, the infection may produce considerable discomfort, local tenderness, and fever. The process may be slow to resolve and may leave internal scarring in its wake. Any of the bacteria normally found in the vagina may be responsible, and without microbiologic studies there is no way to make a definitive choice of antibiotics.

infections of the uterus The endometrium is the portal of entry for most serious postpartum infections.* All have the potential of spreading through the wall of the uterus, to the pelvic peritoneum, and into the local blood vessels. From the latter, dissemination to distant organs may occur, with disastrous consequences.

Endometritis is the first inflammatory reaction that occurs, regardless of the infecting organism. The subsequent course of events is shaped by an interplay of host and parasite in which resistance and virulence both play important parts. The role of excessive trauma and hemorrhage in predisposing the mother to infection has already been pointed out. The role of bacterial virulence is illustrated by three very different syndromes.

HEMOLYTIC STREPTOCOCCAL SEPSIS This infection is characterized by the rapid spread of bacteria through soft tissues with relatively little tissue reaction, necrosis, or suppuration. The lymphatic vessels are favorite channels of extension. The infection may be accompanied by extreme constitutional reaction, such as toxic delirium and shock. General peritonitis may occur, and bacteremia may result in metastatic infection.

This is undoubtedly one of the most virulent

---

*For practical purposes, septic abortion is simply a variant of postpartum uterine infection, except for the underlying circumstances.

infections of the puerperium; its early onset (within the first day or two) and rapid progression are clinical clues to its etiology. The responsible organisms are beta-hemolytic streptococci belonging to group A or, less commonly, group B. Group A streptococci were formerly often implicated in epidemics of childbed fever, because they were carried from one patient to another on the hands or in the pharynx of hospital attendants. If the patient is suffering from a streptococcal sore throat at the time, she herself may be the source of uterine infection. These epidemiologic considerations do not apply to group B streptococci, which are often normal inhabitants of the vagina, but uterine infections due to them are equally dangerous.

Penicillin G is the antibiotic of choice; in patients with severe penicillin allergy, erythromycin or clindamycin may be used. Tetracycline is not advised because some group A and most group B streptococci are resistant to it.

MIXED AEROBIC-ANAEROBIC INFECTIONS In addition to its normal bacterial flora, various fecal organisms are frequently present in small numbers in the vagina. Against healthy tissues these organisms are harmless, but they may cause considerable trouble when introduced into open wounds. Their relatively low virulence (compared with hemolytic streptococci) is associated with two clinical phenomena: (1) the tendency for two or more species to be present simultaneously, as though one alone were not powerful enough to cause disease; and (2) the tendency for infections to be contained locally rather than to disseminate rapidly. Local tissue reaction usually establishes an effective barrier so that, even if infection penetrates the uterus, it is likely to be confined to the pelvic peritoneum and may be walled off in the form of an abscess. Such infections develop more

slowly and are not as threatening as those due to hemolytic streptococci. However, fever and leukocytosis are always present and in some cases may be the only signs of infection. Etiologic organisms include aerobes (such as *Escherichia, Klebsiella,* and *Proteus* species) and anaerobes (such as *Peptostreptococcus* and *Bacteroides* species) in various combinations.

Infections of this type, especially those involving anaerobes, are often associated with pelvic thrombophlebitis. Under these circumstances bacteria will gain access to the bloodstream, and septic pulmonary embolism is an important and possibly serious complication. The effect of such embolism may be pneumonia, lung abscess, or acute right ventricular failure.

Surgery is usually required for drainage of pelvic abscesses, which characteristically do not respond to even the best antibiotic regimens. Anticoagulation has been known to reduce fever which persisted in the face of other remedies; in these cases, thrombophlebitis was evidently an important part of the pathologic process. Ligation of thrombosed veins may be necessary to control recurrent pulmonary embolism (see Chap. 23).

The choice of antibiotics is difficult for several reasons: (1) both the identity and the antibiotic susceptibilities of the bacteria are unpredictable; (2) the anaerobes are difficult to culture and their antibiotic susceptibilities are difficult to determine; and (3) the fact that the pathogens are also members of the normal perineal flora raises doubts as to which wound isolates are truly significant. (Organisms cultured from the blood are always considered significant.) Recommendations change from time to time. At this writing, a combination of gentamicin (for the gram-negative aerobes), ampicillin (for enterococci), and clindamycin (for the anaerobes) is acceptable pending a reliable bacteriologic diagnosis.

CLOSTRIDIAL MYOMETRITIS Uterine infections caused by *Clostridium perfringens* have special characteristics because of the unique properties of the organism. Normally a harmless inhabitant of the intestine and occasionally the vagina, its introduction into devitalized tissues turns it into a life-threatening menace. The conditions for its invasiveness have often been met in unprofessional attempts at abortion, which combined tissue mutilation with unclean techniques; however, any unusually traumatic labor may likewise set the stage.

Under these circumstances, the organisms produce a series of powerful toxins which cause tissue necrosis or gangrene; this permits further invasion, and a vicious circle is set up that, all too often, requires hysterectomy for control. The exudate from such infections usually contains a good deal of gas, and gas shadows may be visible on a pelvic x-ray. The term *gas gangrene* has been given to clostridial infections of this severe type, although the gas itself is incidental, being a product of bacterial metabolism and without known toxicity.

The most serious complication results from the entry of large numbers of clostridia into the circulation. The effects may be similar to hemolytic streptococcal septicemia (see above) with high fever, delirium, and shock. In addition, there may be massive intravascular hemolysis, with more than half the red blood cells being destroyed in a few hours. The hemoglobin released into the plasma is useless as an oxygen carrier and is, further, toxic to the kidneys. Complete renal shutdown may occur, with total cessation of urine formation. Metabolism of free hemoglobin in the liver may lead to deep jaundice. Telltale laboratory signs are gross red discoloration of the urine and plasma; the latter is visible on examination of sedimented blood in a tube.

Large doses of antibiotics (preferably penicillin) are essential in management. Gas gangrene antitoxin may also be given, although its value is not firmly established. The outcome, however, depends at least as heavily on supportive therapy, which includes measures to counteract shock, transfusion of red blood cells, and appropriate surgery; days to weeks of dialysis may follow the crisis, until the kidneys regain their function.

mastitis and breast abscess Infection of the breast is a complication of lactation and nursing. Entry of bacteria is facilitated by cracking or fissuring of the nipples, and it is plausible that tissue resistance is lowered by the pressure associated with vascular engorgement. Before lactation actually begins, breast engorgement itself may be associated with low-grade fever, usually on the second or third postpartum day. Infection, however, is a much later event, so that there is little cause for confusion.

Symptoms vary from mild local pain and tenderness to a severe constitutional reaction with fever and leukocytosis. If not appropriately treated, what starts as diffuse cellulitis may localize in an abscess, which then requires open drainage or needle aspiration of pus.

These infections are almost always caused by gram-positive cocci, usually coagulase-positive staphylococci. In selecting an antibiotic, it is well to remember that most staphylococci are resistant to penicillin and, frequently, also to other antibiotics. Agent of choice is one of the semisynthetic antistaphylococcal penicillins, such as oxacillin, cloxacillin, dicloxacillin, or nafcillin. Ampicillin should never be used, because against staphylococci it is no more effective than penicillin G. For penicillin-allergic patents, clindamycin is recommended. Nursing is generally discontinued on the affected side until the lesion has healed, a breast pump being used to withdraw the milk in the interim.

study questions

1 What special precautions should a pregnant woman observe when she is exposed to the following infectious diseases during pregnancy?
   a Gonorrhea
   b Poliomyelitis
   c Rubella
   d Syphilis
   e Toxoplasmosis
   f Upper respiratory infection
2 Differentiate between asymptomatic bacteriuria and cystitis. What measures should the patient take to prevent infection? How can you, the nurse, prevent infection during labor and in postpartal care?
3 Venereal diseases are often hidden in women. What screening tests are provided during prenatal care (see Chap. 5)?
   a Is it possible to become reinfected after treatment during pregnancy?
   b How does the mother's treatment affect the fetus?
   c If the baby is born with the disease, what are the symptoms, treatment, and prognosis for (1) gonorrhea, and (2) syphilis?
4 Serology may still remain positive after treatment. What is the basis for this statement?
   a If the baby is born *seropositive*, does that mean the child has syphilis?
   b What does it mean if the baby is seronegative when the mother has syphilis?
5 A pregnant woman may ask you about toxoplasmosis.
   a What preventive measures can she take?
   b When is infection most damaging to the fetus?
   c What are the adverse results in the fetus?
6 Be able to explain to a patient the immunization precautions during pregnancy.
7 List the precautions necessary to obtain a satisfactory lab specimen for a septic workup when a patient has symptoms of infection.
   a Urine culture
   b Blood culture
   c Wound culture
   d Smear of vaginal or cervical secretions
8 Note the number of sites for infection before and after delivery. For each of the sites, list the following:
   a Symptoms
   b Signs
   c Usual bacteria (if specified)

   d Route of transmission of infections, or predisposing factors
   e Treatment/nursing support
9 Be prepared to counsel a woman who is breastfeeding about signs and symptoms of mastitis and usual methods of alleviating these.

bibliography

INFECTIONS DURING PREGNANCY

Reviews
Barrett-Connor, E.: "Infections and Pregnancy: A Review," *Southern Medical Journal*, **62**:275–284, 1969.
Hardy, J. B.: "Immediate and Long-range Effects of Maternal Viral Infection in Pregnancy," *Birth Defects*, **12**(5):23, 1976.
Monif, G. R. G. (ed.): *Infectious Diseases in Obstetrics and Gynecology*. Harper & Row, New York, 1974.

Cytomegalovirus
Birnbaum, G., J. I. Lynch, A. M. Margileth, W. M. Lonergan, and J. L. Sever: "Cytomegalovirus Infections in Newborn Infants," *Journal of Pediatrics*, **75**:789–795, 1969.
Hanshaw, J. B., A. P. Scheiner, A. W. Moxley, L. Gaev, V. Abel, and B. Scheiner: "School Failure and Deafness after 'Silent' Congenital Cytomegalovirus Infection," *New England Journal of Medicine*, **295**:468–470, 1976.
Sterner, H., and S. M. Tucker: "Prospective Study of Cytomegalovirus Infection in Pregnancy," *British Medical Journal*, **2**:268–270, 1973.

Gonorrhea
Barsam, P. C.: "Specific Prophylaxis of Gonorrheal Ophthalmia Neonatorum," *New England Journal of Medicine*, **274**:731–734, 1966.
Charles, A. G., S. Cohen, M. B. Kass, and R. Richman: "Asymptomatic Gonorrhea in Prenatal Patients," *American Journal of Obstetrics and Gynecology*, **108**:595–599, 1970.

Hepatitis
Mollica, F., S. Musumeci, and A. Fischer: "Neonatal Hepatitis in Five Children of a Hepatitis B Surface Antigen Carrier Woman," *Journal of Pediatrics*, **90**:949–951, 1976.

Herpes Simplex
Nahmias, A. J., W. E. Josey, Z. M. Naib, M. G. Freeman, R. J. Fernandez, and J. H. Wheeler: "Perinatal Risk Associated with Maternal Genital Herpes Simplex Virus

Infection," *American Journal of Obstetrics and Gynecology*, **110**:825–837, 1971.

Influenza
Widelock, D., L. Csizmas, and S. Klein: "Influenza, Pregnancy, and Fetal Outcome," *Public Health Reports*, **78**:1–11, 1963.

Listeriosis
Gray, M. L., H. P. R. Seeliger, and J. Potal: "Perinatal Infections Due to *Listeria monocytogenes*. Do These Affect Subsequent Pregnancies?" *Clinical Pediatrics*, **2**: 614–623, 1963.
Ray, C. G., and R. J. Wedgwood: "Neonatal Listeriosis, Six Case Reports and a Review of the Literature," *Pediatrics*, **34**:378–392, 1964.

Malaria
Lewis, R., N. H. Laverson, and S. Birnbaum, "Malaria Associated with Pregnancy," *Obstetrics and Gynecology* **42**:696, 1973.
McQuay, R. M., S. Silberman, P. Mudrik, and L. E. Keith: "Congenital Malaria in Chicago. A Case Report and a Review of Published Reports (U.S.A.)," *American Journal of Tropical Medicine and Hygiene*, **16**:258–266, 1967.

Mycoplasma
McCormack, W. M., P. Braun, Y.-H. Lee, J. O. Klein, and E. H. Kass: "The Genital Mycoplasms," *New England Journal of Medicine*, **288**:78–89, 1973.

Rubella
Plotkin, S. A., F. A. Oski, E. M. Hartnett, A. R. Hervada, S. Friedman, and J. Gowing: "Some Recently Recognized Manifestations of the Rubella Syndrome," *Journal of Pediatrics*, **67**:182–191, 1965.
Rudolph, A. J., M. D. Yow, A. Phillips, M. M. Desmond, R. J. Blattner, and J. L. Melnick: "Transplacental Rubella Infection in Newly Born Infants," *Journal of the American Medical Association*, **191**:843–845, 1965.
Sallomi, S. J.: "Rubella in Pregnancy. A Review of Prospective Studies from the Literature," *Obstetrics and Gynecology*, **27**:252–256, 1966.

Syphilis
Curtis, A. C., and O. S. Philpott: "Prenatal Syphilis," *Medical Clinics of North America*, **48**:707–720, 1964.

Toxoplasmosis
Couvreur, J., and G. Desmonts: "Congenital and Maternal Toxoplasmosis. Review of 300 Congenital Cases,"

Developmental Medicine and Child Neurology, **4**: 519–530, 1962.
Williams, H., "Toxoplasmosis in the Perinatal Period," *Post graduate Medicine*, **53**:614, 1977.

Tuberculosis
Avery, M. E., and J. Wolfsdorf: "Diagnosis and Treatment: Infants of Tuberculous Mothers," *Pediatrics*, **42**: 519–522, 1968.
Committee on Drugs, American Academy of Pediatrics: "Infants of Tuberculous Mothers: Further Thoughts," *Pediatrics*, **42**:393, 1968.

Urinary Infection
Heineman, H. S.: Urinary Infection in Pregnancy, in J. H. Moyer and C. D. Swartz (eds.), "Symposium on the Management of Pyelonephritis," *Modern Treatment*, **7**: 349, 1970.

Immunization
Public Health Service Advisory Committee on Immunization Practices: "General Recommendations on Immunization," *Morbidity and Mortality Weekly Report*, **25**: 355, 1976.

INFECTIONS DURING THE PUERPERIUM

Collins, C. G.: "Suppurative Pelvic Thrombophlebitis," *American Journal of Obstetrics and Gynecology*, **108**: 681–687, 1970.
Gibbs, R. S., T. N. O'Dell, R. R. MacGregor, R. H. Schwarz, and H. Morton: "Puerperal Endometritis: A Prospective Microbiologic Study," *American Journal of Obstetrics and Gynecology*, **121**:919–925, 1975.
Greenhalf, J. O.: "The Problem of Pelvic Infection," *Practitioner*, **216**:513–518, 1976.
Roser, D. M.: "Breast Engorgement and Postpartum Infections," *Obstetrics and Gynecology*, **27**:73–77, 1966.
Rotheram, E. B., and S. F. Schick: "Nonclostridial Anaerobic Bacteria in Septic Abortion," *American Journal of Medicine*, **46**:80–89, 1969.
Swenson, R. M., T. C. Michaelson, M. J. Daly, and E. H. Spaulding: "Anaerobic Infections of the Female Genital Tract," *Obstetrics and Gynecology*, **42**:538–541, 1973.
White, C. A.: "β-Hemolytic Streptococcus Infections in Postpartum Patients," *Obstetrics and Gynecology*, **41**: 27–32, 1973.

26

PROBLEMS COMPLICATING LABOR AND DELIVERY

MÄRRETJE JELLES BÜHRER
ELIZABETH J. DICKASON

PRETERM BIRTH

Preterm birth is the chief factor in neonatal morbidity and mortality. Although neonatal intensive care facilities have reduced the mortality rates, the prevention of preterm birth will continue to be a major obstetric problem for research in the 1980s.

The prevention of preterm labor is a problem because of the incomplete understanding of the factors that begin true labor. The prevention of labor demands a knowledge of how to interrupt the cycle of factors that allow the labor to begin early.

maternal factors

What maternal factors seem to precipitate early labor? Very early after 20 weeks, the cause may be an incompetent cervix or a complication, such as placenta previa or abortion resulting from lowered fertility with low progesterone levels, the same factors that cause labor to start prematurely after the age of viability.

Some researchers think that one factor is an alteration of uterine blood supply, since premature contractions occur in connection with heavy smoking, high altitudes, severe hypertension and preeclampsia, and over-stretching of uterine muscles by multiple pregnancy or polyhydramnios.[1] All these situations have in common a reduction in blood flow to the uterine muscle. See Chap. 10 for other factors in the initiation of labor which are interdependent and complex. Once the process of labor begins, it usually goes through to completion. If it starts before 38 weeks of gestation, or preterm, the outcome is an infant compromised by immaturity.

prevention of preterm labor

Labor can be halted only if diagnosed in the latent period, before the cervix has dilated to 4 cm or is 75 to 100 percent effaced (in a primipara).[2] The presence of ruptured membranes in this period usually means that labor must be allowed to progress because the natural barrier against infection has been breached.

At present, therapy involves several pharmacologic agents plus bed rest. Physicians vary in their choice of these agents but agree on the need to diagnose first the existence of true labor. Even with drug availability, sedation and bed rest are sometimes the only choices selected by the obstetrician.

nursing care When a patient is admitted to the hospital in preterm labor, the nurse will need to prepare for the possibility of a low-birth-weight infant. Several observations and actions are necessary on admission. After gentle vaginal examination, the mother is placed on complete bed rest, on her side.

The enema is omitted, and further vaginal exams are kept at a minimum. Since future therapy will be based on observations during the first few hours after admission, baseline fetal heart tones and maternal vital signs are taken and labor is monitored. An external labor monitor is applied so that even mild conractions unfelt by the mother can be recorded. During this period of diagnosis, x-ray pelvimetry or ultrasound measurements can aid in determining fetal size.

Usually several hours pass before a decision regarding treatment is made because the decision depends upon the predicted size and condition of the infant. The mother will be very apprehensive and need continuing support and clear explanations of the decisions as to the method of treatment.

pharmacologic therapy Several types of agents are used to reduce contraction rate and intensity. Other agents are still under investigation in research centers, and pregnant women receiving these research drugs should be fully informed as to the risks and benefits prior to institution of therapy.

BETA$_2$-RECEPTOR STIMULANTS Beta$_2$-receptor stimulants are widely used for asthmatic patients and are inhaled as a powder or an aerosol for local effect to relieve bronchospasm. For inhibition of uterine contractions, such a smooth muscle response is best obtained when the drug is given intravenously. Once action has been effective, the dose can be lowered and given orally or intramuscularly.

Major adverse effects are the result of smooth muscle dilatation: postural hypotension, dizziness, trembling, nervousness, and weakness. An average increase of heart rate of 30 beats per minute and a decrease in blood pressure of 10 to 15 mmHg are expected during initial stages of treatment.

Beta$_2$-receptor drugs include ritrodrine, fen-

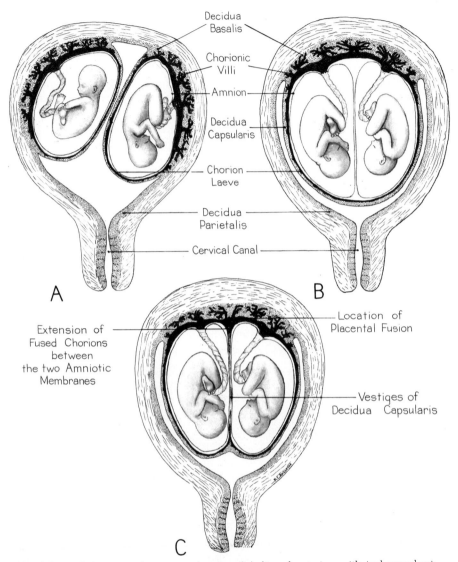

Decidua
Basalis

Chorionic
Villi

Amnion

Decidua
Capsularis

Chorion
Laeve

Decidua
Parietalis

Cervical Canal

A

B

Extension of
Fused Chorions
between
the two Amniotic
Membranes

Location of
Placental Fusion

Vestiges of
Decidua Capsularis

C

fig. 26-1   Schematic diagrams showing (a) diovular twins with independent membranes; (b) monovular twins; and (c) diovular twins implanted close to each other, resulting in fusion of their membranes. (*From Bradley M. Patten, Human Embryology, 3d ed., McGraw-Hill, New York, 1968.*)

oterol, metaproterenol, salbutamol, and terbutaline. The most widely used drug, and the only one currently approved for use outside of research settings, is isoxsuprine (Vasodilan).

ISOXSUPRINE   Titration of the isoxsuprine dose with maternal blood pressure and uterine contraction response will determine the dosage. The average dose is 0.25 to 0.5 mg/min, IV, diluted in 5 percent dextrose in water and administered by an infusion pump. After contractions diminish, 5 to 20 mg IM or PO q3 to 6 h for 3 to 10 days is a common dosage.

Nursing care Place the patient in a slight left lateral tilt, with a small pillow behind her back to maintain the side-lying position. Careful monitoring must be carried out in this position but may be difficult. Watch for fetal responses to contractions or for the maternal tachycardia and hypotension. Watch for and assist the patient if reactions of weakness, vomiting, or nervousness occur. Maintain bed rest. In some settings, once contractions are stabilized, the patient may take oral medication and return home. In such cases, the patient should be given careful instructions about postural hypotension and the possibility of returning intensity of contractions. In other cases, the patient is hospitalized until treatment is completed and contractions cease.

ETHANOL Ethyl alcohol has been used effectively to delay preterm labor (70 percent success rate). The drug appears to act on the hypothalamus to inhibit oxytocin release, but ethanol does not seem to hinder injected oxytocin. Labor is best delayed if treatment is begun in the latent phase.

Blood levels of 0.09 to 0.16 per 100 mL are necessary to inhibit contractions. This rather high level will cause symptoms of mild to moderate intoxication in the patient, and nursing care must be focused on protecting the patient from injury as well as monitoring contraction responses. Slurred speech, headache, sedation, flushed face, elevated pulse, lack of control, mood swings, and vomiting are special problems in the initial period. Some physicians order an antiemetic to reduce symptoms of nausea. There are many interactions with other drugs, and tables should be consulted, especially if the patient has been receiving anticoagulants, diuretics, or insulin (severe hypoglycemia).

Transfer across the placenta causes fetal levels to equal maternal levels within a few minutes. If treatment is ineffectual, the infant will be born with these high levels. Since the young infant has a much slower rate of metabolism as a result of immaturity of the liver, the infant will show dose-dependent effects in the transitional period. The symptoms will include CNS depression, hypotonia, hiccups, hypothermia, hypoglycemia, and changes in acid-base balance.

Dosage Using a 9.5 percent ethyl alcohol solution, 15 mL/kg per hour for 2 h is given intravenously by infusion pump. The dose is then reduced to 1.5 mL/kg for the next 6 h. (Some continue it for 10 h.) The infusion is stopped if labor progresses more than 4 cm or if membranes rupture.

Nursing care Close observation is of primary importance, with safety as a focus. Expect nausea and vomiting, diuresis, and perhaps incontinence. Have emesis basin and bedpan available. The patient should be given nothing by mouth (NPO), and mouth care should be performed as necessary. The patient should remain in bed, with side rails up if drowsy. Try to maintain her in a lateral tilt position. If the patient becomes restless, continous monitoring will be difficult.

The aim is to reduce contraction rates to below three per 10-min interval and reduce their intensity until they finally cease. Close observation is continued when the patient is transferred back to the antepartum unit, since labor may begin to intensify as alcohol is excreted. The recovery period may take up to 12 h and may include signs and symptoms of a "hangover." Administer comfort measures as necessary.

MAGNESIUM SULFATE Infusions of magnesium sulfate have been used to halt premature labor. Contractions have been stopped in 70 to 80 percent of the cases where an initial dose of 4 g was injected slowly, followed by 2 g/h.[3] It is important to note that the same precautions must be observed regarding magnesium sulfate as are followed in the treatment of preeclampsia (see Chap. 23).

premature rupture of membranes

One-third of all premature labors appear to be related to premature rupture of membranes (PRM). The cause of early rupture is often unknown, but some of the factors leading to this event are infection of the cervix or vagina, cervical incompetency, multiple pregnancy, hydramnios, and malpresentation.

Occasionally, a traumatic amniocentesis with multiple attempts to tap fluid may succeed in rupturing membranes. The risk of infection is mainly for the fetus, as the mother can usually be effectively treated with antibiotics. Normal respiratory movements in utero serve to pull amniotic fluid into the trachea, but if fetal hypoxia occurs, deep grasping respiratory movements are triggered which move fluid deep into the alveoli. The infant is then born with the likelihood of amnionitis pneumonia or perinatal aspiration syndrome (PAS). Swallowing movements also occur in utero, and infected fluid can be taken into the gastrointestinal tract, causing gastroenteritis after birth.

gestational age and PRM The latent period, from rupture until labor begins, is usually prolonged when the infant is preterm; labor begins within 24 h in only about 50 percent of these cases.[4] The longer the latent period, the higher is the potential risk of ascending infection, since the barrier (cervical mucus and fetal membranes) has been breached.

Although infection in the fetus secondary to amnionitis is a major cause of death in term infants, preterm infants most often die from respiratory distress syndrome. For preterm infants, a side benefit of early membrane rupture has been noted. If membranes are ruptured for 16 h or more prior to birth, such a stressor acts to speed lung maturation and surfactant production (see Chap. 29) and thus reduces the mortality from respiratory distress. Thus the outcome depends primarily on gestational age at time of rupture. Berkowitz has outlined a treatment regimen based on current findings.[5]

Under 33 weeks: No intervention to hasten labor. The mother is followed closely for signs of infection while being maintained on bed rest. If infection occurs, or if the fetus reaches 33 weeks' gestation, intervention begins.
33 to 36 weeks: A period of 16 h is allowed to elapse to obtain the potential benefit of increased lung maturity.
37+ weeks: Labor is induced if not active by 12 h, since infection rate is serious cause of mortality.

treatment After a speculum exam of the vagina and cervix is done, the pH of vaginal fluid should be determined with nitrazine paper. Normal vaginal pH is 4.5 to 5.5, and amniotic fluid is 7.0 to 7.5. Thus the presence of fluid will turn the litmus paper toward alkaline. False-positive results may occur if cervical mucus, blood, urine, or antiseptic solution are inadvertently tested. In addition, amniotic fluid shows a ferning pattern if allowed to dry on a glass slide.

Signs of infection are a cloudy fluid, with white blood cells and microorganisms. Occasionally the odor will be foul. Maternal pyrexia may or may not be present.

Antibiotics are usually withheld if delivery is imminent so that cultures of the infant can be obtained. If labor is slow, however, intravenous antibiotics will be started after blood, amniotic fluid, and cervical cultures have been obtained.

MULTIPLE PREGNANCY

A multiple pregnancy carries a higher risk of perinatal morbidity and mortality, because the incidence of preterm delivery of low-birth-weight infants is much higher than that with single gestations. Infants may be "small for date" or preterm or both. Medical care is aimed at maintaining the pregnancy as long as possible to give the infants the best chance of survival.

types of multiple pregnancy

monovular twins Monovular twins (monozygous) are the result of a single fertilized ovum (zygote) which has divided exactly in two before implantation. This process of "twoing," or twinning, may occur from 2 to 7 days after fertilization. The time of division affects whether the two fetuses have separate amnions and chorions, but there will always be a single placenta. Each of the blastocysts develops into an individual with similar intelligence, physical characteristics, and sex. Monovular, or identical, twins are intensely interesting to study from the psychosocial, biologic aspects, as these two individuals have the same genetic constitution.

diovular twins Diovular, or fraternal, twins stem from two ova, released at the same time, that have been fertilized. They may have placentas fused together or ones that develop absolutely separately (Fig. 26-1). Even if the placentas fuse, each has an individual chorion and amnion. Fraternal twins (dizygous) may look so much alike that they can be thought identical, or they may be as different in size, coloring, personality, and ability as brothers and sisters in a family can be. Twinning chances increase with increasing parity, but so far no hereditary causes have been

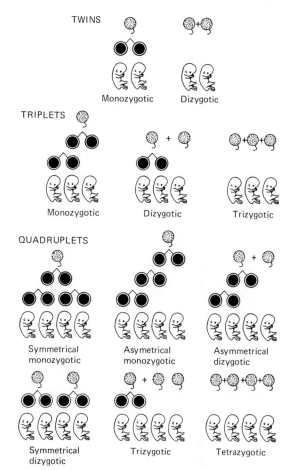

fig. 26-2 Diagrammatic illustration of the possible embryological origin of multiple pregnancy. (*From E. S. E. Hafez, "Physiology of Multiple Pregnancy," Journal of Reproductive Medicine,* **12:**88, 1974, with permission.)

found to predispose toward monovular twinning. Fraternal twinning appears to be a hereditary tendency for the woman to mature more than one ovum during the ovulatory period (Fig. 26-2).

triplets and quadruplets Triplets and quadruplets may be either diovular or monovular, but single-ovum pregnancies are least frequent. There may be mixed groups, with a set of monovular infants and one or two diovular infants.

quintuplets and sextuplets   It is very rare for single-ova pregnancies to produce so many infants. In most cases, either two or three distinct placentas or masses of two or three have fused together. These pregnancies are most often linked to drugs that stimulate the ovary, resulting in hyperovulation (Fig. 26-3).

Siamese twins   One of the odd accidents which can occur only with identical twinning is the failure, in some cases, to separate completely during early development. The infants are born as *conjoined* or "Siamese" twins. Nursing care of these infants is interestingly outlined by Dickson.[6]

test for twin type

Blood factors must be identical in monovular twins, as must be the chemical substances such as haptoglobins and gamma globulins.

Footprints and fingerprints will be nearly the same. "Ear prints" can assist in identifying identical twins, since ear formations are distinctive from birth onwards. Often an identical twin appears to be a mirror image of the other, for instance with the whorl of hair on the crown of the head on the opposite side. Skin grafts from one identical twin will always be accepted by the other twin. The placental structure is studied as well for relationships of the chorion and amnion, searching for one or two chorionic membranes, (Monochorionic must equal a monovular twinning). In the United States, approximately 28 percent of the twins are monozygous and 72 percent are dizygous.[7]

multiple pregnancy caused by drugs

In recent years, treatment for infertility has led to an increased incidence of multiple gestation. Because of this, the statistics for naturally occurring multiple pregnancies are somewhat changed. Prior to this change, multiple births

fig. 26-3   Ultrasound scan of quintuplets showing only three heads. (*Courtesy of B. Reaney and B. Kaye, "Delivering the Chicago Quints," Contemporary OB/GYN, March 1973.*)

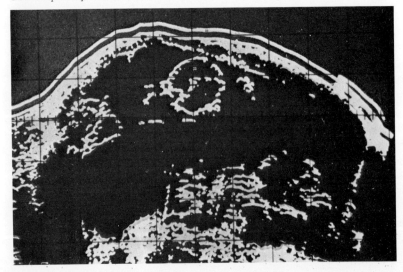

occurred most frequently in the black population and least often in the Oriental. Identical twinning occurs at much the same rate in every racial group.

Two major drug therapies are in use for lowered fertility. Clomiphene citrate and menotropins plus human chorionic gonadotropin (HCG) are very specifically used to stimulate ovulation in a woman who is subfertile.

clomiphene citrate (Clomid) In women who have adequate estrogen output but ovulate rarely, Clomid appears to stimulate increased output of pituitary gonadotropins, which in turn affects the growth of the graafian follicle. Ovulation occurs in about 80 percent and pregnancy in about 60 percent of those treated.[8] The multiple pregnancy rate is about 8 percent.

The drug is very potent and can cause abnormal ovarian enlargement. Side effects are related to enlargement of the ovary. Vasomotor symptoms, "hot flashes," resembling menopausal symptoms, and blurred vision disappear soon after the drug is discontinued.

Dosage is usually 50 mg po for 5 days beginning on the fifth day of the cycle. If treatment is unsuccessful with properly timed coitus, repeated cycles of treatment are given for 6 to 8 months, and the dose is raised to 100 mg and then to 150 mg. A single injection of HCG (5000 to 10,000 IU) 5 to 7 days after the last dose of each cycle (day 16 or 17), may be used to stimulate a luteinizing hormone (LH) surge and thus ovulation.

If the drug is inadvertently taken during a very early pregnancy, malformation is possible. Therefore careful basal temperature readings are essential every day after beginning the first 5-day course. The woman is instructed in the method and is asked to report any changes suggestive of pregnancy.

menotropins Human menopausal gonadotropin and human chorionic gonadotropin are administered intramuscularly in sequence to obtain ovulation in patients with low fertility. Thirty percent of those taking this drug conceive more than one fetus.[9]

Pergonal is a combination of FSH (follicle-stimulating hormone) and LH obtained from the urine of postmenopausal women. When administered intramuscularly for 9 to 12 days, it produces ovarian follicle growth only. To cause *ovulation*, HCG must be given intramuscularly 24 h after the last HMG dose. Clomid may be added to this combination in difficult cases. Administration of this therapy requires daily visits to the physician and, after day 14, follow-up every other day until success or failure is evident.

Side effects include ovarian enlargement, causing abdominal distension and pain in some cases. Urinary estrogen levels are used to monitor effective levels and warn of hyperstimulation.

diagnosis of multiple pregnancy

Twins often came as a surprise when confirmation depended only on palpation and auscultation of fetal heartbeat. Even now, diagnosis is difficult before 20 or 24 weeks, when the signs become more evident that there is more than one fetus developing. The most accurate method of diagnosis is ultrasound. The gestational sacs can be visualized between 5 and 10 weeks after fertilization.[10] Occasionally, when more than two babies are present, diagnosis may be complicated by overlapping outlines and at birth time, there is one more baby than predicted (Fig. 26-3)!

prematurity and low birth weight

The great majority of multiple pregnancies follow a normal course but delivery comes early. The length of gestation from the onset of the last menses to birth is about 22 days

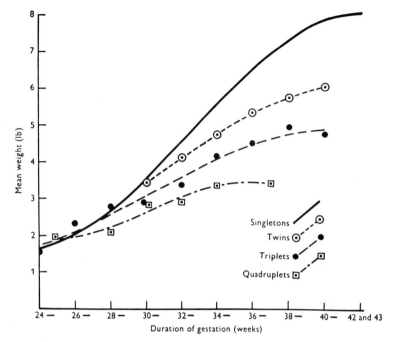

fig. 26-4 Duration of gestation and mean weight for single infants, twins, triplets, and quadruplets. (*From Frederick C. Battaglia et al., "Birth Weight, Birth-Weight-Low Gestational Age Infants," Pediatrics,* **37:**418, 1966.)

less than in a single birth, averaging birth at 37 weeks. Even if there are identical twins, they may differ considerably in weight. Especially in fraternal girl-boy pairs, girls often weigh less than the boy partner at birth. Sometimes one infant has dominated because of better placement of the placenta nourishing it. The small infant is called the discordant twin and may have severe intrauterine growth retardation and postnatal problems (Figs. 26-4 and 26-5).

prenatal course

Pregnancy proceeds normally during the first trimester when the embryos are small. The only problem noted for some is increased nausea and vomiting, which may reflect in-

creased levels of HCG produced by the larger placenta. As the growth rate increases, however, the major physiologic problems will be caused by *pressure* of the overlarge uterus on the surrounding organs, *anemia,* and *fatigue.* There may be an increased incidence of *polyhydramnios* and *preeclampsia* for some women. There are increased risks of an early complex delivery. Prenatal care for the mother includes precautions against these problems, and therapy is directed toward maintaining the pregnancy as long as possible.

pressure effects The uterus causes pressure on the ureters, bladder, intestines, vena cava, and renal vasculature, and later, on the diaphragm. Increased pressure may lead to varicose veins of the rectal, saphenous, or

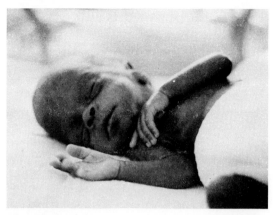

fig. 26-5 Premature, low-birth-weight infant.

vulvar veins. Constipation and digestive problems may be accentuated during the second and third trimesters. Pressure on the ureters may favor urinary stasis and chronic infection. Pressure in each case is relieved by a side-lying position whenever the mother rests. Toward the end of the third trimester, she may have to use a semi-Fowler's position for sleep. During the day she may have to wear a well-fitted maternity corset to provide some support for the abdomen.

anemia Maternal anemia can be prevented by a diet rich in iron and the addition of supplemental iron and folic acid, since the iron requirement is increased for a multiple pregnancy. Complicating intake is the fact that the mother usually can tolerate small meals only, because of increased pressure on the stomach.

rest Rest for the mother carrying a multiple gestation is the most important single factor in preventing preterm delivery. In a Colorado series, perinatal mortality was 6 percent in a bed-rest group compared with 23 percent in a non-bed-rest group.[11] The average weight of each baby in the bed-rest group was 250 g more, and the pregnancies averaged about six more days in duration.

Along with bed rest and limited activity, many physicians are now using medication (Vasodilan) in hopes of preventing premature labor. Once the cervix begins to efface, the mother is admitted to the hospital in order to give the infants a few more days to mature.

major problems in multiple pregnancy

hydramnios Polyhydramnios, the production of an abnormally large amount of amniotic fluid, can precipitate premature labor and may for a period cause the appearance of multiple gestation. Hydramnios is more common in multiple pregnancies and where there are renal or gastrointestinal anomalies in the infant.

Normally, the amnion circulates and reabsorbs about 350 mL of amniotic fluid per hour in later pregnancy. If even a 1- or 2-mL imbalance occurs, the buildup of pressure can be quite dramatic. The uterus enlarges more rapidly than normal in the second half of pregnancy, and the pressure symptoms experienced by the mother may be quite severe. An amniocentesis may be one way of relieving pressure, but there is a definite risk connected to repeated tapping of the amniotic sac. As a further complication, when membranes rupture prior to or during labor, there is a much greater risk of a prolapsed cord.

preeclampsia The chances of preeclampsia are more common in multiple gestations, but the reasons for this increased incidence are unknown. The regimen of bed rest should help to diminish the incidence of hypertension, edema, and albuminuria.

hemorrhage Because of the enlarged placental site, the internal os may be completely or partially covered. The warnings signs of bleeding prior to labor should be noted carefully. During delivery, a lower uterine or a cervical tear is not uncommon. After delivery the mother may have postpartum hemorrhage because of uterine atony and the large placental site.

labor   With therapy, the mother may approach nearer to term than has been customary in the past. She is observed carefully, and the condition of the cervix checked each week. She is instructed to notify the physician when the contractions begin regularly. Usually, considerable dilatation and effacement of the cervix have already taken place during prelabor, so that it appears that the active phase of labor is shortened.

Problems during labor are those of uterine overdistension, with resultant ineffective contractions. Abnormal presentations of one fetus may cause special hazards to the second twin. The first infant may have a vertex presentation, but the second twin often is in a transverse or breech position, with the attendant problems of difficult delivery and possible prolapse of the cord.

Preparation for a multiple delivery requires a multidisciplinary approach. Neonatologists, anesthesiologist, obstetrician, and nurses must coordinate activities. Resuscitation equipment for several infants must be available, and the premature nursery must be ready to receive the infants. Each cord is tagged at the maternal side, and each infant is identified in order of birth. After delivery, the placenta is examined to aid in the diagnosis of zygosity.

problems in care of the infants

Mothers who expect the arrival of more than one infant have time to prepare psychologically and financially to receive them. How much of a problem their arrival causes depends on many factors. Fortunately the birth of more than one infant often rallies the whole family to help. Usually, such an event is expensive, with extended hospitalization for the preterm infants. Every possible referral to supportive agencies may be needed.

Since multiple births occur more often in women who have had children, they already may have some skill in child care. Most parents find that in the first year it makes no difference whether the infants are fraternal or identical. What is important is their birth weight, as well as their gestational age at birth. One infant may be behind the other and, if responses differ, the parents may suffer undue anxiety. Nurses can assist in helping the parent recognize the uniqueness of each infant.

Twins may be so engrossed with each other that they may delay speech until later than a single child. Their growth pattern depends upon their gestational age at birth. The mother should be familiarized with the delay in maturation caused by preterm birth and be alert for the differences in growth which will emerge fairly soon.

INDUCTION

Under normal circumstances, most women need no stimulus to begin labor. The popularity of "babies by appointment," elective induction, has waned since the advent of fetal monitoring, and most obstetricians now use induction of labor only for those situations in which a problem indicates that the normal body processes need to be augmented. *Induction,* or the use of agents to bring on the onset of labor, and *stimulation,* the use of agents to increase the speed and intensity of labor, should require a situation that demands artificial intervention in the body timing. Recently, the use of oxytocin for elective induction has been discouraged by the FDA. The following are the *major indications for induction:*

Placental insufficiency with chronic fetal distress
Premature rupture of fetal membranes
Prolonged pregnancy (+41 weeks)
Preeclampsia
Rh sensitization
Diabetic mother
Hypertensive mother
Fetal death

Since oxytocin was first accepted in 1948, several agents have been studied for their effective physiologic action on the uterine muscle: sparteine sulfate, buccal and subcutaneous oxytocin, and now, intravenous oxytocin and prostaglandins. The first three have been largely discarded; prostaglandins are the subject of intensive studies and promise to be quite satisfactory in optimum doses.

Nonpharmacologic methods have been used: exercise, enemas, castor oil, and more recently, amniotomy (rupture of the membranes) and "stripping of the membranes" (digital separation of the membranes from the lower uterine wall). Of these methods, walking stimulates labor once it has begun, an enema in early labor clears the lower intestinal tract and may slightly stimulate contractions, and castor oil makes the woman miserable. Rupturing the membranes before labor begins places the mother at risk of acquiring infection (see above), as does stripping the membranes.

Although there is no completely safe way to change the speed of labor or initiate it, yet with careful observation, regulated dosage, and fetal monitoring, induction and stimulation with oxytocin and perhaps with prostaglandins can be used effectively where indicated.

Under ordinary circumstances, the blocks to uterine contractility are extremely effective.

Therefore the readiness of the body for labor has always been a key factor in the success of induction. The Bishop score is one of several scores which have been constructed to evaluate readiness.[12] A value is assigned each criterion—0, 1, 2, or 3 points (Table 26-1). The higher the number, the better is the condition for labor. A score of 9 or more indicates a ready patient who will have an average induced labor of 4 h.[13]

The processes during prelabor which normally take several weeks prior to the beginning of regular contractions and dilation must be effected within a few hours during induction. These changes are movement of the head into the pelvic inlet to engagement station, stretching of the lower uterine segment and upper vaginal wall, and softening (ripening) of the cervix. If induction is begun before the cervix is ready, there will be a time lag before true labor begins. An oxytocin infusion may be administered for 8 to 12 h and then discontinued so that the patient can sleep. The next morning marked changes may be seen in the progressive cervical effacement. Contractions during this period are painless and yet have an effect and can be monitored by the external sensor.

table 26-1 Bishop score

	0 ⟶ 3 points	
Dilation of the cervix	Closed ⟶	5 cm dilated
Effacement of the cervix	Zero ⟶	80 percent effaced
Station of the presenting part	−3 ⟶	+1, +2
Consistency of the cervix	Firm ⟶	soft
Position of the cervix	Posterior, anterior	

Note: A score of 0 to 5 is considered unfavorable for induction.

If induction is used, the nurse must understand that the patient goes through the same "work of labor" only over a shorter span of time. Thus, the total pressure needed (measured in Montevideo units) (see Fig. 10-2) to dilate the cervix completely and to cause the descent and expulsion of the fetus is the same as for spontaneous labor, but the contractions may be more intense, more frequent, and longer in duration.

As the body responds to oxytocin, the contractions should be physiologic, i.e., normally effective. However, the individual sensitivity to oxytocin changes from phase to phase of labor and from woman to woman, so that the dosage must be *titrated,* adjusted by her response to the infusion. It is important to avoid *hypertonus,* or excessively strong, long contractions with inadequate periods of relaxation because the compromised blood supply to the fetus may lead to tragedy (hypoxic baby, ruptured uterus).

method of oxytocin administration

The pharmacologic effect of oxytocin is explored in Chap. 20. Because of its short half-life, it is safest to administer the drug by the intravenous route. One ampul (10 units) diluted in 1000 mL Ringer's lactate solution or dextrose and water yields 10 milliunits/mL of solution. Although different concentrations are ordered, the drug is always administered in terms of *milliunits per minute.* The only way accurately to regulate flow is to use an infusion pump, with the solution being added by a "piggyback" line to an infusion containing a solution of 5 percent dextrose in water. In this way, should hypertonus occur, the intravenous flow can be stopped immediately.

precautions

Nurses often react negatively to oxytocin use because they have seen abuses and know the real dangers of fetal distress if labor is not carefully monitored. However, knowledge of the way in which oxytocin changes in normal labor pattern will help to objectify nursing care. There are some important factors to remember.

1. Very few patients can tolerate oxytocin-augmented contractions and remain "in control" in the true Lamaze sense. Therefore, patients usually will need some analgesia.
2. Oxytocin sensitivity varies markedly from person to person, and sensitivity varies from phase to phase of labor. The patient may indicate her progress in labor by a change in her response to oxytocin.
3. The setup, observation, and maintenance of a problem-free infusion fall within nursing measures, but the obstetrician is responsible for beginnning the intravenous infusion and for titration of the dosage (which includes remaining with the patient for a sufficient period after each change in rate or dosage to ensure a problem-free administration). The physician must be within call for unexpected problems.
4. An infusion pump is the preferred means of controlling the rate of flow; second best is a microdropper setup. Both are used as a piggyback addition to a plain infusion.
5. Labor may be substantially shortened and may move toward delivery more rapidly than expected. Therefore close observation is mandatory.
6. Because the labor is speeded up, there will be more pressure on the head (presenting part), less recovery time between contractions, and greater possibility of fetal distress. Therefore, fetal heart tones must be regularly observed. (Hon recommends a minimum of every 10 min in normal labor.) External or internal monitoring of each patient is highly recommended and may become mandatory in the future (see Chap. 27).

table 26-2 Diagnostic criteria for the six major dysfunctional labor patterns (DLPs)*

	nullipara	multipara
Prolonged latent phase	$\geq$ 21 h	$\geq$ 14 h
Protracted active phase dilation	< 1.2 cm/h	< 1.5 cm/h
Secondary arrest of dilation	No change for $\geq$ 2 h	No change for $\geq$ 2 h
Prolonged deceleration phase	$\geq$ 3 h	$\geq$ 1 h
Protracted descent	< 1 cm/h	< 2 cm/h
Arrest of descent	No change for $\geq$ 1 h	No change for $\geq$ 0.5 h

Source: From R. J. Sokol et al., "Normal and Abnormal Labor Progress," *Journal of Reproductive Medicine,* **18** (1): 48, January 1977.
*Based on Friedman.

7 The nurse may shut off the infusion at the first indication of a hypertonic, or *tetanic,* contraction. The nurse must never flush the IV tubing or manipulate a poorly running IV infusion in such a way as to inject larger doses of oxytocin into the vein.

DYSTOCIA

Difficulty with any aspect of labor is termed *dystocia.* A major cause of dystocia is cephalopelvic disproportion (CPD) in which, depending on pelvic bone structure (see Fig. 10-8), the fetal head may not fit well into the inlet, through the midcanal, or through the outlet. When the fetal head is too large, or pelvic measurements are contracted, vaginal delivery becomes difficult, if not impossible.

Labor contractions also may be a cause of dystocia if they are ineffectual or erratic and thus unable to achieve the work of labor. Six dysfunctional patterns are shown in Table 26-2. Each phase of labor, as identified by Friedman, has a usual rate of progress. When delay occurs, some underlying reason is usually present. Figure 26-6 is a graphic illustration of the patterns that indicate abnormal progress.

delayed latent phase

A prolonged latent phase, according to Friedman, is that which lasts for more than 21 h in a nullipara or 14 h in a multipara. Counseling of the patient regarding the time of entry into the hospital may prevent false labor being mistaken for a prolonged latent phase. However, if the latent phase is truly prolonged, stimulation of labor will be started after pelvimetry is obtained.

fig. 26-6 Prolongation of phases of labor. (*a*) Prolongation of latent phase; (*b*) prolongation of active phase; (*c*) secondary arrest of dilation. (*From E. W. Page, C. A. Villee, Human Reproduction: The Core Content of Obstetrics and Gynecology and Perinatal Medicine, Saunders, Philadelphia, 1972.*)

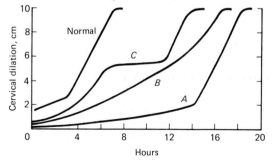

delayed active phase

The active phase (4 to 8 cm) should last no longer than 2 to 4 h because the cervix should be dilating at a rate of more than 1.2 cm/h in the nullipara and 1.5 cm/h in the multipara. Slower rates may be caused by lack of dilation resulting from CPD, malposition, or ineffectual contractions. Pelvimetry will be obtained to assess feto-pelvic relationships. If disproportion is present, a cesarean delivery is planned without delay. In other cases, oxytocin stimulation may be used.

delayed descent

The normal rate of descent in the pelvic phase should be 1 cm/h in the nullipara and 2 cm/h in the multipara. A prolonged deceleration or pelvic phase (9 cm through delivery) or slower than normal descent are causes for concern. Again, the size of the fetal presenting part in relationship to the canal may inhibit progress. Bony structure may have borderline measurements, or finally, contractions may be ineffective.

abnormal presentations of the head

brow presentation Unless a brow presentation changes, in the process of descent, to a vertex or face presentation, the head at its largest diameter will be coming through the birth canal. A persistent brow presentation usually cannot be delivered except by cesarean section (Fig. 26-7a).

face presentation To present the face first, the fetal head must be extremely hyperextended. There is a smaller diameter presenting than with the brow, but the trauma to the tissues and the extreme molding of the head are injurious to the fetus. Unless the chin will rotate so that it can be delivered under the symphysis pubis, the face presentation is very difficult to deliver vaginally. Face presentations are hard to diagnose, as the face becomes very edematous and landmarks are indistinct. Although the face will resume normal appearance within a week or two, the mother's first sense of shock after seeing the bruising and swelling may be very difficult to overcome (Fig. 26-7b).

occiput posterior position When the vertex presentation changes to an occiput posterior position during internal rotation, the

fig. 26-7 (a) Brow presentation. (b) Types of face presentation. (*Courtesy of Ross Laboratories, Columbus, Ohio, Clinical Education Aid.*)

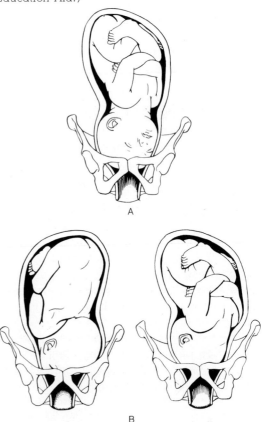

A

B

process of delivery will be prolonged. To convert to an anterior position, a 180° arc must be traversed across the sacral curve. The nurse can remind the mother how to deal with "back labor." The woman may walk around, if she is in the active phase. She may push on her hands and knees, squatting, or lying on her side if in the second stage. More than once, a woman has been required to lie supine because of a monitor, when any of these other positions would have facilitated rotation of the fetal head. It is during such a difficult laboring process that *informed* nursing intervention is most important. However, in this rotational process, a transverse arrest does sometimes occur, and the rotation does not complete the turn. There will be increased sacral pressure felt by the mother, and rarely can she cope with this complication of labor without some analgesia or regional anesthesia. If the occiput posterior persists, the delivery is more difficult. Cesarean section may then be considered a wise choice.

breech presentation

When engagement of the buttocks takes place it may occur in three ways: (1) *frank breech:* thighs flexed and knees extended so that feet are beside the head; (2) *complete breech:* the infant appears to be sitting in a yoga position, cross-legged; and (3) *incomplete, footling breech:* where one leg is extended so that the foot is the leading part (Fig. 26-8).

Breech presentations can be delivered vaginally, but they do carry a higher risk. Often a preterm or the second or third infant of a multiple pregnancy will present in this way. Small infants do not have as much mechanical difficulty as larger infants (> 8 lb). The larger infant may have shoulder or head dystocia, as the cervix may allow the body to protrude before full dilation. The head then becomes trapped by the tight cervical rim.

A mortality of 10 to 20 percent is related to these mechanical problems as well as to prematurity. (The overall incidence of breech presentation is about 3 to 4 percent. If the infant weighs less than 2500 g, however, the incidence rises to 10 to 20 percent.) In addition, there is a higher rate of cord prolapse, premature rupture of membranes, trauma to the infant (see Chap. 29), and fetal distress. Because of these complications, currently, about 20 to 30 percent of breech presentations are delivered by cesarean section, and in

fig. 26-8 Breech presentation. (*a*) Frank breech; (*b*) complete breech; (*c*) incomplete breech (footling). (*Courtesy of Ross Laboratories, Columbus, Ohio, Clinical Education Aid.*)

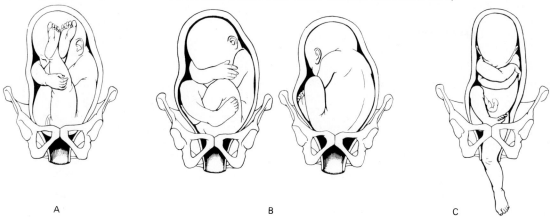

A   B   C

some institutions, up to 80 percent are delivered operatively.[14]

shoulder presentation

A transverse lie or oblique lie cannot be delivered vaginally. In some instances, external manipulation prior to labor can turn the fetus into a cephalic or breech presentation. Otherwise, a cesarean must be done (Figs. 26-9 and 26-10).

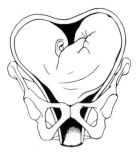

fig. 26-9 Shoulder presentation. (*Courtesy of Ross Laboratories, Columbus, Ohio, Clinical Education Aid.*)

OPERATIVE DELIVERY*

When problems occur during labor, the availability of surgical intervention can save both mother and infant from damage or even death. Judicious intervention in cases of fetal distress, for instance, has markedly reduced damage from anoxia. In the past, such anoxia had been one of the major causes of cerebral palsy and mental retardation.

Historically, before cesarean delivery was available, women who could not give birth vaginally died during childbirth. In addition, deep lacerations of the perineum were not uncommon, often going unrepaired. Women who had traumatic births experienced prolapse of the bladder (cystocele), the rectum (rectocele), or the uterus itself.

episiotomy

Today, in order to prevent these potential problems, most women giving birth to first or second infants or to very large infants are considered candidates for an episiotomy, a surgical incision enlarging the introitus. There is, however, an increasingly large group of women who refuse such surgical intervention. The controversy stems from the *routine use* of

*This section is based on the chapter by James H. Lee, Jr., in the first edition

fig. 26-10 Graphic display of cervical-dilation-time patterns based on computer-derived data from 10,293 patients studied. The variations from the curves from that occurring in association with occiput anterior fetal positions (heavy line) are apparent. Nearly uniform slowing with occiput posterior (light line) and occiput transverse (heavy broken line), and modified normal pattern with breech presentation (light broken line) are shown. (*Used by permission of Emanuel A. Friedman and Bernard H. Kroll, "Computer Analysis of Labor Progression: V. Effects of Fetal Presentation and Position," Journal of Reproductive Medicine **8**(3):121, 1972.*)

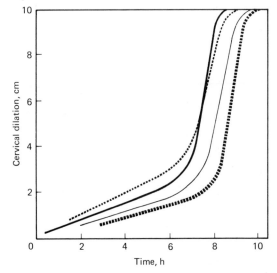

the intervention rather than from any argument with its use when there are definite reasons for enlarging the introitus. It appears that under the consumer pressure of educated women, such a procedure must be carefully reevaluated.[15]

As the infant's head crowns, perineal tissues are stretched to the maximum limit. With slow, careful guidance of the head, it is possible to deliver without a *perineotomy*, a surgical incision into the tissues between the vaginal introitus and the anus. Most western obstetricians today feel that damage to the deeper tissues can best be avoided by performing a clear surgical cut, rather than risking a jagged tear (laceration).

types A surgical cut to enlarge the opening is done when the infant's size appears to be large in relation to the introitus or when a premature infant is born, to prevent pressure on the head. Two types of incisions are made. A median episiotomy (perineotomy) is easier to cut and repair but carries the risk of extension into the rectal wall and anus if the fetal head is larger than expected. For a large infant, a mediolateral episiotomy (*episio*-Labium) is done. This approach is safe, but cuts through more tissue and therefore is more painful during the healing process. The two types are contrasted in Table 26-3. Local anesthetic is necessary for an episiotomy unless a median is done when the head is tightly crowning. It is safer to make the incision before that point, however, to avoid being rushed. Repair can be delayed until the placenta is delivered, unless there is extra bleeding. The wound is closed from the inner layers toward the outer. Usually, no sutures show on the skin surface as stitches are made with fine (00 or 000) absorbable catgut suture.

care of the wound Observation of episiotomy suture line should be included in assessment during the first 24 h after birth. Any swelling, redness, purulent exudate, or gaping of the wound edges should be reported. The patient should be instructed to report any swelling or pain after the initial recovery period. Comfort measures include placing an "ice glove" on the perineum. (Fill a nonsterile examining glove with chipped ice, secure by a rubber band, and wrap in a disposable bed pad with the clean paper side against the wound.) It is understood that the wound cannot be kept sterile, but good perineal hygiene will usually allow healing to progress without infection. Other comfort measures are detailed in Chap. 11.

lacerations

Even with an episiotomy, it is possible for tissues of the birth canal to tear because of overdistension (see Table 26-4). Signs of hidden lacerations are excessive vaginal bleeding and formation of hematomas, especially

table 26-3 Tissues incised for episiotomy

median episiotomy (perineotomy)	mediolateral episiotomy
Posterior fourchette	Posterior fourchette
Median raphe of perineal body	Bulbocavernosus muscle
External anal sphincter fibers	Urogenital diaphragm
	Transverse perineal muscles
	Fasciae covering levator ani muscle

table 26-4   Types of lacerations

Perineal lacerations	
First degree	Skin, mucous membrane of posterior fourchette and proximal vagina
Second degree	Muscles and facia up to anal sphincter, plus above tissues
Third degree	Laceration of above tissues continuing through anal sphincter
Fourth degree	In addition to above tissues, anterior rectal wall is torn
Sulcus tear	Folds of the vagina are torn, often over the ischial spines
Periurethral tear	Tissues around the urethra are torn, sometimes the urethra itself
Cervical tear	Any degree, from small shallow tears to deep lacerations through entire cervix into lower uterine segment
Uterine tear	Usually in lower uterine segment, which is thinner during later pregnancy; especially possible if multifetal gestation, or site of placenta previa, or precipitate labor

over the ischial spines or into the lower vaginal wall or labia. Tears around the clitoris or urethra will form hematomas and cause extensive edema, which will inhibit voiding. The patient will need a Foley catheter for 12 to 24 h and special assistance with analgesia prior to spontaneous voiding.

forceps operation

In some instances, the force of uterine contractions and maternal expulsive efforts are inadequate to cause rotation and descent of the head through the pelvic canal. The application of specially shaped metal forceps can assist in descent and rotation, acting as a "shoehorn" to facilitate movement through a "tight fit."

The use of such instruments has a long history. In early times, forceps were used only to extract a dead fetus. In the sixteenth century,

Peter Chamberlen the Elder invented the first set used for live births. Tragically, these instruments were kept a professional secret for more than 100 years, while innumerable women died because of dystocia. Finally, Edmund Chapman introduced and publicized forceps in the middle of the eighteenth century, and subsequently many types have become available. Figure 26-11 illustrates four major types currently in use.

A delivery requiring forceps is now called a *forceps operation*. It is considered an operative procedure because the application and use of such instruments, *without skill,* can damage the mother or the infant. Conversely, it is important to note that skillfully applied forceps have probably saved more lives than any other surgical instrument.

types of forceps operations   Forceps operations are classified in relation to the station and position of the fetal head. The

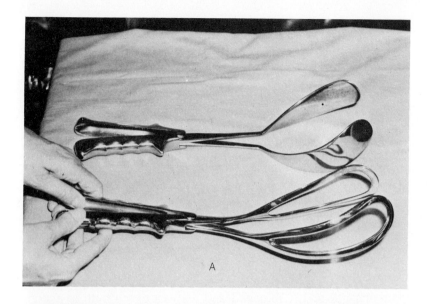

A

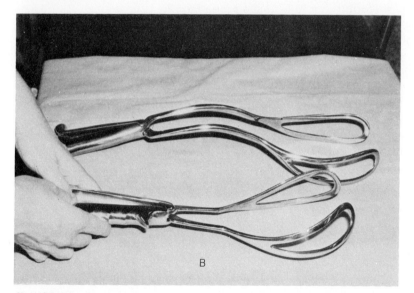

B

fig. 26-11 Forceps in common usage. (*a*) Top: Tucker-McLean forceps, with solid, smooth blades. Bottom: Elliot forceps. (*b*) Top: Piper forceps for breech deliveries; note curve of shank. Bottom: Simpson forceps.

following classifications are utilized by the American College of Obstetrics and Gynecology:[16]

1 *Low forceps operation:* Forceps are applied after the scalp has been or is visible at the introitus, without separating the labia, when the skull has reached the pelvic floor, and the sagittal suture is in the anteroposterior (*AP*) diameter of the outlet.

2 *Midforceps operation:* Forceps are applied after the head is engaged but the conditions for low (outlet) forceps have not been met, i.e., rotation has not yet occurred to the *AP* diameter or station is less than +3 (on pelvic floor).

3 *High forceps operation:* Forceps are applied before the head is engaged. Such a maneuver is almost never justified, for cesarean section would be a safer choice.

Before forceps are applied, several requirements must be met: the cervix must be completely dilated, the head must be engaged and its position known, the pelvic canal and outlet must be large enough to pass the head and shoulders, and the membranes must be ruptured. In addition, bladder and rectum must be empty. Finally, no patient should have forceps applied *without* adequate anesthesia. Indications for use are given in Table 26-5.

dangers of forceps Unskilled application may cause injury to cervix, vaginal wall, rectum, and bladder. The infant may be damaged by fracture of the skull or by pressure from a badly located forceps pressing on ear or eye. (Superficial bruises on cheeks caused by pressure are not uncommonly seen, but these heal rapidly.) Prior to the application of forceps, it is mandatory for the physician to carefully locate the sides of the infant's head and apply the forceps so that the curved, spoon-shaped area is over the cheekbones. After application is checked and position verified, pressure is applied in a downward direction to bring the head under the symphysis pubis. As the head rotates around the pubic bone and crowns, the forceps are gently removed and the rest of the birth is accomplished (see Fig. 26-12).

vacuum extraction operation

The use of a suction cup attached to the fetal head has been substituted for forceps. Vacuum from a suction pump is applied to keep the cup in place and a steady pull is applied to the cup. The scalp is pulled by vacuum into the cup and, depending on the duration and extent of pulling, an edematous ring (caput) will develop with some bruising. Some

table 26-5 Indications for use of forceps

fetal problems	maternal problems
Arrested descent	Uterine inertia in late second stage
Arrested rotation	Inability to push effectively as a
Abnormal presentation	result of:
Face or brow	Exhaustion
Breech (forceps for head)	Regional or general anesthesia
Fetal distress in late second	Mild CPD
stage	Poor position for pushing
Preterm infant (to protect	Chronic disease requiring the least
fragile head)	possible stress during delivery:
	e.g., cardiac, chest disease, hypertension

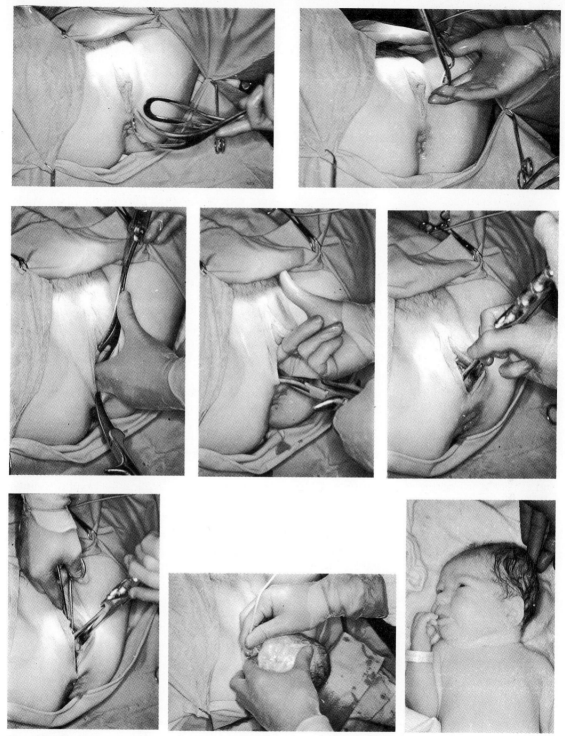

fig. 26-12 Delivery using outlet forceps in occiput anterior position. (*From A. L. Haskins, "Use of Outlet Forceps in Occiput Anterior Position," Modern Medicine, copyright © The New York Times Media Company, Inc., Sept. 4, 1972.*)

physicians think that the vacuum cup is a safer method of delivery in spite of this caput, since no pressure is applied to the fetal skull. Others, dismayed at the bruising and feeling that parents will be alarmed, have avoided use of such an instrument. Vacuum extraction operations are used frequently in Europe and are classified in the same manner as forceps operations.

cesarean delivery

The goal for operative delivery is the same as that for an unassisted vaginal delivery: the safe birth of a healthy infant. Birth by *cesarean section* has become a safer procedure in the last decade because of improved use of analgesia and anesthesia, as well as a clearer recognition of when to intervene surgically. As a result, operative delivery is done much more frequently. Statistics vary in different settings; some institutions caring for high-risk women now have a rate over 50 percent, whereas the average rate across the country is 10 to 20 percent. The rate is rising for at least two reasons: (1) physicians are aware of the adverse results of severe fetal distress, and (2) they are concerned with preventing lawsuits over possible birth injury resulting from a difficult birth.[17] It has been pointed out by Donovan that the movement to home births on the part of well-educated couples stems in part from the fear of unwarranted surgical intervention. Obstetrical intervention is accepted uncritically by many in the nursing and medical profession, because of known "rescues" of compromised infants. However, it is also true that intervention is often done on fairly slim grounds, such as a slight delay in one phase of labor.

The nurse assisting the laboring woman can utilize many skills in working through the labor phases: providing support, coaching, positioning for best effect, and most of all, demonstrating a confidence in the woman's ability to come through the experience positively. If the trend toward operative delivery is to be slowed or reversed, all such positive support will be needed. In the meantime, when a woman has a cesarean delivery, the nurse must work with her to minimize the problems. A rate of one cesarean out of four or five deliveries indicates that the cesarean birth mother (and father) is present in large numbers on the postdelivery unit and in the delivery area.

indications The abdominal route for delivery is chosen when additional hypoxic stress must be prevented, when pelvic dimensions are inadequate, or when some pathologic condition is causing excessive maternal or fetal distress. Table 26-6 lists indications for cesarean delivery.

Today, the most common reason for surgery is a repeat cesarean section, for, on rare occasions, the force of labor contractions may rupture the uterine scar. Most obstetricians follow the practice of repeating surgery once a first cesarean has been done. A few physicians will allow a trial of labor if the reason for the initial section was temporary, not structural, i.e., caused by an unforeseen problem, such as cord prolapse or an adverse response to oxytocin. In addition, the type of initial incision is considered before a trial of labor. An incision into the body of the uterus, since it cuts across major contracting muscles, is thought to be more likely to break open under the stress of labor. A transverse incision into the lower uterine segment is considered much safer, since this portion is fairly passive during labor.

types of incisions The type of uterine incision is determined by the fetal presentation and by the exigencies of surgery (i.e., emergencies, where every minute counts). It is important to note that the abdominal incision does not indicate the type of uterine incision. One of the first questions asked after an unexpected cesarean is "Do I always have to have a cesarean birth, now?" Only by checking on the type of *uterine incision* can a correct response be made.

ABDOMINAL INCISION   To approach the uterus, a vertical-subumbilical or midline incision is done most frequently. If a transverse incision is made, it may be either a *Pfannenstiel* or *Cherney* type. In the former, skin and rectus fascia are opened transversely but the peritoneum is opened vertically. The Cherney incision is a transverse one for skin, muscle, and peritoneum.

UTERINE INCISION   The choice is made to cut into either the upper or lower segment. Today, a *classical* incision, where the upper segment is incised vertically, is only done when an emergency exists and rapid access to the fetus is necessary or when placenta previa covers the lower segment. Lower segment incisions may be made vertically, or transversely in a curved line. The advantages include less bleeding and less tissue repair; in addition, after the bladder has been reaffixed over the suture line, the wound is outside the peritoneal cavity.

Some physicians utilize an *extraperitoneal* section, in which the lower segment is approached without entering the peritoneal cavity. When there is actual or potential uterine infection, such an approach may prevent spread into the cavity.

Finally, after the baby is delivered, some women will have a *cesarean hysterectomy*. In emergencies, removal of the uterus itself is done when there is uncontrollable bleeding or severe rupture. This operation is planned if disease is present, such as cancer or multiple myomas (fibroid tumors).

preparation   Most childbirth preparation classes have usually given some orientation

table 26-6   Indications for cesarean delivery

Delay in labor
1. In preparatory period
   No response to pitocin, postmaturity
2. In active phase
   Arrest of dilatation, prolonged active phase, or uterine inertia
3. In descent phase
   Cephalopelvic disproportion, cervical dystocia, uterine inertia

Abnormal presentations
1. Brow, mentum, poor flexion of head, occiput posterior position in a primipara
2. Transverse
3. Breech

Fetal distress
1. Chronic—poor environment demonstrated by falling estriols or presence of erythroblastosis
2. Acute—during labor—demonstrated by changes on monitor of uteroplacental insufficiency (UPI), cord compression (CC), and loss of fetal heart tone, or pH changes

Maternal illness
1. Placental dysfunction, placenta previa, abruptio placenta, herpes progenetalis (active)
2. Diabetes, (delivery before 37 weeks is usual)
3. Chronic hypertension, severe preeclampsia
4. Cancer of cervix or uterine fibroids
5. Repeated stillbirths for no known cause
6. Elderly primigravida with other problems
7. Massive obesity

Repeat cesarean delivery
Must repeat if incision on uterus is a classical one on the uterine body. Doctor may allow labor with careful observation if first incision is into the lower uterine segment (less danger of rupture of scar)

to a possible cesarean delivery, but in many cases, there has been an implication that a cesarean is somehow the result of failure of the couple's determination. Such an implication is patently wrong and harmful, since no couple *elects* to have an operative birth. Rather, surgery results from a combination of factors previously discussed.

Parents need to be oriented according to the two patterns of cesarean delivery. Those couples having planned surgery because of repeat sections or known factors causing dystocia should be grouped together for classes. In all other classes, the possibility of emergency surgery as an alternative method must be discussed and reasons for it explored.

When a cesarean delivery is necessary, support for the parents should be as thorough as possible. The process of labor and delivery should be discussed, as well as methods of anesthesia and preoperative preparation. In this way as each step is explained, fear of the unknown can be reduced.

Wherever possible, the father should be beside the mother. In a few settings, he can remain in the delivery room, seated facing the woman to share the moment of birth. In other settings, he must wait outside, unsure and often uninformed about the status of the mother or newborn. (Change is being sought by prepared couples as they protest exclusion of the woman's partner.)

Several groups have formed to assist the couple, notably the *Cesarean Birth Method,* "a comprehensive approach for enhancing the childbirth experience of cesarean families."[18] This group recommends specific techniques of support during the preparation and delivery periods: (1) full information as soon as a decision for surgery has been reached; (2) step-by-step explanations of preoperative procedures (see Table 26-7); (3) recognition of fears and feelings; (4) support during actual surgery (if awake) with a running commentary; (5) use of an instant-picture camera for the moment of birth and for the first few minutes, especially if the father is not present or if mother is under general anesthesia.

the recovery period Bonding is perhaps the most frequently cited problem in the recovery period. If there has not been preparation delineating the steps in recovery, on awaking from general anesthesia the mother

table 26-7 Preoperative care for cesarean delivery

planned surgery	emergency surgery
Admission prior to surgery, usually the evening before; NPO for 12 h	In labor area already; NPO
Surgical consent must be signed Be sure ID band is correctly made out	Consent signed on admission to labor; check identification carefully
Physical examination Lab tests done and recorded on chart:CBC, Hgb, Hct, type and cross-match, urinalysis	Physical exam done briefly, if at all. Reliance on prenatal chart. Lab tests done, ask for fast results. Urinalysis done on admission to labor
Abdominal-perineal prep	Abdominal prep
Enema	No enema, unless done early in labor
Baseline vital signs on chart including fetal heart rate	Already on chart, record latest vital signs, maintain fetal monitor until moved to OR.
Explanation of all steps of preparation	Involve partner in all explanations; anxiety level will be very high; keep person informed
Foley catheter inserted, usually before preoperative medication	Foley catheter inserted while other preparation is being carried out
Preoperative medication on time, only after everything else is done, charted, and patient properly identifed	No preoperative medication may be given; varies according to condition and if continuous regional anesthesia is already being utilized
Intravenous started in OR	Intravenous already in place; oxygen may also be given if fetal distress is cause

may feel overwhelmed by the presence of an IV or a Foley catheter. She certainly cannot anticipate the abdominal discomfort and may have to focus on her pain to the exclusion of the infant or father. If regional anesthesia has been used, she should see the infant wet and dripping just after delivery and hold the infant once its basic care has been completed. If the infant's condition is satisfactory, the same bonding steps should be taken as for any new parent, i.e., in the recovery room, under a radiant heater, there should be time for quiet acquaintance with mother and father and early breast-feeding, if chosen. If there is any problem, and the infant must be in the special care nursery, the father should be carefully oriented to the procedures and infant's condition. Then he and the nurse can interpret the baby's condition to the mother. With early ambulation or via a wheelchair, a visit to the nursery should take place within 12 h if the infant cannot be brought to the bedside. The old custom of not allowing mother–infant contact until the intravenous was removed (fear for safety) can be overcome easily by having the nurse stay with the mother while she meets her infant.

When emergency surgery has taken place, women need special help with their reactions. Donovan and Allen have identified five reactions that may need therapeutic intervention:[19]

1 Relief, at least initially, is a common reaction. If the labor was long and difficult, a cesarean section offers the promise of an end to this painful, stressful stage.
2 Anxiety, apprehension, and fear that something will happen to mother or baby because of anesthesia. The father is often excluded from surgery without any assistance with these feelings.
3 Guilt is the least likely reaction to be mentioned but is a common feeling, i.e., questioning any bad effect of taking medication, gaining too much weight, not doing enough exercise, etc. If couples have had positive experience in preparation or prior births, both may feel cheated out of this delivery. The mother may also feel bewildered, angry, sad, and lonely unless an effort is made to support and reassure her. The father may also feel left out, angry, sad, and lonely.
4 Varying depths of anger may be experienced but not expressed. Often a mother will later speak of feelings of anger against the baby for being too small, too big, getting "itself into trouble." Later also, discomfort may be expressed in angry feelings against the baby who "put me through all this." Guilt over such unacceptable feelings is common but unexpressed.
5 Helplessness and the question, "Why did this happen to me?" is almost universal.

Donovan and Allen suggest that the nurse establish rapport and assist the mother to express these feelings. Such therapeutic intervention can be very helpful as the mother receives reassurance that such feelings follow normally after such a stress.

planning care during recovery The postcesarean mother must proceed through the rapid involutional changes just as a woman does after a vaginal delivery. Factors changing the pattern of normal recovery are associated with the reasons for which the surgery was done. If a long, exhausting labor without progress or descent preceded delivery by cesarean section, one should be alert for uterine atony (exhaustion) with extra vaginal bleeding. If the reason was fetal distress or cord prolapse, unexpected emergencies, the maternal recovery should be smooth. If the reason was placental dysfunction or separation, postpartum hemorrhage is a real possibility. If a cesarean delivery was done after

table 26-8 Postoperative care of mother after a cesarean delivery

goals	intervention
A. Promote recovery from surgery	
1. Maintain fluid and electrolyte balance	Usually IV fluids for 24 h. Monitor intake and output for 24 h, especially after Foley catheter removed. Diaphoresis, diuresis common. Encourage intake of fluids, especially if breast-feeding.
2. Encourage adequate nutrition	PO intake resumed gradually. Sometimes patient can go back to regular diet within 12 h, but diet varies according to type of anesthesia and reason for surgery. Should have high protein intake. Stool softener may be ordered beginning 24 h after surgery.
3. Provide wound care	Observe for signs of infection, intact suture line. Dressing removed in 2 to 3 days, stitches out by 5 to 6 days. No dressing changes usually required.
4. Plan supportive physical care	Encourage postoperative regimen of turn/cough/deep breath for 24 h. Give complete care for first 24 to 48 h, using opportunity to encourage patient to express feelings over surgery. Then encourage independence and self-care. Shower after dressing removed.
5. Early ambulation	Up, walking (not sitting in chair) by 12 to 18 h after surgery. Sometimes support hose indicated prior to ambulation (check prenatal history). Include nursery visits in early walks.
6. Monitor vital signs	Depending on type of anesthesia, recovery should be complete by 6 to 8 h. Be alert for drug-induced postural hypotension or hypertension. Expect some elevation of temperature in the first 18 to 24 h. Watch hydration.
B. Provide relief from discomfort	
1. Analgesia as necessary	Begin with stronger narcotic, switch to milder after first 48 h. Provide relief before voiding or bathing and enough time before ambulation to avoid postural hypotension.
2. Prevent abdominal distension	Encourage activity and ambulation. Apply abdominal binder as necessary. Observe for return of bowel sounds, flatus.
3. Prevent engorgement of breasts	If ordered, be sure milk suppressant is administered correctly. Provide relief measures to lactating mother: breast pump, supportive bra, analgesics, ice packs to axilla and breasts, frequent nursing opportunities to ensure establishment of lactation.
C. Assess involution	Check bleeding, lochia. Note reason for surgery, and adapt care according to presence of infection, history of hemorrhage, etc. Check fundus only if signs of subinvolution are present, and then only very gently.
D. Orient patient to procedures and progress	
1. Encourage expression of feelings about surgical delivery	Be alert to cues of hostility or depression over "failure." Encourage independence after the first 24 to 48 h.
2. Identify for the patient the steps in her recovery	Orient her to expected progress and self-care at home. Discuss plans for assistance in the first weeks, her need for rest, and timing of resumption of usual activities.

E. Foster parent–infant bonding
   1. Promote skill in feeding   Expect her to be fatigued in first 24 h, but persist in positive assurance that she wants to feed baby. Feed at bedside in early hours if mother is medicated and groggy. Encourage father's participation, since he will take most responsibility in first few days at home.

   2. Supply information about infant care   Support attendance at ward/unit classes on infant care. Provide literature.

   3. Refer to visiting nurse for home visit   All mothers delivered by cesarean should be referred for a home visit by a health professional.

F. Evaluate interventions, identify problems, and plan for resolution.

prolonged period of ruptured membranes, uterine infection may result. Thus, recovery is particularly affected by the prenatal and delivery course, and planning for care must be based on that data. (Refer to chapters detailing complications, as well.) The age of the patient, her support system, whether this was an initial or repeat experience, the preparation received, and the type of anesthesia must all be considered.

Once the data base has been obtained and the problems identified, it is possible to begin formulating a specific plan for recovery care. Table 26-8 outlines the care that is needed by an uncomplicated postoperative patient.

EMERGENCY DELIVERY*

A delivery becomes an emergency when it is outside the usual planned, prepared setting. The mechanism of labor remains the same, of course. Four main settings will be considered: home delivery, en route in car or taxi, somewhere in the hospital, and in a disaster situation.

The woman who delivers so rapidly is usually a person who has a relatively painless labor, one who does not feel her contractions until the transition stage or until actually bearing down. Often the patient goes to the bathroom because the urge of bearing down is an overwhelming sensation; she then realizes that the delivery is imminent.

asepsis

Basic medical asepsis can be observed even in an emergency delivery. The home environment is a safe place for a delivery because the mother is used to her own environmental bacteria. (Indirectly, so is the fetus.) The baby is being born through a passage that is not

*This section was written by Marretje Bührer.

aseptic; because of this, no delivery is really sterile. Once you understand that fact, it is easier to proceed with a home delivery, doing your best with soap and water or whatever is on hand.

assessment and preparation

If one or more persons are present, the most knowledgeable one handles the delivery while directing the others to seek help by calling the number of the police, ambulance, or fire department. Utilize the family to get equipment and assist with the delivery.

Assess the situation. If the patient is in the bathroom and the baby is ready to be born, lower her to the floor. (It is difficult to deliver a baby while the mother is standing up.) Place several towels under her buttocks to allow some height for delivering the shoulders. If there is time, transfer her to her bed and proceed by placing her crosswise on the bed with her buttocks slightly hanging off the mattress. Instruct her to place her hands under her thighs, to support herself. One can also use a table and the patient can rest her feet on the backs of two chairs. A person's possessions are valuable to her, protect the mattress, floor covering, or furnishings with a plastic shower curtain, plastic tablecloth, newspapers, towels and old sheets. A dishpan can be used to catch the flow of amniotic fluid and blood.

While all these preparations are being made, give emotional support to the patient. Comfort her, tell her that she is doing beautifully, and reassure her that everything is going well. In order to win time, ask the cooperation of the mother during a bearing-down contraction to blow instead of push. Short blows, or panting, prevent the mother from bearing down. Remember! One less push gives you 3 to 5 min more to prepare.

If there is time, wash your hands and wash down the perineum. A wet towel and dishwashing liquid are quick cleansing tools.

the delivery

Once the head crowns, ask the mother not to push but to use the pant-blow respiration pattern. Place one hand fully on the baby's emerging head and give very gentle counter-pressure while the head is being born. Sudden popping out of the head should at all times be prevented, since it may cause intracranial hemorrhage. The gentle counter-pressure lets the head emerge slowly through the vaginal opening. There is no hurry. When the child's head emerges from the vagina, gently stroke the child's nose downward to expel mucus and amniotic fluid. (This is the way the nose is blown by people unaccustomed to Kleenex or handkerchiefs.) "Milk" the throat by an upward stroking movement on the neck and under the chin. Then "milk" the nose to expel excess mucus. This method enables the child to have a fairly clear oral and nasal pharynx. Feel for the cord. If there is a loose cord around the neck, slip it over the head. If it is fairly tight, a gentle pull may allow more to come forth and enable you to slip it over the head.

The mechanism of labor at this point is that the child is still enclosed by the vaginal wall with great pressure on the thorax, pressure which is part of the preparation for respiration. Some amniotic fluid will still be bubbling through the trachea because of the squeezing of the chest. Therefore, while you wait, continue milking the nose and stroking the neck and chin.

Take the head in two hands, press it gently downward and ask the mother to push. This will enable you to deliver the anterior shoulder under the symphysis pubis. When the beginning of the upper arm appears, lift up the head gently, all the while looking under the baby to see the posterior shoulder emerge. Correct delivering of the shoulders may prevent upper vaginal or perineal lacerations. Remember the vagina is not a straight passage but is almost J-shaped. The head comes down under the symphysis pubis; so must the shoulders. When the shoulders are born, slide a hand along the back and legs and grab the feet, while the other hand supports the neck and head. Release the hand around the neck and rub the back with that hand. Then place the baby, wrapped in a towel, head downward on the mother's abdomen. There's no hurry. If no ambulance service is coming, complete the delivery.

If the delivery takes place with no chance of transport, you may tie the cord. Resist dramatic nonhygienic methods. Through eons of time different means have been used, from a sharp stone to chewing the cord through. The latter method is not recommended because the human mouth contains more organisms than almost any other instrument you could find. Most homes have some sewing notions—wool, heavy cotton thread, string, or button thread. Never use silk or fine thread as it will sever the cord in the tying act. Tie the cord in two places, 3 in from the baby's abdomen, then about 2 in farther up. To cut, you can use a kitchen knife, scissors, or a new razor blade. If fire is available, you can hold the cutting tool over a flame; if alcohol is available, wipe it off well.

If you know that no help is available to complete the delivery, wrap the baby in a baby blanket or a soft old sheet and then a blanket, and proceed to wrap that part of the cord hanging from the vagina in a clean towel or cloth and wait for separation of the placenta. When it separates, ask the mother to push and deliver the placenta. Never pull the cord, for the cord may snap or part of the placenta may come away. The placenta can remain in the uterus for 24 h without injury to the mother.

post delivery care

Once separation has occurred, however, post-delivery care is identical to that in the hospital. Keep the patient warm, watch her pulse, check for signs of bleeding or shock, and check the fundus frequently. If the uterus has a tendency to relax, massage it very gently. Other methods include, besides the massage, use of ice cubes wrapped in a cloth, a heavy weight such as a big book placed just above the fundus, and breast stimulation. For breast stimulation, one can either put the child to the breast or use manual stimulation.

Be careful about letting the patient see her blood loss. Estimated blood loss in a normal delivery is anywhere from 250 to 500 mL. Remember that this blood is mixed with a large amount of amniotic fluid. Estimate the amount for a later report.

If the mother is not going to the hospital, she needs fluid replacement. Hot tea with honey, salty broth, or whatever she can drink can be prepared by the family. If transport is available, do not give fluids orally. There may be a need in the hospital for general anesthesia for exploration of the uterus and repair of lacerations.

infant care

If you have to stimulate breathing, do not *hit* the child or slap the back or buttocks. (One does not hit an unconscious patient to make him breathe.) A gentle slap or flicking on the soles of the feet or rubbing the back is often enough stimuli. Quickly assess the response of the infant to birth. If the infant does not spontaneously cry or breathe, place the child on a flat surface, roll up a towel and place it under the baby's shoulders, extend the head downwards and give mouth-to-mouth resuscitation. Your priority after establishing res-

piration is maintaining the infant's temperature. Dry the baby, use whatever is available (something clean and warm) as a wrap, and place the child either in a crib or in the mother's arms.

preterm infant Unfortunately, many precipitate deliveries result in preterm infants. Your problems are then multiplied. Gentle handling and a warm environment are especially crucial to the small baby. A good environment for the preterm baby is a small cardboard box within a larger one. In the outer box, place warm water bottles and newspapers; use lightweight baby blankets to cover the baby. One can also use a box near an open oven door, with the oven on low heat. The environmental temperature for the preterm infant must be in the low 90° range to prevent cold stress. If no other aid is available, placing the infant next to the mother's skin and wrapping them both will be the safest method of maintaining temperature.

If all is well and no transport is available, you may, when the status of the full-term infant is stabilized, wash it in warm water with mild soap. Since the cord is still wet, you can immerse the baby in the water. After all, water has been the neonate's usual environment. The precaution here is to prevent chilling. The infant may nurse as soon as possible, for sucking will assist the mother, as well.

delivery en route to the hospital

Delivery in a car or taxi is perhaps the most complicated in terms of setting, lack of equipment, and assistance. If there is enough time, place the patient on the back seat of the car. Place the mother's skirt or pants under her to provide a screen against the much-used seat. Since we are dealing only with the actual delivery, the focus is on protecting the baby. Support the head, ease out the shoulders, and clear the airway. Wrap the baby in anything available, and place it in the mother's arms. If necessary, put the baby next to the mother's skin and then wrap her and the baby in whatever is available. The car should be kept idling to provide heat, but in any event, watch the infant for chilling.

At the hospital, a mother who delivers en route will be taken directly to the delivery room, where the cord will be cut. She is then prepared for the removal of the placenta and manual exploration of the uterus, and is examined for cervical and vaginal lacerations. An infusion will be started, and oxytocin will be given, either directly intravenously or added to the infusion. The infant will be routinely taken care of, placed in an observation nursery, and observed for signs of trauma, low temperature, intracranial hemorrhage, and infection.

The physician may place both mother and infant on prophylactic antibiotics.

precipitate delivery in the hospital

A precipitous delivery may also occur in a labor room! The same rules apply as in an emergency delivery. Give the mother emotional support, have her breathe correctly (pant-blow), and ask for her cooperation.

A portable emergency kit in the labor room contains the following: two Kelly clamps, one plastic cord clamp, one scissor, a bulb syringe, two red-top tubes, a receiving blanket, four towels, 4- by 4-in gauze sponges, and a placenta basin (Fig. 26-13).

After the cord has been cut, the baby and the mother are both transferred to the delivery room, where the usual procedures—delivery of the placenta, and examination for lacerations—take place. Care to the baby is given as after a normal delivery.

delivery during disaster

Much has been written about disaster nursing. The type of care that can be provided in

fig. 26-13 Emergency delivery pack.

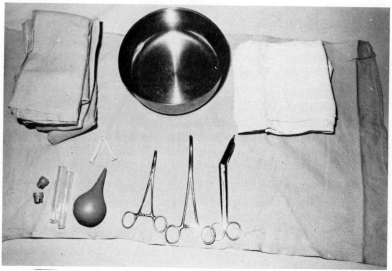

disaster conditions depends on whether there has been any prior planning for or warning of disaster. With prior planning, people are prepared to manage an emergency delivery and delivery kits are available. Should you be the *one* doing the planning, and the drug store, dime store, or home is your only resource, remember to provide:

Something for cleansing	alcohol, liquid soap
Something to clear an airway	ear bulb syringe, meat basting syringe
Something for the cord	strong cotton thread or yarn, new razor blade, scissors, or knife
Something for padding or protection	newspapers, brown paper, large plastic bags, old sheets, towels
Something to warm the baby	blanket, towel, clean sheet, shirt, diapers
Something to put the baby in	carton, box, padding
Something to feed the baby	bottles, milk powder, etc., should mother not be able to nurse

In an unpredictable major disaster, rules may be unusable. It is those at the periphery of a disaster who may help in the ways listed above. A woman delivering alone will instinctively try to preserve herself and the child.

The rules for emergency situations are well outlined in Mahoney's *Emergency and Disaster Nursing* (see Bibliography). Panic will interfere with clear thinking, and since information and experience are the best tools to quell panic, it is usually up to the person with the most medical experience to take charge. When panic is reduced, people will usually work together to deal with crises in quite sensible, remarkable ways.

study questions

1 In order to halt preterm labor, therapy must be started before what phase of labor? What basic pharmacologic action is sought from drugs currently in use?
2 Describe the nursing supportive care for a woman receiving
   a Ethanol IV
   b Isoxsuprine IV
   c Magnesium sulfate IV
3 Identify for each of the above drugs the special observations of the infant that must be made in the nursery if treatment is not successful and labor proceeds to delivery.
4 Differentiate between identical and fraternal twins in at least three ways.
5 When a woman is receiving therapy for infertility, special observations must be made for signs of ovarian hyperstimulation. What are these signs?
6 How does the presence of more than one fetus change the usual course of pregnancy? Identify physiologic reasons for at least five problems.
7 What intrinsic factors make oxytocin the drug of choice for induction?
8 Calculate the numbers of milliunits in 1 mL of a mixture containing 10 units of oxytocin in 500 mL of 5 percent dextrose in water. How many milliliters per minute should be given if the patient is ordered to receive 10 milliunits per minute?
9 Identify the safety measures which must be practiced when oxytocin is used during labor.
10 Define dystocia and give examples of dystocia in major phases of labor.
11 Study Figs. 26-7, 26-8, and 26-9 and describe why birth from these presentations would be injurious to the infant.
12 What special care should be planned for a patient with a fourth-degree perineal laceration or one with a periurethral laceration?
13 What factors must be present before forceps are applied to the fetal head? In which situations are forceps essential to a safe delivery? Refer to Table 26-2 and note the adverse effects which could occur from lack of intervention.
14 Compare forceps and vacuum extraction operations as to possible effects on the newborn infant.

15 Identify at least six ways a couple can be supported as they prepare for a cesarean delivery.

16 Plan ways of including the father in the process of birth and recovery when your hospital setting does not allow him to be in the OR with the mother.

17 Talk to a mother who has had a cesarean delivery because of pregnancy complications and modify the plan in Table 26-8 for her.

18 A home delivery may be planned for or may be an "unplanned" emergency. List the differences. Read two references on planned home deliveries.

19 Identify four basic principles governing safety of delivery in any setting.

references

1 P. Barden, "Premature Labor: Its Management and Therapy," *Journal of Reproductive Medicine,* **9**(3): 113, 1972.

2 R. Landesman, "Premature Labor: Its Management and Therapy," *Journal of Reproductive Medicine,* **9**(3): 95, 1972.

3 C. M. Steer and R. H. Petrie, "A Comparison of Magnesium Sulfate and Alcohol for the Prevention of Premature Labor," *American Journal of Obstetrics and Gynecology,* **129**(1):2, September 1977.

4 R. L. Berkowitz, "Premature Rupture of Membranes; a Review and Treatment Plan," *Contemporary OB/GYN,* **10**:36, November 1977.

5 Ibid., p. 39.

6 W. S. Dickson and D. T. Meilieke, "Surgical Separation of Conjoined Twins," *Canadian Nurse,* May 1973, p. 26.

7 D. M. Purohit et al., "Management of Multifetal Gestation," *Pediatric Clinics of North America,* **24**(3): 482, August 1977.

8 *AMA Drug Evaluations,* 3d ed., Publishing Sciences Group, Littleton, Mass, 1977, p. 581.

9 Ibid., p. 572.

10 Purohit, op cit., p. 487.

11 J. Delaney, "Immediate Bedrest in Multiple Gestation Cases," *ObGyn News,* **8**:6, 1973.

12 E. H. Bishop, "Pelvic Scoring for Elective Induction," *Obstetrics and Gynecology,* **24**:266, 1964.

13 M. J. Hughey, T. W. McElin, and C. C. Bird, "An Evaluation of Preinduction Scoring Systems." *Obstetrics and Gynecology,* **48**(6):367, December 1976.

14 T. P. Barden, "Perinatal Care," in S. L. Romney et al. (eds.), *Gynecology and Obstetrics: Health Care of Women,* McGraw-Hill, New York, 1975, chap. 37, p. 677.

15 D. Haire, *The Cultural Warping of Childbirth,* International Childbirth Education Association, Hillside, N.J., 1972.

16 American College of Obstetrics and Gynecology, *Obstetric-Gynecologic Terminology,* Davis, Philadelphia, 1970, p. 408.

17 Romney, op. cit., p. 678.

18 B. Donovan and R. M. Allen, "The Cesarean Birth Method," *Journal of Obstetric, Gynecologic and Neonatal Nursing,* **6**:37, November/December 1977.

19 Ibid., p. 40.

bibliography

Preterm Birth

Liley, A. W.: "Disorders of Amniotic Fluid," in N. Assali (ed.), *Pathophysiology of Gestation: Fetal Disorders,* Academic Press, New York, 1972, vol. 11.

Ostergard, I. K.: "The Physiology and Clinical Importance of Amniotic Fluid. A Review," *Obstetrical and Gynecological Survey,* **25**:297, 1970.

Multiple Pregnancy

Faroqui, T. O., et al.: "A Review of Twin Pregnancy and Prenatal Mortality," *Obstetrical and Gynecological Survey,* **28**: 144, 1973.

Hafez, E. S. E., "Physiology of Multiple Pregnancy," *Journal of Reproductive Medicine,* **12**:88, 1974.

Gause, W.: "Multiple Pregnancy, Diagnosis, Delivery and Problems of Development," *Journal of Obstetric and Gynecological Nursing,* **1**(3): 22, 1972.

"Multiple Pregnancy," *New England Journal of Medicine,* **288**:1239–1336, 1973.

Pernoll, T. L., and R. W. Carnes: "Electronic Fetal Monitoring of Twin Gestation," *American Journal of Obstetrics and Gynecology,* **115**:582, 1973.

Scheinfeld, A.: *Twins and Supertwins,* Lippincott, Philadelphia, 1965.

Induction

Christie, G. B., and D. W. Cudmore: "The Oxytocin Challenge Test," *American Journal of Obstetrics and Gynecology,* **118**(3): 327, 1974.

Friedman, E. A., and A. Sachtleben: "Oral Prostaglandin E_2 for Induction of Labor at Term," *Obstetrics and Gynecology,* **43**(2): 178, 1974.

Leake, R. D., R. Gunther, and P. Sunshine: "Perinatal Aspiration Syndrome: Its Association with Intrapartum Events and Anesthesia," *American Journal of Obstetrics and Gynecology,* **118**(2): 271, 1974.

Suspan, G. (ed.): "Induction of Labor: An Invitational Symposium," Parts 1 and 11, *Journal of Reproductive Medicine,* **6**(1): 17–34, 1971; **6**(2): 17–31, 1971.

Cesarean Delivery

Anderson, S. F., "Childbirth as a Pathological Process. An American Process. An American Perspective." *American Journal of Maternal Child Nursing*, **2**(4):240, July/August 1977.

Bampton, B. A., and J. M. Mancini: "The Cesarean Section Patient Is a New Mother, Too," *Journal of Obstetric, Gynecologic, and Neonatal Nursing*, **2**(4):58, 1973.

Diddle, A. W., J.R. Semmer, and J. F. Slowey: "Cesarean Section: A Changing Philosophy," *Postgraduate Medicine*, **53**:3, 1973.

Friedman, A.: "The Functional Divisions of Labor," *American Journal of Obstetrics and Gynecology*, **109**: 274–280, 1971.

———: "Patterns of Labor as Indicators of Risk," *Clinical Obstetrics and Gynecology*, **16:** 172–183, 1973.

Mevs, L.: "The Current Status of Cesarean Section and Today's Maternity Patient," *Journal of Obstetric, Gynecologic, and Neonatal Nursing*, **4:**44, July/August 1977.

Reynolds, C. B.: "Updating Care of Cesarean Section Patients," *Journal of Obstetric, Gynecologic, and Neonatal Nursing*, **4:**48, July/August 1977.

Emergency Delivery

Disaster Manual for Nurses, 3d. ed., rev., Massachusetts Civil Defense Agency, Framingham, 1966.

Mahoney, Robert F.: *Emergency and Disaster Nursing*, 2d ed., Macmillan, New York, 1969.

27

FETAL STUDIES

ELIZABETH J. DICKASON

5

THE HIGH-RISK INFANT

INTRODUCTION

In recent years, it has become possible to study the developing fetus and to determine a fairly reasonable estimation of its status. Fetal studies are utilized for four major purposes: diagnosis of (1) genetic disease or (2) congenital defects, and determination of (3) fetal maturity or (4) fetal condition.

genetic studies

Many defects cannot as yet be prevented, but modern techniques allow early diagnosis where the possibility of problems might exist. Early diagnosis is recommended when one or both parents have chromosomal abnormalities or carry genetically sex-linked diseases. In addition, when one child is affected with a genetic defect, the family is considered to be more likely to have a second child so affected.

detection of congenital defects

Congenital defects can occasionally be identified if they interfere with organ function or involve limb, cranial, or spinal deformities. Radiographic studies can identify obstruction in the GI tract or kidneys, or outline skeletal abnormalities. Ultrasound can pick up some cardiac problems, as well as identify fetal soft tissue abnormalities or disproportionate head size, i.e., hydrocephaly, ancephaly.

assessment of fetal condition or maturity

Fetal condition can be assessed in a number of ways, all of which compare findings to a set of normal values. Both the interpretation of normal growth patterns and the definitions of what is normal function have become much clearer in the past few years. Fairly narrow distinctions can be made, and no longer do physicians have to rely upon rough estimates when decisions about method and time of delivery must be made.

Two of the major causes of infant mortality and morbidity are early labor with resultant prematurity and a poor uterine environment with resultant fetal distress. Fetal studies can help to reduce infant problems by identifying the best time to deliver a baby who is stressed or by predicting the gestational age of the fetus and its need for supportive care once birth takes place.

Numerous methods have been utilized, but those currently of most value in determining fetal maturity or condition will be discussed in this chapter.

TESTING FOR FETAL STATUS

amniocentesis

Utilizing amniotic fluid, cast-off fetal cells can be cultured, i.e., grown in a medium over a period of 10 days to 2 weeks. Cell division occurs, and growth can be stopped at just the right point to obtain a clear microscopic view of the chromosomes. These are photographed under a high-power microscope, arranged in pairs, and studied for abnormalities. This karyotype is useful in determining the infant's sex and the presence of autosomal trisomies, translocations, or mosaicisms (see Chap. 28).

Biochemical studies of enzymes of these growing cells can inform the physician of genetically transmitted metabolic diseases; i.e., inborn errors of metabolism (IEM). Currently, about 40 of these metabolic disorders can be detected before birth.

Amniocentesis for suspected genetic problems is done ideally at the sixteenth week of pregnancy, since before this time, there appears to be too little amniotic fluid. Scheduling it at the sixteenth week allows time for the 2 to 6 weeks needed for karyotyping and biochemical studies. There remains time for the parents and the genetic counselor to discuss the alternatives open to them. If a therapeutic abortion is chosen, it should be done before the end of the twentieth week of pregnancy.

Amniocentesis later in pregnancy is most often done to determine the conditions of the fetus or the degree of fetal maturity. Amniocentesis is performed to determine fetal age and fetal pulmonary maturity in high-risk pregnancies, when the effects of waiting until term with a poor intrauterine environment have to be balanced against the handicap of prematurity resulting from early delivery. Ultrasound is done just prior to amniocentesis to determine placental location and fetal position.

procedure The nurse will assist in the amniocentesis:

1   Have the patient void to empty her bladder.
2   Position and drape the patient in supine position; place a rolled towel for slight lateral tilt if she is affected by supine hypotension.
3   Apply external fetal monitor for baseline recordings for 10 min.
4   Take mother's vital signs.
5   Gather equipment:
    Sterile gloves, drape
    Antiseptic for skin-prep swabs
    Local anesthetic
    5-mL syringe with 25-gauge needle
    1½-in 20-gauge needle with stylet—for first insertion
    5-in 22-gauge needle with stylet—threaded through 20-gauge needle (Fig. 27-1)
    Labeled tubes for fluid specimen, amber colored.
    3- and 20-mL syringes (Fig. 27-2)
6   Assist physician as necessary.
7   Arrange for specimen to be taken to lab.
8   Take mother's vital signs, and reapply monitor for 30 min.
9   Observe for untoward effects:

    Bleeding   Increased fetal activity
    Premature labor
    Pain   Infection (fever)
    Contractions   Amnionitis

10 Instruct the mother in follow-up care as prescribed by the physician. She is discharged once it has been determined that there are no untoward effects.

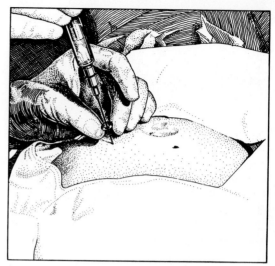

fig. 27-1 Aseptic technique of transabdominal amniocentesis. A short needle with stylet for first insertion through maternal tissue makes it possible to avoid contact of the amniocentesis needle with maternal skin. (*Redrawn, courtesy of Bernard Mandelbaum, M.D.*)

The risks of amniocentesis must be explained to the mother without unduly alarming her. In very rare instances morbidity occurs. The fetus may be punctured and may hemorrhage. Abruptio placentae or amnionitis may also occur. Maternal morbidity—hemorrhage, abdominal pain, or peritonitis—has been reported. Labor may be precipitated, causing abortion or, if later in pregnancy, premature delivery. A consent must be signed after a complete explanation has been given to the patient. All patients must have blood type and Rh recorded. If the patient is Rh negative and not sensitized, she receives 1 mL Rhogam after the procedure (see Chap. 29).

summary of uses Aminocentesis is a technique used in the following circumstances:

Sites of insertion

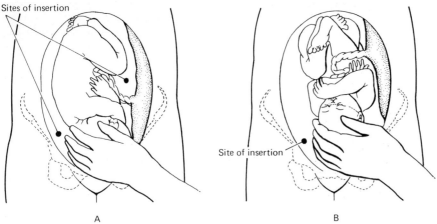

Site of insertion

A
B

fig. 27-2 Sites of insertion into amniotic fluid. (*Redrawn, courtesy of Bernard Mandelbaum, M.D.*)

Diagnosis of genetically carried diseases
Determination of the sex of the fetus
Determination of some congenital defects
Determination of condition and maturity of the fetus
Introduction of radiopaque liquid for amniography
Induction of abortion by salinization or by instillation of prostaglandins, urea.
Reduction of intrauterine pressure in cases of polyhydramnios

radiologic methods

x-ray Radiation dosage should be carefully controlled in potentially pregnant women. The only safe days for x-rays are the first 10 days after the menstrual period. Otherwise, before a pregnancy is discovered a woman might receive an excessive dose, affecting a highly radiosensitive embryo. The first 3 months of development—the period of *organogenesis*—are the most important. However, as is well known, dosage may be cumulative, and high doses of radiation to the mother have been correlated with an increased incidence of malignant diseases in the child, such as leukemia. Therefore, x-rays are used only when it is essential to aid a diagnosis[1]

Since bony structure can be visualized on x-ray, *pelvimetry,* the measurement of the pelvic size and shape, is one of the uses of x-ray in obstetrics. Fetal position, size, and head diameters in relationship to pelvic size can be determined. Pelvimetry is usually done when the patient is in labor to aid in diagnosis of cephalopelvic disproportion.

In suspected placenta previa, soft-tissue x-rays can show the vague outlines of the placenta in a low-lying position if the head is displaced. The most accurate and benign method of localizing the placenta is ultrasonography.

For *amniography* an amniocentesis is performed, removing 20 to 25 mL of fluid. An equal amount of contrast material is introduced into the amniotic sac. The contrast material mixes through the fluid, outlines the fetus and is swallowed by the fetus. Absence of swallowing or obstruction of the intestinal tract can be seen in malformed infants. A timed series of x-rays is taken to demonstrate the distribution of the contrast material.

biochemical assessment

tests for fetal maturity The amniotic fluid can be studied for bilirubin, creatinine, color, turbidity, cell content, and in some cases, hormonal content. The gestational age of the infant can be predicted by four parameters:

1 In normal infants, bilirubin disappears from the fluid by 36 to 37 weeks' gestation. There is a predictable curve, which can be analyzed. If the fluid shows no bilirubin, the infant is usually mature enough to survive outside the uterus. Rarely used, this is the least accurate method of estimating fetal age.
2 Creatinine increases with age after 32 weeks' gestation. This rising curve is correlated with a value of 2 mg/100 mL as usually indicating a mature infant (1.8 mg/ 100 mL = 36 weeks or more).
3 Staining the cells found in the amniotic fluid with Nile blue sulfate causes "fat cells" to turn orange. If 20 percent or more of the cells found in the specimen are orange-stained, the infant is usually more than 36 weeks' gestation and more than 2500 g in weight.[2]
4 Lecithin/sphingomyelin ratio. Lecithin and sphingomyelin are surface-active phospholipids found in the amniotic fluid which reflect the maturity of the fetal lung. By evaluating the concentration of these substances, and the ratio between them, a determination can be made as to the readiness of the fetus for respiratory independence.

A ratio of 2:1 L/S shows that the lung is mature enough to function. A ratio of 1:1 indicates immaturity. Ratios in between show variable outcomes. The lower the L/S ratio, the more severe is the respiratory distress that can be anticipated in the neonatal period.[3]

Mature L/S ratios indicate that respiratory distress is unlikely. They also correlate fairly well with central nervous system and liver maturity. If membranes rupture early, the L/S ratio may mature more rapidly than expected. Care must be taken in obtaining the sample, as any blood in the sample will give false-positive values. A quick "shake test" has been developed to obtain a general indication more rapidly than the laboratory method needed for the L/S ratio. Such a test can be done at the bedside but is not considered as accurate in borderline cases.

fetal blood sampling

Fetal status during labor can be assessed by obtaining fetal capillary blood from the presenting part—scalp or buttocks. After membranes are ruptured, the fetal scalp is sprayed with a silicone jelly so that a bead of blood will form when the scalp is punctured. Drops of blood are collected in a long glass capillary tube (Fig. 27-3). By microanalysis of small amounts of blood, it is possible to test the fetal pH, P_{CO_2}, P_{O_2}, glucose, and base deficit values. Hematocrit and hemoglobin values can also be determined. Note that if there is marked caput or edema of the buttocks, the pH results may be more acidic than current status indicates.

procedure The mother is positioned in dorso-recumbent or Sim's position and draped. The perineal area and vagina are cleansed of all blood, mucus, and amniotic fluid. Sterile equipment is used:

Gloves, long forceps, cotton swabs, antiseptic
Endoscope for visualizing the cervix

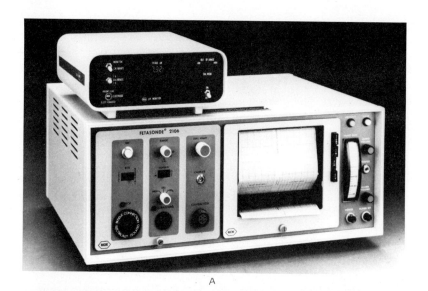

A

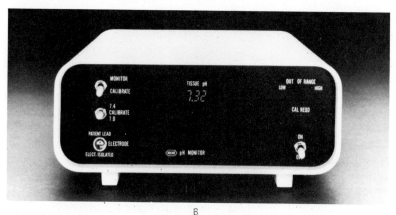

B

fig. 27-3 Continuous fetal pH monitoring is possible using readings conveyed from a scalp attachment. Pictured is (a) the Roche Fetasonde Fetal Monitor Model 2106 with the pH monitor (b) on top of it. Note the reading of 7.32 tissue pH. (*Photographs courtesy of Roche Medical Electronics, Inc., Cranbury, N.J.*)

Ethyl chloride spray to cause hyperemia of scalp
Knife blade with long handle
Long heparinized glass capillary tubes
Cotton swabs and swab holders
Silicone jelly

The time of sampling must be noted as a correlative factor with current fetal and ma-ternal condition. If indicated, blood may be drawn from the mother at the same time to be measured for her pH, P_{O_2}, P_{CO_2}, glucose, hematocrit, and hemoglobin. All such specimens must be analyzed at once, since the fetal condition may be deteriorating.

Fetal capillary blood samples from the scalp are normal if above 7.25. Early in labor, most infants have a pH similar to the adult,

7.35 to 7.40. Under the stress of active labor, especially in the transitional period, oxygen transfer may be reduced by strong contractions with inadequate periods of relaxation of the uterine muscle. With increasing hypoxia, the fetus enters a state of mild and then, if uncorrected, severe acidosis.

During the second stage of labor, a pH of 7.28 is considered normal, and such a state of mild acidosis appears to contribute to the maintenance of respiratory effort after birth. When abnormal heart rate patterns are seen on the fetal monitor, concurrent scalp samples will clarify if these heart rate differences are associated with increasing acidosis.

Until recently, scalp samples had, of necessity, to be intermittent. The time of sampling had then to be correlated with the contraction and heart rate pattern, since analysis took time. There is now available a continuous fetal pH analyzer which is attached to the fetal scalp. Unfortunately, not many delivery units have this sophisticated equipment. With either method, however, a falling pH in the presence of abnormal fetal heart rate patterns is an indication for interruption of the labor process, usually by cesarean section. Values listed below are guidelines:

Normal = a value over 7.25
Borderline = a value of 7.20 to 7.25; should be repeated within 20 min
Acidosis = a value of less than 7.2; the fetus should be delivered promptly

sound

auscultation For many years the only methods of evaluating fetal condition were by palpation and sound, i.e., feeling for size and position and listening to the fetal heartbeat. The fetal position, the amount of fluid, and the position of the placenta affect the transmission of sound, as does the quality of the stethoscope. The method of ausculation is described in Chap. 5. By means of the stethoscope, the fetal heart can be heard by about 20 weeks post-LMP.

Auscultation is useful in pregnancy but has been shown to be much less accurate than the newer methods of monitoring the fetus. However, until all labor rooms are equipped with monitors, and ultrasonography becomes more widely available, nurses must still become skilled in listening with a stethoscope to the fetal heart sounds.

phonocardiography A microphone enclosed in a soft cover is placed over the abdomen at the site of best fetal heart sounds. When the fetus shifts position the microphone must be shifted. Additional sounds may be picked up, and external noise, maternal sounds, and fetal movements limit the accuracy of this technique.

ultrasonography The application of sound waves at very high frequencies appears to be noninjurious to human tissue within the range of 1 million to 9 million cyles per second. The normal audible limits are 20 to 20,000 cycles per second. Utilizing the principle of sonar, sound pulses are beamed into the body. Echoes bounce back from the interface between two types of soft tissue and are converted into electrical energy, which can be seen in various display modes on the oscilloscope. *A-mode* utilizes pulse-echo information to move the oscilloscope sweep upward in an amount proportional to the intensity of the echo. Thus, A-mode will look like various degrees of peaks and valleys from a baseline. In *B-mode* (brightness mode) the strength of the echo determines the brightness of the dots displayed, and a two-dimensional display is possible (Fig. 27-4). Real-time sonography shows motion, e.g., respiratory movements of the fetus.

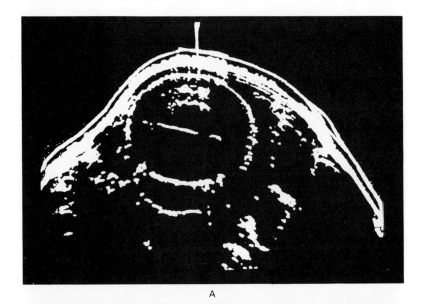

A

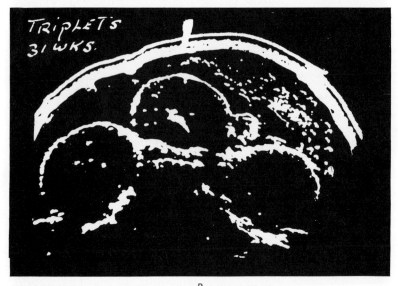

B

fig. 27-4 Ultrasound diagnosis. (*a*) Transverse cross section showing fetal head at 32 weeks. (*b*) Triplets at 31 weeks. (*Courtesy of Picker Corporation.*)

A new development is *gray-scale imaging* in which echo amplitudes (strengths) are related to varying intensities of gray, somewhat like a black and white television. Strong echoes are brighter, and less intense ones a

are softer gray. Dot density may also be used on the display. Similar to newsprint photos, the closer the dots, the darker the gray (and the more intense the echo). With these techniques, observation of numerous details of placental or fetal characteristics is now possible.

Since ultrasonography is noninvasive, there is no preparation for obtaining an image other than offering fluids to the patient, since a full bladder is often used as a marker.

The Doppler effect has been applied to a transducer which utilizes a continuous beam of sound in contrast to pulse-echo of the above modes. The echoes returning from different types of soft tissue are compared for their differences from the parent sound. These differences are translated into audible signals. The higher the speed of the object reflecting the sound, the higher the pitch of the sound heard. Using such a modified device, sounds of the fetal heart, flow of umbilical cord blood, placental flow, and maternal venous or arterial flow can be distinguished (see Fig. 27-5)

USES Ultrasound is a very accurate method for detecting problems in pregnancy; for instance, the location of implantation of an embryo can be determined after the eighth week, although the embryo may weigh only 1 g and be only 2.8 cm in length. There are many obstetric situations in which ultrasonography can be of use (Table 27-1). Among these are placental localization, detection of abnormal implantation, detection of abnormalities of fetal development, and determination of fetal maturity by accurate measurement of the biparietal diameter of the fetal head.

HEAD SIZE Measurements of the biparietal diameter (BPD) of the fetal head can be used to estimate fetal age and normal growth rates. Beginning in the second trimester, a baseline measurement is obtained. Serial measure-

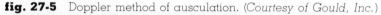

fig. 27-5 Doppler method of ausculation. (*Courtesy of Gould, Inc.*)

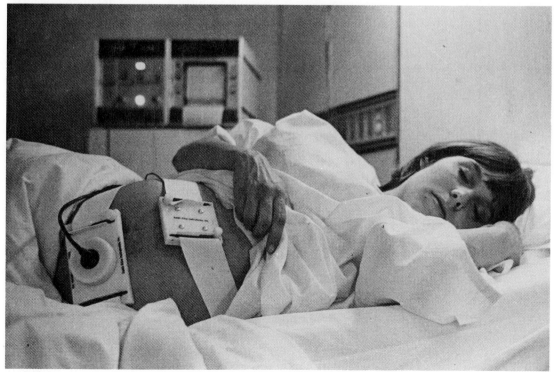

table 27-1 Ultrasound evaluation recommended for problems in pregnancy affecting fetal status

I.   Abnormal fetal growth may occur
     First trimester viral infection
     Hydatidiform mole
     Drug addiction
     Chronic hypertension
     Preeclampsia
     Diabetes
     Multiple pregnancy
     History of small babies
     History of congenital defects
     Poor nutrition or weight gain
     Hydramnios

II. Gestational age is uncertain or needs to be
     known
     Irregular menses, unknown LMP
     Obesity
     Previous cesarean section
     Primigravida 35 years or more
     Preterm delivery anticipated
          Diabetes
          Rh sensitization
          Hypertension
          Cardiac disease
          Previous stillborn

ments at 2- to 3-week intervals are then made and the findings compared to a graph of normal patterns (Fig. 27-6). It can be determined whether the infant falls into a low or high percentile in measurements, and later observations can then identify if growth retardation is taking place (Table 27-2).

The fetal head should grow at a steady rate of about 3 mm per week between 20 and 32 weeks. Measurements at 30 weeks can usually identify the *sonar EDD*, the estimated date of delivery, within ±9 days.[4] In the third trimester, the rate of head growth slows and is variable, approximating 1.8 mm per week.[5] Poor growth from the measurements of the second trimester can identify an infant in difficulty. To make the diagnosis more precise, transthoracic measurements are also used and the ratio compared.

RESPIRATORY MOVEMENTS   Real-time ultrasonography (utilizing serial transducers with B-scan display) demonstrates that movements of the fetus are present early in gestation.

fig. 27-6 Biparietal diameter averages by weeks of gestation. (*From S. N. Werner, et al., "A Composite Curve of Ultrasonic Biparietal Diameters," Radiology,* **122:**781, 1977.)

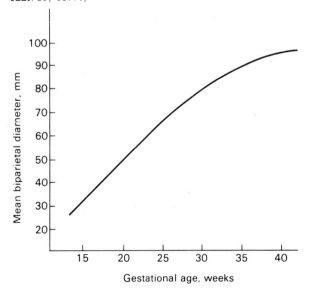

table 27-2 Biparietal diameter percentile values from 16 to 40 weeks (diameters measured in centimeters)

fetal age, weeks	BPD percentiles						
	5	10	25	50	75	80	95
16	3.1	3.2	3.4	3.7	4.0	4.1	4.5
17	3.4	3.5	3.7	4.0	4.3	4.4	4.7
18	3.7	3.8	4.0	4.3	4.5	4.6	4.9
19	3.9	4.2	4.3	4.5	4.8	4.9	5.1
20	4.2	4.5	4.6	4.7	5.0	5.1	5.3
21	4.5	4.8	4.9	5.0	5.3	5.4	5.5
22	4.9	5.0	5.2	5.3	5.6	5.7	5.8
23	5.2	5.3	5.5	5.6	5.9	6.0	6.2
24	5.5	5.6	5.8	5.9	6.2	6.3	6.6
25	5.8	5.9	6.0	6.2	6.5	6.6	7.0
26	6.1	6.2	6.3	6.6	6.8	6.9	7.3
27	6.4	6.5	6.7	6.9	7.1	7.2	7.6
28	6.6	6.7	7.0	7.2	7.4	7.5	7.9
29	6.8	6.9	7.3	7.5	7.8	7.9	8.3
30	7.1	7.2	7.6	7.8	8.0	8.2	8.6
31	7.3	7.4	7.8	8.0	8.2	8.4	8.8
32	7.5	7.6	8.0	8.3	8.4	8.6	9.0
33	7.7	7.8	8.3	8.5	8.6	8.8	9.1
34	7.9	8.0	8.5	8.7	8.9	9.1	9.3
35	8.2	8.3	8.7	8.8	9.1	9.3	9.6
36	8.3	8.5	8.9	9.0	9.3	9.4	9.7
37	8.4	8.8	9.0	9.2	9.4	9.5	9.8
38	8.5	8.9	9.1	9.3	9.5	9.6	9.9
39	8.7	9.0	9.2	9.4	9.6	9.7	10.0
40	8.9	9.3	9.4	9.5	9.7	9.8	10.1

Source: R. Sabaggha, "Biparietal Diameter: An Appraisal," *Clinical Obstetrics and Gynecology,* **20**(2):301, June 1977.

After the twentieth week, from these generalized movements, respiratory movements have been observed to be present at a rate of 30 to 70 breaths per minute.

Prior to 36 weeks of gestation, four types of normal chest wall movements have been identified:[6]

1 Rapid, shallow movement, increasing in depth to a peak and then declining. These breaths usually precede or follow fetal movements.
2 Irregular, shallow breaths mixed with slower deeper breaths. These deeper breaths may be felt by the mother.
3 Rarely, there occur rapid, deeper breaths at 10 to 15 times a minute, usually felt by the mother as hiccups.
4 Finally, the normal fetus may have short periods of apnea (6 s).

After 36 weeks the fetus breathes very much like the newborn, diaphragmatically, exchanging fluid in movements which are irregular in rate, rhythm, and depth. A circadian rhythm with an approximately 8-h cycle has been observed.

It is postulated that a normal fetus will have breathing movements present 60 to 90 percent of the time. A few studies have observed that infants in difficulty, who later had low Apgar scores at birth, have had movements less than 30 percent or more than 90 percent of the time.[6]

Cigarette smoking depresses fetal breathing movements up to 1 h, as do other hypoxic stresses. When a fetus is stressed by hypoxia or acidosis, prolonged apnea and isolated gasps (slow, deep breaths) occur, with movement of fluid more deeply into the respiratory tract. Conversely, when hypercapnia occurs, tachypnea with deeper breaths will result.

fetal electrocardiography (FECG)

indirect FECG   An indirect fetal electrocardiogram may be obtained during the prenatal period by means of electrodes placed on the mother's abdomen. The resulting record is a mixture of maternal and fetal cardiograms. This procedure has been especially useful in the past in diagnosing multiple pregnancy or intrauterine death in the antepartal period.

direct FECG   Direct fetal electrocardiography is possible with a fine coil or clip electrode attached to the presenting part of the fetus, after membranes have been ruptured. The resulting tracing on the monitor records the accurate heart rate and variability. The direct method of monitoring the fetal heart rate is preferable in any case of suspected fetal distress, because a more precise evaluation can be made of fetal condition. Most often, a simultaneous intrauterine pressure is also recorded so that uterine contraction pressure can be evaluated for its effect on fetal functioning. To do this, a fluid-filled Teflon catheter is passed through the cervix (Fig. 27-7), and changes in amniotic fluid pressure are then recorded continuously.

PROCEDURE   The patient is placed in the Sim's or lithotomy position and the perineum is

fig. 27-7   Procedure for attaching internal monitor. (a and b) After membranes are ruptured, the catheter is introduced past the fetal head into the uterus. (With permission of Corometrics Medical Systems, Inc., Wallingford, Conn. Copyright, 1974.)

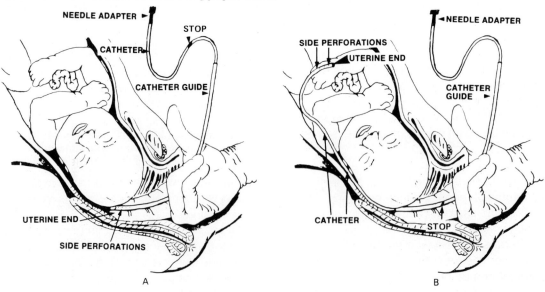

cleansed. Surgical asepsis is used for the following equipment:

Gloves, forceps, cotton swabs, antiseptic
Disposable scalp electrode
Teflon catheter with tubing attached to a three-way stopcock
Introducer for catheter (see Fig. 27-8*a–h*)
10-mL syringe filled with saline solution to remove air from the tubing and cathether.

Nonsterile equipment includes tapes to attach the leg plate securely, Velcro strap, and ECG jelly applied to the leg plate.

ELECTRONIC MONITORING OF THE FETAL HEART

Utilizing various methods, information about fetal condition is obtained, especially in the periods before and during labor. It is important to know what the current status of the fetus is in order to assess its ability to withstand the stress of labor.

The uterine contraction record is helpful in assessing the quality of labor. It is invaluable in following the course of patients who are receiving oxytocin for the induction or stimulation of labor.

Which patients should be monitored electronically during labor? The condition of any patient in the high-risk category should be monitored during labor. Electronic monitoring answers the question: Can this very important fetus tolerate the stresses imposed by uterine contractions which temporarily reduce blood flow to the fetus? As long as the record is normal, labor can be permitted to continue and a normal baby can be anticipated. An abnormal tracing which cannot be corrected implies a poor tolerance for labor in that fetus, and labor should be terminated; this often is done by cesarean section.

In all patients receiving oxytocin during labor, electronic monitoring should be performed. It allows for the earliest detection of excessive uterine activity and the resultant fetal anoxia secondary to impairment of circulation of blood through the uterus to the placenta.

In normal labor patients, not requiring oxytocin, monitoring will allow for improved observation of the fetal heart (a continuous recording) and the quality of labor. It will detect episodes of umbilical cord compression and usually allow for their correction, permitting optimal circulation to the fetus. Electronic monitoring should prevent the sudden intrapartum death of an apparently normally formed fetus. These deaths may be due to previously unrecognized umbilical cord compression or intolerance to labor contractions and decreased uterine circulation.

normal patterns

Learning to interpret fetal monitoring records requires time and practice. Records showing the following features are within a normal pattern:

1 Rate between 100 and 180 beats per minute, with the averages between 120 to 160 beats per minute.
2 Good beat-to-beat variation of 5 to 10 beats per minute.
3 Accelerations of the heart rate with uterine contractions or fetal movements.
4 Early decelerations: Moderate slowing of the fetal heart rate (FHR) at the time of contractions, which are uniform in shape, begin with the onset of the contraction, and end with the return of the contraction to the baseline. Early decelerations are caused by head compression and characteristically appear late in labor, when contractions are intense and frequent, and

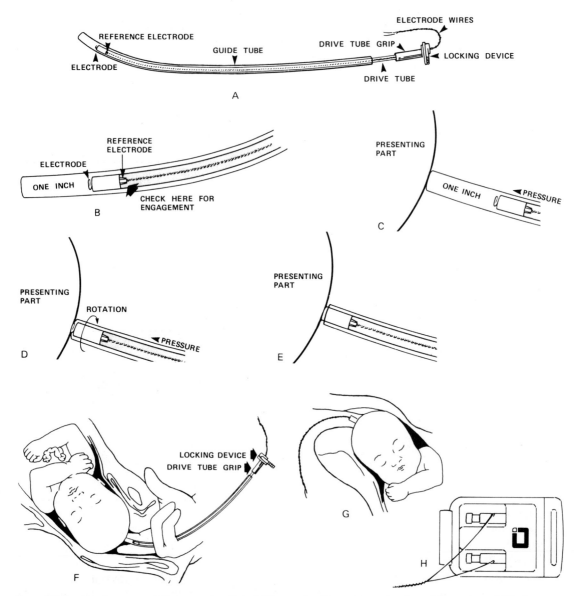

fig. 27-8 Application of Corometrics Spiral Electrode. The patient is placed in a dorsal lithotomy position, and the fetal presenting part is identified. The electrode (*a, b*) is to be applied only to scalp or to fetal buttocks. Green and red wires end in a spiral electrode, which is attached in a circular motion while pressing against the presenting part (*c, d, e*). Once in place, the guide tube can be removed (*f, g*) and the wires attached to the color-coded pushposts on the leg plate (*h*). (*Diagram courtesy of Corometrics Medical Systems, Inc., Wallingford, Conn., 1977.*)

the head is applied to an almost fully dilated cervix.

5 No other decelerations during labor.

All the above features in the record correlate very well with a healthy fetus equipped to tolerate the stress of uterine contractions during labor (Fig. 27-9).

abnormal findings

Abnormal findings in monitoring records are as follows:

1 *Late decelerations* show a pattern of slowing of the FHR beginning during the peak of a uterine contraction and persisting after the contraction is over. Late decelerations are due to fetal hypoxia and are serious indications that the fetus is potentially in distress. Any factor which interferes with the arrival of oxygen to the fetus will cause late decelerations. Some examples are partial separation of the placenta, hyperactive uterine contractions without relaxation intervals (usually due to excessive oxytocin dosage), maternal hypotension with resultant poor circulation to the uterus, preeclampsia with severe hypertension and poor placental perfusion.

2 *Variable deceleration* is the most common pattern seen in monitored patients. As its name implies, the pattern of slowing bears less relationship to contractions than the more uniform early and late deceleration. The deceleration is more rapid in onset and recovery, and each deceleration may differ from those before and after. It is the most dramatic of the patterns, with dips in rate of 60 beats per minute being common. Variable decelerations are usually caused by compression of the umbilical cord. Since the umbilical cord is highly sensitive to compression, variable decelerations do not always mean fetal difficulty. Variation

in the pattern (i.e., decelerations that last longer, become greater in amplitude, and are unresponsive to treatment) usually signifies fetal anoxia.

3 *Loss of beat-to-beat variation* in fetal heart rate is a serious sign of fetal anoxia. A straight line on the fetal heart recording is the most serious index of anoxia to the fetal heart itself. The interpretation of such a record must be cautious, because certain drugs administered in labor, such as Scopolamine, magnesium sulfate, and diazepam may significantly reduce beat-to-beat variation.

Familiarity with reading a monitoring record takes considerable practice. Further discussion of these patterns can be found in Hon and Martin (see Bibliography).

FETAL DISTRESS

Fetal distress may be chronic, occurring all during the course of pregnancy, or acute, usually manifested during labor but also appearing when the mother is deprived of oxygen (e.g., when anesthesia is poorly administered) or with a bleeding complication, such as placenta previa.

acute fetal distress

The classic definition of fetal distress included abnormalities in fetal heart rate, a rate under 120 or over 160 beats per minute, and the appearance of meconium in the amniotic fluid. Unfortunately these signs correlate very poorly with the actual condition of the fetus, and the management of labor with only these criteria often results in the emergency delivery of babies who were never in jeopardy and failure to recognize the truly hypoxic fetal state.

Fetal distress results from the failure of

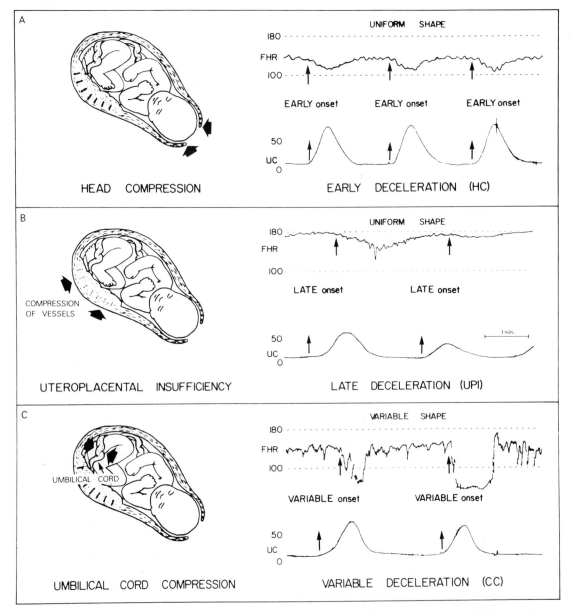

fig. 27-9 Chart of mechanisms of fetal heart rate patterns. (*a*) Head compression (HC), usually observed during transition and second stage. (*b*) Uteroplacental insufficiency (UPI), present when blood flow to the fetus is compromised. (*c*) Cord compression (CC), returning to normal heart rate only when pressure is relieved. (*From Edward P. Hon, An Introduction to Fetal Heart Monitoring, Harty Press, 1968.*)

oxygen to be delivered in adequate supply to the fetus. The most obvious interference with the baby's oxygen supply would result from compression of the umbilical cord. Such compression can be caused by prolapse of the cord with pressure by the presenting part against the pelvic wall, tight loops of cord around the fetal neck or trunk, short cords, or true knots in the cord. Cord compression produces *variable decelerations*. If the obstruction to blood flow through the cord increases, the duration of the decelerations will also increase, lasting 20 to 30 s after the contraction is over, adding a *late component* to the variable deceleration.

Other causes of inadequate oxygen delivery to the fetus are related to uteroplacental blood flow. Abnormally strong or long uterine contractions will temporarily shut off blood flow to the placenta. A poor "head of pressure" in the blood supply to the uterus which may result from maternal hypotension (e.g., supine hypotensive syndrome, epidural anesthesia, or maternal blood loss) will cause fetal anoxia. Uteroplacental insufficiency results in *late decelerations* in the fetal heart rate record. These decelerations may be very subtle at first, and represent a change in the rate of only 5 to 10 beats per minute. Any deceleration which persists after a uterine contraction ends must be considered to represent fetal hypoxia.

Thus, all late decelerations and progressively severe variable decelerations as well as a loss of beat-to-beat variation in fetal heart rate indicate acute fetal distress.

treatment of acute fetal distress   When signs of fetal distress appear, the following steps should be taken:

1 Discontinue administration of oxytocin. Uterine contractions may be too long or strong for optimal placental circulation.
2 Change the patient's position to (a) relieve pressure on the umbilical cord and (b) take the weight of the pregnant uterus off the vena cava, correcting hypotension due to supine hypotensive syndrome. Try both the right and left lateral positions or the Trendelenburg position. This simple maneuver will often correct an abnormal fetal heart rate pattern.
3 Administer oxygen 8 to 10 L/min to mother by mask.
4 Examine the patient to rule out umbilical cord prolapse.
5 Check maternal blood pressure.

If an abnormal pattern of fetal heart rate persists despite these measures, fetal scalp sampling should be performed, if this technique is available. If fetal acidosis, with pH below 7.20, is present, labor must be terminated. If fetal scalp sampling cannot be done, and after 20 min there is no improvement in the pattern, delivery should be performed by the most expeditious method, usually cesarean section.

If the abnormal fetal heart rate pattern is corrected, labor may be allowed to continue. Thus, electronic monitoring has the advantage of displaying the results of therapy to correct fetal anoxia, and allows a more intelligent and scientific decision to be made regarding the management of labor.

In the presence of an abnormal fetal heart rate pattern and a normal fetal scalp pH, fetal scalp sampling must be repeated in 20 to 30 min. If pH remains normal, the fetal condition is considered good enough to allow labor to progress. The reason for this is that fetal scalp sampling is a more reliable index of fetal well-being than fetal heart rate patterns.

Electronic monitoring is an excellent screening test to select those babies whose management will be improved by measurement of their acid-base balance. The combined use of both procedures is the ultimate in accurate assessment of fetal condition.

chronic fetal distress

Chronic fetal distress arises during the course of pregnancy and results from any condition which interferes with fetal nutrition and oxygenation. It may be present for several months. The common causes of chronic fetal distress are as follows:

1 Maternal diseases such as chronic hypertension, preeclampsia, congenital heart disease, diabetes, Rh incompatibility, severe anemia.
2 Underdevelopment of the placenta, resulting in a placenta too small to nourish the growing fetus adequately. This results in the "small-for-dates" fetus, which may weigh as little as 2 to 3 lb at full term. The causes for this condition are not fully understood.
3 Chronic infections of the fetus which interfere with development. Most common of these are rubella, toxoplasmosis, syphilis, tuberculosis, herpes, and cytomegalic inclusion disease.

The condition of the fetus that survives to term, in spite of chronic distress, must be carefully monitored in labor, since this stressful interval often produces more damage and even death (see Table 27-3). Acute fetal distress is a very common complication in labor of these previously jeopardized fetuses.

diagnosis of chronic distress The diagnosis of chronic fetal distress requires a very careful maternal history to discover known factors interfering with fetal growth. Frequent prenatal visits to discover and treat complicating illnesses (e.g., ketosis or infection in a diabetic patient) are mandatory. Clinical and ultrasound determination of fetal growth during the course of pregnancy will often detect the "small-for-dates" baby.

Especially useful is the plasma or urinary estriol determination performed on maternal blood and urine. A rising estriol level from the twenty-eighth week of gestation to term is normal. A flat estriol curve on repeated weekly determinations indicates suboptimal growth. A falling level often precedes intrauterine death by 48 to 72 h. A falling level is an indication for termination of pregnancy, if the fetus is viable (Fig. 27-10).

Unfortunately, at present, recognition of chronic fetal distress, rather than its prevention or treatment, is all that is possible. What is possible, however, is its recognition and the removal of the baby from its hazardous environment in the uterus at the time when the infant is most likely to survive. Very often the fetus suffering from chronic distress will do much better in the nursery than in the uterus. Until that optimal delivery date arrives, most of the fetuses will benefit from maternal bed rest, which will allow maximal uterine circulation.

antepartal monitoring of the fetus

The ability of the fetus to withstand the stress of labor can be tested prior to active labor by recording the characteristics of the fetal heart during the last trimester of pregnancy. There are currently three methods in use : (1) determining a reactive/nonreactive baseline response; (2) the nonstress test; and (3) the oxytocin challenge test (Fig. 27-11).

reactive baseline response A tracing of the fetal heart is obtained for at least 20 min. The signs of a healthy reactive fetus are as follows:[7]

1 The presence of accelerations of the FHR of 15 beats per minute in response to contractions, fetal movements, or upon stimulation (e.g., vaginal exams or abdominal palpation for position)

table 27-3 Problems of chronically distressed postmature infants (severe cases)

problem	observation	etiology	detection and treatment
Meconium staining and aspiration	Meconium in amniotic fluid. Yellow-green staining of skin, nails, and cord. Increased AP diameter of chest. Decreased size of abdomen. Rales and rhonchi over entire lung. Retractions, flaring nostrils. Lowered P_{O_2} due to intrapulmonary shuntings and reestablished shunting through DA and FO. Increased AP diameter of chest.	Placental insufficiency causes hypoxic insult to fetus. Result is relaxation of anal sphincter. Hypoxia causes deep gasping fetal respiratory movements. Amniotic fluid with cells, fetal hair, vernix, and meconium drawn into tracheobronchial tree—acts as a ball-valve, as thick material is not expelled in early respiration. Air is trapped in smaller branches, increasing the volume of the chest.	Prenatal detection—presence of chronic distress, late decelerations, deep variables, condition of amniotic fluid. At birth—physician will perform tracheal intubation and suction trachea under direct laryngoscopic visualization. Resuscitation will continue with oxygen, circulatory support, and buffering of acidotic pH; IV fluids will be started. May require assisted ventilation in nursery. Antibiotics usually ordered, as aspirated material is a good medium for bacterial growth, both gram-positive and gram-negative.
Polycythemia Central hematocrit, more than 70	Infant appears ruddy, color changes to cyanosis when crying. May become jaundiced quickly if condition not corrected. Renal vein thromboses may occur.	Intrauterine stress causes increase in red blood cells to increase oxygen-carrying capacity.	Central hematocrit taken (peripheral is always at least 5% less). Partial exchange transfusion. Remove certain amount of blood and replace with plasma
Hypoglycemia, below 30 g/100 mL	Asymptomatic or may be jittery, apneic, or have increased respiratory difficulty.	Decreased fat stores, recent intrauterine weight loss. Polycythemia, red blood cells use glucose.	Dextrostix at ½, 1, 2, 4, and 6 h of age, then q6h × 72 h. IV of 10% dextrose in water, with bolus of 15 or 20% dextrose. Early oral fluids if possible.
Hypocalcemia, less than 8 mg/100 mL	Same symptoms as hypoglycemia.	Unknown.	Assess serum calcium levels and administer calcium gluconate; dose is dependent on weight and condition.
Hypothermia, less than 37°C	Cyanosis, apnea.	Lowered fat stores, result of resuscitative efforts, poor attention to environmental temperature, cerebral damage to temperature-control center.	Continuous skin temperature sensor. Correct cause of environmental stress.

Source: Bonnie Silverman, R.N., P.N.C., with permission.

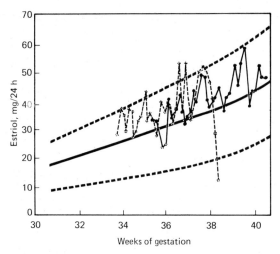

fig. 27-10 Drop in urinary estriol concentration indicates fetal distress late in pregnancy. (*From Contemporary OB/GYN, 1(1):15, 1972.*)

2 A baseline variability of 5 to 20 beats per minute
3 A heart rate within 120 to 160 beats per minute

If one or more of these characteristics is absent, or if decelerations occur during the tracing, the fetus is thought more likely to have acute distress during labor.

nonstress test Near the time of labor, when mild contractions are present, the FHR is monitored for a period of about 60 min. During this period, if three contractions within 10 min occur without any decelerations, the fetus is thought to be able to withstand the stress of labor. (In some borderline instances, oxytocin will need to be used, in addition, to ascertain a poor response.) These two tests without oxytocin have the advantages of taking less time and costing less than the oxytocin stress test.

oxytocin challenge test (OCT) The additional stress of an infusion of dilute oxytocin to augment contraction intensity will usually identify a fetus at risk of distress during labor. A fetus already suffering from placental insufficiency will show signs of late or variable decelerations.

PROCEDURE FOR OCT   After being informed of the purpose and expected duration of the test, a consent is signed by the patient. Since most women selected for such an evaluation have high-risk pregnancies, anxiety about the infant's condition may be high. The nurse, therefore, should explain each step and answer questions fully.

The patient is asked to void and usually is allowed no food or fluid before the test. Maternal vital signs are recorded every 15 to 30 min. She should be positioned in semi-Fowler's, with a left lateral tilt to prevent caval compression. A baseline reading is obtained for a period of 15 to 30 min. During this period, if strong enough contractions occur, the oxytocin challenge is not initiated. If there are no strong contractions, the intravenous infusion is begun. Dilute oxytocin, via infusion pump is added to the mainline IV. The rate of flow is very slow to begin with, since some women are hypersensitive to oxytocin. (usual initial rate of 0.5 milliunits/min to 1.0 milliunits/min) Observation is crucial! The rate of flow is increased every 10 to 15 min until three moderately strong contractions occur within 10 min. If there is no adverse effect, the test is then finished. The duration of the test is therefore quite variable, and a patient should be so informed.

Signs of problems will be late or variable decelerations, a change in fetal heart rate into tachycardia or bradycardia, or uterine hypertonus. Any abnormally long contractions should be noted at once and the infusion stopped. If the OCT is positive, showing adverse responses, the fetus is considered to be in a borderline balance. If an OCT is negative, the fetus is considered to be in a safe state for 5 to 7 days.

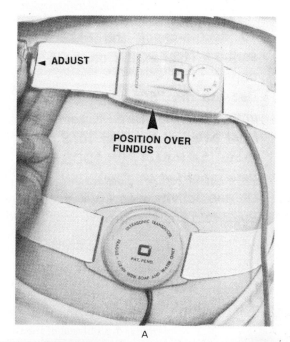

A

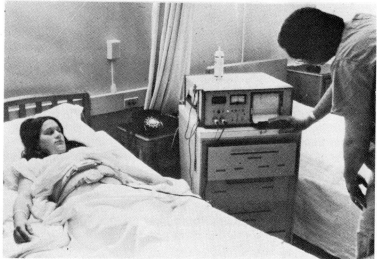

B

fig. 27-11 (a) Positioning of fetal external monitor. (b) External monitor used for OCT. (*With permission of Corometrics Medical Systems, Inc., Wallingford, Conn. Copyright, 1974.*)

nursing interventions

Nurses are being asked to monitor maternal and fetal responses in challenge tests. Umbeck has outlined a protocol used in one setting.[8] Each hospital will, of course, determine its own criteria for nursing management. No matter what the criteria, the patient must be supported through the procedure with careful explanations of each change. Her privacy should be protected and her anxiety level reduced. It is also beneficial to offer her reading material to help her pass the time.

The nurse should be aware that women have had a variety of responses to the use of a monitor during labor. Starkman identified from such responses the perceived benefits and problems listed in Table 27-4.[9-10]

To reduce problems and enhance benefits the nurse must protect the patient's privacy and orient staff to these studies of patient response. In addition, the nurse should give explanations of each change and procedure, allowing the patient's questions and comments to guide the depth of information provided. Finally, the nurse can emphasize the ways in which the patient and the supportive person with her can utilize monitor information to enhance the labor experience.

table 27-4   Responses of women after fetal monitoring

perceived benefits of monitor	perceived problems of monitor
1. A protector of the fetus: elaborating its status to the watchers.	1. A competitor for attention: staff and husband focused on monitor instead of patient.
2. An extension of the mother: providing information on contractions.	2. A "mechanical monster": discomfort of position, straps, insertion of internal monitor, dangling wires.
3. An aid in communication: as a point of common interest with the physician.	3. A cause of enforced immobility: being afraid or being told not to turn or the machine would "be upset."
4. An extension of the baby: the heart sounds reassured the mother (especially when there had been a prior stillbirth).	4. A poorly functioning machine: breakdowns, poor recordings, odd sounds caused increased anxiety.
5. A positive reinforcement of the husband's role: women felt husbands worked with them better when they could see contractions on monitor.	5. A noisy machine: the constant emission of sound was perceived as highly irritating to some women, especially in the transition phase.
6. A distraction: something to watch during long hours of labor.	6. A source of increased anxiety: each minor change in sound caused the anxious mother more problems as she fantasized the baby in trouble.
7. An aid in mastery: Lamaze patients could prepare for onset and identify peaks of contractions.	7. A source of injury to the baby: incomplete explanations caused women to think the internal electrode was "into the baby's head or soft spot." (Scalp infections after internal electrode use are a possibility.)
	8. A cause of lack of privacy: a constant stream of people in and out, often with the patient uncovered to see connections, etc.

Source: Adapted from M. N. Starkman, "Fetal Monitoring: Psychologic Consequences and Management Recommendations," *Obstetrics and Gynecology,* **50**(4):500, 1977.

study questions

1 When is amniocentesis first utilized for genetic studies? How is it utilized later in pregnancy?

2 Describe the instructions for preparation and follow-up which the mother should receive from the nurse before the amniocentesis.

3 What four tests are used to indicate fetal maturity using amniotic fluid? Which is the most significant predictor of survival after birth?

4 Name four steps in fetal blood sampling for which the nurse is responsible.

5 The last serial measurements of biparietal diameter were done on March 25. If the infant falls into the twenty-fifth percentile with a BPD of 7.6 cm, at what calendar date would you expect the infant to be mature (+37 weeks): (a) April 25, (b) May 15, (c) June 10?

6 Review the normal patterns of the fetal heart rate and rhythm. What nursing interventions are required if you note on the monitor the following:

a From a baseline of 124, the FHR is now 150. The mother has just received an epidural.

b After membranes were artificially ruptured, the FHR changed to 90 from a baseline of 124.

c Recovery from a 20-beat deceleration takes place before the decrement of a contraction is over.

d The baseline variability is erratic (20 to 40 beats) and sometimes there is no record marked on the moving paper. The mother is restless and turning from side to side.

7 How do the reasons for chronic distress differ from those for acute distress? What measures are useful in promoting fetal health in diagnosed chronic distress?

8 Study Table 27-4 and compare responses to a laboring woman you have observed while the fetal monitor is in place. How many of these negative responses could have been changed or been more positive if nursing intervention had been effective?

references

1 J. Sternberg, "Irradiation and Radiocontamination During Pregnancy," *American Journal of Obstetrics and Gynecology,* **108**:3, 1970.

2 L. Gluck, and M. V. Kulovich, "Lecithin/Sphingomyelin Ratios in Amniotic Fluid in Normal and Abnormal Pregnancy, "*American Journal of Obstetrics and Gynecology,* **115**:14, 1973.

3 R. Perkins, "Antenatal Assessment of Fetal Maturity:

A Review, *"Obstetrical and Gynecological Survey,* **29**(6):369, 1974.

4 R. E. Sabbagha, "Biparietal Diameter: An Appraisal, *"Clinical Obstetrics and Gynecology,* **20**(2):301, June 1977.

5 M. J. O'Sullivan, "Acute and Cronic Fetal Distress," *Journal of Reproductive Medicine,* **17**(6):320, 1976.

6 F. A. Manning, "Fetal Breathing Movements as a Reflection of Fetal Status," *Postgraduate Medicine,* **61**:116, 1977.

7 A. M. Flynn, and J. Kelly, "Evaluation of Fetal Well-being by Antepartal Fetal Heart Monitoring," *British Medical Journal,* **1**:936, 1977.

8 K. Umbeck and F. Diamond, "An Oxytocin Challenge Test Protocol," *Journal of Obstetric, Gynecologic, and Neonatal Nursing,* **6**(1):29, January/February 1977.

9 M. N. Starkman, "Fetal Monitoring: Psychologic Consequences and Management Recommendations," *Obstetrics and Gynecology,* **50**:(4):500, 1977.

10 M. N. Starkman, "Psychological Responses to the Use of the Fetal Monitor During Labor, *"Psychosomatic Medicine,* **38**:269–277, 1976.

bibliography

Clements, J. A., A. C. G. Platzker, and D. F. Tierney.: "Assessment of Risk of RDS by a Rapid Test for Surfactant in Amniotic Fluid," *The New England Journal of Medicine,* **298**:1077, 1972.

Daw, E.: "Fetography," *American Journal of Obstetrics and Gynecology,* **115**:5, 1973.

Grimwade, J. C.: "The Management of Fetal Distress with the Use of Fetal Blood pH," *American Journal of Obstetrics and Gynecology,* **106**:2, 1970.

Hon, E. R.: *An Introduction to Fetal Heart Rate Monitoring,* Harty Press, New Haven, Conn., 1969.

"Intrapartum Evaluation of the Fetus," *Journal of Obstetric, Gynecologic, and Neonatal Nursing, Supplement,* **5**:5, September/October 1976.

Martin, C. B., and B. Gingrich: "Factors Affecting the Fetal Heart Rate: Genesis of FHR Patterns," *Journal of Obstetric, Gynecologic and Neonatal Nursing, Supplement,* **5**(5):30, September/October 1976.

Nitowsky, H. M.: "Prenatal Diagnosis of Genetic Abnormality," *American Journal of Nursing,* **71**:8, 1971.

Perkins, R. P.: "Antenatal Assessment of Fetal Maturity, A Review," *Obstetrical and Gynecological Survey,* **29**(6): 369, 1974.

Sabbagha, R. E. (ed.): "Ultrasound in Obstetrics; A Symposium," *Clinical Obstetrics and Gynecology,* **20**(2): 229–351, June 1977.

28

GENETIC PROBLEMS

DOLORES LAKE TAYLOR

Each person is unique, different from anyone else who has ever lived. Yet, as human beings belonging to the species of Homo sapiens, we all have certain common features. The question that has puzzled scientists and anthropologists for centuries is what the natural forces are that interact to give all humans a general likeness as a species and at the same time such distinct differences.

More personally, this question puzzles and perhaps worries every expectant family as they patiently await the arrival of their newborn infant. Almost from the time the child is conceived, parents cannot help but wonder what it will be like. Will it be a boy or a girl? Will it have brown or blue eyes? And will it look like father or more like mother? More importantly, will it be all right, or by some odd fate will it be defective or malformed? If there is a history of seizures, mental retardation, cystic fibrosis, cancer, diabetes, alcoholism, or mental illness in the family, how might this affect the unborn child? No family, if its history is examined carefully enough, is entirely free of some type of inherited disease. What are the chances, then, that disease or defect, rather than health, will be inherited?

These questions and many others like them are asked frequently, with the expectation that the nurse will be able to provide satisfactory answers. Wherever the nurse works, patients will want to know answers to questions regarding the heredity of their children. The lay public expects a nurse to know and to give appropriate answers and guidance toward preventive health resources.

A basic understanding of the laws of heredity and the nature of hereditary material is a good place to begin. Environmental factors which help to promote genetic endowment or influence genetic change must also be considered, since human beings, like all living things, are products of both heredity and environment. Often it is the interaction of heredity and environment, rather than either one separately, which determines the outcome of any one situation.

The idea that characteristics are inherited has been present for thousands of years. However, Darwin's theories of evolution[1] and Mendel's observations of hereditary traits in plants[2] were among the first contributions to modern genetics. Since 1955, our knowledge of molecular biology has rapidly expanded the horizons of genetics.

As a nurse, you may be surprised to find that though your knowledge of genetics can be applied most directly in maternal and child health nursing, there will be many other instances in which it can also be utilized. Caring for many other kinds of patients, such as those who have diabetes, heart disease, and cancer, will entail at least a basic understanding of the genetic concept so that supportive family health care may be given.

THE NATURE OF HEREDITY

genes: carriers of hereditary traits

A gene is a unit of heredity material, *deoxyribonucleic acid* (DNA), which has a specific function. Sometimes this specific function is to determine a certain trait, such as eye color. More often the specific function is to determine a particular step in some complex process of the body's chemistry. Genes control protein synthesis, the formation of enzymes and antibodies, and the structure of hormones; they influence almost every chemical process in the body. Some of these activities are dictated directly by the genes. Other actions are made possible through the indirect genetic regulation of feedback responses. In some instances, two or more genes work together to determine precisely how the molecules of the body, such as hemoglobin, are made. There are also *operator* genes and *regulator* genes which start and stop the release of hormones and enzymes. Interacting with processes in the endocrine system through feedback signals, operator and regulator genes help to maintain homeostasis in the body. Thus, through gene action, the various enzymes and hormones can be turned on or off as needed.

If you recall how the egg and sperm are formed during gametogenesis (see Chap. 3) and how they unite when fertilization takes place, you will remember that half the genetic material comes from the mother's 23 chromosomes and half from the father's. The hereditary characteristics of the new infant are determined by the genes strung together in beadlike chains along these chromosomes. Within the chromosomes, each gene has its own particular place, or *locus*. Just as the chromosomes each have a matched partner, so the genes within them occur in pairs. One member of the pair occupies its locus on one chromosome while its partner, or *allele*, occupies the corresponding place on the matched chromosome.

The alleles in a gene pair may be identical or slightly different. The slight difference in one allele as compared with its partner in the pair is one factor accounting for differences between parents and their children. If a person has both members of a gene pair absolutely alike, he or she is a *homozygote.* On the other hand, sometimes the genes in a pair might be slightly different because the one inherited from one parent may be slightly different from the one inherited from the other parent. The person who has two genes in a pair which are slightly different from each other is called a *heterozygote.*

Sometimes one of the alleles in a gene pair is more dominant, while its partner is recessive. The type of gene (genotype), whether dominant or recessive, influences the overt characteristics (phenotype) of the individual according to Mendel's laws. See Table 28-1 and note that the first two examples are homozygotes, while the last one is a heterozygote.

Eye color is but one of the thousands of examples illustrating Mendel's laws of heredity (Table 28-2). By applying these laws, one can see how dominant or recessive genes can influence body chemistry and metabolism. If a person has inherited a defect in gene action involving body chemistry, that person has a metabolic problem which is

table 28-1 Mendel's laws of dominance

genotype		phenotype expression
gene	allele	
Dominant (D)	Dominant (D)	Dominant (DD)
Recessive (r)	Recessive (r)	Recessive (rr)
Dominant (D)	Recessive (r)	Dominant (Dr)

table 28-2 Inheritance of eye color*

parent	parent	children
Brown (B, B)	Brown (B, B)	Brown (B, B)
Blue (bl, bl)	Blue (bl, bl)	Blue (bl, bl)
Brown (B, B)	Blue (bl, bl)	Brown (B, bl)
		Brown (B, bl)
Brown (B, bl)	Blue (bl, bl)	Brown (B, bl)
		Blue (bl, bl)
Brown (B, bl)	Brown (B, bl)	Brown (B, B)
		Brown (B, bl)
		Brown (B, bl)
		Blue (bl, bl)

*According to Mendel's laws, brown (B) is dominant and blue (bl) is recessive.

inborn. PKU, Tay-Sachs disease, and muscular dystrophy are a few of the many hundreds of these kinds of problems.

In summary, the genes control body chemistry because they contain within them the specific instructions necessary for the body to build molecules of protein, to utilize energy, to grow, to change, and to carry on all of life's processes. How the body receives the vastly complex information about how to maintain itself is determined largely by the nature of the genetic material DNA (deoxyribonucleic acid). Life is passed on from one generation to the next through the DNA in the genes, just as chromosomes are passed on from parent to child. Life maintains itself after birth as old cells wear out, die, and are replaced by new cells with the ability to function as they should because of the remarkable DNA within them.

DNA: the molecule of life

Considering that DNA possesses all the hereditary information necessary to maintain life, it is a remarkably simple molecule. Coiling around itself, the molecule forms a double helix which looks like a twisted ladder. It has two side chains held together by cross rungs. The side chains are long, alternating links of sugar, or *deoxyribose*, bound to alternating phosphates. The chain is bent in such a way that the sugars lean inward while the phosphates lie along the outermost parts of the helix. The cross rungs are formed by nitrogen bases called *nucleic acids*. There are four nucleic acids: *adenine, thymine, guanine,* and *cytosine*. Thus, DNA is *deoxyribonucleic acid* formed by sugar (deoxyribose) and base (nucleic acid). Sugar is always the sides of the ladder, and nucleic acids make up the rungs (see Fig. 28-1).

base-pairing laws The Watson-Crick base-pairing laws state that adenine (A) always pairs with thymine (T), while guanine (G) always pairs with cytosine (C (Fig. 28-2). The reason why the nucleic acids pair in this manner is that this is the only way in which they fit together chemically. (A more detailed, but readable, explanation can be found in *The Genetic Code* by Isaac Asimov.)

The Watson-Crick base-pairing laws are universal. Whether applied to a plant, bug, cow, cat, elephant, mouse, or man, these base-pairing laws hold true. Life everywhere has within it the same structure in its DHA. You might ask, then, "If the basic structure of DNA is the same for all life, how is it possible for living things to take so many forms and for individuals in the same species to be so different from one another?" The answer to this difference among the various species of plants and animals is that the *ratio* of the base pairs differs (not the pairs themselves). The amount of guanine must equal the amount of cytosine, and the amount of adenine must equal the amount of thymine, but the ratio of the former group to the latter is species-specific. Some animals have more adenine and thymine; other animals have more guanine and cytosine.

In addition to the ratio of base pairs from the four nucleic acids found in the DNA, animals (and human beings) differ from one

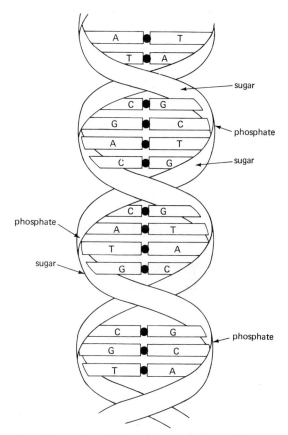

fig. 28-1 The DNA molecule is shaped like a ladder that is twisted into a helix. The sides consist of alternating phosphate bonds (outside) and sugar molecules (inner twists). The rungs are composed of nucleic acids: adenine (A), thymine (T), guanine (G), and cytosine (C).

another in the nature of the specific kinds of protein which form their body structure. DNA acts as an instructional pattern for making proteins. The information in the DNA map is in coded form. It is often called the genetic code, or the code of life.

RNA: the messenger

Information in DNA regarding how to make body protein and carry on all life processes

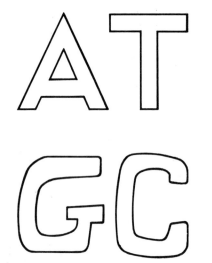

fig. 28-2 Watson-Crick base-pairing laws:
adenine always pairs with thymine (A-T),
guanine always pairs with cytosine (G-C).

remains useless if it does not have some way
of getting out of the helix to the ribosomes of
the cell where proteins are made. DNA itself
does not go directly to the ribosomes. Instead,
RNA (*ribonucleic acid*) reads the information
in DNA, interprets it, takes the message to the
ribosomes, and supervises the making of the
proteins in the proper manner.

There are several kinds of RNA. First there
is messenger RNA (mRNA), which reads the
message in DNA and carries the message to
the ribosomes. When the information is
needed by the cell, mRNA moves to DNA and
lines up along the one helix so that the bases
of RNA pair up with the bases in DNA. RNA
contains adenine, guanine, and cytosine, but
uracil replaces thymine: A, G, C, U. They line
up thus:

RNA			DNA
Uracil	U	A	Adenine
Guanine	G	C	Cytosine
Cytosine	C	G	Guanine
Adenine	A	T	Thymine

After having matched up with DNA, the
bases are ready to read the DNA message.

Always, three RNA bases work as triplets. The
triplets are called *codons*. Thus, UGC in the
example above forms a codon. In all, there
are 64 codons. Each codon specifies the
message for making an amino acid. Since
there are only about 20 amino acids, several
codons can carry instructions for one amino
acid. Some codons give the signals to start
and stop, since RNA cannot begin just anywhere. It must have specific instructions about
where and when to begin to read which amino
acids are needed. It also must know when to
stop working. For all living things, the code
for making amino acids is the same.

The sequence of amino acids along a protein chain is what determines the nature of
the protein molecule. Proteins are made by
stringing together hundreds of amino acids
in proper sequence. After mRNA takes the
message to ribosomes, soluble RNA (sRNA)
sees that the proper amino acid is gotten and
placed in correct position on the ribosome as
the links of amino acids are hooked together.
When all links are finished, the new protein
falls off the ribosome and goes to the spot
where it is needed in the cell.

Each minute of life from conception onward,
thousands of DNA molecules become active
at the appropriate second they are needed.
RNA reads the message in the DNA coded
form and oversees the manufacturing of protein to maintain life. Each step in the links
required to make protein requires a particular
enzyme, without which that step cannot take
place. At the exact moment needed, the correct enzyme must arrive to act as a catalyst
in order for the step to occur. Genes carry the
information for making and releasing those
enzymes.

The one gene–one enzyme theory was first
proposed by Beadle.[3] He states that so many
genes are packed into the 46 chromosomes
of each cell that the information would fill 500
volumes of encyclopedias if it were typed out
on an ordinary typewriter. All this information

operates through the genetic code to produce billions of precisely made complex molecules, properly arranged and structured into appropriate tissue forms composing a newborn 7-lb bundle of healthy baby! Think how many times a molecule of DNA must duplicate itself to grow, by mitosis, the millions of cells needed to form each organ. How many messages RNA has to carry and how many molecules of protein are made on the cytoplasmotic ribosomes in 9 months of gestation! By the same genetic code, the baby grows into a toddler, grade-school child, adolescent, and adult who may, in time, reproduce his or her own offspring.

mutations

Considering all this, it is quite remarkable that genetic mistakes are rarely made. Mutations, or genetic changes, do occur, however, from time to time. Sometimes the mutations are produced spontaneously; at other times, they are caused by environmental factors. How often mutation occurs remains unknown, since we see only the result of mutation, not the molecular change in the DNA directly. Naturally, then, if the mutation produces no observable change, it goes unrecognized. Since our powers of observation are limited, there are probably many changes which we do not see. Helpful mutations especially are unrecognized. Harmful genetic changes are the ones upon which we tend to focus, because they are the most recognizable of natural changes in people.

Harmful mutations in human beings have been found in several types of disorders. *Point mutations* involve a single nucleotide or gene; therefore, each point mutation in the affected homozygote produces a specific inborn error in metabolism. Two examples of point mutations are sickle-cell anemia (see Chap. 22) and PKU.

Chromosomal abnormalities involve more than a single pair of genes. They involve either an entire chromosome or at least a major part of a chromosome.

THE CHROMOSOMES

Genes are carried in the chromosomes, and their arrangement is very precise. The chromosomal pattern is called a *karyotype*. It was not until 1959 that the correct number of chromosomes in human beings was known to be 46 in each living normal cell except the egg and the sperm, which have 23. Since chromosomes occur in matched pairs, there are 22 pairs of autosomes and two sex chromosomes. The normal female karyotype is therefore, 44 autosomes and 2 sex chromosomes, 44XX. The normal male has one X chromosome, plus a Y chromosome. The normal male karyotype, shown in Fig. 28-3, is 44XY.

Chromosomes are classified according to their size and shape and the position of the *centromere*.[4] Figure 28-4 gives a schematic representation of sizes and shapes of chromosomes. Those most alike are grouped under the same letter, according to the Denver classification, an international system for designating normal as well as abnormal chromosomes so that medical men everywhere will have a standard approach to communication in genetics. The Denver classification is shown in Table 28-3.

Although almost any tissue of the body may be used for determining the karyotype of that body, skin cells or leukocytes are usually used. The entire process is too complex to be discussed fully; in brief, the cells are put under the microscope, the laboratory technician looks for a cell in metaphase when all the chromosomes are lined up at the equator, and that cell is stained and photographed. Later, the photograph is enlarged, and the chromosomes are cut out and pasted on a

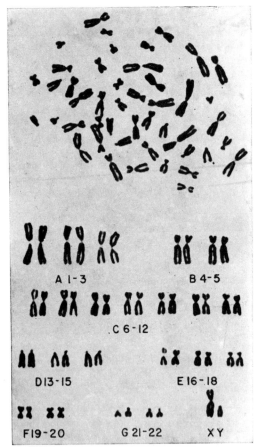

fig. 28-3 *Male karyotype. (From Ian Porter, Heredity and Disease, McGraw-Hill, New York, 1968.)*

sheet of paper according to their size and shape. More precise methods for determining karyotype are now available with the aid of a computer.[5]

chromosomal abnormalities

About once in every 1000 live births, an infant arrives in the world with a chromosomal abnormality. Many types of chromosomal disorders are known. Only part of a chromosome may be passed on, as in chromosomal *dele-* *tion*. A piece of one chromosome may be improperly hooked to another so that there is a *translocation* of chromosomal material. The two ends of a chromosome may reach around and "grab hold" of each other (like a dog chasing its tail), resulting in *ring* formation. Probably the most common chromosomal error that can be compatible with life is the presence of an extra chromosome in one of the pairs, or a *trisomy*.

trisomy 21 The characteristics of the person with trisomy 21 were described by Down many years before Lejeune discovered in 1959 that three chromosomes 21 appeared in all the cells of an infant with this condition.[6] The syndrome (formerly called mongolism) is now called Down's syndrome or trisomy 21.[7]

NONDISJUNCTION The extra chromosome in trisomy 21 usually results from an error in meiosis called *nondisjunction*. Meiosis is the process by which *reduction division* takes place from 46 to 23 chromosomes in the mature ovum. During normal meiosis, one member of each of the chromosome pairs goes to form the mature ovum. The matched partner in the pairs is discarded in the polar body, which is nonviable. In nondisjunction, however, both members of the twenty-first pair of chromosomes go to the ovum; they fail to disjoin, or separate. When the sperm fertilizes the ovum, it contributes the third chromosome 21, resulting in trisomy 21 (Fig. 28-5).

In the female, meiosis begins during her own fetal life long before she herself is born. Then the process of meiosis stops before reaching completion, and a long resting stage takes place from before birth to puberty. During ovulation the ovum finishes its final stages of maturity. The older a woman is, the longer the resting stage of any particular ovum will have been before it becomes ready for fertilization during the normal female ovarian cycle. The long resting stage appears to have

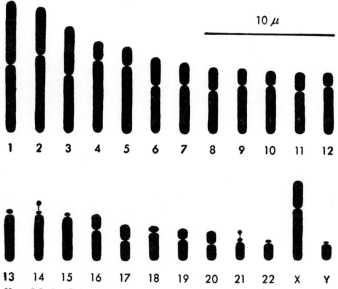

1 2 3 4 5 6 7 8 9 10 11 12

13 14 15 16 17 18 19 20 21 22 X Y

fig. 28-4 Schematic representation of chromosome. (*From Patten, Human Embryology, McGraw-Hill, New York, 1968.*)

something to do with the incidence of trisomy 21.[8] A child has a 50 times greater chance of being born with trisomy 21 if the mother is over 40 years of age than if she is her twenties. In fact, 95 percent of all children with Down's syndrome (Table 28-4) are born to older mothers.

TRANSLOCATION In contrast to the nondisjunction type of trisomy 21, a rare form of

table 28-3 Classification of chromosomes

group	autosomes	sex chromosomes	characteristics of chromosomes	no. of chromosomes	
				men	women
A	1–3		Large with median or slightly submedian centromere	6	6
B	4–5		Large with submedian centromere	4	4
C	6–12	X	Medium with submedian and median centromere	15	16
D	13–15		Medium, acrocentric	6	6
E	16–18		Shore with median or submedian centromere	6	6
F	19–20		Shore with median centromere	4	4
G	21–22	Y	Short, acrocentric	5	4
Total				46	46

Source: From Ian Porter, *Heredity and Disease*, McGraw-Hill, New York, 1971.

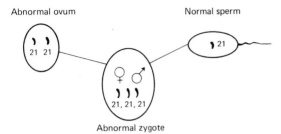

Abnormal ovum   Normal sperm

Abnormal zygote

fig. 28-5 Nondysjunction of chromosomes. The abnormal zygote has an overdose of chromosome 21, which causes Down's syndrome. (*Courtesy of The National Foundation—March of Dimes.*)

Down's syndrome is sometimes found among young mothers but may not be as closely related to age as once believed. This is *translocation,* in which part of chromosome 21 sticks to another chromosome before the ovum is mature. In addition, there is also a fully normal chromosome 21 in the ovum. The sperm brings in the third, so that there are still three chromosomes at 21. This type of Down's syndrome is found in mothers whose chromosomal patterns show by karyotype that they themselves are carriers of the problem. Translocation trisomy is extremely rare.[9] Because these children are likely to be born to younger parents and because the disorder is familial and may therefore affect other siblings, genetic counseling is of high priority.

PHYSICAL CHARACTERISTICS Children with Down's syndrome have a characteristic

table 28-4 Risk of trisomy 21 resulting from nondisjunction, in relation to mother's age

mother's age, yr	risk
Less than 29	1 in 3000
30–34	1 in 600
35–39	1 in 280
40–44	1 in 70
45–49	1 in 40

Source: From Ian Porter, *Heredity and Disease,* McGraw-Hill, New York, 1968.

appearance[10] whether their condition is of the translocation or of the nondisjunction type (see Fig. 28-6 with description). Because an entire chromosome is involved in Down's syndrome, malformations have been found in almost every organ and enzyme system (Fig. 28-7). Not every child has all of them, but each affected child has many. Cardiac defects and a tendency to develop rheumatic fever are common. Children with Down's syndrome have a genetic intolerance to atropine.[11] Therefore, the nurse who works with such a child must take special precaution to look for unusual effects produced by medications and anesthesia (Fig. 28-8a, b).

The single most universal characteristic of Down's syndrome is mental retardation. Usually, the degree of retardation is severe enough to prevent the child from learning skills beyond the elementary school level (if even this much can be accomplished). An occasional child has the ability and the opportunity to reach fifth- or sixth-grade levels in some areas of learning.

Inherited potential is only one of the factors involved in determining how much any given child will be able to achieve. Motivation, attention span, level of anxiety, parental attitude, community facilities, and proper guidance are extremely important to the retarded child, just as they are to the normal child. Simple tasks which the normal child learns quickly will often be major accomplishments for the child with Down's syndrome. Self-help skills, such as toilet training and learning to dress, may take years to learn as each task is broken down into specific, clearly defined steps programmed into a pattern of learning responses. Routine, structure, and clear expectations are vital to learning. Love, patience, consistency in expectations and in limit setting are essential to the success and happiness of the child with Down's syndrome.

At best, children with this disorder can be expected to work under the close supervision of an understanding adult when they are given clear, simple, repetitive tasks to perform. As adults, they may become employable in a sheltered, workshoplike setting. They may be semi-independent, but they will require some outside supervision all their lives. In view of this, the question of institutionalization or residential placement will probably arise at some time in infancy or childhood as the family tries to decide what is best to do. No quick answers can be given. Usually, the longer these children are able to be with their natural family in a home situation, the greater advantage they have of feeling loved, wanted, and part of a family.

In some situations where family tension is great, where there are other pressures of additional children or relatives, poor com-

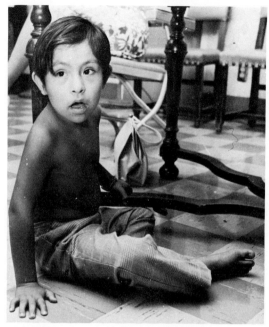

fig. 28-7 Boy with Down's syndrome. Sometimes light speckles in the iris, called Brushfield's spots, can be seen. The child's vision is often poor because of eye muscle imbalance or because of a refractory error. (*Courtesy of The National Foundation—March of Dimes.*)

fig. 28-6 Girl with Down's syndrome. Note the small round head with a flat broad face and flat nasal bridge. Epicanthic folds at the inner corner of the eyelids give a slanting appearance to the eyes, resulting in the misnaming of the syndrome "mongolism." (*Courtesy of The National Foundation—March of Dimes.*)

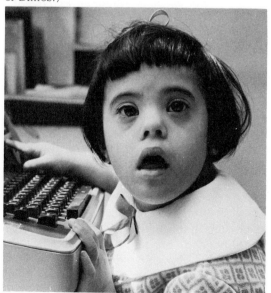

munity facilities, or other problems, foster care or residential placement may be the best answer. Each child's situation must be handled on an individual basis.

COMMUNITY RESOURCES Community agencies, parents' groups and the local chapter of The American Association for Retarded Children can provide considerable support and guidance. The local school system in almost every county can make arrangements for school attendance in special classes within the community. Special education teachers trained in working with retarded persons are often available for consultation. Nurses, whether in the doctor's office, in the hospital, or in the home, can provide considerable help to the family

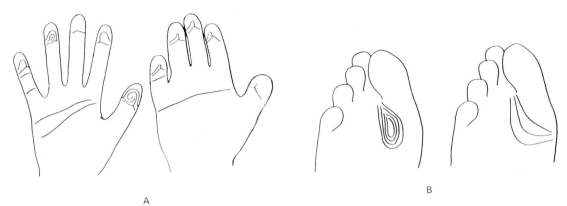

A   B

fig. 28-8 (a) Comparison of handprints and footprints. The left handprint of a normal child shows whorls on the thumb, a radial loop in the index finger, and ulnar loops on the ring and little fingers. There are two flexures in the little finger and two palmar creases. Hands of children with Down's syndrome show many more ulnar loops and most have a single ("simian") palmar crease. The hands of Down's syndrome patients are often short and stubby, with little fingers curving inward. (b) The left foot of a normal child shows characteristic whorls or loops in the "ball" of the foot, called the hallucal area. Foot of Down's syndrome child shows tibial arches instead of whorls or loops in the same area. (Courtesy of The National Foundation—March of Dimes.)

because of their knowledge of growth and development and their communication skills.

trisomy 18 About one in 3000 infants born alive has trisomy 18.[12] The karyotype shows either a complete or partial extra chromosome 18, making three rather than two chromosomes 18 and resulting in a total chromosomal count of 47, rather than the normal 46. Babies with trisomy 18, like those with trisomy 21, tend to be born to older mothers. Infant girls seems to be affected by this syndrome more than boys. Low birth weight, hypotonia, weak cry, a severely receding chin (which makes sucking difficult), and low-set, malformed ears are characteristic. Because the ears and the kidneys develop at the same period in embryonic life, frequently kidney abnormalities are also noted. Extra fingers, overlapping fingers, and rocker-bottom feet are very typical of children with trisomy 18.

The nurse working in the newborn nursery is sometimes the first person to discover a chromosomal abnormality such as trisomy 18. It may be possible to miss the clues to abnormality in the initial delivery room check of the newborn infant, but in the nursery, the infant may fail to suck well, may have a peculiar cry, or may be hypotonic. Since not all newborn infants with trisomy 18 appear grossly deformed, this condition could possibly go undetected without alert observation. Babies with trisomy 18, like all infants with genetic and congenital abnormalities, present difficult nursing-care problems. Intake of nourishment poses a problem because sucking is poor and the infant tires before having eaten enough. Intravenous administration of fluids is frequently necessary. Respiratory failure is also likely, because of hypotonia.

The nurse must also cope with her or his own feelings about the birth of an atypical infant who is doomed to have lifetime problems. The life expectancy of babies with trisomy 18 is usually short, and most infants with this condition die before reaching their first birthday. Some live through the first few years of life but require residential placement because of severe mental and physical retardation.

trisomy 13 to 15   Another chromosomal disorder is trisomy 13 to 15, so named because chromosomes 13, 14, and 15 look so much alike that it is hard to distinguish one from another. In trisomy 13 to 15, there is an extra chromosome of this group, so that the total chromosomal count is 47 rather than 46, but just which one is present in triplet form is uncertain. Infants with this syndrome are frequently severely deformed, with gross abnormalities involving the eyes, head, or any of the major organs.[13]

Two-thirds of these infants have severe cleft palate and cleft lip (Fig. 28-9). The nurse must recognize that cleft palate does not always mean that the infant has a trisomy of this type, but a trisomy cannot be ruled out because the cleft palate is not present.

Most often infants having trisomy 13 to 15 die in the first few months of life because so many major organs are abnormal. Should the infant live, medical and ethical problems sometimes arise about what treatment measures should be undertaken, especially whether surgical intervention and cosmetic reconstructions should be attempted. Is it morally right to go to great length to attempt to perform plastic repairs and organ transplants, for example, on an infant who is destined to be severely retarded and deformed? On the other hand, is it humane to allow an infant, no matter how different from normal, to survive with difficulty in eating or some other major discomfort when intervention could relieve the distress? Such questions as these come to mind and must be carefully considered. In most circumstances, if medical or surgical intervention promotes comfort or helps the parents to feel less anxiety without creating false hope, it is undertaken.

cri-du-chat syndrome   In 1963, several infants and children were found to have been born with severe psychomotor retardation, small head, hypertelorism (widely separated eyes), small face, and low-set ears. The cry

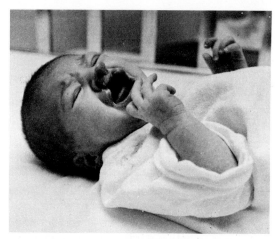

fig. 28-9   Severe cleft lip and palate. (*Courtesy The National Foundation—March of Dimes.*)

of such a child is a characteristic meowing like the sound of a hungry lost kitten. Hence the name *cri-du-chat* (French for "cry of the cat") is given to this syndrome, which results from a missing part (deletion) of chromosome 5. Although cute at birth and in early childhood, these children often grow to become less attractive or even severely enough handicapped in appearance by facial disproportions to require later surgery for cosmetic purposes. The catlike cry is lost after a year or two, but mental retardation persists throughout life.

nursing support of the mother   In the past, it frequently was the practice not to allow mothers to see their newborn infants if they were deformed. Nurses and physicians thought it was kind to spare the mother. This practice has changed in recent years after recognition that not permitting a new mother to see her deformed infant may create greater anxiety than she would have if she had seen the child. The imagination is sometimes much more cruel than the reality. Careful preparation and support are necessary before bringing such a baby to the awaiting parents. It is important to listen with quiet empathy and to accept their reactions and feelings, no matter what they may be.

Nurses must be careful not to impose their own feelings and values on the already burdened parents. They must provide reassurance when it is realistic to do so, but they should not give false hope. With the permission of the physician, referral can be made to agencies such as the National Foundation, local parent groups, and other resources, including religious affiliations. An understanding of the parents' reaction to the birth of a defective child, as well as an understanding of the grief and mourning process, is essential to the nurse who works with parents and their handicapped children or who in any way is involved with genetic counseling.[14]

sex chromosomal abnormalities

Turner's syndrome   Changes in the sex chromosomes have different effects from those of autosomal defects. An error involving the X or Y chromosomes results in a sex chromosomal abnormality. *Turner's syndrome* is a chromosomal disorder in which one of the X chromosomes is missing (see Fig. 28-10). Total chromosomal count is therefore on 45 instead of 46, and the karyotype is 45XO. The affected female is short, squat, and obese, with a thick neck, shieldlike chest with widely-spaced nipples, and very poor breast development (Fig. 28-11). The ovaries, if present, are poorly formed and usually do not function normally, so that usually the patient is not fertile.

These little girls generally grow into adults unless they have a cardiac defect, which sometimes accompanies Turner's syndrome. Mental retardation is lifelong, and most persons with Turner's syndrome are found in institutions by the time they become adults.

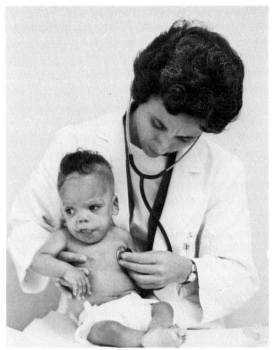

fig. 28-10   Turner's syndrome, 7-month-old infant. (*Courtesy of The National Foundation— March of Dimes.*)

This trend may change in the future as better community facilities for special education become available and as the public becomes more informed about and tolerant of individuals who are in need of special guidance at some point in their lives. Other atypical forms of Turner's syndrome exist but will not be discussed here.

triple X syndrome   About one in 1200 newborn girls has 47XXX. Since there appear to be no clinical symptoms, the condition usually goes undetected. In general, the more X chromosomes there are, the more likely it is that there will be mental retardation.

Klinefelter's syndrome   In one study, about 1 in 200 boys was born with an extra X chromosome and a karyotype of 47XXY.[15]

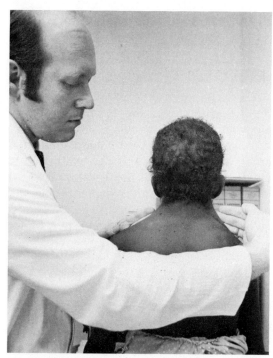

fig. 28-11 Turner's syndrome at 11 years of age, showing webbed neck. (*Courtesy of The National Foundation—March of Dimes.*)

Other studies indicate an incidence of 1: 1000.[16] The 47XXY karyotype is called Klinefelter's syndrome, a condition not usually very apparent until puberty. At that time the boy begins to develop secondary female sex characteristics such as breast enlargement, wide hips, high-pitched voice, and absence of typical male hair distribution (Fig. 28-12). The penis is usually normal, but the testes remain undeveloped at less than 2 cm diameter. Testosterone levels do not reach adult values, sperm is not produced, and the boy remains unfertile. However, ejaculate is formed, and the young man is usually not impotent.

The youth with Klinefelter's syndrome has a lanky appearance with long arms and legs but has poor muscle development. Although many with the syndrome may be somewhat

retarded, there is a wide range of IQ noted in such persons. Hormones may improve general male appearance but will not alter the underlying chromosomal abnormality. It should be noted that these individuals should not be assumed to have homosexual behavior, which is most likely psychosocial in orgin.

XYY syndrome Another disorder of the male sex chromosome is the 47XYY or "Superman" syndrome. In the first studies, a number of tall, well-coordinated, muscular, and aggressive men were found to have the XYY syndrome. Since these studies were done on

fig. 28-12 Klinefelter's syndrome. (*Courtesy of The National Foundation—March of Dimes.*)

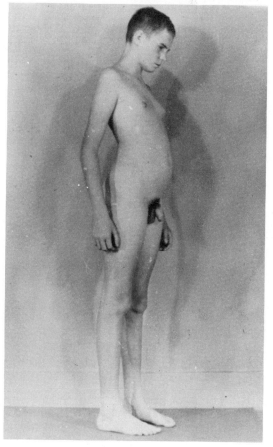

men in prison for aggressive crimes, the first assumption was that criminal behavior might be influenced by the extra Y chromosome. Further studies have shown that there is no indication that such behavior is at all related to the extra Y.

The incidence is thought to be one in 1000. Screening for the Y chromosome became possible after a portion of the cell bearing the Y chromosome was found to receive a fluorescent stain. Thus the name *F body*. When two F bodies are found in one cell, two Y chromosomes will be found on analysis (Table 28-5).

AUTOSOMAL RECESSIVE DISORDERS OF MOLECULAR ORIGIN: SINGLE GENE DEFECTS

An increased understanding of molecular biology and the genetic code has led to current knowledge and discovery of hundreds of disorders which result either from the failure to inherit particular genes required to make specific enzymes or from irregularities in the enzyme function itself. These disorders, called *inborn errors in metabolism*, IEM, (or

table 28-5 Chromosomal disorders and their characteristic symptoms

chromosomal disorder	characteristic symptoms

Trisomy 21 (Down's syndrome)	Flat, round face
	Depressed nasal bridge
	Protruding tongue
	Epicanthal folds and
	  Brushfield's spots
	Short neck
	Thick trunk and short stature
	Broad hands with simian
	  crease
	Hypotonia
	Mental retardation

Trisomy 18 (Edwards's syndrome)	Failure to thrive Difficulty in sucking Small face, receding chin Low-set, malformed ears Kidney or cardiac abnormalities Overlapping fingers Rocker-bottom feet Hypotonia Mental retardation
Trisomy 13-15 (Patau's syndrome)	Failure to thrive Microphthalmia Cerebral dysgenesis Cleft palate and lip Congenital heart condition Polydactyly Deformed extremities (Note: Symptoms vary; gross deformities are common.)

disorders of molecular origin), are transmitted by the *autosomal recessive* mode of Mendel's laws of inheritance, with a few sex-linked exceptions.

Autosomal recessive transmission means that both parents are carriers (heterozygotes) of the disorder but appear normal themselves. Since they each have one of the genes in a given pair, they have enough of the genetic information necessary for making a particular enzyme. Hence, phenotypically, they themselves have no overt signs of disease, and without symptoms of illness, they lead normal lives. A problem only arises if two carriers of the same defect mate. Then, for every pregnancy, the statistical probabilities are that one in four will have the disorder, two in four will be carriers, and one in four will be unaffected (see Table 28-2).

Since most people do not know if they are carriers of a disorder, the chances of having an affected child is usually not known until after the birth. The probabilities of two carriers mating is only about one in 12,000 for the general population, but since people tend to mate with those who have similar racial, religious, and cultural backgrounds, the chances are higher for some groups and

chromosomal disorder	characteristic symptoms
Deletion of short arm of chromosome 5 (cri-du-chat)	Failure to thrive Round face with low-set ears Hypertelorism Microencephaly Mental retardation "Cat cry" Sucking difficulty
Turner's syndrome (45XO)	Often not detected until puberty Sort stature Lack of secondary female sex characteristics Shield chest Web neck Infertility Mental retardation (mild)
Klinefelter's syndrome (47XXY)	Often not detected until puberty Secondary female characteristics in male Infertility Poor development of male characteristics Mild mental retardation (?)
Superman syndrome (47XYY)	Tall, muscular build Aggressiveness Acne persisting into adulthood Fertility unaffected

Source: Adapted from Ian Porter, *Heredity and Disease*, McGraw-Hill, New York, 1968.

conditions. For example, the incidence of PKU is extremely high among Pennsylvania Amish and fair-skinned northern Europeans, while Cooley's anemia is common among southern Europeans. Sickle-cell disease follows geographic lines as well and is more common in those whose ancestry is from central Africa (see Chap. 22). Finally, Tay-Sachs disease occurs predominately in Ashkenazic Jews throughout the world.

Many of these inborn errors of metabolism can be detected during the newborn period. The alert nurse in the nursery is usually the first to note changes or differences in the affected infant. Typical symptoms of many, but not all IEM, include vomiting, poor weight gain, failure to thrive, tremors, seizures, and strange-smelling urine or feces. Careful observation must be continued in well baby supervision, since some defects do not become evident until the infant is somewhat older or has changed diet.

Space does not permit a detailed discussion of inborn errors. The student should refer to Porter,[7] Stanbury and Wyngaarden,[17] and Nyhan[18] for further information. The important thing to remember is that many of the inborn errors involve the chemistry of proteins, lipids, or carbohydrates and, if detected early, are treatable so that gross defects can often be prevented.

inborn errors of amino acid metabolism

phenylketonuria The child who has phenylketonuria (PKU) is missing the enzyme *phenylalanine hydroxylase,* which converts the amino acid phenylalanine to tyrosine. Because this conversion cannot take place, excess phenylalanine accumulates in the blood. In an attempt to get rid of the excess, the body converts it to phenylpyruvic and phenylacetic acid, which are excreted in the urine. The nurse can test for these substances in the urine with Phenistix or by the ferric chloride test; if present, a bright blue-green spot will appear. Such a urine test is usually not positive in the early days, since adequate milk intake is necessary before buildup of metabolic products occurs.

In all but a few states, PKU blood testing in the nursery is mandatory before discharge. Fair-skinned infants should regularly be retested at the first pediatric visit since, occasionally, a test will become positive after the first week of life. PKU is present if blood phenylalanine levels are above 8 mg/100 mL by any of the three methods of testing: Guthrie, La Due, or McCann Robins.

Treatment involves reducing phenylalanine intake by using *Lofenalac* formula, never giving regular milk or protein foods, and carefully measuring all fruits and vegetables, since almost no food is free of this amino acid. Without proper treatment the probability is very great that the child will become severely retarded.[19] Rigid dietary treatment is absolutely essential, and places a great demand on the family. A supportive, well-informed nurse can be very helpful to the family during this time. In late childhood, it is possible to allow more freedom in the diet, but the woman who has PKU should again be careful in phenylalanine intake if she becomes pregnant.

maple sugar urine disease Another inborn error involving amino acid metabolism is a disorder in which infants excrete urine which has a characteristic "maple syrup" smell. Because of problems involving the metabolism of amino acids *leucine, isoleucine,* and *valine,* failure to thrive, seizures, and metabolic imbalance are apparent in the newborn. Unless this disease is detected early, the infant will die. Blood levels for these amino acids must be measured several times a day, and a special formula, calculated by the pharmacist to replace each amino acid, must be given. After several months, a few new foods can be slowly added. Fortunately, with proper dietary treatment, mental retardation and seizures can be prevented.

histidinemia and homocystinuria Histidinemia involves a defect in the metabolism of histidine and is characterized by mild mental retardation and hearing and speech defects. Homocystinuria causes mental retardation and defects in the lens of the eye, plus other eye problems. Failure to thrive, seizures, and hepatosplenomegaly also indicate its presence. A diet low in *methionine,* an amino acid precurser of homocystine, has been used in some children, but there is still insufficient data to assess the value of the results. In some types of homocystinuria, vitamin B_6 in large doses appears to be helpful.

inborn errors of lipid metabolism

Defects in lipid metabolism are also called lipid storage diseases or cerebral-macular degenerative disorders. Inherited as autosomal recessive defects, they involve some abnormality in the production or storage of lipid in the viscera, the brain, or both. While there are many similarities among all these disorders, each has its own specific facets and particular enzyme defect. In general, the storage of an abnormal amount or form of lipid is responsible for the damage to the brain and other involved tissues.

In addition to the classical form of Tay-Sachs, there are three variants of the disease which have a later onset. All involve a cherry-red spot in the macula, seizures, loss of mental and motor abilities, and eventually death.

Until recently, little could be done for the affected individuals. Within the last few years, advances have been made in the detection of carriers, and the affected fetus can now be identified, using amniotic fluid. Treatment in terms of cure is not possible yet for infants with Tay-Sachs disease, but there is some hope of arresting symptoms in Gaucher's disease.[20]

Tay-Sachs disease Found primarily among Ashkenazic Jews throughout the world, this disease does occasionally occur in other races. The infant appears normal at birth and develops normally for the first few months. By 6 months to 1 year, failure to thrive becomes apparent, and a regression occurs, with inability to sit or do any of the previously developed activities. Progressive degeneration continues, with blindness, seizures, and paralysis. Death occurs within 1 to 5 years because there is no treatment.[21]

Carriers can be detected by blood levels of the enzyme *Hexosaminidase A,* commonly called Hex A. Amniocentesis is then advisable for the pregnant woman when both parents are carriers. In many communities, screening is being done under the auspices of the National Foundation-March of Dimes, the Tay-Sachs Association, or other community groups. Genetic counseling can be made available for those who discover that they are carriers.[22]

Gaucher's disease Gaucher's disease is really a group of four varieties of autosomal recessive disorders and is diagnosed by the deficiency of the enzyme *β-glucoside.* As a result the lipid *glucocerebroside* is stored in abnormal amounts in brain, bone, liver, and spleen. In children, the brain and liver are most involved. In adults, the bone is most likely to be involved. Treatment has become possible within the last few years through injection of a human enzyme obtained from aborted fetuses. This enzyme prevents the development of symptoms for many years.

Thus the recent advances in understanding Gaucher's disease offer a real breakthrough in the future of treatment for such genetic disorders.

inborn errors of carbohydrate metabolism

galactosemia Because an enzyme, *galactose L-phosphate uridyl transferase,* is missing, the infant cannot tolerate lactose, a disaccharide milk sugar. To be utilized, lactose must be converted to the monosaccharides, glucose and galactose. This step is accomplished in the affected child, but the next step is hindered. The enzyme is necessary for galactose to be converted to glucose. Only glucose can enter the Kreb's cycle to be converted to ATP, CO_2, and H_2O; consequently, galactose builds up in the blood and finally spills into the urine. High levels of galactose produce severe vomiting and refusal to eat, with resulting failure to thrive, weight loss, dehydration and severe seizures, hepatosplenomegaly, and cataracts. Symptoms may begin after the first feeding of almost any milk formula, but especially after breast milk because of its higher lactose content.

If the symptoms are recognized early and treatment is initiated, brain damage, mental retardation, and blindness can be prevented. Treatment consists of a low-galactose formula at first. As the infant matures, puddings, cake mixes, cream soups, meat from milk-fed animals (veal), or any commercial foods containing galactose (or lactose) must be avoided. It is important to teach the mother to read labels carefully. Again as the child grows up, foods with low levels of these substances can be introduced carefully.

congenital carbohydrate malabsorption problems There are several genetically related problems of carbohydrate malabsorption in which too much sugar given to the infant produces severe vomiting, diarrhea, and colic. Symptoms are often most severe about 3 months of age but may certainly occur earlier. These disorders are caused by specific enzymatic problems in the absorption or utilization of disaccharides. It is the combination of genetic predisposition and dietary habits that produces overt symptoms. The treatment is to reduce carbohydrate in the diet with CHO-free formula and CHO-modified diet in later infancy and childhood.

glycogen storage disorders When the body has elevated glucose levels, it converts the glucose and stores it as glycogen. As energy is required, glycogen is converted back to glucose. Problems may occur anywhere in this process, and the ten or more disorders are all carried as autosomal recessive traits. Symptoms include seizures, mental retardation, and developmental or learning disabilities. To date, there is no specific treatment for Von Gierke's syndrome, Pompe's syndrome, and glycogenoses, types I through IX.

MULTIFACTORIAL POLYGENIC INHERITANCE

There are many conditions which "run in families." Until recently, it was thought that this occurred by chance, but now it is known that some types of birth defects, such as cleft lip and palate (CLP), hydrocephaly with spina bifida, congenital hip dislocation, and pyloric stenosis, are produced by polygenic inheritance. In this type of inheritance, more than one pair of genes, and probably several different genes on several different chromosomes, play a role in the presence or absence of the defect. In addition, specific environmental factors also contribute to the development of the entity. In some instances, nutrition, poor intrauterine environment, toxins, medications, hormones, and pollution are important variables which either foster or inhibit the expression of gene potential, leading then to normality or pathology.

Because so many factors are involved, there is no clear-cut absolute probability for the development of the defects, but for any specific family, there are statistical methods that the genetic counselor can use to predict the likely risk of a repeated occurrence. In general, the more close relatives who have the condition, the greater is the probability of recurrence in future offspring. For example, if two children in a family are already affected with spina bifida, the probability of a third child with this defect is twice that of a family that has only one child with such a disorder (see Fig. 29-8).

Given an accurate, detailed family history and data to work out a pedigree, the genetic counselor can predict the likely probabilities of having another defective child. For example, in the general population, there is a one in 1000 risk of having a child with cleft lip and palate, and yet the child with the CLP has a 3 percent chance of having another sibling and a 10 percent chance of having offspring with the defect.

In addition to birth defects, there are many acquired chronic conditions which are of polygenetic multifactorial inheritance. Diabetes, arthritis, hypertension, and most probably, cancer are included.

AUTOSOMAL DOMINANT INHERITANCE

Some conditions involving body structure, such as extra fingers or some types of dwarfism, are passed down from generation to generation with a 1:2 probability of inheriting the defect if one parent has the condition (Fig.

28-13). These are autosomal dominant conditions and always involve morphology. Usually these disorders are minor, for if they were major, there would be poor chances of survival to reproductive age.

Even if such conditions involve more extensive structure, e.g., achondroplasia, it is still usually possible for affected individuals to cope satisfactorily with their environment. The achondroplastic dwarf is capable of making the necessary adjustments to survive physically, emotionally, and socially. Such dwarfs participate in society and would go unnoticed except for their size and shape.

One exception to the usually minor nature of autosomal dominant conditions is Huntington's chorea, a neurologic degenerative disorder developing in middle adulthood. The disease progresses to eventual paralysis and death. Since symptoms do not develop until later in life, it is highly probable that a person

fig. 28-13 Mendel's inheritance pattern. In this tracing of a family's inheritance pattern the dominant (D) gene would be passed from the heterozygous father to two out of four possible offspring. The mother is homozygous for a recessive trait (r).

	D (dominant)	r (recessive) ♂
r	Dr	rr
r	Dr	rr
♀		

with Huntington's chorea will have children before symptoms develop. There is a 50 percent chance that the affected genetic material will be passed to the offspring. Currently, research is being done to attempt to diagnose this condition much earlier so that both treatment and genetic counseling will be of greater value.

SEX-LINKED GENETIC DISORDERS

Another group of inherited disorders comprises those which are *sex-linked*. Sex-linked conditions are transmitted by mothers to sons. The woman is a heterozygote in the sex-linked conditions. The genes for these disorders are located on the X chromosomes. Since a woman has two X chromosomes, if a gene on one of them is missing, one-half of her sons will have the disorder. If a son inherits the X chromosome with the missing gene, he will have the disorder because the male karyotype is XY. If he inherits the normal chromosome, he will be normal. Naturally, half the daughters of a woman heterozygous for sex-linked disorders will be carriers. No daughters will have the disorder, since the father will have contributed a normal X chromosome. Sex-linked conditions include classic hemophilia, Duchenne's muscular dystrophy, and Lesch-Nyhan syndrome.

ENVIRONMENTAL FACTORS INFLUENCING GENETIC HEALTH AND FETAL GROWTH

We now know that many factors in the environment produce mutation through a change in the genes themselves, as dictated by a "mistake" or change in the DNA itself. A genetic change, i.e., a change in the genetic material itself, in turn alters body chemistry and metabolism. It is conceivable that a mutation could in some instances be positive, i.e., helpful. In human beings at least, such changes are difficult to detect. The mutations that are noticed and are of concern are the harmful ones. As stated previously, they may result in inborn errors of metabolism which could be passed on to offspring.

A defect in body structure and form that is due to environmental problems which alter the growth of the fetus after fertilization is termed a *congenital defect* or *anomaly*. Those chemicals or viruses which cause damage are called *teratogenic* agents. The same kinds of agents which produce damage to an egg or a sperm prior to fertilization (resulting in genetic defects) can also produce damage to somatic cells of the developing baby after fertilization (resulting in congenital defects). Let us look at some of the agents which produce genetic change and congenital abnormalities.

radiation

Radiation of all types presents a potential hazard. The risk is proportional to the amount of radiation and the length of exposure, as well as to the nature of the particular tissue involved. Rapidly growing and immature cells are particularly vulnerable to radiation. Thus ova, sperm, fetal cells, and blood cells are most susceptible to radiation damage. This was demonstrated unfortunately by the hundreds of survivors of two atomic bomb attacks, who show more chromosomal breaks and have a higher incidence of leukemia than the general population. X-rays in the early weeks of pregnancy can damage the developing fetus: thus x-rays for diagnostic purposes should be avoided if at all possible and should be considered only with careful precaution.[23] Prior to pregnancy, a person (either male or female) should avoid overexposure to x-rays. Lead aprons should be worn by nurses and technicians who are frequently exposed to radiation in the x-ray department when they assist patients during the taking of x-rays.

Emissions from microwave ovens, cosmic radiation, ultraviolet radiation, and perhaps even radar and sonar may pose potential hazard. Often cells damaged by such agents repair themselves before producing offspring, but under some circumstances mutations can be induced by the types of radiation mentioned, and then the mutant cell will produce abnormal offspring. Much of this radiation is present in our natural environment from solar and other astronomic sources independent of humans. We are more concerned with human-made radiation hazards and other dangerous sources of genetic change in the environment as a result of poor control of industrial and other wastes.

industrial pollution

In the long run, atomic power may be less of a potential hazard than some forms of chemical and industrial pollution. Hydrocarbons, plastics, insecticides, and metals such as lead, copper, and mercury are known to be associated with birth defects. Birth defects among children born to parents who work in lead mines have been reported in Germany and elsewhere. Styrene and other chemicals used in the making of plastics have been known to induce leukemia in fetuses and in adults.

nutritional deficiency

Nutritional deficiency during pregnancy may be the cause of some birth defects. Spina bifida, meningomyelocele, and cleft palate with harelip have been produced in laboratory animals lacking vitamin C in their diet. On the other hand, Cooke[24] reports that excessive vitamin A and also lack of vitamin B may produce similar results in rats and mice. McKibbin and Porter[25] report vitamin C deficiency in human children with myelomeningiocele which seems to be related not to poor diet but to failure to use vitamin C in the body once it is ingested. What relationship the faulty vitamin C metabolism may have in terms of cause or effect remains unclear.

drugs

Any drug given during pregnancy, especially in the early weeks, could endanger the fetus. LSD, barbiturates, caffeine, and cyclamates have been known to cause chromosomal breakage, which could result in severe birth defects of the skeletal, nervous, and cardiovascular systems. Thalidomide, used as a mild tranquilizer by pregnant women in Europe, is known to have been responsible for the production of hundreds of children without arms or legs. It is ironic to think that the very drug that was intended to help their mothers maintain better equilibrium during pregnancy results in a lifetime of misfortune for them. Steroids rank high among the problem drugs. A single dose of testosterone given to a mother who is spotting early in pregnancy may produce ambiguous genitalia and adrenal cortical hyperplasia in the female fetus. Additional examples of how drugs may affect the fetus are given in Chap. 20, where drug implications for the infant are discussed.

viruses

Viruses are great inducers of genetic change. Since a virus is either RNA or DNA enclosed in a protein coat and contains no ribosomes or mitochondria, it injects its genetic material into the living cell it invades, then takes over the cell to reproduce itself. In doing so, it alters the normal arrangement of the cellular DNA. If the cell lives, it grows and reproduces abnormal cells altered by the virus. Mutant cells may be involved in some malignant disorders and may contribute to the uncontrolled carcinogenic process. Viral infections may well prove to be a contributing factor in some forms of leukemia. Rubella virus, cytomegalic inclusion virus, and herpes virus are especially detrimental to the human fetus (see Chap. 25).

GENETICS, THE NURSE, AND THE FUTURE

Prenatal care and family health care can contribute much to the prevention of congenital and genetic defects. If one knows a person's whole family and understands something about the family background and history, it is possible to make some speculations about the kinds of health (and especially gene associated) disorders most likely to develop. Communication skills and a basic nurse-patient relationship which involves trust are essential for gathering much of the data required about a family in order to give appropriate genetic counseling of a more involved nature. Current techniques in amniocentesis and cytology have contributed methods for detecting problems during early fetal life with little risk to mother or fetus. During these procedures the nurse must give support and understanding to help alleviate fear.

As knowledge about enzyme structure and activity increases, it may become possible in the future to make artificial enzymes, just as insulin is given as a substitute in the diabetic. These enzymes may then be used to treat individuals with inborn errors of metabolism, just as diabetics are currently being given

medical treatment and nursing guidance. Genetic engineering may come about in the future, though man probably will never control intelligence or make a "super race" in test tubes as the science fiction writers would have us expect. Psychologic characteristics are either multigenetic (meaning that they involve complex interaction of many genes which man cannot duplicate) or they are influenced greatly by environment. Future treatment of a number of diseases (hemophilia, cystic fibrosis, sickle-cell anemia, and possibly even Tay-Sachs disease, leukemia, and other malignancies induced by interactions of heredity and environment) does fall within the potential reality of genetics in the near future. What role nurses will have in this exciting future depends upon their own willingness to become invloved.

study questions

1 Differentiate between a gene and a chromosome.
2 Define the following terms:

allele	locus
operator gene	regulator gene
homozygote	heterozygote
phenotype	genotype

3 Chart the probabilities of inheritance for the child for the following characteristics (use the sample in Fig. 28-13):
  a The father is heterozygous for brown eyes, and the mother has blue eyes (see Table 28-2).
  b The father carries a recessive gene for PKU and so does the mother.
  c The father is not a carrier at all, but the mother has an autosomal recessively carried disease (such as sickle-cell anemia).
4 Describe the function of enzymes in the body. What does the statement "one gene–one function" or "one gene–one enzyme" describe?
5 List the signs of Down's syndrome which would be observed in a newborn infant. As the child grew, what further problems would appear?
6 Differentiate between trisomy 18, 13 to 15, and cri-du-chat syndrome as far as observable signs in the nursery.
7 Read an article by either Drotar, Floyd, or Young,

and identify the nursing interventions you would use in caring for a mother whose infant has a birth defect.

8 What are the typical IEM symptoms that can be noted in the newborn nursery.

9 Differentiate between autosomal recessive and dominant inheritance. Compare these types with multifactorial polygenetic inheritance patterns.

10 Read current newspapers for items about environmental factors which adversely influence fetal health. How would you counsel a pregnant woman on exposure to these agents?

references

1 Julian Huxley and H. B. Kettelwell, *Charles Darwin and His World,* Random House, New York, 1965.

2 J. M. Barry, *Molecular Biology and Chemical Control of Living Cells,* Prentice-Hall, Englewood Cliffs, N.J., 1964, pp. 44–56.

3 George Beadle, *The Language of Life,* Doubleday, Garden City, N.Y., 1966.

4 Victor McKusick, *Human Genetics,* Prentice-Hall, Englewood Cliffs, N.J., 1965, p. 10.

5 Alex Fraser, *Computer Genetics,* McGraw-Hill, New York, 1970.

6 Victor McKusick, op. cit., p. 5.

7 Ian Porter, *Heredity and Disease,* McGraw-Hill, New York, 1968, pp. 42–50.

8 Kay Corman Kintzel and Delores Lake, "Medical Genetics and the Nurse," in Kay Corman Kintzel et al., *Advanced Concepts in Clinical Nursing,* 2d ed., Lippincott, Philadelphia, 1977, pp. 109–163.

9 *Chromosome 21 and Its Association with Down's Syndrome,* The National Foundation—March of Dimes, New York, N.Y.

10 Ian Porter, op. cit., pp. 42–43.

11 Ibid., p. 244.

12 Ibid., p. 53.

13 Ibid., pp. 54–55.

14 R. K. Young, "Chronic Sorrow: Parents Response to Birth of a Child with a Defect," *MCN,* **2**(1):38, January/February, 1977.

15 F. Sergovich, et al., "Chromosomal Aberrations in 2,159 Consecutive Births," *New England Journal of Medicine,* Apr. 17, 1969, pp. 851–855.

16 I. Porter, "The Clinical Side of Cytogenetics, *Journal of Reproductive Medicine,* **17**(1):10, July 1976.

17 J. B. Stanbury and J. B. Wyngaarden, *The Metabolic Basis of Inherited Disease,* McGraw-Hill, New York, 1969.

18 W. L. Nyhan, *Amino Acid Metabolism and Genetic Variation,* McGraw-Hill, New York, 1967.

19 D. Lake, "Nursing Implications from an Investigation of Diet, Development and Mothering to Two Groups of Children with Phenylketonuria," in *ANA Clinical Sessions, 1968,* Appleton-Century-Crofts, New York, 1968.

20 A. Gerbie et el., "Amniocentesis in Genetic Counseling," *American Journal of Obstetrics and Gynecology,* **109**(5):765–768, 1971.

21 H. L. Nadler, "Intrauterine Detection of Genetic Disorders," in J. P. Greenhill (ed.), *Yearbook of Obstetrics and Gynecology,* Yearbook, Chicago, 1972.

22 Porter, op. cit., p. 418.

23 J. Sternberg, "Irradiation and Radio Contamination during Pregnancy," *American Journal of Obstetrics and Gynecology,* **108**(3):490–495, 1970.

24 R. Cooke, *The Biologic Basis of Pediatric Practice,* McGraw-Hill, New York, 1968.

25 B. McKibbin, and R. Porter, "The Incidence of Vitamin C Deficiency in Meningomyelocele," *Developmental Medicine and Child Neurology,* **9**:338–344, 1967.

bibliography

Asimov, I. *The Genetic Code,* Signet Books, New American Library, New York, 1962.

Becker, K.: "Successful Use of Therapeutic Androgenization in Klinefelter's Syndrome," *Modern Medicine,* Nov. 13, 1972, p. 57.

Brady, R.: "Hereditary Fat Metabolism Diseases," *Scientific American,* August 1973, pp. 88–97.

Brown, D.: "The Isolation of Genes," *Scientific American,* August 1973, pp. 20–30.

Drotar, D., A. Baskiewicz, N. Irvin, J. Kennell, and M. Klaus: "The Adaptation of Parents to the Birth of an Infant with a Congenital Malformation: A Hypothetical Model" *Pediatrics* **56**(5):710, November 1975.

Eppink, H.: "Genetic Causes of Abnormal Fetal Development and Inherited Disease," *Journal of Obstetric, Gynecologic, and Neonatal Nursing,* **6**(6):14, 1977.

Ferreira, A. J.: *Prenatal Environment,* Thomas, Springfield, Ill., 1969.

Floyd, C. C.: "A Defective Child Is Born: A Study of Newborns With Spina Bifida and Hydrocephalus," *Journal of Obstetric, Gynecologic, and Neonatal Nursing,* **6**(4): 56, July/August 1977.

Hecht, F.: "Genetic Diagnosis in the Newborn," *Pediatric Clinics of North America,* **17**:1039, 1970.

Marshall, D.: "Congenital Cytomegalovirus Infection" *Nursing Mirror,* **142**:49, January 3, 1976.

Nadler, H.: "Prenatal Diagnosis of Inborn Defects," *Hospital Practice,* June 1975, p. 41.

Nitowsky, H. M.: "Prenatal Diagnosis of Genetic Abnormality," *American Journal of Nursing,* **71**:1551, 1971.

Reisman, L. E.: "Chromosomal Abnormalities and Intrauterine Growth Retardation," *Pediatric Clinics of North America,* **17:**101, 1970.

Rennert, O. M.: "Irradiation and Radiation Exposure", *Clinical Obstetrics and Gynecology* **18**(4):177, 1975.

Sparkles, R. S., and B. F. Crandall: "Genetic Disorders Affecting Growth and Development," chap. 4 in N. Assali (ed.), *Pathophysiology of Gestation: Fetal-Placental Disorders,* vol. 2, Academic Press, New York, 1972, pp. 208–64.

Watson, J.: *The Double Helix,* Signet Books, New American Library, New York, 1969.

Wilson, J. G.: "Environmental Effects on Development and Teratology," in Nicholas Assali (ed.), *Pathophysiology of Gestation: Fetal-Placental Disorders,* vol. 2, Academic Press, New York, 1972, chap. 5, pp. 270–314.

Winchester, A. M. *Human Genetics,* Merrill, Columbus, Ohio, 1971.

OTHER RESOURCES

National Foundation—March of Dimes
P. O. Box 2000, White Plains, N.Y. 10602

Ross Laboratores (Formula)
Columbus, Ohio 43216

Mead Johnson Company (Formula)
Evansville, Ind. 47721

Mental Retardation Abstracts
Department of Health, Education and Welfare
300 Independence Avenue, S.W.
Washington, D.C.

National Institutes of Health
Bethesda, Md.

National Society for Crippled Children and Adults
2023 West Ogden Ave.
Chicago, Ill. 60612

National Association for Retarded Children
420 Lexington Ave.
New York, N.Y. 10017

National Cystic Fibrosis Research Foundation
3379 Peachtree Road N.E.
Atlanta, Ga. 30326

29

THE HIGH-RISK FULL-TERM INFANT

MARVIN L. BLUMBERG

From the time that the ovum is fertilized until the fetus is delivered and the umbilical cord severed, this fetus has a parasitic existence inside the mother's uterus, where she nourishes it, breathes for it, and carries off its waste products. Yet, during that time the fetus must gradually mature in its structures and internal functions to utilize properly the nutrients and oxygen furnished to it and be able to convey away its waste products through the proper organs. Cerebral centers that control proper functioning, enzymes that affect digestion, absorption, and excretion of metabolic by-products, lungs that exchange carbon dioxide for oxygen, and a host of other mechanisms and structures must be mature enough and ready at the instant of birth to take over for the independent existence of the newborn.

Immaturity, dysfunction, or lack of any of the normal control functions may result in temporary or permanent damage to vital structures, especially to the brain. In recent years, medical research in the fields of neonatal physiology, biochemistry, and pharmacology has brought about sufficient expertise to help the prematurely born infant to survive by correcting, treating, or compensating for certain defects and deficiencies (see Chap. 30). This chapter discusses the medical problems of the full-term newborn that arise whenever there is difficulty in establishing and maintaining respiration, circulation, neurologic function, metabolic function, excretion, and immunologic defenses.

ESTABLISHING AND MAINTAINING RESPIRATION

The metabolic functions of all living cells are basically dependent upon an oxidation-reduction cycle. Oxygen from air inspired into the pulmonary alveoli osmoses into the surrounding capillaries, where it becomes united in a loose chemical bond with the hemoglobin of the circulating erythrocytes to form *oxyhemoglobin*.

fetal oxygenation

During fetal life, the oxygen enters through the mother's lungs, into her bloodstream to the placenta, where oxygen separates from the maternal oxyhemoglobin, passes through the maternal-fetal placental membrane, and is picked up by the fetal erythrocytes. In turn, carbon dioxide in the fetus is transported by the fetal erythrocytes and transferred to the maternal circulation through the placenta.

It must be quite apparent that the concentration of oxygen furnished to the fetus by the mother via the umbilical arteries is lower than the original arterial oxygen blood concentration in her circulation, for she has already used a considerable amount for her own needs. Two mechanisms enable the fetus to function at an average oxygen blood saturation of *40 to 60 percent*, whereas the newborn infant after several hours requires an average oxygen saturation of *85 to 90 percent*.

1   The fetus has a relative *polycythemia*, or increase in red blood cells, ranging from 4.5 to 6.5 million per cubic millimeter, with a hemoglobin content of 17 to 20 g/100 mL of blood. The number will drop off gradually in the postnatal period to a norm of 4 to 5 million red blood cells per cubic millimeter and 12 to 14 g hemoglobin per 100 mL. This *polycythemia* affords more erythrocytes for transport of the oxygen to the fetal body cells, to compensate for the reduced concentration of oxygen.
2   Fetal hemoglobin has a greater affinity and, therefore, a greater carrying capacity for oxygen, as well as a lower dissociation constant for fetal oxyhemoglobin than for postnatal oxyhemoglobin. The rate and the ease of reduction of fetal oxyhemoglobin are greater, thus furnishing oxygen more readily and more completely to the body cells.

Before 26 weeks of gestation the fetal lung is still very immature. Between 26 and 30 weeks, the lung is still weak and has only a small surface area for the exchange of gases. It is, however, rapidly developing an adequate capillary system. Between 31 and 36 weeks, there is considerable improvement in gas exchange ability and in total lung surface area. By 37 weeks there is enough mature alveoli formation for the lungs to function adequately for a term baby. Prior to 27 weeks of gestation it is difficult to sustain human independent life because of the poor ability of the existing alveolar functioning surface to oxygenate the blood, no matter how much oxygen is furnished to the infant. After 27 to 28 weeks of gestation, if no other abnormalities or severe dysfunctions exist, pulmonary aeration can more readily be accomplished.

initiation of respiration

As the mature fetus is about to be thrust into a postnatal independent existence, the combination of tactile and thermal stimuli upon the infant's skin produces an afferent-efferent reflex which causes a deep gasping breath and crying. Once established in the normal term baby, respiration will continue spontaneously through a combination of chemical stimulus to the respiratory center of the medulla by blood carbon dioxide level. Other regulatory mechanisms come into play as well, such as in the Hering-Breuer reflex, by which afferent branches of the vagus nerve situated in the pleura sense the degree of stretch of the lung. Inflation of the lung causes arrest of inspiration and allows expiration to follow. Then deflation of the lung stops expiration and initiates inspiration.

The first breath normally requires very high intrathoracic pressures in order to expand the totally collapsed alveoli. After the first expiration, the lungs retain up to 40 percent of the total lung volume as residual air. Subsequently, inspiratory pressures are far lower. Lung inflation can be demonstrated in a simple fashion by blowing up a round toy rubber balloon. It requires more effort to start the first expansion than to continue to expand the balloon with subsequent blowing breaths.

The phenomenon which enables an alveolus or a gas bubble of liquid to maintain its round shape and expansion is known as surface tension. In the mature alveolus expansion is maintained by a thin film of fluid, *surfactant*, a phospholipid, which reduces surface tension as the alveolar radius decreases during expiration, thus preventing collapse and retaining residual alveolar volume.

respiratory distress

Respiratory distress is a broadly descriptive term meaning increased effort of breathing. It may result from a number of causes, often interrelated, such as developmental immaturity, pharmacologic depression, and birth trauma.

respiratory distress syndrome Respiratory distress syndrome (RDS), often referred to as hyaline membrane disease, is a frequent cause of respiratory difficulty. Although RDS occurs most frequently in premature infants under 33 weeks of age, there are factors predisposing a full-term neonate to this condition, such as delivery by cesarean section, especially from a diabetic mother.

The incidence is estimated to be about 40,000 per year and until recently the mortality rate was about 30 percent. Today, if the infant is able to receive intensive care in neonatal centers, death rates have dropped to about 10 to 20 percent.[1] Infants who weigh less than 1500 g are most vulnerable.

Although small infants may have surfactant in their lungs at birth, a sufficient level and a rapid rate of synthesis must be maintained, at least at the start, or else alveoli will collapse after each breath. Alveolar collapse with each expiration causes hypoxemia, or lower oxygen concentration in the blood, which in turn will lead to acidosis and hypoglycemia. Reflexly, constriction of the pulmonary vasculature and diminished blood flow to the lungs occur with the result of further hypoxemia. Surfactant formation is further inhibited by hypoxemia, acidosis, and hypoglycemia, and transudation, or movement of fluid into the alveolar spaces, takes place. Respiratory exchange is progressively blocked and, if untreated, is likely to result in death. Postmortem microscopic examination of the lungs reveals an eosinophilic-staining amorphous hyaline membrane lining many of the alveoli. Thus, hyaline membrane is a result of the respiratory distress syndrome, not the cause.

PREVENTION OF RDS Since the small, immature infant is most likely to be affected, delaying preterm labor is the best preventive measure (see Chap. 26). Recently, treatment of the mother with corticosteroids just prior to preterm delivery has been proven somewhat effective in reducing RDS incidence. Such treatment is based on the empirical observation that in response to stress the fetal adrenals produced glucocorticoids, which in turn acted to speed lung maturity. To mimic this effect, betamethasone is administered to the mother. If enough time elapses prior to birth, e.g., more than 24 h, the benefit of speeded lung maturity and surfactant production seems to take place.

Liggens and Howie recommended the regimen of 12 mg betamethasone IM q24h × 2 at least 24 h before expected delivery.[2] If more than 24 h elapse, the incidence of RDS appears to be even lower. This effect is especially evident in infants weighing less than 1250 g.

other causes of respiratory distress Respiratory difficulty may also be caused by intrinsic pulmonary factors or extrinsic problems. Intrinsic disorders include primary *atelectasis*, or failure of a large number of alveoli to expand, *emphysema*, or overexpansion of a lung segment caused by a ball-valve type of obstruction of a bronchiole, *pneumatocele*, or cystic area within the lung, and pneumonia from aspiration of amniotic fluid or of an early oral feeding. These all produce difficulty in breathing because they diminish the gas-exchange ability by direct effect or by indirect compression effect.

Extrinsic disorders produce respiratory distress primarily by compression and displacement of a lung and/or the mediastinal structures. These include *herniation* of abdominal viscera into the thoracic cavity through a congenital defect in the diaphragm, *pneumothorax* (air in the pleural space), and *chylothorax* (free lymphatic fluid in the pleural space).

Congenital *choanal atresia* (Fig. 29-1), blockage of the nasal passages posteriorly due to a membrane or to a solid bony plate, may produce respiratory distress and suffocation. The affected infant, in trying to breathe through the obstructed passages, becomes more and more hypoxic and develops all the symptoms of progressive deterioration.

Respiratory depression in the neonate may produce hypoxia, hypoxemia, and acidosis if it does not subside spontaneously or by the application of stimulant drugs. The two main causes of respiratory depression are (1) heavy recent maternal sedation or narcosis that crosses the placenta and strikes the infant's respiratory center just about the time of delivery and (2) prolonged cerebral hypoxia resulting from fetal distress during labor or delivery. The *major causes of respiratory distress* are shown in Table 29-1.

signs and symptoms of respiratory distress The nursery nurses are the front-line professionals in the care of the newborn. Learning to observe and assess the infant in

fig. 29-1 Choanal atresia. (Note blockage of the nasal passage posteriorly.)

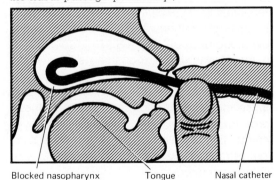

Blocked nasopharynx   Tongue   Nasal catheter

distress is an essential aspect of care for such babies. The signs of distress stem mainly from lowered oxygen levels and from the resultant fatigue caused by the effort to exchange air.

These signs are listed in the following outline:

I. Changes in respiratory rate and rhythm
   A. Rising respiratory rate
   B. Tachypnea
   C. Periods of apnea
II. Presence of respiratory sounds
   A. Grunting, expiratory sound (RDS)
   B. Stridor, inspiratory sound, (upper airway obstruction)
   C. Wheeze (obstruction within thorax)
   D. Rales (moisture in lungs)
   E. Feeble cry (fatigue)
III. Use of accessory respiratory muscles
   A. Flaring nostrils
   B. Retractions
      1. Suprasternal
      2. Sternal
      3. Substernal
      4. Intercostal
IV. General condition
   A. Central cyanosis
      1. Circumoral
      2. Head and trunk
   B. Poor muscle tone
   C. Poor reflex responses
   D. Hypothermia

Persistent *tachypnea*, with a rate over 50 to 60 times per minute, may be an early sign of low blood oxygen level. Obstructive difficulty in the airway, atelectasis, or hyaline membrane disease will cause the infant to have grunting respirations. An infant grunts because the epiglottis is closed in an effort to force expiration against pressure, thereby maintaining some residual air in alveoli. Chest wall retractions will also occur with drawing in of the intercostal areas between the ribs

table 29-1 Major causes of respiratory distress

I. Intrinsic problems
   A. Primary atelectasis
   B. Emphysema
   C. Pneumatocele
   D. Pneumonia
      1. Perinatal aspiration syndrome
      2. Amnionitis pneumonia
II. Congenital anomalies of respiratory tract
   A. Choanal atresia
   B. Tracheoesophageal fistulas
   C. Laryngeal or tracheal stenosis
   D. Agenesis of lung
III. Extrinsic problems
   A. Diaphragmatic herniation
   B. Pneumothorax
   C. Chylothorax
   D. Diaphragmatic (phrenic nerve) paralysis
IV. Respiratory depression
   A. Hypoxia
   B. Narcosis
V. Hyaline membrane disease (RDS)
VI. Immaturity
   A. Exhaustion

and the subcostal area beneath the ribs on each inspiration. Because the immature infant has somewhat pliable bones, the whole sternum can be seen to retract. Cyanosis may also be present and is significant if it extends beyond the hands and feet to the face and trunk (central cyanosis). (See Chap. 30).

treatment of depressed respiratory responses The first consideration in supporting respiration must be to establish a clear airway. Pharyngeal secretions must be removed by gentle suction, either by mouth by means of a DeLee catheter with a trap, or by machine with low negative-pressure suction. In the presence of obstructive anomalies of nose, tongue, pharynx, or larynx, it is often necessary to insert a pharyngeal airway to depress and extend the tongue, or even an endotracheal tube, to maintain pulmonary air exchange. When the infant's respiratory effort is too weak or when the lungs cannot expand properly, it may be necessary to assist ventilation. Direct intermittent positive pressure accomplishes oxygenation at varying concentrations through a firmly but gently applied face mask or through an endotracheal tube (Fig. 29-2). For alternative methods of providing oxygen, see Chap. 30.

USE OF OXYGEN   If the airways are clear and if sufficient alveolar surface is available, it is usually unnecessary to supply oxygen at a concentration higher than 35 to 40 percent. (Air at sea level contains 20 percent oxygen by volume.) In severe depression it may be necessary to introduce up to 100 percent for short periods of time. The dangers inherent in exposing the neonate to excessive concentrations of oxygen for any length of time have been well documented as oxygen toxicity. The eyes of the small premature infant are particularly vulnerable to the effects of elevated plasma oxygen concentrations for prolonged periods. Damage to the retinal

fig. 29-2   Resuscitation of the newborn: equipment for endotracheal intubation. After the larynx has been visualized with the laryngoscope and the fluid, mucus, or other obstruction suctioned out, the endotracheal tube may be left in place while intermittent positive-pressure breathing is carried out. Sometimes a small airway is inserted after the endotracheal tube is removed. Oxygen, humidity, warmth, careful handling, and observation are critical in the follow-up period.

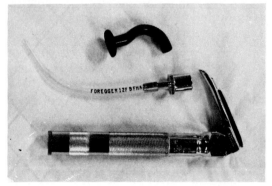

blood vessels by fibrosis and the subsequent formation of a membrane within the eye result in a condition known as *retrolental fibroplasia* that can produce permanent blindness.

Another potentially serious effect of overoxygenation is *hyperoxemia,* or too high a blood oxygen level, that may interfere with the enzymatic pathway responsible for the formation of surfactant in the neonate. Any reduction of an adequate amount of mature surfactant may aggravate an already existing situation of respiratory distress.

In addition, hyperoxygenation can produce serious damage to the lungs if it is prolonged. Proliferative changes develop in the pulmonary vascular endothelium and in the alveolar and bronchiolar epithelium, leading to fibrosis. This diminishes the oxygen diffusion into the blood and makes the infant dependent on higher oxygen supplies, thus creating a vicious cycle and further lung damage.

Another major consideration in maintaining oxygen levels is body temperature. If the infant's body temperature falls below normal range, the rate of metabolism increases, and this increase causes an increase in oxygen consumption. (See thermoneutral ambient temperature, Chap. 14.)

USE OF RESPIRATORY STIMULANTS AND NARCOTIC ANTAGONISTS   Pharmacologically, respiratory stimulants and narcotic antagonists are not necessarily synonymous. Drugs such as caffeine sodium benzoate and nikethamide (Coramine) stimulate the respiratory center in the floor of the fourth ventricle of the brain and are mainly effective in counteracting the effect of depression by barbiturates. Rarely used for infants, these respiratory stimulants counteract cerebral hypoxia of mild to moderate degree. Narcosis and its attendant respiratory depression usually require a more specific narcotic antagonist that does not further depress respiration. Such a drug is naloxone (Narcan), which lacks the morphinelike properties of the two other narcotic antagonists. Nalorphine (Nalline) and levallorphan (Lorfan) may potentiate respiratory depression and so should preferably not be used in the neonate. The dose of naloxone is 0.01 mg/kg, administered intravenously, intramuscularly, or subcutaneously.

USE OF PLASMINOGEN FOR HYALINE MEMBRANE DISEASE   A second method for the prevention and treatment of hyaline membrane disease has been described recently. One milliliter of human plasminogen, a blood derivative and precursor of plasmin, is injected intravenously, usually via the umbilical vein, within 1 h after birth, into prematures or other infants considered to be at risk for the development of hyaline membrane disease. Plasmin dissolves fibrin as it forms in the pulmonary alveoli and thus prevents its inhibiting surfactant activity. Plasminogen administration has been shown to reduce the incidence and mortality of severe respiratory distress syndrome.

CORRECTION OF ACIDOSIS AND HYPOGLYCEMIA   Hypoxemia, if uncorrected, can lead to a build-up of carbon dioxide and a consequent lowering of pH of the blood, causing acidosis and the development of hypoglycemia. The administration of sodium bicarbonate in glucose solution intravenously by way of the umbilical vein or a peripheral vein can prevent these serious chemical imbalances. The concentrations utilized are usually 5 meq/kg in mildly acidotic infants to 10 meq/kg in severe cases. The sodium bicarbonate is hyperosmolar and must be diluted in a 5 percent glucose solution. Rate of administration depends on the infant's condition and is titrated with response. The use of the same solutions administered via a nasogastric tube instead of intravenously has been described as effective prevention and treatment in mildly to moderately acidotic neonates, without the

risk of infection or thrombosis from intravenous administration. With any route, administration must be monitored by blood tests in order to avoid overalkalinization while bringing the pH out of the acidotic range.

If airways are patent, normal chemistries are maintained, and body structures are mature enough, an infant can be supported through respiratory depression and distress and recover.

Anomalous deformities such as diaphragmatic hernia and pneumatocele, and conditions such as pneumothorax and chylothorax, of course require prompt surgical intervention.

MAINTAINING CIRCULATION

normal fetal circulation

The structure of the normal fetal cardiovascular system is essentially what it will be after birth, with the exception of two main shunts or shortcuts that enable more efficient direction of oxygenated blood, and the presence of the umbilical vessel lifeline from the placenta. Since the fetal lungs are not functional, the pulmonary blood flow is needed only to nourish the lung tissue, not for gaseous exchange. A large amount of the blood that leaves the right ventricle of the heart through the pulmonary artery is, therefore, shunted directly into the aorta and the systemic circulation through the ductus arteriosus between the two vessels. This duct normally closes shortly after birth as the systemic blood pressure builds up.

The second important shunt that exists before birth and closes, at least functionally, after birth is the foramen ovale between the left and right atria of the heart. In fetal life, this allows a portion of the maternally oxygenated blood returning to the fetal right atrium via the vena cava to shunt through to the left atrium, down to the left ventricle, and out to the aorta, thus again bypassing the pulmonary circuit.

At birth the umbilical two arteries and one vein cease their functions of carrying blood for the purpose of gas exchange, nutrition, and waste exchange. Their division is followed by atrophy of their connections from umbilicus to the systemic arteries and veins.

circulatory abnormalities

In the complex mechanism of chambers, conduits, and function of the cardiovascular system, it is a marvel that structural anomalies occur as infrequently as they do (Fig. 29-3). Structural deviations may be manifest in both intracardiac and extracardiac areas. They may vary from defects that are not immediately life-threatening, requiring no early treatment, to severe anomalies that are incompatible with life.

Structural defects often involve a shunt or communication between parts of the heart or great vessels. If the shunt or communication is large enough or so situated that enough venous or deoxygenated blood is spilled back into the systemic or left-sided vascular system, the infant will be *cyanotic*. Otherwise, the anomaly is described as *acyanotic*. Heart murmurs may or may not be audible, depending on the location and size of the anomaly.

Among the less severe defects are persistent *patent ductus arteriosus* (Fig. 29-4), *coarctation,* or narrowing of a segment of aorta, *stenosis* of the pulmonary artery, *intraventricular septal defect* (Fig. 29-5), *auricular (atrial) septal defect* (Fig. 29-6), i.e., persistence of a patent foramen ovale between the two auricles. Among the more severe anomalies, some that are incompatible with life can be helped by emergency surgery in the neonate. Later, if the child survives, revision surgery may improve chances for prolonged survival. Among these conditions are transposition of the aorta and pulmonary artery to the reverse ventricles, and total anomalous

fig. 29-3 Normal heart (adult). *(From Ross Laboratories, Columbus, Ohio, Clinical Education Aid No. 7.)*

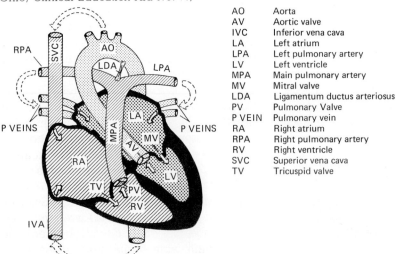

AO	Aorta
AV	Aortic valve
IVC	Inferior vena cava
LA	Left atrium
LPA	Left pulmonary artery
LV	Left ventricle
MPA	Main pulmonary artery
MV	Mitral valve
LDA	Ligamentum ductus arteriosus
PV	Pulmonary Valve
P VEIN	Pulmonary vein
RA	Right atrium
RPA	Right pulmonary artery
RV	Right ventricle
SVC	Superior vena cava
TV	Tricuspid valve

venous drainage with reversal of the venous return to the auricles. *Cor triloculare,* or three-chambered heart (two auricles and one ventricle), is, of course, impossible to correct surgically at present. The anomalies of heart and great vessel structures known as *tetralogy of Fallot* (Fig. 29-7) and *Eisenmenger's syndrome,* though not incompatible with life, will impair efficient cardiac function as the infant grows.

While the cardiac electrical impulse is initiated within the heart itself at the sinoatrial (SA) node, extracardiac neurogenic effects may play a role in regulating heart rate and action by way of the vagus nerve. Central effects on the circulatory center in the medulla of the brain from anoxia, circulating drugs, intracranial pressure from birth trauma,

fig. 29-4 Patent ductus arteriosus. The patent ductus arteriosus is a vascular connection that, during fetal life, short-circuits the pulmonary vascular bed and directs blood from the pulmonary artery to the aorta. Functional closure of the ductus remains patent after birth; the direction of blood flow in the ductus is reversed by the higher pressure in the aorta. (*From Ross Laboratories, Columbus, Ohio, Clinical Education Aid No. 7.*)

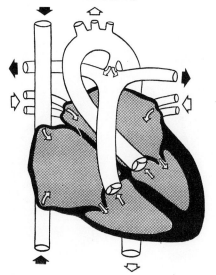

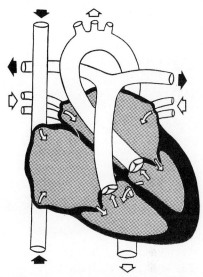

fig. 29-5 Ventricular septal defect. A ventricular septal defect is an abnormal opening between the right and left ventricles. Ventricular septal defects vary in size and may occur in either the membranous or the muscular portion of the ventricular septum. Because of higher pressure in the left ventricle, a shunting of blood from the left to right ventricle occurs during systole. If pulmonary vascular resistance produces pulmonary hypertension, the shunt of blood is then reversed from the right to the left ventricle, resulting in cyanosis. (*From Ross Laboratories, Columbus, Ohio, Clinical Education Aid No. 7.*)

edema, or hemorrhage into the vital centers may indirectly affect the activity of the cardiovascular system.

signs and symptoms Signs and symptoms of circulatory abnormalities in an infant are similar in some respects to those of respiratory distress. An inefficient heart or anomalous great vessels may manifest signs and symptoms of poor oxygenation of the infant's blood supply in the form of cyanosis. Tachypnea will result from the body's effort to absorb more oxygen by more rapid breathing. If the strain on an anomalous heart is too great, heart failure may develop. In this case,

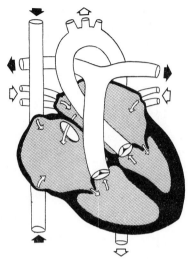

fig. 29-6 Atrial septal defects. An atrial septal defect is an abnormal opening between the right and left atria. Basically, three types of abnormalities result from incorrect development of the atrial septum. An incompetent foramen ovale is the most common defect. The high ostium secundum defect results from abnormal development of the septum secundum. Improper development of the septum primum produces a basal opening known as an ostium primum defect, frequently involving the atrioventricular valves. In general, left-to-right shunting of blood occurs in all atrial septal defects. (*From Ross Laboratories, Columbus, Ohio, Clinical Education Aid No. 7.*)

in addition to signs of air hunger, the infant will be extremely restless and fretful and will be unable to feed because of inability to suck and swallow as a result of respiratory difficulty.

Some cardiovascular anomalies are asymptomatic in the neonatal period except for the presence of a murmur that can be heard only with a stethoscope on the infant's chest. Experienced nurses can, of course, detect unusual chest sounds when they observe vital signs.

supportive care In the presence of a heart that is beating continuously and consistently too rapidly (i.e., at a ventricular rate over 180 beats per minute), it is necessary to slow the heart rate and to increase the force of each beat by administering digoxin, usually intramuscularly. In emergency situations, the drug may be administered intravenously, at least initially.

The first line of treatment for a cardiovascular anomaly of the cyanotic type is the use of oxygen at a sufficiently high concentration to alleviate the cyanosis. Emergency surgical procedures are basically designed to channel enough oxygenated blood into the systemic circulation to sustain life as efficiently as possible.

As with any infant, normal or not, nutrition and fluid intake must be provided by the most

fig. 29-7 Tetralogy of Fallot. This disorder is characterized by the combination of four defects: (1) pulmonary stenosis, (2) ventricular septal defect, (3) overriding aorta, and (4) hypertrophy of right ventricle. It is the most common defect causing cyanosis in patients surviving beyond 2 years of age. The severity of symptoms depends on the degree of pulmonary stenosis, the size of the ventricular septal defect, and the degree to which the aorta overrides the septal defect. (*From Ross Laboratories, Columbus, Ohio, Clinical Education Aid No. 7.*)

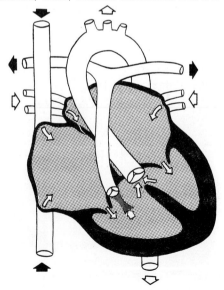

practical method—oral, nasogastric tube, or intravenous routes.

MAINTAINING NEUROLOGIC FUNCTION

The very complexity of higher forms of animal life makes it essential that there be a governing and directing system, in essence a switchboard control, to organize all the specialized functions into a synchronous, reciprocating operation. This system is the nervous system, the brain at the center, the spinal cord as the trunk line, and the peripheral nerves beyond.

Anomalies, malformations, and destructive injuries within the nervous system will affect its functions and, therefore, the function of other systems or organs that it controls in variable fashion and degree, depending on the location and extent of the defect.

neurologic abnormalities

The etiology of nervous defects in the neonate is essentially threefold—developmental, infectious, and accidental. Developmental defects may be genetic (usually a recessive trait and usually part of a more general syndrome) or they may be due to *dysgenesis* (faulty development at some stage of early embryonic development). Among the developmental anomalies is *microcephaly*, or totally small cortex.

Hydrocephalus, or an excessively enlarged head, results when circulation and reabsorption of cerebrospinal fluid are prevented by absence or stenosis of the normally existing channels or foramina by which the ventricles of the brain communicate with the subdural space (Fig. 29-8). *Spina bifida*, an inherited defect in which part of the spinal cord and meninges extrude through an opening in the lower back, often accompanies hydrocephalus. A rare anomaly is *cerebral agenesis*, resulting in what is commonly, and unfortunately, referred to as anencephalic monster—a condition in which the entire brain is absent except for the medullary brainstem with its centers of circulation and respiration control. The entire cranium is open, exposing the rudimentary primitive brain segment.

Certain maternal viral infections occurring especially in the first trimester can be devastating to the developing brain. The principal viral agents are rubella virus and cytomegalovirus. The toxoplasma and spirochete can damage the brain even later in gestation (see Chap. 25).

Accidental damage to the brain may be caused by anoxia or hemorrhage. Frequent or appreciable maternal (placental) bleeding during the second or even the third trimester, after the brain has been basically formed, may produce sufficient cerebral anoxia to damage the cerebral cortex. During labor, damage may result from prolonged deprivation of oxygen to the brain caused by obstruction of the umbilical vessels by knotting or pressure, by premature separation of the placenta (abruptio placentae), a relatively long period before the head is delivered, or possibly even by excessive hypoxic anesthesia to the mother (Chap. 20).

traumatic birth injuries

trauma to the head   In addition to labor accidents, there are a number of injuries that can jeopardize the newborn. These can be divided broadly into two categories: noniatrogenic (not caused by the treatment) and iatrogenic (caused by the treatment). They may affect either the brain or peripheral nerves or may simply cause bruising of tissues. Noniatrogenic injuries to the head include the following: (1) cephalhematoma, a localized subperiosteal hemorrhage at the area where

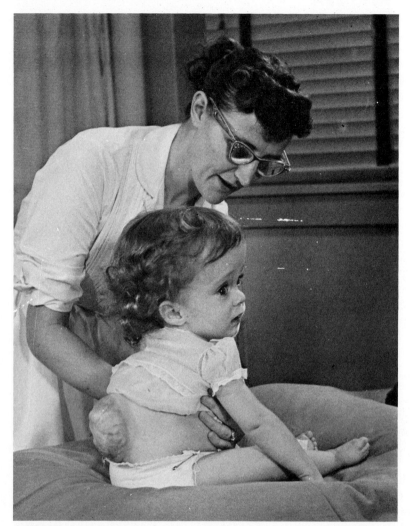

fig. 29-8 Hydrocephalic child with spina bifida. (*Courtesy of The National Foundation—March of Dimes.*)

the skull was pressed by strong uterine contractions for considerable time against either the partially dilated cervix or against the ischial spines; (2) very severe molding of the infant's skull in a narrow or constricted pelvis may cause a linear or even a depressed fracture or tears in the major cerebral vessels as a result of excessive stretching. Small hemorrhages may cause damage indirectly through an anoxic effect on the affected areas, as blood and, thus, oxygen supply are cut off. Major hemorrhages are usually fatal.

peripheral nerve trauma Occasionally peripheral nerves are injured during delivery. The blade of obstetric forceps may sometimes compress the facial nerve in the area anterior to the ear and below and lateral to the eye, producing a peripheral type of facial paralysis which usually resolves, since the continuity of the nerve is usually not disrupted.

More serious is injury to the brachial plexus where it originates from the spinal cord at the base of the neck and runs to the arm through the axilla. This injury occurs when the head is markedly extended laterally to the opposite side, with the arm extended and the shoulder depressed. The effect of this maneuver is occasionally to *avulse,* or tear away, the plexus of nerves from the spinal cord, an irreparable and irreversible damage. If the lower part of the plexus only is avulsed, the result is Erb's palsy, or partial paralysis of the arm with inability to supinate or elevate it. If the entire plexus is avulsed, the result is total flaccid paralysis of the arm, or Klumpke's paralysis. There is usually accompanying damage to the contiguous stellate autonomic ganglion at the level where the brachial plexus emerges from the cord, producing a Horner's syndrome of *ptosis,* or drooping of the eyelid, and *enophthalmos,* or retraction of the eyeball. Finally, in very rare instances, there is spinal cord injury from undue torsion and stretching of the spine.

hypoglycemia and brain damage

The brain is sensitive to chemical changes in the blood, in addition to the concentrations or partial pressures of oxygen and carbon dioxide. Lack of glucose in the blood can be especially damaging to brain cells. *Hypoglycemia* may occur when the infant's blood sugar level drops too low. Normally the newborn will have and will tolerate glucose levels as low as 40 mg/100 mL even though fetal glucose levels are thought to be between 60 and 80 mg/100 mL. In the first 4 to 6 h after birth, normally available glycogen stores are

mobilized to maintain levels of 50 to 60 percent. Hypoglycemia is defined as occurring when, for two consecutive readings 1 h apart, the blood glucose levels fall below 30 mg/100 mL in the full-term infant and below 20 mg/100 mL in the preterm infant. Hypoglycemia can be expected in any high-risk infant and probably occurs more often than realized in the term infant. Early feedings are essential, glucose/water or plain water, then with milk, to stabilize blood sugar. The outdated custom of withholding fluids and milk from the infant for 8 to 16 h precipitated many problems. Hopefully, this custom will be reversed as the effects of hypoglycemia are taken more seriously.

Hypoglycemia will be present in any severe hypoxic or acidotic state, when glycogen stores are inadequate (low-birth-weight infants), or when there is some obstructive or nonabsorptive pathologic condition. The infant of a diabetic mother (IDM) can be expected to demonstrate hypoglycemia for another reason. Born with an overactive pancreas because of constant exposure to high blood glucose levels from the mother, the infant produces higher than normal levels of insulin. Levels below 20 to 30 mg/100 mL may occur early, 2 to 4 h after birth, and treatment should be instituted at once.

supportive care When blood sugar is found to be very low, treatment may require intravenous glucose. From 15 to 25 percent glucose is infused for a period, and then concentrations are reduced to 5 to 10 percent. By 3 days of life the infant should be stabilized unless further pathology develops.

Infusion of glucose should clear up symptoms, which, in order of frequency, include tremors, cyanosis, convulsions, apnea, apathy, abnormal cry (weak or high-pitched), lethargy, temperature instability, refusal to eat, and eyes rolling up toward forehead. Such nonspecific symptoms may result from numerous other problems, and diagnosis may be difficult to determine.

Before blood is drawn for glucose levels, the extremity should be warmed. Otherwise, an underestimation may occur. In addition, if not used correctly, the screening test, Dextrostix (Ames), can overestimate glucose levels. Dextrostix may deteriorate with light and humidity. Therefore a sample stick from the bottle being used should be tested. Using a drop of 5 percent glucose in water, there should be a strong positive reaction.

results of neurologic damage

Cerebral anomalies, infections, and some teratogenic drugs early in gestation will virtually always result in some degree of mental deficiency. Sometimes damage from trauma, anoxia, or hemorrhage may be mild enough not to be destructive of brain cells, thereby causing only transient effects or minimal brain effects. Some of these effects are related to later learning disabilities.

The extent of severe damage depends on the location of the damage. Involvement of the prefrontal or frontal cortex results in impairment of intelligence. Involvement of the motor area of the brain will probably cause neuromuscular *spastic cerebral palsy*. Anoxic damage to the more deeply located basal ganglia that relay and control motor impulses usually leads to *athetoid cerebral palsy,* with its uncoordinated involuntary movements of gross muscle groups.

Cerebral palsy may be defined as a condition of gross neuromuscular defects resulting from widespread damage to the cortex or the basal ganglia of the brain or both during the immature stages of their development after the time that their primitive differentiation is completed. Damage to the embryonic brain during the first trimester usually results in death or anomaly rather than cerebral palsy. Prenatal cerebral damage after the first trimester accounts for an estimated 20 percent of cases of cerebral palsy. Intrapartum cerebral injury is the main cause of cerebral palsy and is responsible for about 60 percent of cases. Finally, cerebral insults during the first 2 or 3 years of life, before all the nerve centers and nerve tracts have matured, account for approximately 20 percent of cerebral-palsied children.

signs and symptoms   Several signs and symptoms should alert the nursery nurse to the existence of neurologic deficits. Severe depression of the infant's responses, with general poor muscle tone, failure to respond to tactile or mildly painful stimuli such as flicking the soles of the feet, brisk rubbing of the trunk, or pulling on a few strands of hair, and a weak brief cry are suggestive evidence of cerebral depressive effects that could be transient, permanent, or even fatal. Cerebral lesions that produce irritation of the brain, such as hemorrhage or anomalies, may cause the infant to cry with a very high-pitched shrill voice almost like the mewing of a cat. Other signs of cerebral irritative lesions are frequent local muscle group tremors or twitching of extremities or face, or even generalized seizure activity of the face, trunk, and extremities. Head measurements should be taken at birth and then at regular intervals to evaluate the rate of head growth. Any deviation from normal must be further evaluated.

A flaccid, limp arm is usually indicative of brachial nerve plexus injury. After a forceps delivery, a one-sided facial weakness, drooping of the mouth, and possibly also of the eyelid, are due to facial nerve injury from the forceps application.

supportive care   Treatment falls mainly into the prophylactic categories of good prenatal care, competent obstetric procedures, and probably, good genetic counseling. Universal vaccination to stop epidemics of rubella must be undertaken. Avoidance of teratologic drugs during pregnancy, the proper usage of sedatives and narcotics during the first stage of labor, and the correct administration of anesthesia during the second stage of labor or during cesarean section, are all important considerations.

Therapy for existing neurologic conditions and effects can be divided into several categories. One is the administration of drugs such as narcotic antagonists, oxygen, and the agents for narcotic withdrawal symptoms. Another is the administration of glucose solution orally or intravenously for hypoglycemic effects. Most other aspects of treatment are rehabilitative and applied beyond the neonatal period for mental and neuromuscular deficits.

transitional drug effects

Many drugs in the maternal system will equilibrate with the fetus by transplacental osmosis or active passage unless the drug is of very large molecular weight or is highly protein-bound. While the placenta is functioning, drug excretion is managed by the mother. Once the infant is born, its own kidneys and liver must manage metabolism and excretion. Overwhelmed by the maternal dosage still in its system, the infant may be affected for an extended period until the drug can be excreted.

Barbiturates, tranquilizers, narcotics, and anesthetics administered briefly during labor and delivery may depress the newborn infant's respirations and ability to adjust to extrauterine life. The outcome depends on the size of the dose and the duration of administration to the mother (see Chap. 20). Of serious concern because of their neurologic effects, which may lead to convulsions and even death if untreated, are the narcotic addicting drugs ingested or injected by the mother during pregnancy.

infant of the drug-dependent mother Drug addiction or dependence is usually thought of in terms of the abuse of narcotic drugs such as heroin or methadone, but withdrawal also occurs from tranquilizers, such as diazepam, and barbiturates, such as phenobarbital. Propoxyphene hydrochloride (Darvon) is also included because its molecular structure is similar to that of methadone. Approximately 80 percent of infants born to drug-dependent mothers will show withdrawal symptoms after birth.[3] The manifestations of such symptoms fall into four categories: (1) CNS symptoms, (2) GI symptoms, (3) respiratory symptoms, and (4) symptoms of autonomic nervous system disturbance (see Table 29-2).

Heroin addiction may vary in intensity, depending upon the quality of drug which has been taken by the mother. Heroin has a short half-life, and therefore withdrawal symptoms are usually evident early, within 24 to 72 h after birth.

table 29-2 Neonatal withdrawal symptoms

Central nervous system
  Irritability
  Tremors
  Convulsions (1–2% heroin, 6–10% methadone)
  Excessive crying
  Poor coordination of suck and swallow
Gastrointestinal
  Vomiting
  Diarrhea
Respiratory
  Tachypnea
  Hyperpnea, leading to cyanosis and apnea
Autonomic nervous system
  Sneezing
  Lacrimation
  Yawning
  Hyperpyrexia
  Sweating

Methadone may have been abused illicitly like heroin or may have been administered under a controlled program as a substitute for heroin, a theoretically more acceptable addiction. Methadone has a longer half-life in the system than does heroin (less frequent doses are required by the addict), and withdrawal takes longer. Symptoms may appear as late as 2 to 3 weeks after birth and are usually more severe.

Phenobarbital (or other barbiturates) may cause symptoms beginning about 5 to 7 days after birth, which may be quite severe, sometimes accompanied by seizures. The infant susceptible to phenobarbital withdrawal would be one whose mother took high doses of the drug regularly. Infants of preeclamptic women on doses for short intervals may or may not show signs. Observation well into the first month of life is essential for any of these infants.

pharmacologic treatment In cases of mild withdrawal, a sedative alone may be effective to control symptoms. All doses must be tapered gradually during the recovery period to avoid recurrence of symptoms.

Phenobarbital (2 mg/kg q 3 to 4 h IM) is given until the infant is clinically stable, and then the dose is given orally. Chlorpromazine (Thorazine) (0.5 to 1.0 mg/kg q 4 h IM, until stable, and then PO) may be an alternative treatment. Doses of both these drugs are tapered after the infant is stabilized, and doses are reduced every 2 to 3 days until the infant is fully recovered.

In severe cases, elixir of paregoric may be used because of its effect in reduction of vomiting and diarrhea. However, vomiting may prevent oral administration, and constipation may result from excessive doses. The dosage is 3 drops (0.2 to 0.3 mL) q 4 h PO, raised by 1 drop each dose until symptoms are controlled. The highest dose may be about 8 drops, or 0.5 to 0.6 mL. After 4 to 7 days of stabilization, each dose is carefully lowered by 1 drop every 2 to 3 days while close observation is maintained for return of symptoms.

supportive care In addition to pharmacologic therapy, supportive care is crucial. The infant must be protected from injury resulting from restlessness, seizures, or friction abrasion on knees, elbows, and head. Fluid and electrolyte balance must be maintained and nutrition provided. Intake and output must be recorded carefully, and stimulation reduced by swaddling the body firmly when tremors are severe and by grouping nursing activities to reduce fatigue of handling. Problems that persist because of delayed bonding may be severe. The infant who is sent home or to foster care with continuing problems may be introduced into a hostile environment. In hospital, it is best to assign the same nurse to the infant as much as possible, so that some continuity of care can be maintained. (See Chap. 21 for care of the drug-dependent mother.)

MAINTAINING GENITOURINARY FUNCTION

Although the gonads and the urinary system develop from adjacent embryonic structures and share some portion of an outlet, the two systems function completely independently. The present discussion is concerned primarily with urinary function.

renal and urinary tract problems

In the neonate there is no concern with renal diseases such as glomerulonephritis, collagen disease, and renal chemical malfunction.

The pathologic conditions affecting the urinary tract of the newborn are principally congenital anomalies and infection (Fig. 29-9).

Anomalies may involve the kidney, the ureter, the bladder, and even the urethra. Some kidney malformations are *horseshoe kidney* (in which the two kidneys are fused across the midline, forming one horseshoe-shaped organ) and *polycystic kidney* (in which a number of the collecting units fail to empty into the renal pelvis so that they form large cysts of unexcreted urine).

Obstructive uropathies include *hydronephrosis*, in which the ureter or bladder outlet is obstructed, causing the entire pelvis and calyces to dilate with urine, and *hydroureter*.

fig. 29-9 Developmental disturbances of the kidneys. (Sketched from museum preparations: *a, c, d*, in the University of Michigan Anatomical Collection; *b*, in the Dypuytren Museum, Paris.) (*a*) Unilateral pelvic kidney; (*b*) horseshoe kidney; (*c*) dystopic left kidney fused to right kidney; (*d*) nearly complete agenesis of the left kidney. (*From B. M. Patten, Human Embryology, 3d ed., McGraw-Hill, New York, 1968.*)

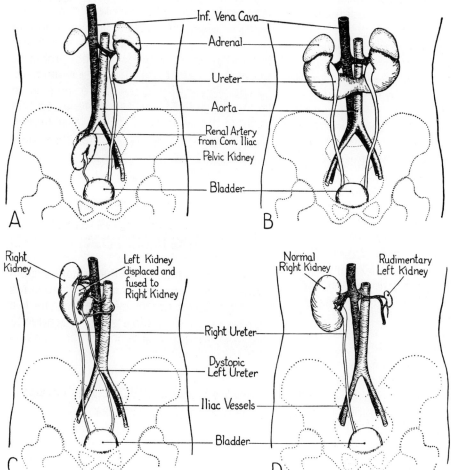

Constriction of the ureter at the ureteropelvic junction, often caused by an aberrant blood vessel, narrowing at the ureter junction with the bladder, stricture or posterior urethral valve at the bladder outlet, or even a constricted urethral meatus at the external opening are obstructive uropathies. A severe anomaly is *extrophy* of the bladder, in which the entire urinary bladder is open onto the lower abdominal surface and the ureters thus are open externally.

Urinary tract infections most often result from bacteria entering the bloodstream of the infant after surface trauma. Ascending infection from the urethra in newborn girls is less common than later in infancy or childhood.

genital abnormalities

Genital abnormalities usually take the form of ambiguous genitalia, making sex determination difficult for the observer. These may be caused by sex chromosomal aberrations, adrenal cortical hyperplasia in the infant, maternal androgenic hormones, and true or pseudohermaphroditism (Fig. 29-10).

Sex chromosomal aberrations may produce a male phenotype (body structure) with an extra female sex chromosome, such as Klinefelter's syndrome, or a female phenotype with an absent female sex chronomosome, such as Turner's syndrome. There are many other types of sex chromosomal aberrations and gonadal dysgenesis. The major types are discussed in Chap. 28.

Adrenal cortical hyperplasia produces excess androgenic hormone, which causes clitoral enlargement suggestive of a penis in the newborn girl. Similar masculinization of the female external genitalia may be observed in infants when the pregnant mother had an androgen-producing adrenal tumor or when the pregnant mother was treated, for whatever reason, with testosterone or other androgenic hormones.

Hermaphroditism is more commonly

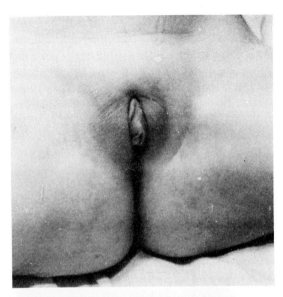

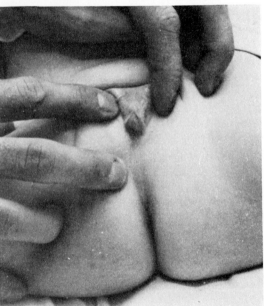

fig. 29-10 Ambiguous genitalia. (*From J. German and J. L. Simpson, "Abnormalities of Human Autosomes: 1. Ambiguous Genitalia Associated with a Translocation 46, XY, t (Cq +; Cq −)," in Birth Defects: Orig. Art. Ser., D. Bergsma (ed.), Part X, The Endocrine System, published by Williams & Wilkins Co., Baltimore, for The National Foundation—March of Dimes, vol. VII, no. 6, 1971, p. 145, with permission of the copyright holder.*)

pseudo- than true. It results from faulty embryologic differentiation of the genital precursor tissues. Pseudohermaphroditism may show atypical external genitalia, but there is normal unisexual internal genitalia and a corresponding sex chromosome pattern. The rare true hermaphrodite has characteristics of both sexes, such as both testes and ovaries, and a mosaic sex chromosome pattern of both male and female genotypes.

Two developmental aberrations in the male that are not produced by genetic or hormonal causes are *hypospadias* and *cryptorchidism*. In the former, the penile urethra may lie open for a segment on the undersurface of the penis proximal to the tip of the glans, or it may end in an orifice or meatus proximal to the normal opening at the end of the penis.

In cryptorchidism, or undescended testes, one or both testes may remain up in the abdomen or in the inguinal canal. It may result from a short spermatic cord preventing its descent through the inguinal canal into the scrotum, or from developmental delay that can be rectified later by the administration of injections of anterior pituitarylike (APL) hormone derived from pregnant mares' urine or by use of human menopausal gonadotropin (HMG) injections. Correction of severe hypospadias or cryptorchidism unresponsive to hormone therapy is generally relegated to the surgeon.

signs and symptoms of urologic problems A normal neonate may void urine at the time of delivery or occasionally not for about 24 h. Persistence of *anuria* beyond that time, however, should be reported by the nurse and should become the concern of the physician. A markedly distended abdomen, especially in the lateral flank areas, should be called to the attention of the physician. A palpable mass in those areas should create suspicion of an anomalous kidney, and x-ray studies should be pursued, with injection of radiopaque renal-excreted dye.

External anomalies, such as extrophy of the bladder or grossly abnormal genitalia, of course are readily apparent.

supportive care Some anomalies are amenable to surgery and others are not. In the former category, some conditions require emergency surgical intervention that is usually palliative initially and that must be followed later by more definitive procedures. In some, surgery will eventually be necessary but it is not an early lifesaving measure. Horseshoe kidney may conceivably have normal function. In any event, no surgery is indicated. Polycystic kidney cannot be corrected or improved surgically. If it is bilateral, neither kidney can or should be removed. If it is unilateral and asymptomatic, the involved kidney may have to be removed later.

Obstructive uropathy presents a surgical emergency in the newborn. Palliative nephrostomy must be performed in the first days of life by inserting tubes into the renal pelvis through a flank incision to drain the urine continuously out of the kidney in order to prevent irreparable damage to the glomeruli from back pressure. Later, when the infant's condition will permit, surgery will be performed to relieve the cause of the obstruction.

Infection, of course, must be treated vigorously with antibiotics. It is best to identify the invading organism by culture of the blood and urine, in order to ascertain the most effective antibiotics.

MAINTAINING METABOLIC FUNCTION

In a sense, a living organism may be regarded as a chemical factory in which life processes are normally maintained by a balance of anabolic synthesis and catabolic degradation of protoplasm. These chemical reactions are carried out largely through the intermediary action of enzymes, organic compounds that enable reactions to occur without themselves being an integral part of the reaction. Often the chemical reactions involve the alteration of a toxic waste substance by several enzymes in a kind of chain reaction. The end product is thus prepared to be excreted through the kidneys or the gastrointestinal tract. Enzymes, in addition, are essential in the transport and metabolism of organic compounds which cannot penetrate cell membranes by osmosis as do simple inorganic ions like sodium and chloride.

enzymatic deficiencies

The delicate balance of normal function can be upset if one enzyme fails to develop or is incomplete. The absence or deficiency of an enzyme may be the result of genetic inheritance or a developmental defect. A number of such enzyme deficiencies have been identified, and more are being investigated. Chapter 28 discusses symptoms and care of infants with major problems.

In each case, the deficiency will demonstrate symptoms which reflect the incomplete metabolic breakdown of organic materials. There will be an accumulation in the bloodstream of unmetabolized or partially metabolized products. When these products can be excreted, even though not completely metabolized, tests on urine can indicate their presence. When products are not excreted, blood tests provide the only information.

Although in most cases, inborn errors of metabolism affect amino acid, lipid, or carbohydrate metabolism, other problems affect enzymes which govern liver transformation of other substances, e.g., the Crigler-Najjar syndrome, a condition in which the liver cells fail to produce the enzyme *glucuronyl transferase*. Such an enzyme is important in bilirubin metabolism, and a deficiency will cause high levels of unmetabolized bilirubin in the bloodstream.

Another problem is a deficiency in glucose-6-phosphate dehydrogenase (G-6-P-D), an enzyme that is normally contained in erythrocytes. When an individual's red cells are deficient in this substance, severe hemolysis and anemia may occur in response to certain drugs or circumstances. (See Chap. 22 for further discussion.)

Routine tests for inborn errors of metabolism are performed by legal mandate before the infant is discharged from the nursery. In New York, for example, blood is tested for phenylalanine, leucine, methionine, histidine, galactose uridyl transferase, adenosine deaminase, and hemoglobin S-S (sickle-cell disease). It is important to note that these early screening tests do not always identify the infant at risk, so that continued observation and assessment are important (see Chap. 28 and Table 29-3).

supportive care   No complete treatment exists for any of these metabolic disturbances. The most important step is to recognize the deficiency as early as possible. If there has been a family history of the disease, the infant should be completely tested. Any signs of failure to thrive, strange-smelling urine, loose smelly stools (indicating undigested milk), excessive mucus, vomiting, jaundice, irritability, and tremors or seizures will alert observers to the presence of some kind of problem.

When the specific deficiency is identified, treatment is to eliminate, as much as possible, the causative organic material. For instance, high levels of phenylalanine can be reduced by eliminating milk from the diet and placing the infant on a controlled amino acid diet. Similarly an infant who cannot digest (metabolize) lactose or galactose must be placed on a milk-free diet. Infants with G-6-P-D should not be given drugs or substances which precipitate hemolytic responses. More difficult to treat are those problems in which enzymes needed in essential body functions are missing; then, only the symptoms can be treated.

table 29-3 Screening tests in the newborn infant

condition	possible symptoms	type of sample			tests available	
		dried blood	serum	urine	Guthrie	other tests
PKU and hyperphenylalaninemia	Mental retardation (MR)	+	+	+	+	Fluorescent methods, amino acid chromatography
Tyrosinemia	MR, liver and kidney damage	+	+	+	+	Fluorescent methods, amino acid chromatography
Histidinemia	? MR, ? benign	+	+	+	+	Fluorescent methods, amino acids chromatography
Homocystinuria (methionine)	MR, bone, eye, liver and arterial damage	+	+	+	+	Amino acid chromatography, urine nitroprusside test
Maple syrup urine disease (leucine)	MR, acidosis, convulsions	+	+	+	+	Amino acid chromatography
Galactosemia	Cataracts, liver, brain and kidney damage	+	+	+	+	Beutler test, blood or urine galactose
Hypothyroidism	Cretinism	+	+		+	T_4 or TSH
Alpha-1-antitrypsin deficiency	Hepatitis in infancy, emphysema in adults	+	+		+	
Hereditary angioneurotic edema	Abdominal pain, evanescent edema	+	+		+	C'1-esterase inhibitor activity
Muscular dystrophy	Progressive muscle disease in children	+	+		+	Creatine phosphokinase
G-6-P-D deficiency and other RBC glycolytic enzymes	Hemolytic anemia	+	+		+	
Hemoglobinopathies	Sickle-cell disease	+	+		+	Electrophoresis
Hyperlipidemia	Arterial disease in adults		+			? Lipoprotein electrophoresis
Adenosine deaminase deficiency	Immunodeficiency disease in infancy	+	+		+	
Hypoglycemia			+			Dextrostix
Aminoacidopathies and organic acidemias	MR, ? acidosis		+	+		Chromatotography of blood and/or urine at several weeks of age
Neuroblastoma				+		VMA
Congenital infections	MR	+	+			Cord blood IgM levels
Cystic fibrosis	Lungs and alimentary tract	Stools				BM meconium test

Source: From N.R.M. Buist, "Metabolic Screening of the Newborn Infant,"*Clinics in Endocrinology and Metabolism*, **5**(1):284, March 1976.

problems preventing intake or absorption of nutrients

Antenatally, all nutrients are furnished through the umbilical vessels from the mother. Postnatally, the infant is dependent upon an intact gastrointestinal tract from mouth through anus and upon the ability to suck and to swallow.

Problems preventing intake or absorption of food fall into two categories, functional and structural. Functional disturbances may be the result of immaturity of the suck and swallow reflexes. They may also be caused by the debilitating effects of respiratory distress, systemic infection, or central nervous system damage. Structural problems are essentially caused by congenital deformities in various areas of the gastrointestinal tract, for instances, *cleft palate* may interfere with sucking (Fig. 29-11).

Gastrointestinal anomalies below the pharynx are more serious and life-threatening. *Esophageal atresia* is a narrowing of the esophagus at any point. *Tracheoesophageal fistula,* a communication between the trachea and the esophagus, may occur in any of five variations. As shown in Fig. 29-12, the type accounting for 87 percent of cases is the blind pouch proximal esophagus with tracheoesophageal fistula distally. In this condition swallowing of liquids will result in regurgitation, with danger of aspiration into the trachea and beyond. Other types are also illustrated in Fig. 29-12.

Intestinal obstruction may be caused by *atresia* anywhere below the stomach. Atresia may occur in the duodenum, the jejunum, or the ileum at any level and may affect variable lengths of intestine. Functional obstruction may result from congenital adhesion bands constricting the intestinal lumen, intestinal malrotation during embryonic formation, me-

fig. 29-11 (a) Cleft lip. (b) Cleft palate. (*From Ross Laboratories, Columbus, Ohio, Education Aid No. 7.*)

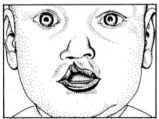
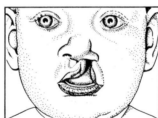
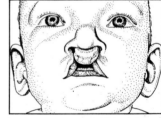

UNILATERAL INCOMPLETE   UNILATERAL COMPLETE   BILATERAL COMPLETE

A

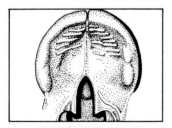
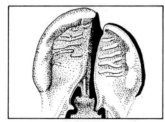
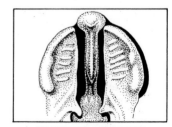

SOFT PALATE ONLY   UNILATERAL COMPLETE   BILATERAL COMPLETE

B

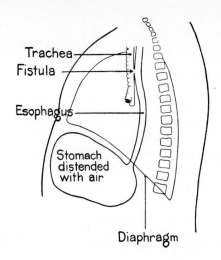

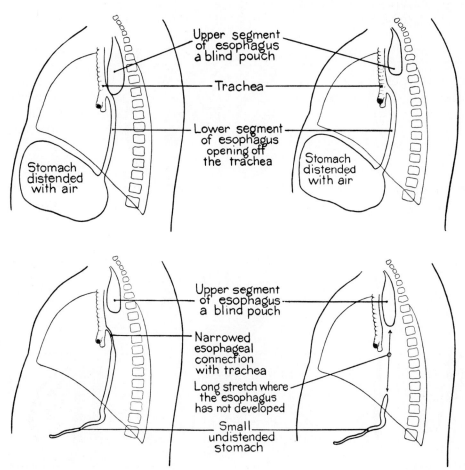

fig. 29-12 Types of tracheoesophageal fistulas. (*From C. E. Corliss, Patten's Human Embryology, 4th ed., McGraw-Hill, New York, 1976.*)

conium ileus and *imperforate anus* (Fig. 29-13). Meconium ileus is a failure of intestinal function caused by blockage by very thick meconium. Such a condition is usually caused by *cystic fibrosis* a genetic disease that prevents normal mucous gland secretion. *Om-*

phalocele is an anomaly in which an abdominal wall defect allows herniation with a membranous covering of a portion of the intestine at the site of the umbilicus. Omphalocele may produce ileus or obstruction.

Pyloric stenosis at the stomach outlet does

fig. 29-13 Imperforate anus (four types of disorder). (Redrawn from Corning.) (a) Anal atresia combined with obliteration of lower part of rectum. (b) Anal atresia combined with a rectovaginal fistula. (c) Uncomplicated anal atresia. (d) Anal atresia combined with rectovesical fistula and agenesis of the rectum. (*From B. M. Patten, Human Embryology, 3d ed., McGraw-Hill, New York, 1968.*)

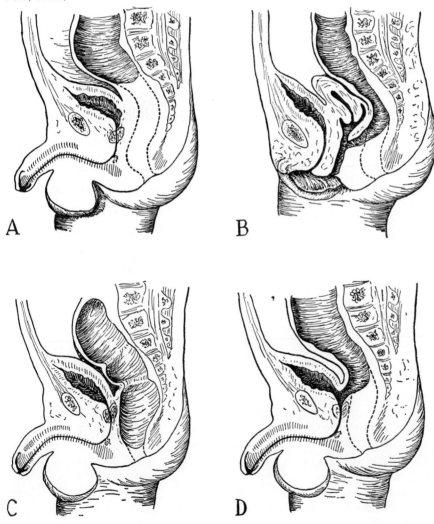

not usually show symptoms until about five to seven weeks of age, when projectile vomiting occurs. Pyloric stenosis occurs mainly in male infants.

supportive care   Treatment must be directed toward surgical correction of any existing obstructive disorder and toward supplying nourishment by one of several routes. Where functional disturbances interfere merely with intake, as in immaturity, sepsis, or cerebral insult, adequate nutrition may be sustained by nasogastric tube feeding. Where chest surgery has been performed to correct tracheoesophageal anomalies, a temporary gastrostomy is performed and a tube sutured into the opening for feedings until the esophageal junction heals. Supplementary intravenous fluids containing glucose and electrolytes or blood transfusions may also be indicated.

Infants with obstruction of the colon or with imperforate anus will require a colostomy or a jejunostomy to bypass the distal surgical repair in order to allow healing. These procedures add to the problems of nursing care, for the more liquid stool is quite irritating to the skin surrounding the stoma.

PARENTERAL HYPERALIMENTATION   In cases of extensive or protracted intestinal obstruction or dysfunction, adequate nutrition cannot be maintained by peripheral vein infusions. Any solution of adequate amounts of nutrients such as amino acids and hypertonic glucose is too viscous and even sclerosing for small veins. Deep intravenous *hyperalimentation* is a technique by means of which a highly enriched solution equivalent in nutritive value to milk can be administered to the infant. A polyethylene catheter is introduced into the external jugular vein at the side of the neck through a small skin incision. The catheter is threaded down through the superior vena cava to the right atrium of the heart. Thus, the

concentrated solution is immediately diluted into the rapidly flushing large volume of blood entering the heart without irritating any vascular walls. The exterior portion of the catheter is tunneled under the skin for several centimeters, from the point of introduction into the jugular vein upward, and brought out through a lateral incision in the scalp. The solution is pumped into the catheter by steady flow by an electric infusion pump with an interposed millipore filter to eliminate any milliparticles of solid matter that could initiate thrombi or otherwise block small blood vessels. Details of feeding methods used for preterm infants are found in Chap. 30.

MAINTAINING IMMUNOLOGIC DEFENSES

The process of immunization is the mechanism by which the body produces antibodies to neutralize or destroy foreign protein substances known as *antigens*. These antigens may be live microorganisms or inert organic structures such as red blood cells and killed bacterial vaccines. The specific antibody structure remains fixed in the "memory" of the plasma cells and other cells of the reticuloendothelial system, so that when the host is again challenged by either the natural disease organisms or a booster dose of vaccine, a rapid rise in level (titer) of the specific antibody will occur. Immunity in response to antigen stimulus is called *active immunity*.

In contrast, if preformed antibodies from another source are injected into the host just before or during an attack of an antigen, the host will have no need to form specific antibodies. The donated antibodies from human serum from another already immunized person or in animal serum (e.g., from a horse) can confer *passive immunity* on the host. The donated antibodies will last in the system about 4 to 6 weeks, after which there is neither protection nor "memory" for recall of antibody formation by future antigen invasions.

humoral defenses

The newborn infant has two humoral defense mechanisms against infections that are both dependent upon the gamma globulin (gg) fraction of the blood known as the immunoglobulins (Ig). These are the antibodies that inactivate invading alien substances like bacteria and viruses by combining with their antigens and destroying them. One source of immunoglobulins is the mother, from whom the fetus acquires smaller molecular immunoglobulins (IgG) by transport across the placenta beginning at the fourth to sixth month of gestation. These confer passive immunity on the infant against such diseases as measles, rubella, and smallpox if the mother has had the diseases or has been immunized against them.

Another source of immunoglobulins of larger molecular weight (IgM) is the fetus' or neonate's own limited production of active antibodies in response to intrauterine or postnatal infection. Thus, for example, a fetus infected in utero by a luetic (syphilitic) mother will have IgM detectable in the bloodstream at birth.

The neonate's supply of IgG against many common perinatal infections, such as gram-negative fecal organisms like *Escherichia coli* and *Klebsiella* and gram-positive vaginal flora like *Listeria monocytogenes* and beta-hemolytic streptococci group B, is virtually nonexistent. Nor is the neonate capable of forming enough immunoglobulins to combat massive bacterial invasion by these organisms, to which older individuals are mainly immune. Neonatal infections are therefore potentially life-threatening because of the newborn infant's immunologic incompetence. (See protection via breast milk, Chap. 16.)

There are certain rare conditions in which the individual lacks immunologic competence because of congenital defects that result in a lack of gamma globulins. Such a condition is called *agammaglobulinemia,* and there are two types. One results from the absence of the thymus gland and, therefore, of T-cell immunity, the DiGeorge syndrome. The other type is exemplified by the Bruton agammaglobulinemia in which plasma cells are lacking, and therefore, there is an absence of humoral immunity and gamma globulins. Other conditions and syndromes of immunologic incompetence develop beyond the neonatal period for various reasons.

supportive care The newborn period and the first few months of infancy require special intervention to protect the infant from infection. Nursery asepsis and instruction to parents regarding ways of protecting the infant must be thorough.

immunologic problems

isoimmunization The mechanism of becoming *sensitized* or of forming antibodies against antigens from the same species is termed *iso*immunization or alloimmunization. Normally, immunization is essential for survival of the host, but in several cases it is a detrimental process. Where there is Rh factor incompatibility or ABO incompatibility, the infant may be jeopardized. Many other incompatible blood groups exist, but problems with Rh and ABO factors are most commonly seen.

When two parents have different blood types, the infant of these parents may inherit a red blood cell group from the father that differs from the mother's group. As a result, specific antibodies that can destroy those erythrocytes may be produced in the mother's serum against the antigen of the fetal red cells when even a few of these enter her bloodstream during gestation or at the time of delivery.

The placenta is usually a very effective barrier between maternal and fetal circulation, so that an antigen-antibody reaction takes place during or after pregnancy only if there is intermingling of fetal cells into the mother's circulation. Movement may go in the mother's direction when minute breaks occur in the placental interface—in cases of infection of the placenta itself, during trauma at delivery or abortion, or when normal small tears occur in the placenta as it separates naturally during the third stage.

By the same antigen-antibody reaction, a nulliparous Rh-negative woman may be immunized and build up anti-Rh antibodies after receiving a transfusion of Rh-positive blood. The antibody buildup in either the gestation or transfusion situation will not harm the woman herself but will be detrimental to future Rh-positive fetuses.

Studies have shown that it takes as little as 0.5 mL blood containing the antigens to cause a significant antibody response.[4] It requires about 72 h for this critical process to be stimulated, an important factor in the application of preventive therapy. Antibody formation may take 6 weeks to 6 months after stimulus. Once there has been an antibody response, however, the maternal antibodies can traverse the barrier to enter the fetal circulation and attack the erythrocytes.

ABO incompatibility Genetic inheritance of one factor from each parent leads to six possible genotypes in the ABO blood group system.

Homozygous	Heterozygous
OO	AO
AA	BO
BB	AB

Depending on which antigen is in the red cell, the opposite antibody is present in the plasma. For example, if a person has type B,

then there will be anti-A antibodies in the plasma (see Table 29-4).

The pathogenesis of ABO incompatibility differs from that operating in Rh incompatibility because the group O mother already possesses a and b agglutinins (i.e., anti-A and anti-B antibodies) which may cross the placental barrier and interact with the A or B factors in the erythrocytes of the fetus. Interestingly, when both Rh and ABO incompatibility coexist, the presence of anti-A or anti-B antibodies in the mother's circulation usually suppresses her production of Rh antibodies. As the incompatible fetal erythrocytes enter her bloodstream, they are destroyed by the anti-A or anti-B antibodies before their Rh antigen can stimulate the mother's formation of anti-Rh antibodies.

ABO may account for about two-thirds of the maternal isoimmunization with consequent neonatal disease,[5] but with milder effects than Rh incompatibility. There are three possible combinations that are incompatible.

Mother	Infant
O	A, B, or AB
A	B
B	A

Problems are most frequent with an O mother and an A infant, less common with the O mother and a B infant, and very rare in the other combinations.

Rh incompatibility The Rh group is made up of several factors of varying strengths. We refer to *positive* factors as to the strongest factors in reaction with a specific

table 29-4 ABO antigen placement

type	antigen in red cell	antibodies in plasma
O	None	Anti-A, anti-B
A	A	Anti-B
B	B	Anti-A
AB	A and B	None

table 29-5 CDE typing of Rh group, with Rh-hr equivalents

Rh 1	= D	= Rh$_o$
Rh 2	= C	= rh′
Rh 3	= E	= rh″
Rh 4	= c	= hr′*
Rh 5	= e	= hr″

*At present Hro(d) is not demonstrable but is considered as part of the scheme.

antiserum test. In this country the Rh group is referred to using the *CDE* typing, but others use the Rh-Hr system. Table 29-5 indicates the equivalents. Factor *D* is the major factor in Rh incompatibility, although in rare instances the infant will be jeopardized by other factor (*C* or *E*) incompatibility (Fig. 29-14).

An Rh-negative person must be homozygous because the Rh-negative cell group is a recessive genetic factor; both the genes involved are lacking the dominant Rh factor and are therefore "negative." An Rh-positive person may be either homozygous or heterozygous, for the dominant gene overshadows the others in the group. The genetic inheritance laws indicate that if both parents are heterozygous for positive, the infant has a 50 percent chance of being heterozygous positive, a 25 percent chance of being homozygous positive, and a 25 percent chance of being homozygous negative (Fig. 29-15). This pattern demonstrates one of the reasons why incompatibility does not always result in problems for the infant.

fig. 29-14 Method of transfer of antigen-antibody. (*Courtesy of Ross Laboratories, Columbus, Ohio, Clinical Education Aid No. 9.*)

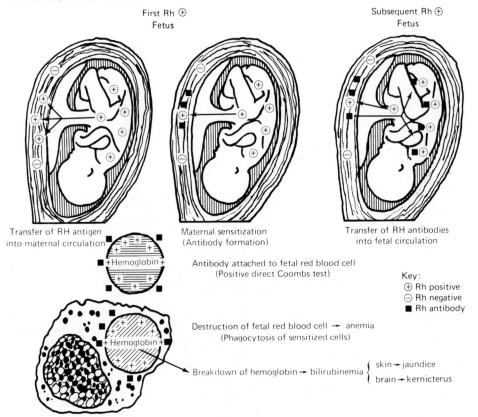

First Rh ⊕ Fetus

Subsequent Rh ⊕ Fetus

Transfer of RH antigen into maternal circulation

Maternal sensitization (Antibody formation)

Transfer of RH antibodies into fetal circulation

+Hemoglobin+

Antibody attached to fetal red blood cell (Positive direct Coombs test)

Key:
⊕ Rh positive
⊖ Rh negative
■ Rh antibody

+Hemoglobin+

Destruction of fetal red blood cell → anemia (Phagocytosis of sensitized cells)

Breakdown of hemoglobin → bilirubinemia { skin → jaundice / brain → kernicterus

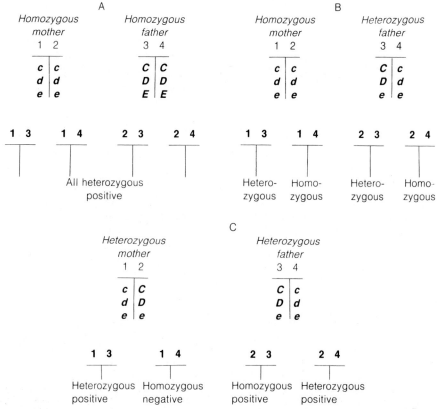

fig. 29-15 Examples of zygosity with the Rh grouping (CDE.) (*Adapted from Obstetrics Illustrated.*)

effects on the fetus and neonate Though there are no clinically apparent effects on the mother as a result of isoimmunization, the consequences for the fetus and infant may range from mild to fatal, if untreated. Depending on the level of the mother's antibody titer and the concentration of her antibodies that entered the fetal circulation before birth, the degree and duration of hemolysis of the infant's blood cells may be more or less severe.

COOMBS' TEST   The most frequently used test to determine antibody presence in fetal or maternal blood, the Coombs' test, uses the serum of rabbits immunized against human globulin. Because the maternal Rh antibodies are globulins, the rabbit immune *antiglobulin* will cause agglutination (direct Coombs' positive) when added to the affected infant's cord blood, the cells of which are coated with maternal antibodies. The *direct* Coombs' test is often negative in the presence of ABO incompatibility, perhaps because of the lack of sensitivity of A or B antigens in the infant's cells.

The *indirect* Coombs' test uses the mother's serum rather than her red cells to demonstrate whether antibodies are present, either from a prior transfusion of incompatible blood or by isoimmunization during pregnancy. A rise in the level or titer indicates that the process is continuing to proceed, more antibodies are forming, and the fetus will be jeopardized. A reaction at a titer of 1:8 is acceptable, but anything stronger than that is a sign of maternal sensitization.[4] A higher titer means that the serum has been diluted several times and still gives an agglutination reaction when placed with the antiglobulin.

ANEMIA   In severe cases of incompatibility, the fetus becomes very anemic. Fluid is pulled into the vascular system, and edema develops in all body tissues. Without treatment, this edematous, anemic infant with *hydrops fetalis* will die in utero or soon after birth. With current therapy the incidence of such severe disease has been much diminished; rarely is such a condition seen.

hyperbilirubinemia

Hemoglobin breaks down into globin (globulin fraction) and heme. The heme fraction then splits into molecules of iron and unconjugated bilirubin. The latter becomes bound to circulating albumin molecules and is transported to liver cells. Slowing or interference with this binding and transport process raises the blood concentration of unconjugated, indirect, fat-soluble bilirubin. In order to be excreted, bilirubin must be conjugated within the liver by an enzymatic reaction with *glucuronyl transferase*. The conjugated form is called direct bilirubin and is water-soluble. It is excreted mainly through the bile into the intestines; some is partially reabsorbed and stored for reuse, and some is excreted by kidneys in the form of urine urobilinogen. Table 29-6 lists the causes of neonatal hyperbilirubinemia.

developmental hyperbilirubinemia

In newborn infants, some elevation of bilirubin stems from the normal process of destruction of excess fetal hemoglobin. Once oxygen is

table 29-6   Causes of neonatal hyperbilirubinemia

I. Elevated unconjugated bilirubin
    A. Iso (or allo) immunization
       1. Rh_o incompatibility
       2. ABO incompatibility
       3. Subgroup incompatibility
    B. Physiologic jaundice
    C. Hemolytic jaundice
       1. G-6-P-D deficiency
       2. Congenital erythrocyte abnormalities
    D. Sepsis
    E. Crigler-Najjar syndrome
    F. Maternal drugs
    G. Hematoma

II. Elevated conjugated bilirubin
    A. Atresia of bile duct
    B. Biliary stasis or inspissated bile syndrome
    C. Neonatal hepatic disease
       1. Hepatitis
       2. Cirrhosis

available through the lungs, the higher fetal hematocrit value is no longer necessary and within a few days the red blood cell count drops to the level of 4.5 to 6 million. This destruction of extra cells temporarily overloads the immature liver beyond its capacity to furnish enough enzyme for glucuronidation (conversion of bilirubin to the conjugated form). Thus, all newborns, unless postmature, are likely to experience an elevation of bilirubin blood level, with a mean peak of about 6 mg/100 mL on the third or fourth day of life. Since jaundice becomes clinically evident at about 5 mg/100 mL, only about half of all newborns will show signs of such physiologic jaundice. The term *developmental hyperbilirubinemia* is now used as a more exact description of the process.

hemolytic jaundice   Hemolysis of red cells, either because of G-6-P-D enzyme deficiency or because of congenital abnormalities of the hemoglobin molecule, such as spherocytosis or, rarely, even sickle-cell disease, may cause a high level of bilirubin in the same manner as does erythrocyte destruction in cases of blood group incompatibility.

sepsis   Sepsis is a condition of generalized infection in the newborn, usually accompanied by bloodstream infection (bacteremia or septicemia), as a result of invading microorganisms. This serious type of infection produces jaundice by hemolysis, liver involvement, or both.

Crigler-Najjar syndrome   The Crigler-Najjar syndrome is a rare inherited autosomal (not sex-linked) recessive condition in which the liver, although otherwise structurally and physiologically normal, does not produce a sufficient amount of glucuronyl transferase. Thus, jaundice is almost always present in afflicted individuals because of their ever-present hyperbilirubinemia.

maternal drugs   As has been previously noted, some drugs administered to the mother prior to labor and delivery, or even to the neonate (notably sulfonamides), will compete with unconjugated bilirubin for albumin-binding sites. This keeps more bilirubin circulating free in the blood and leads to jaundice or an increase in the already elevated levels.

hematoma   In a large hematoma that has been produced by trauma during delivery, there is an appreciable amount of extravasated blood. As this is broken down and resorbed into the bloodstream, it raises the level of circulating unconjugated bilirubin.

elevated conjugated bilirubin   Unlike the unconjugated form, conjugated bilirubin is not fat-soluble and is, therefore, not toxic for the brain cells. Nevertheless, elevated levels do indicate serious underlying pathology within the liver, and it does produce jaundice. Causes of elevated levels of conjugated bilirubin are *congenital atresia* or obstruction of the bile duct, *inspissated bile syndrome* or stasis of thickened bile in the bile passages within the liver, hepatitis acquired from an infected mother, and, very rarely, congenital cirrhosis of the liver.

kernicterus

When bilirubin levels rise too high, brain damage may occur because of deposit of the fat-soluble, indirect-reacting bilirubin in brain cells. This event, *kernicterus,* is to be avoided because it leads to permanent damage of the brain cells. Symptoms of kernicterus are lethargy, poor feeding, opisthotonus, and hypertonus. Kernicterus may result in the child having chorioathetoid cerebral palsy, deafness, and mental retardation. In lesser degrees it results in minimal brain dysfunction, with clumsiness and learning disabilities.

Between developmental hyperbilirubinemia with levels under 10 mg/100 mL and kernicterus, there lies a range of bilirubin levels that are serious but treatable. Keeping bilirubin levels below 18 to 20 mg/100 mL has fairly consistently prevented kernicterus. However, a compromised, sick infant can be damaged more easily. Premature infants are especially vulnerable because of immaturity of body systems. If the baby is anoxic or has acidosis, hypoglycemia, or infection, it is much more vulnerable to kernicterus at lower levels of bilirubinemia.

supportive care   Until the early 1960s the only treatment available for use in serious cases of hemolysis and jaundice was an exchange transfusion. A fetus severely affected with erythrocyte destruction from incompatibility early in gestation was virtually doomed to fetal death and stillbirth or to a very premature birth. Now, in severe cases, when the infant is deemed too small to survive and is suffering from severe anemia because of red cell destruction, an intrauterine transfusion can be done.

INTRAUTERINE TRANSFUSION   After correct placement of the transfusion cannula through the mother's abdominal wall into the uterus, Rh-negative, type O packed red cells are administered into the fetal peritoneal cavity. Amazingly, the red cells can be absorbed intact across the peritoneal wall into the circulation of the infant.

Intrauterine transfusions may have to be administered as early as the twenty-first week of gestation and may have to be repeated several times to maintain an adequate hemoglobin and hematocrit level. Although there is a high risk of complications, many cases are on record in which a jeopardized infant has been carried to a safe delivery and become a normally thriving infant.

It is possible to predict if the infant will have trouble by testing two factors; the mother's antibody titer (rising titers mean increasing antibody production) and the level of bilirubin excreted into the amniotic fluid by the fetus (rising levels mean increasing hemolysis).

The physician may have to estimate the best time for delivery, balancing immaturity against a rising titer (maternal indirect Coombs' test) and bilirubin level (amniotic fluid density). Delivery as early as 4 weeks preterm may prevent a considerable amount of hemolysis and hyperbilirubinemia, but the resultant immaturity may handicap the infant in other serious ways in addition to inadequate bilirubin metabolism.

EXCHANGE TRANSFUSION   When there is a serious degree of jaundice in the first 24 h of life or low levels of hemoglobin because of hemolysis, an exchange transfusion may be the most effective way to rescue the infant. The process involves removing and replacing about 20 mL at a time, by way of an umbilical vein catheter and a three-way stopcock connected to a syringe, a blood container, and the catheter, usually until as much as 500 mL of blood has been exchanged. A low-birth-weight baby might be given less blood.

In order to prevent the clotting of the donor blood in the container, sodium citrate is added to it at the time of collection. When this citrated blood is given to the infant, it tends to deplete his serum calcium by combining with it. Since low calcium levels can cause tetany with convulsions, and possibly even death, 1 mL of 10 percent calcium gluconate should be injected slowly through the venous catheter after each 100 mL of blood has been exchanged.

The goal of an exchange transfusion is the removal of about 80 percent of the infant's Rh-positive antigenic red cells along with the maternal anti-Rh antibodies, and replacement with Rh-negative nonantigenic red blood cells. The infant's own type (A, B, or O) with Rh-negative blood is used. The donor blood is also cross-matched against the mother's serum to test for serologic compatibility. When ABO incompatibility is severe enough to call for an exchange transfusion, the infant is given type O, Rh-negative blood. In very severe cases of either, there may be enough circulating antibodies that a second or even a third transfusion may be required.

PHOTOTHERAPY   For a long time it was known that when blood was drawn from a patient for bilirubin determination, the specimen had to be shielded from light. Light produced a chemical change, causing a false low reading. Then some observers noted that there seemed to be a lower incidence of jaundice among newborns on the sunny side or in the brightly lighted areas of the nursery than among those infants in the less bright areas. It took a while for these observations to be synthesized into a hypothesis that could be tested and proved.[6]

The chemical reaction is a photic one, dependent on light intensity at the blue-short-wavelength end of the visible spectrum. It was originally thought that the therapeutic effect of phototherapy was the result of the transformation of the fat-soluble unconjugated bilirubin, a tetrapyrole compound, into a dipyrole water-soluble compound that was excreted by the kidneys. The current concept, however, is that the unconjugated bilirubin molecule is somehow altered by phototherapy to enable it to pass through the liver cells unaltered by glucuronyl transferase and to be excreted in the bile.

During treatment, which lasts about 3 days, the baby's eyes must be shielded from the light. Eye pads covered by a light-proof outer bandage or pad protect the delicate retina from prolonged exposure to bright light. Nurses should remove the baby from the lights and remove the eye shield during feeding times in order to permit early visual stimulation for the infant and to cleanse the eyes (Fig. 29-16).

Complications of therapy should be noted. Insensible water loss is increased to two to three times that of infants not receiving therapy. There is an increase in stooling, sometimes with the consistency of diarrhea, probably as a result of the increase of unconjugated bilirubin in the stool. Rash may occur, and the possibility of increased speed of absorption of intramuscular medication has been explored. Since a large surface must be exposed while the infant is unclothed, temperature regulation may be a problem.[7] Although these problems are less significant than the effect of severe jaundice, they still require observation and intervention before they become major problems. Removing the infant from lights is the remedy.

Though phototherapy has become widely accepted, there is some lingering doubt about its complete safety. Questions exist about the possible long-range toxicity of bilirubin breakdown products and about the effect of light energy on the chemical elements of the blood and other body cells. Therefore, some limitations and guidelines for the application of phototherapy are important. It is not used prophylactically to prevent physiologic jaundice but is used only after bilirubin levels have risen above 12 to 14 mg/100 mL, and the duration of use is only long enough to drop the blood level back down below 10 mg/100 mL. When properly employed, phototherapy is a useful tool to prevent damaging hyperbilirubinemia.

OTHER THERAPIES   Other therapeutic modalities are sometimes used to prevent or to lower hyperbilirubinemia. Phenobarbital is a com-

fig. 29-16   (a) Phototherapy. (b) Eyes must be bandaged to protect against light. (*Photographs by Ruth Helmich.*)

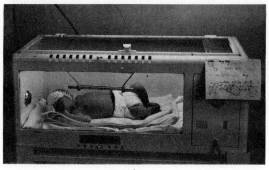

A

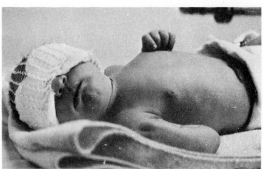

B

pound that enhances enzyme production in the liver cells and so induces (speeds up) glucuronyl transferase activity. When it is administered to the gravida in the last weeks of her pregnancy or to the newborn after birth when there is expected risk of hyperbilirubinemia, the drug has been shown to lessen or even to prevent its occurrence. However, when the medication is administered to the infant after the occurrence of jaundice, it does not seem to reduce it appreciably.

Another treatment procedure to prevent or treat jaundice is the intravenous injection of human albumin into the jaundiced infant or the neonate at risk. This affords more binding sites for the unconjugated bilirubin molecules on the increased number of albumin molecules and thus enhances transport to the liver for glucuronidation.

Thus, while other treatments are available for the treatment of hemolytic disease and hyperbilirubinemia and are able to obviate the need for exchange transfusions in many cases, there are instances when transfusions are mandatory. Where there is an initial or early high blood bilirubin level, where the level is rising rapidly, or where the level has reached dangerous levels, exchange transfusion must not be delayed or deferred lest kernicterus develop.

prevention of isoimmunization

The mechanism of passive immunization forms the rationale for preventing isoimmunization of Rh-negative mothers who bear Rh-positive infants. Rh-negative gamma globulin (RhoGAM) is a serum concentrate containing pooled anti-Rh D antibodies. These antibodies, if injected within 72 h after delivery or abortion, will destroy any Rh-positive fetal cells that may have entered the mother's circulation at the time of delivery. Because these fetal cells are destroyed, the mother

then has no stimulation to form her own antibodies with cells that are imprinted with "memory" for the next occasion. Just *after* each subsequent pregnancy the mother who is not isoimmunized must be *passively reimmunized*. In this way any development of hemolytic disease for the newborn can be completely prevented. Once she becomes sensitized, RhoGAM can no longer be of any value. Therefore, before administration, both her and her infant's Coombs' test reactions must be checked. If the response is already positive, antibodies have already formed and it is too late to begin prevention. Since the gamma globulin has been cross-matched with her blood, the cross-match numbers must also be carefully checked before intramuscular administration.

So far, no similar procedure exists for preventing ABO incompatibility. There are no amniotic fluid tests or blood tests to distinguish between naturally present a or b agglutinins in an O mother's serum and an augmented titer due to the introduction of fetal A or B erythrocytes into her blood. Nor has there been developed an antiserum for passive immunization if such tests were available. Fortunately, ABO incompatibility is usually less severe and rarely requires exchange transfusion.

Prevention is the key to future elimination of Rh-negative problems. Every woman who is typed as Rh-negative with a homozygous or heterozygous mate should be educated about prevention. Anti-D gamma globulin should be administered to her within 72 h of any delivery, abortion, or stillbirth, to provide protection against active isoimmunization.

study questions

1 Review the difference in oxygenation in the fetal and neonatal period. What factors will cause hypoxia prior to birth? (See Chaps. 26 and 27.) How does hypoxia after birth occur?

2 Outline the causes underlying the respiratory dis-

tress syndrome. Describe which infants are more likely to experience this difficulty after birth.

3 Describe the signs of respiratory difficulty a nursery nurse could observe. What major supportive care should be provided?

4 What is the difference between a cyanotic and an acyanotic cardiac anomaly?

5 How is it possible to prevent brain injury to the developing fetus? List four preventive measures which should be included in prenatal care or in care during labor and delivery.

6 Some traumatic birth injuries are unavoidable. Describe those injuries to the head and peripheral nerves which are minor and quickly healed and compare them with the major injuries.

7 How can a nurse identify the signs of hypoglycemia in the newborn? What is the best treatment for a full-term infant? How does care for an IDM differ?

8 What are signs of neurologic damage which a nurse can observe in the nursery?

9 Why does the newborn take longer than an adult to show withdrawal signs? Contrast methadone and heroin withdrawal patterns.

10 Identify nursing care based on each of the symptoms in Table 29-2. How does pharmacologic treatment assist the infant through withdrawal? Why is it important to taper drugs at the end of treatment?

11 Anomalies of the genitourinary tract may or may not be visible. Renal or ureter problems most usually show as disturbed voiding patterns. What are these signs?

12 What steps must be taken before the infant with ambiguous genitalia is sent home? (See Chap. 28, too.)

13 List the major signs and symptoms and interventions for four major inborn errors of metabolism. (Pick the four most commonly seen in your area.) Also refer to single-gene defects as discussed in Chap. 28.

14 Obstructive problems in the GI tract usually require surgical repair. What signs and symptoms would make a nursery nurse aware that there was a baby with such a problem? (List defects and usual signs.)

15 Why is the newborn so susceptible to infection? (Refer also to breast-feeding benefits in Chap. 16.)

16 Although with the wide use of the preventive effect of Rh gamma globulin, the problem of incompatibility has diminished, nurses need to be aware that immigrants, patients from poorer areas of the country, or those who have delivered or aborted without medical supervision may be sensitized. If a pregnant woman is to be tested for Rh sensitization, what three tests are used?

17 Describe the differences between ABO and Rh incompatibilities as to:

a Severity
b Incidence
c Who is high risk
d Results on infant
e Preventive treatment

18 Why is hyperbilirubinemia a serious concern in the newborn infant? Which physiologic factors aggravate its effect?

19 Compare developmental hyperbilirubinemia with severe and kernicteric states.

20 Describe the methods of treatment for excess bilirubin, and identify when each would be selected.

21 What precautions must be taken before you administer Rh_oD gamma globulin to a newly delivered mother? Should the woman know the purpose of the injection? How would you explain it to her?

references

1 P. M. Farrell and R. E. Wood, "Epidemiology of Hyaline Membrane Disease in the United States: Analysis of National Mortality Statistics," *Pediatrics*, **58**:167, 1976.

2 G. C. Liggins and R. N. Howie, "The Prevention of RDS by Maternal Steroid Therapy," in L. Gluck (ed.): *Modern Perinatal Medicine*, Year Book, Chicago, 1974, pp. 415–424.

3 S. R. Kendall, "Transitional Drugs and the Newborn," in E. J. Dickason et al. (eds.), *Maternal and Infant Drugs and Nursing Intervention*, McGraw-Hill, New York, 1978, p. 271.

4 E. R. Jennings, "Fetal-Maternal Hemorrhage: Its Detection, Measurement and Significance," *RhoGam Symposium*, New York City, Apr. 17, 1969.

5 L. M. Gartner and M. Hollander, "Disorders of Bilirubin Metabolism," in N. Assali (ed.), *Pathophysiology of Gestation: Fetal and Neonatal Disorders*, vol. 3, Academic Press, New York, 1972, chap. 8, p. 466.

6 J. F. Lucey, "Neonatal Jaundice and Phototherapy," *Pediatric Clinics of North America*, **19**(4):827, 1972.

7 J. W. Seligman, "Management of Hyperbilirubinemia," *Pediatric Clinics of North America*, (24):522, July 1977.

bibliography

Ambrus, C. M., Choi, T. S., Cunnanan, E., et al.: "Prevention of Hyaline Membrane Disease with Plasminogen," *Journal of the American Medical Association*, **237**:1837–1841, 1977.

Ampola, M. G.: "Symposium on Early Detection and Management of Inborn Errors," *Clinical Perinatology* **3**: 1–2, March 1976.

Buist, N. R., "Metabolic Screening of the Newborn Infant," *Clinics in Endocrinology and Metabolism* **5**(265): 88, 1976.

Ellis, M. I., "Haemolytic Diseases of the Newborn," *Nursing Times*, **71:**2050–2052, 1975.

Fluge, G., K. F. Stoa, and D. Aarskog: "Endocrinological Aspects at Follow-up Studies in Neonatal Hypoglycemia," *Acta Paediatrica Scandinavica*, **64:**280–286, 1975.

Harris, H.: Cardiorespiratory Problems in the Newborn. *Postgraduate Medicine* **60:**92–97, 1977.

Hirschhorn, K.: "Human Genetics," *Journal of the American Medical Association*, **224:**597–604, 1973.

Kelly, V. C. (ed.): *Practice of Pediatrics*, Harper & Row, New York, 1976.

Klugo, R. C., J. H. Fisher, and A. B. Retik: "Management of Urogenital Anomalies in Cloacal Dysgenesis," *Journal of Urology* **112:**832–835, 1974.

Levy, H. L.: "Newborn Metabolic Screening: Past-Prospect," *New England Journal of Medicine*, **293:**824–825, 1975.

Madden, J. D., J. N. Chappel, F. Zuspan, et al.: "Observation and Treatment of Neonatal Narcotic Withdrawal," *American Journal of Obstetrics and Gynecology*, **127:**199–201, 1977.

Mamunes, P.: "Newborn Screening for Metabolic Disorders," *Clinical Perinatology*, **3:**231–250, 1976.

Meloni, T., S. Costa, A. Dore, et al.: "Phototherapy for Neonatal Hyperbilirubinemia in Mature Newborn Infants with Erythrocyte G-6-PD Deficiency," *Journal of Pediatrics*, **85:**560–562, 1974.

Morrow, G.: "Nutritional Management of Infants with Inborn Metabolic Errors," *Clinical Perinatology*, **2:** 361–372, 1975.

Ostrea, E. M., C. J. Chavez, M. E. Strauss: "A Study of Factors That Influence the Severity of Neonatal Narcotic Withdrawal," *Journal of Pediatrics*, **88:**642–645, 1976.

Pierog, S., O. Chandavasu, and I. Wexler: "Withdrawal Symptoms in Infants with the Fetal Alcohol Syndrome," *Journal of Pediatrics*, **90:**630–633, 1977.

Rosta, J., Z. Makoi, D. Bekefi, et al.: "Time-Limited Phototherapy of Term Newborns in ABO Hemolytic Disease and Hyperbilirubinemia," *Journal of Perinatal Medicine*, **3:**198–203, 1975.

Rudolph, A. M., H. L. Barnett, and A. H. Einhorn (eds.): *Pediatrics*, 16th ed., Appleton-Century-Crofts, New York, 1977.

Ruhbar, F.: "Observations on Methadone Withdrawal in 16 Neonates," *Clinical Perinatology*, 369–371, 1975.

Schaffer, A. J., and M. E. Avery (eds.): *Diseases of the Newborn*, 4th ed., Saunders, Philadelphia, 1977.

Stern, L.: "The Use and Misuse of Oxygen in the Newborn Infant," *Pediatric Clinics of North America*, **20:** 447–464, 1973.

Strauss, M. E., R. H. Starr, Jr., E. M. Ostrea, et al.: "Behavioral Concomitants of Prenatal Addiction to Narcotics," *Journal of Pediatrics*, **89:**842–846, 1976.

Vaughn, V. C., R. J. McKay, and W. E. Nelson: *Textbook of Pediatrics*, 19th ed., Saunders, Philadelphia, 1975.

Walker, W.: "Haemolytic Anemia in the Newborn Infant," Clinical Haematology **4:**145–166, 1975.

———: "Management of RH Isoimmunization," Lancet, **1:**256–257, 1976.

Zawodnik, S. A., G. D. Bonnard, A. E. Gautier, et al.: "Antibody-dependent Cell-mediated Destruction of Human Erythrocytes Sensitized in ABO and Rhesus Fetal-Maternal Incompatibilities," *Pediatric Research*, **10:** 791–796, 1976.

30

THE PRETERM INFANT

ARLENE RITZ

The death toll among babies born too soon and too small has been appallingly high. Even with intensive research and advances in the medical and nursing care of such infants, they account for approximately 63 percent of the infants that die every year. Not only does preterm birth carry with it a high death rate, but studies have repeatedly confirmed the increased frequency of sequelae such as mental retardation, neurologic diseases, and visual handicaps.

CLASSIFICATION

In recent years the terminology regarding fetal growth and birth weight has become more precise. The term *low birth weight* is presently defined as a birth weight of less than 2500 g regardless of gestational age. The use of birth weight alone is misleading in diagnosing prematurity. For example, a newborn may weigh under 2500 g but may be a mature neonate without any physiologic underdevelopment. Because of this confusion, both the American Academy of Pediatrics Committee on the Fetus and the Newborn[1] and the Expert Committee of the World Health Organization have recommended that a clear distinction be made between the terms *low birth weight* and *prematurity,* as follows:

Low-birth-weight infant—any live-born infant with a weight at birth of 2500 g or less.
Premature infant—a live-born infant with a gestation period of less than 37 weeks regardless of weight. (Now referred to as a preterm infant.)

Gestational age is now recognized as the quantitative indicator of fetal growth, and the following nomenclature is used:[2]

Preterm or premature infant is one with a gestational period of less than 37 weeks.
Term or mature infant is one with a gestational period of 38 to 42 weeks.
Postterm or postmature infant is one with a gestational age greater than 42 weeks.

Special problems are posed by infants whose birth weights are below average for their gestational age. This group makes up approximately 30 to 50 percent of all low-birth-weight infants. It is now recognized that the relationship between birth weight and gestational age is very important, since it reflects the quality of fetal growth and, at present, is the standard for defining deviant fetal growth. Battaglia and Lubchenco have formulated charts which enable one to plot birth weight in relation to fetal growth percentile curves.[3] Ideally, each neonate should be compared with a population of similar ethnic, racial, and perinatal backgrounds, but such charts are not currently available. When birth weight is plotted on growth percentile curves,

these neonates are divided into three groups, each of which presents different clinical problems:

AGA: Average-for-gestational-age — Neonates falling between the tenth and ninetieth percentile who are believed to have normal fetal growth. Such infants born before 37 weeks' gestation are considered true preterm neonates.
LGA: Large-for-gestational-age — Neonates falling on or above the ninetieth percentile who are believed to have growth acceleration or excess.
SGA: Small-for-gestational-age — Neonates falling on or below the tenth percentile who are believed to have intrauterine growth deficiency or retardation (Fig. 30-1).
These SGA neonates account for a large proportion of perinatal mortality, particularly in the intrauterine period. The difficulties encountered by these infants are generally caused by maternal or fetal problems such as malnutrition, multiple births, placental circulation insufficiency, endocrine disorders, and congenital anomalies (Fig. 30-2).
The SGA neonates also may be further divided into SGA preterm, term, and postterm infants. The neonates who are both SGA and preterm suffer the double handicap of being both premature and disadvantaged by maternal or fetal disease which contributes markedly to their exceedingly high mortality.

This chapter is limited to the study of the preterm infant whose survival is at considerable risk because of anatomic and physiologic immaturity. However, reflecting the nomenclature used in the vast literature on the

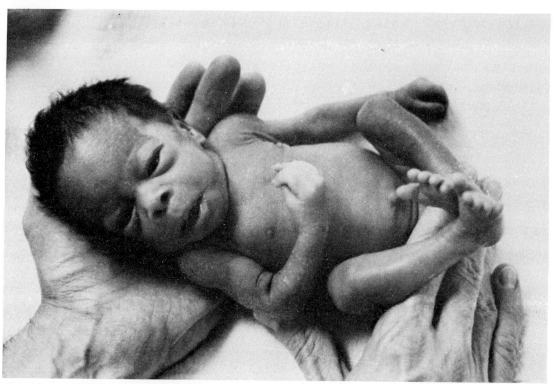

fig. 30-1 Small-for-gestational-age infant. Infant weighing 960 g at birth in the thirty-sixth week of gestation shows the effect of severe intrauterine malnutrition. (*From Pedro Rosso, "Nutrition and Abnormal Fetal Growth," Contemporary OB/GYN, 2(3):54, 1973.*)

subject, in this chapter the word *preterm* is used interchangeably with the words *premature*, *immature*, and *low birth weight*.

INCIDENCE

Using weight as the criterion for prematurity, there is a wide variation in the general incidence throughout the world, which ranges from approximately 4 to 15 percent.

In the United States, approximately 7.2 percent of white infants weigh 2500 g or less at birth.

A significantly higher premature birth rate exists among nonwhites, reportedly as high as 12 to 15 percent. Many etiologic factors have been implicated in this intolerably high incidence—e.g., poor socioeconomic considerations, inadequate nutrition, heavy physical labor, prolonged employment during gestation, and inadequate antepartum care.

MORTALITY

The size and gravity of the problem are reflected in the wastage associated with premature birth. The overall mortality rate of these immature infants reportedly ranges from 20 to 30 percent, which is 30 times that found in mature infants. Studies indicate that approximately 60 to 85 percent of premature neonatal deaths occur in the first 2 days of life. Im-

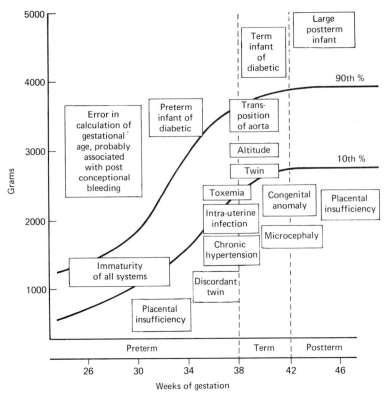

fig. 30-2 Conditions associated with intrauterine growth—related to birth weight and gestational age classification. (*From L. O. Lubchenco, C. Hausman, and Leena Backstrom, "Factors Influencing Fetal Growth," in Nutricia Symposium: Aspects of Prematurity and Dysmaturity, H. E. Stenfert Kroese B. V., Leiden, 1968.*)

maturity accounts for about two-thirds of all infant deaths in the first month of life, and remains the major cause of death throughout infancy. Death is most frequently attributed to immaturity of body systems, intracranial hemorrhage, and infection.

Survival rate is directly proportional to the birth weight. The weight of the fetus increases from 700 g at the end of the second trimester to 3500 g at full term. It is this prodigious growth in the last trimester which influences the ultimate survival rate. For each 500-g group below the 2500-g level, the mortality rate increases fourfold.[4] Mortality reaches almost 90 to 100 percent in the newborn weigh-

ing 1000 g (2 lb) or less, although some centers report survival rates of about 20 percent for infants in this category. As the newborn's weight approaches 2500 g, the survival rate approximates that found in full-term babies.

There is ample evidence that gestational age—if correct—is a valid diagnostic criterion for prematurity. A major difficulty in using this parameter is the reliability of the menstrual history in the average patient.

The nurse can predict the survival possibility of the high-risk infant by looking at the classification chart in Fig. 30-3. Here, weight plus the gestational age is used to predict

NEWBORN CLASSIFICATION AND NEONATAL MORTALITY RISK
BY BIRTH WEIGHT AND GESTATIONAL AGE

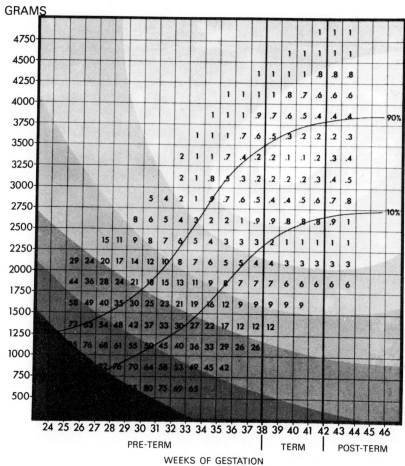

From Lubchenco, Searls, Brazie, J Pediat, 81:814, 1972

Interpolated data based on mathematical fit from original data University of Colorado Medical Center newborns, 7/1/58 – 7/1/69

fig. 30-3 Newborn classification and neonatal mortality risk by birth weight and gestational age. (*From L. O. Lubchenco, D. T. Searls, and J. V. Brazie, "Neonatal Mortality Rate: Relationship to Birth Weight and Gestational Age," Journal of Pediatrics, 81:814–822, 1972.*)

survival. Investigations indicate that the use of both factors is a more significant determinant of survival than use of either weight or age alone. For example, if an infant is admitted to the nursery weighing 1300 g and having an estimated gestational age of 29 weeks, the baby will have about a 50 percent chance of survival. But if the same infant had a gestational age of 33 weeks, the chance of survival would be as high as 70 percent.

MORBIDITY

In addition to this tragic human loss, there is a dreadful risk of morbidity of the infants who survive. During the neonatal period, the preterm infant is especially liable to cerebral hemorrhage, respiratory problems, anemia, dehydration, infections, failure to thrive, and kernicterus.

In general, the lower the birth weight, the greater the incidence of disability in the various aspects of growth and development such as weight, height, and teething. Preterm infants surviving the first year are much more likely to have neurologic and psychologic abnormalities than infants born at term. In a long-term follow-up study on infants weighing under 1500 g at birth, Lubchenco and coworkers reported two out of three infants with central nervous system or visual damage, 50 percent with spastic diplegia, and 40 percent with an IQ under 90.[5]

Social and cultural deprivation so frequently found with these children compounds and complicates the neurologic problems. Emotional immaturity is commonly found during childhood, and prognosis in this regard depends upon the degree of parental emotional stability or distortion.

With the significant improvements in the medical and nursing care of premature infants, survival of very low-birth-weight (under 1500 g) infants has increased. Follow-up studies on these infants have confirmed the pessimistic view that a large number (ranging from 33 to 70 percent) of survivors inevitably suffer from serious abnormalities. This raises an ethical question. Are such extraordinary efforts toward survival justifiable unless there is promise of lessening the incidence of severe handicaps? Rawlings and coworkers point out that modern methods of care aimed at preventing and treating such critical abnormalities as hypoxia, hypoglycemia, and hyperbilirubinemia should not only result in increased survival but also lead to a marked lessening of brain damage in the surviviors.[6] Their contention is supported in an initial study of infants weighing 1500 g or less born at University College Hospital in London between 1966 and 1969. Although this study is limited and incomplete, it offers a new outlook for these infants from the established association of improved survival and increased handicap. Let us hope future studies will confirm this optimism.

CHARACTERISTICS

The physicial appearance of the preterm infant startlingly reflects the deprivation suffered as a result of preterm birth. Figure 30-4 shows a 1300-g, thin, fragile infant suffering from a host of problems common to such babies.

The preterm infant's physical characteristics correlate with gestational age at birth, and classically the infant presents a majority of the features listed in Table 30-1. The more immature the baby, the more exaggerated will be the external differences from the term infant (Fig. 30-5a through e).

Two main parameters are used in the Dubowitz Score to assess gestational age.[7] The first is a series of 10 neurologic signs reflecting postures and primitive reflexes,(Table 30-2) and the second is a series of 11 external characteristics. Figure 30-6 illustrates the neurologic responses with the scores assigned to each, and the procedures for evaluating the postures and reflexes. The external features and their scores are described in Table 30-3. A score of 35 is assigned both to the neurologic signs and to the external criteria, comprising a maximum total score of 70. The graph in Fig. 30-7 correlates this total score with the estimated gestational age. For example, a score of 50 corresponds to a gestational age of 38 weeks; a score of 20 corresponds to 30 gestational weeks.

It is important that the neonatal nurse be

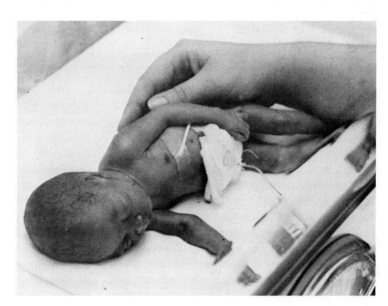

fig. 30-4 A 1300-g infant with estimated gestational age of 31 weeks. This small infant has an arterial catheter in the umbilical cord (to provide fluids and to monitor blood gases) and, attached to the skin of the chest, a temperature-sensing device which leads to the incubator and regulates the environmental temperature according to the infant's variations. (*Photograph courtesy of Long Island Jewish-Hillside Medical Center, New York.*)

table 30-1 Common characteristics of the preterm infant

skin

Thin, delicate, loose, wrinkled
Blood vessels readily seen
Presence of lanugo on face and shoulders
Ecchymosis from trauma or handling at birth
Color reflects baby's condition
First 24 h—smooth, wrinkle-free soles of feet

trunk

Broad and long
Very small chest—wide in transverse, but narrow in anterior-posterior plane
Abdomen round, full, and larger than the chest
Absence of breast nodules

genitalia

Small
Labia majora are open and gaping, and labia minora and clitoris are prominent
Scrotum small; rugal folds and pigmentation absent; testes may be undescended

neurologic status

Minimal activity
Feeble, whining, muted cry
Facial grimacing
Uncoordinated, jerky, asymmetric movements
Gagging, swallowing, and sucking reflexes are weak or absent
Moro reflex is incomplete—throws out arms but does not fist-clench and return arms

face

Head round and relatively large
Eyes prominent
Tongue large
Ears soft and flabby; hug scalp; easily pushed into different shapes
Neck short

extremities

Short in relation to trunk
Fingernails and toenails are soft and extend to the ends of the digits

measurements

Length—less than 47 cm (18 in)
Head circumference—less than 33 cm (13 in)
Disproportion between circumferences of head and thorax; head usually 3 cm or more larger than the chest

position

Lies flat in frog-leg position with shoulders, elbows, and knees all touching mattress. Head is on one side or the other

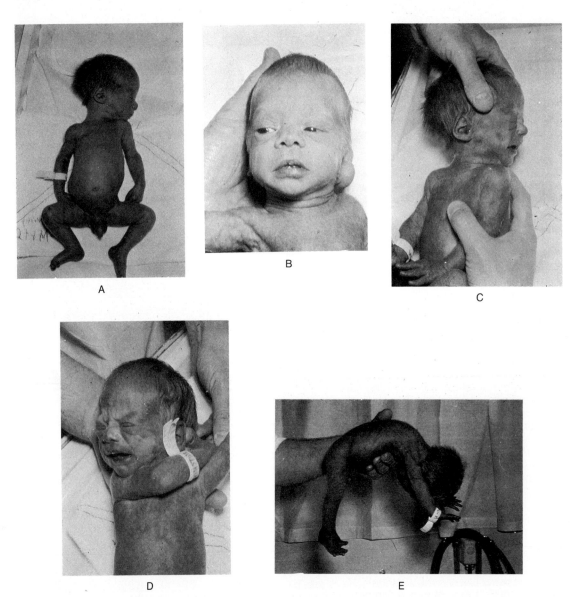

fig. 30-5 Characteristics of the preterm infant. (a) Preterm infant lying supine; note lack of muscle tone, resulting in froglike position with extremities flat on the bed. (b) Preterm infant facies; note lack of subcutaneous fat. (c) Head turned beyond the point of the shoulder. Full-term newborn does not turn head as far as shoulder. (d) Scarf sign: the arm can be pulled around the neck much farther than the arm of a full-term infant. (e) Ventral suspension: the preterm infant hangs limply with straight legs and arms when tested for strength of back and neck muscles. (*Photographs courtesy of Kenneth Holt, M.D., from tape-slide program, "Neurologic Examination of the Newborn," London, England. 1970.*)

table 30-2 Some notes on techniques of assessment of neurologic criteria

posture Observed with infant quiet and in supine position. Score zero—arms and legs extended; 1—beginning of flexion of hips and knees, arms extended; 2—stronger flexion of legs, arms extended; 3—arms slightly flexed, legs flexed and abducted; 4—full flexion of arms and legs.

square window The hand is flexed on the forearm between the thumb and index finger of the examiner. Enough pressure is applied to get as full a flexion as possible, and the angle between the hypothenar eminence and the ventral aspect of the forearm is measured and graded according to diagram. (Care is taken not to rotate the infant's wrist while doing this maneuver.)

ankle dorsiflexion The foot is dorsiflexed onto the anterior aspect of the leg, with the examiner's thumb on the sole of the foot and other fingers behind the leg. Enough pressure is applied to get as full flexion as possible, and the angle between the dorsum of the foot and the anterior aspect of the leg is measured.

arm recoil With the infant in the supine position the forearms are first flexed for 5 s, then fully extended by pulling on the hands, and then released. The sign is fully positive if the arms return briskly to full flexion (score 2). If the arms return to incomplete flexion or the response is sluggish, it is graded as score 1. If they remain extended or are followed only by random movements, the score is 0.

leg recoil With the infant supine, the hips and knees are fully flexed for 5 s, then extended by traction on the feet, and released. A maximal response is one of full flexion of the hips and knees (score 2). A partial flexion scores 1, and minimal or no movement scores 0.

popliteal angle With the infant supine and his pelvis flat on the examining couch, the thigh is held in the knee-chest position by the examiner's left index finger and thumb supporting the knee. The leg is then extended by gentle pressure from the examiner's right index finger behind the ankle and the popliteal angle is measured.

heel-to-ear maneuver With the baby supine, draw the baby's foot as near to the head as it will go without forcing it. Observe the distance between the foot and the head as well as the degree of extension at the knee. Grade according to diagram. Note that the knee is left free and may draw down alongside the abdomen.

scarf sign With the baby supine, take the infant's hand and try to put it around the neck and as far posteriorly as possible around the opposite shoulder. Assist this maneuver by lifting the elbow across the body. See how far the elbow will go across, and grade according to illustrations. Score zero—elbow reaches opposite axillary line; 1—elbow between midline and opposite axillary line; 2—elbow reaches midline; 3—elbow will not reach midline (Fig. 30-5d).

head lag With the baby lying supine, grasp the hands (or the arms if the infant is very small) and pull him slowly toward the sitting position. Observe the position of the head in relation to the trunk, and grade accordingly. In a small infant the head may initially be supported by one hand. Score zero—complete lag; 1—partial head control; 2—able to maintain head in line with body; 3—brings head anterior to body.

ventral suspension The infant is suspended in the prone position, with examiner's hand under the infant's chest (one hand in a small infant, two in a large infant). Observe the degree of extension of the back and the amount of flexion of the arms and legs. Also note the relation of the head to the trunk. Grade according to diagrams (Fig. 30-5e). If score differs on the two sides take the mean.

Source: From L. M. Dubowitz et al., "Clinical Assessment or Gestational Age in the Newborn Infant," *Journal of Pediatrics,* **77**:1, 1970.

table 30-3 Scoring system for external criteria

external sign	score*				
	0	1	2	3	4
Edema	Obvious edema of hands and feet; pitting over tibia	No obvious edema of hands and feet; pitting over tibia	No edema		
Skin texture	Very thin, gelatinous	Thin and smooth	Smooth; medium thickness. Rash or superficial peeling	Slight thickening	Thick and parchment-like; superficial or deep cracking
Skin color	Dark red	Uniformly pink	Pale pink; variable over body	Pale; only pink over ears, lips, palms, or soles	
Skin opacity (trunk)	Numerous veins and venules clearly seen, especially over abdomen	Veins and tributaries seen	A few large vessels clearly seen over abdomen	A few large vessels seen indistinctly over abdomen	No blood vessels seen
Lanugo (over back)	No lanugo	Abundant; long and thick over lower part of back	Hair thinning	Small amount of lanugo and bald areas	At least half of back devoid of lanugo
Plantar creases	No skin creases	Faint red marks over anterior half of sole	Definite red marks over > anterior half; indentations over < anterior third	Indentations over > anterior third	Definite deep indentations over > anterior third
Nipple formation	Nipple barely visible; no areola	Nipple well defined; areola smooth and flat, diameter < 0.75 cm	Areola stippled, edge not raised, diameter < 0.75 cm	Areola stippled, edge raised diameter < 0.75 cm	

Breast size	No breast tissue palpable	Breast tissue on one or both sides, 0.5 cm diameter	Breast tissue both sides; one or both 0.5–1.0 cm	Breast tissue both sides; one or both < 1 cm
Ear form	Pinna flat and shapeless, little or no incurving of edge	Incurving of part of edge of pinna	Partial incurving of whole of upper pinna	Well-defined incurving of whole of upper pinna
Ear firmness	Pinna soft, easily folded, no recoil	Pinna soft, easily folded, slow recoil	Cartilage to edge of pinna, but soft in places, ready recoil	Pinna firm, cartilage to edge; instant recoil
Genitals: Male	Neither testis in scrotum	At least one testis high in scrotum	At least one testis right down	
Female (with hips half abducted)	Labia majora widely separated, labia minora protruding	Labia majora completely cover labia minora		

*If score differs on two sides, take the mean.

Source: Adapted from Farr and Associates, *Developmental Medicine and Child Neurology*, **8**:507, 1966. Reproduced from Dubowitz.[7]

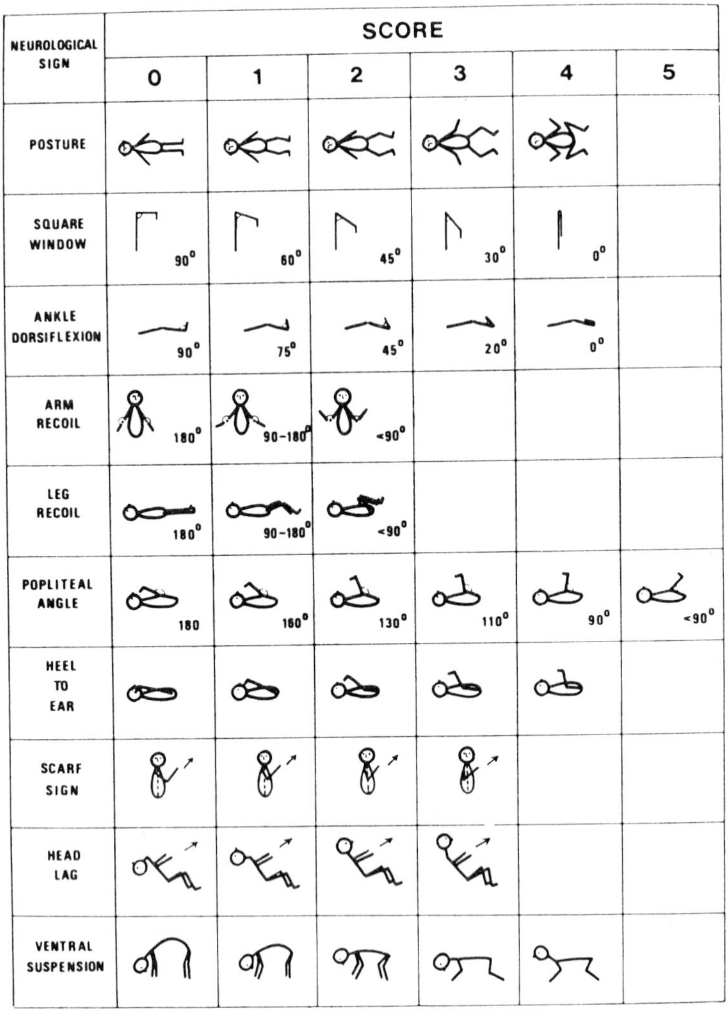

fig. 30-6 Scoring system of neurologic signs for assessment of gestational age. (*From Victor Dubowitz et al., "Clinical Assessment of Gestational Age in the Newborn Infant," Journal of Pediatrics,* **77:***1–10, 1970.*)

familiar with these signs and characteristics. Experience will permit the nurse to complete the whole procedure in approximately 10 min. If possible, the assessment should be made within 24 h after delivery. Using this system, the estimated gestational age is reported to be accurate within about 1 week.[7]

PHYSIOLOGIC HANDICAPS

respiratory adjustments

Crucial to the baby's survival is the adjustment of the vital physiologic systems to extrauterine

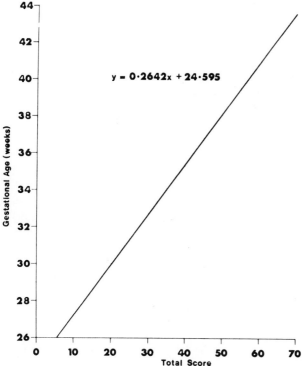

$y = 0.2642x + 24.595$

fig. 30-7 Graph for reading gestational age. The score from Table 30-3 is added to the score from Fig. 30-6. A line is drawn from the horizontal axis to the diagonal line; then from the intersecting point, a line to the perpendicular axis will indicate the age in weeks. (*From Victor Dubowitz et al., "Clinical Assessment of Gestational Age in the Newborn Infant," Journal of Pediatrics,* **77:**1–10, 1970.)

life. The immediate difficulty that the preterm infant encounters is maintaining respirations. By the twenty-seventh week of life, an infant's lungs may be able to function to sustain life (see Chap. 29). However, many factors contribute to impair respirations in these infants with a precarious hold on life—instability of the rib cage, weak chest muscles, soft and collapsible bronchi, incomplete development of alveoli and capillary blood supply, small surface area for the exchange of gases, and inadequate production of surfactant. The high incidence of respiratory distress syndrome in preterm infants is related to this last factor. Aspiration resulting from absent or poor gag or cough reflexes may further embarrass respirations. The nurse must be alert for signs of respiratory distress, which are elaborated on later in the chapter.

temperature adjustment

Maintaining stability of body temperature is extremely difficult for the preterm infant. Because of weak, underdeveloped muscles and inactivity, the baby cannot produce adequate heat. Excessive loss of heat results from the infant's large surface skin area in relation to body weight, and the inadequate supply of fat needed for heat production and insulation.

Since lipid accumulation occurs late in gestation, the preterm infant suffers from insufficient stores of fat in both white and brown adipose tissues. For the mature neonate, white adipose tissue in the subcutaneous areas not only provides energy, but also serves as an insulation against heat loss. Brown adipose tissue, which is unique to the neonate, possesses a greater thermogenic activity than ordinary fat. This mechanism of increased heat production, termed *nonshivering thermogenesis,* is particularly effective during periods of cold stress. Brown fat is located around the heart, kidneys, adrenals, and great vessels, and superficially is deposited around the neck, between the scapula, and behind the sternum. Although starvation reduces the stores of white fat, and cold stress depletes the reserves of brown fat, there is probably some overlap of function. In the normal maturing infant, the progressive replacement of brown with white adipose tissue approximates the development of the ability to shiver.

The preterm infant is incapable of adjusting to environmental changes. The temperature-regulating center in the brain is immature. The infant cannot shiver in response to cold stress; nor can the baby perspire, so that his or her entire body becomes red and flushed when overheated. Problems related to overheating infants have only recently received attention. Perlstein and coworkers reported on the frequent occurrence of apneic spells in premature infants kept in incubators where automatically controlled heating suddenly increased the ambient temperatures.[8]

In order to enable the preterm infant to stabilize body temperature with minimal effort, a controlled environment must be provided through the use of an incubator. Environmental temperature control is intended to maintain the preterm infant's metabolism at the lowest effective rate. Cold stress increases the baby's metabolic rate, necessitating increased oxygen consumption. If thermal stress remains unchecked, glycogen is broken down and the preterm infant's very limited stores are rapidly consumed, resulting in hypoglycemia. This anaerobic breakdown of glycogen also results in an increased production of lactic acid, contributing to metabolic acidosis. *Critical* temperature refers to that temperature below which the infant's metabolic rate and oxygen consumption will increase in an effort to raise body temperature. Should the baby's temperature drop below this critical point, the child's survival will be impaired by a host of metabolic difficulties, including oxygen deprivation, depletion of glycogen stores, reduced blood glucose level, and metabolic acidosis.

nutritional adjustment

Preterm infants present many feeding and nutritional problems. The sucking and swallowing reflexes are often absent or weak, necessitating gavage feeding, and contributing to the easy aspiration of fluids. Storage of glycogen is affected by the immaturity of the liver and the small muscle mass. Small, frequent feedings are essential in order to compensate for the very small stomach capacity, and to prevent hypoglycemia. Digestion and absorption are impeded by low gastric acidity, an immature enzyme system, and incomplete absorption of nutrients such as fats and vitamins.

The rapid growth rate of these infants conflicts with the anatomic and physiologic handicaps that interfere with nutrition. Distension often results from sluggish peristaltic activity. Vomiting and regurgitation are frequently encountered as a result of the small stomach capacity and the weak cardiac sphincter in the stomach (Fig. 30-8).

CARE OF THE HIGH-RISK INFANT IN NEONATAL INTENSIVE CARE CENTERS

In the last decade a revolution has occurred in the care of babies at high risk. A greater understanding of the pathophysiology of the neonate, along with advances in electronics and biochemistry, has drastically altered the complexity of ideal care. The practices of isolation, minimal handling, delayed feeding, and limited oxygen therapy have yielded to more aggressive approaches.

Neonatal specialists in the fields of medicine and nursing have emerged to care for these babies. The demands made on the nurse caring for these infants are great. She must be extremely knowledgeable in perinatology, intensely committed, able to work under stress, and skilled in executing all activities with great attention to detail. Nursing responsibilities include (1) close observation; (2) physical care of the infant; and (3) the use and management of incubators, oxygen and resuscitative equipment, respirators, monitors, infusion pumps, radiant heaters, and phototherapy lamps. Obviously, providing the highest quality of nursing care requires specialized education and experience. Presently, educational programs are being offered by many neonatal intensive care centers on an in-service basis.

Since there is sufficient evidence to show that mortality rates decrease when infants at high risk are cared for in intensive care units, it is now recommended that infants in need be given this advantage. It is unrealistic to expect all hospitals to have the facilities, equipment, and specially trained personnel to establish this type of service. The ultimate solution is to have special care units operate as regional centers. Many hospitals and communities have moved in this direction, and

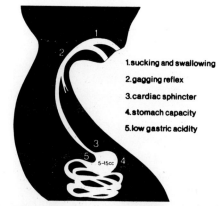

fig. 30-8 Anatomic and physiologic handicaps interfere with nutrition in the small infant. (*From E. J. Dickason and A. Ritz, Care of the Normal Premature Infant, McGraw-Hill, New York, 1970.*)

offer excellent transport services to infants in jeopardy requiring specialized care.

IMMEDIATE CARE IN THE DELIVERY ROOM

The first minutes of life are critical for the preterm infant, and survival and prognosis depend upon the quality of early treatment. It is essential that a physician and nurse adept in the care of prematures be on hand to devote complete attention to the baby. It is the nurse's responsibility to ensure that all equipment needed in caring for the infant is available and in good working condition.

As soon as the infant is delivered, the physician holds the head down and suctions the nostrils and oropharynx with a bulb syringe. Every effort must be made to avoid chilling the baby, since cold stress complicates birth asphyxia and depletes the stores of fat and glycogen. Heat loss occurs from exposure to cool ambient temperature, and from evaporation of amniotic fluid on the baby's skin. The baby should be dried immediately with a warm towel, wrapped in a

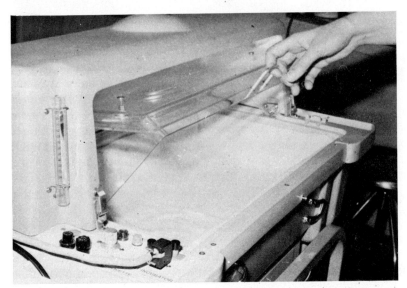

fig. 30-9 Portable incubabor with battery-operated heat source, humidity, and oxygen supply to transport infant from delivery room to intensive care nursery. (*Courtesy of Booth Memorial Medical Center, Flushing, N.Y.*)

warm blanket, and placed in a warm incubator. Examination of the infant, eye treatment, and identification can all be done after the infant has been placed in the incubator. Babies subjected to cold stress often have unrecorded temperatures, and develop cyanosis and shock. Asphyxia occurs more often in the premature than in the full-term infant, and resuscitation procedures should be performed under a radiant heat lamp.

The nurse should appreciate that the Apgar score not only identifies high-risk infants but also provides a widely understood quantitative evaluation of the infant's condition. The scoring system should be used to evaluate the status of the infant at 1 and 5 min after delivery. The procedure has proved most accurate when performed by an impartial nurse or physician not involved in the delivery.

As soon as possible, the infant should be transported to the intensive care nursery in an incubator equipped with a battery-operated heat source (Fig. 30-9). Hospitals not equipped to offer specialized services should make immediate arrangements for transfer of the infant to an appropriate institution. Until transfer is accomplished, efforts are directed at maintaining the infant's respirations and applying external heat. Modern transport facilities are equipped to provide the infant with heat, oxygen, intravenous infusions, and drug therapy (Fig. 30-10).

fig. 30-10 Transport ambulance equipped with every possible type of assistance for the small infant during the trip from a community hospital to the regional neonatal intensive care unit. (*Courtesy of the Long Island Jewish-Hillside Medical Center, N.Y., photographed by Herbert Bennett.*)

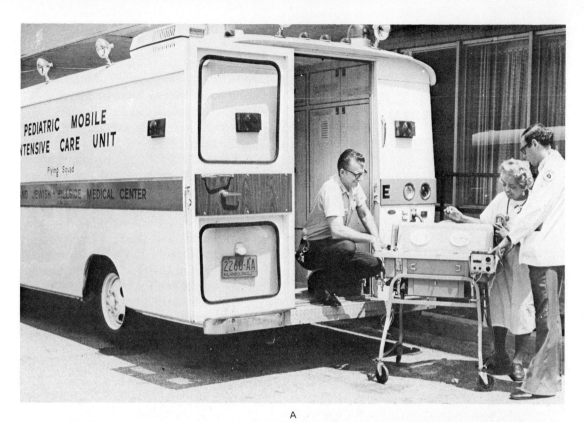

A

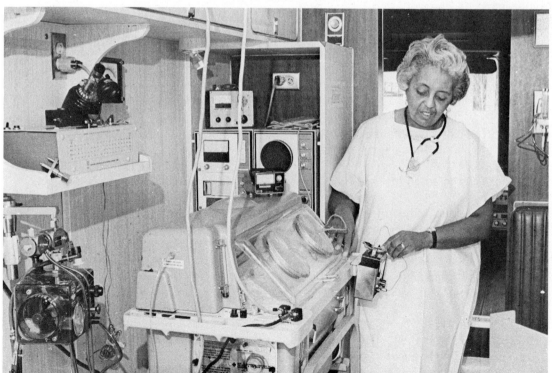

B

ADMISSION TO THE INTENSIVE CARE NURSERY

Since the nursery personnel are generally notified that a patient is in premature labor or that a baby is arriving via transport service, they have the advantage of being prepared for the infant's arrival. A clean incubator must be prepared, heated, and humidified. The incubator is heated to a temperature of between 32.8 to 33.8°C (91 to 93°F), and the relative humidity set at approximately 60 to 85 percent. The incubator temperature is adjusted according to the needs of the baby. The nurse must have all items and equipment needed to care for the infant at hand; i.e., linen, measuring tape, a sling and scale, thermometer and tape to apply the electrode if an automatically controlled machine is used, suction apparatus, resuscitative tray, and intravenous equipment. The supply of oxygen must be checked, and tubing available to deliver it to the incubator.

The major responsibilities of the nurse regarding admission of the infant to the nursery are summarized below.

1 Notify the pediatrician of the infant's arrival.
2 Before removing the infant from the transport carrier, check the oxygen concentration and the baby's temperature.
3 Transfer the infant to the prepared incubator.
4 Verify the identification of the baby with the transport or delivery room nurse. Ensure that:
   a The infant has been properly tagged and foot-printed.
   b The birth record is available and complete.
   c The name of the hospital sending the infant, as well as the name, address, and telephone number of the mother, are available.
   d Correct identification of the infant is marked on the incubator, chart, etc.
5 Check to see that eye prophylaxis and vitamin K_1 were administered. (Most hospitals have a policy of administering 0.5 to 1 mg vitamin K_1 to the infant in the delivery room or nursery to prevent hypoprothrombinemia. It is now known that large doses given to the newborn or to the mother at term may result in hyperbilirubinemia and kernicterus.)
6 Weigh the infant in a sling inside the incubator (Fig. 30-11). The scale must be set to compensate for the weight of the empty hammock.
7 If an automatically controlled incubator is used, attach the electrode to the infant's skin (Fig. 30-4).
8 Keep the infant nude so that she or he may be carefully observed in regard to the following:
   a Excess secretions which require removal by suctioning.
   b Rate and type of respirations, and signs of respiratory distress.
   c Color—particularly ashen appearance of pallor, cyanosis, and jaundice.
   d Activity and cry
9 Investigate the maternal history for early rupture of the membranes, traumatic delivery, diabetes, infection, sterility of delivery. These may serve as clues in identifying an infant in serious jeopardy.
10 Assist the physician with the physical examination. (If no obvious problems were observed in the delivery room, a thorough and careful examination should be delayed until the infant's temperature is stabilized.)
11 If possible, all specialized procedures peformed on the infant should be done in the incubator. If the baby must be removed in order to receive treatment, the infant should be cared for on a table warmed by an overhead heater.

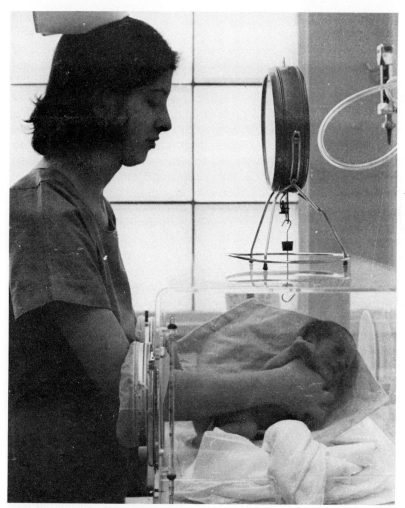

fig. 30-11 Weighing infant in a sling inside the incubator.

12 Record all pertinent information on the baby's chart.

CONTROL OF THE INFANT'S ENVIRONMENT

temperature

Incubators range from those offering only such features as heat and humidity control to so-phisticated machines which provide a totally controlled environment for the infant. Small preterm infants generally require incubators constructed to provide a filtered circulation of air, optimal *ambient* (surrounding) temperature, desirable oxygen and humidity concentrations, and an ingress through portholes so that the baby can be cared for in the incubator. Since the baby remains naked in the incubator, very close observation is possible.

Despite the high temperature of air in the

incubator, radiant heat loss will occur in the infant if the incubator walls become cold. Therefore, incubators should not be placed near cold windows or in the direct path of cool air. Generally, the nurse can make a judgment in this regard simply by feeling the outside of the incubator walls. Ideally, the temperature should not be more than 2°C (3.5°F) below the temperature of incubator air, but such precision would require electronic testing.

Incubators are often livesaving instruments for infants whose thermal stability is precarious. The thermal state of the infant is indicated by his or her temperature, and the machine is either manually or automatically adjusted to regulate the environmental temperature in accordance with the baby's needs.

If the machine is manually controlled, axillary temperature readings are taken. However, the very first reading on admission should be taken rectally to check the patency of the anus. The incubator thermometer reading should be noted before opening the portholes to take the baby's reading. In preterm infants, axillary temperature readings have been found dependable, and the thermometer should be held in place for 1 to 3 min. The infant's axillary temperature readings should be between 36.5 to 37°C (97.7 to 98.6°F). Significant changes in the infant's temperature require that the nurse adjust the incubator temperature by gradually raising or lowering the thermostat. The infant's temperature should be checked every ½ to 1 h until stabilized. It is generally recorded at 3- to 4-h intervals thereafter. The nurse should remember, however, that once the baby's temperature is stabilized, the incubator temperature dial should not be changed. After stabilization, a change in the baby's temperature may be a sign of disease, and this sign could be confused by constant changes in the incubator temperature.

Most incubators used in intensive care cen-

ters are equipped with automatically controlled regulators that respond to a temperature *thermistor probe* which is taped to the baby's skin—generally on the abdomen. The control is set to maintain the skin temperature at the desired level—about 36.1 to 37.2°C (97 to 99°F). Through a control mechanism, the incubator is regulated to increase or reduce heat output in accordance with the predetermined setting. Paper tape is usually placed under the probe to protect the skin, and over it to secure proper placement. If the baby is placed in a prone position with the abdominal probe attached, erroneously high readings will be registered by the thermistor. The machine will respond to the high probe reading although the infant's skin temperature may be sufficiently low to require increased heat output.

For all infants, the critical temperature is higher during the first 2 days of life. Listed below are the ranges of incubator temperatures generally required by infants during the first 2 days and thereafter in relation to weight (Table 30-4).

humidity

The relative humidity should be approximately 85 percent during the first 2 days, and should then be reduced to about 60 percent. A *hygrometer* can be used to check humidity in the incubator. Studies indicate that a humidi-

table 30-4 Desirable temperature ranges of incubator

infant's weight	temperature range	
	days 1 and 2	thereafter
−1500 g	33.8–35°C (93–95°F)	32.8–33.8°C (91–93°F)
1500–2500 g	32.8–33.8°C (91–93°F)	31.7–32.8°C (89–91°F)
2500 g+	32–33°C (89.6–91.4°F)	31.1–32°C (88–89.6°F)

fied atmosphere helps the baby to maintain body temperature, thus reducing oxygen consumption. When humidity is low, loss of heat through evaporation is increased.

Humidity is always administered with oxygen or when high incubator temperatures are used in order to prevent drying of the mucous membranes and dehydration. The nurse must ensure that the incubator humidifier is maintained at a high water level; that the chamber is filled with distilled water to prevent rusting; and that either a disinfectant is added to the water or sterile water is used to prevent bacterial growth. The humidified chamber should be drained, cleaned, and refilled daily.

Mist is not used because it has been found to cause maceration of the infant's skin, thereby increasing the possibility of infection.

MAINTENANCE OF ADEQUATE RESPIRATION

respiratory distress

One of the major problems encountered by preterm infants is respiratory distress. Normally, the respiratory pattern of such infants is one of diaphragmatic breathing, fluctuations of respiratory rates, and sporadic episodes of apnea lasting up to 10 s—*periodic breathing*. Periodic breathing does not result in generalized cyanosis and should not be confused with true apneic episodes. Generalized cyanosis is indicative of severe distress.

Nurses must be constantly alert for indications of respiratory distress. They are in the best position to recognize that a baby is having difficulty and are also excellent judges of the effectiveness of therapy. A baby suffering from air hunger usually exhibits a number of the following abnormal signs. The respiratory rate is sustained in excess of 50 to 60 per minute, and cyanosis may become evident. In some cases, the infant appears ashen or pale. Flaring of the nostrils during inspiration is also indicative of difficulty.

Retraction of the chest during inspiration results from an obstruction to the flow of air into the lungs which may occur at any point in the respiratory tract. Since the lungs do not inflate adequately during inspiration, the pressure in the pleural space between the chest wall and the unexpanded lungs remain negative. The flexible chest wall is therefore pulled inward to fill the space, resulting in retraction of the chest. The thoracic wall may retract between the ribs (intercostal), below the ribs (subcostal), beneath the sternum (substernal), or above the clavicles. In severe distress, there is a simultaneous rising of the abdomen with depression of the chest—a pattern termed *see-saw* breathing.

A sigh or grunt on expiration is a clear sign of distress. By temporarily closing the glottis, the baby attempts to improve alveolar expansion by obstructing the outflow of air. The "back pressure" created increases functional residual capacity, and grunting infants are capable of significantly increasing their arterial oxygen saturation.

suctioning

In the preterm infant, obstruction of the airway often results from the accumulation of mucus and secretions in the mouth and pharynx, or from regurgitation of stomach contents. In such circumstances, suctioning becomes a lifesaving technique.

Suctioning can be accomplished with a rubber bulb syringe, but this method is limited in use since the syringe cannot be passed beyond the baby's pharynx if deeper suction is necessary. Generally, aspiration is performed with the use of a catheter attached to a suction source. The suction may be provided by the operator's mouth on a mucus trap type of apparatus or by a machine. Many pediatricians feel mechanical suction is too traumatic for the baby.

Depending upon the size of the infant, a No. 8 or 10 soft rubber French or plastic catheter is lubricated with sterile water and introduced through the infant's nose or mouth. It is advanced into the oropharynx or trachea, and then suction is applied while the catheter is slowly rotated and withdrawn.

The baby should be properly positioned during the procedure. The infant should be supine with the head lowered to facilitate drainage, and the neck slightly hyperextended to straighten the airway and bring the tongue forward to clear the posterior pharyngeal wall.

If suctioning is not done briefly and gently, it can result in trauma and edema of the tissues, increased production of mucus, and laryngeal spasm. It should be performed in less than 1 min, since air, as well as secretions, is aspirated, which could exaggerate the distress of the infant. There is always danger of stimulating the vagus nerve, resulting in bradycardia. If possible, suctioning should not be done after feedings, since it frequently stimulates the gag reflex. To avoid the danger of introducing infection, a fresh catheter must be used whenever the infant requires suctioning (Fig. 30-12).

problems involved in the use of oxygen therapy

During the 1940s, an intensive search took place to determine the cause of the high incidence of retinopathy (retrolental fibroplasia) in premature infants resulting in complete or partial blindness. By the early 1950s, valid evidence was presented showing hyperoxemia to be the primary etiologic factor. An era followed when oxygen concentrations were limited to 40 percent—even in the presence of cyanosis. Since then the restrictive policies governing the administration of oxygen have been held accountable for an increased mortality in infants in severe respiratory distress, as well as an increased morbidity as a result of brain damage and cerebral palsy.

In the late 1960s, the use of more aggressive approaches in the treatment of preterm infants resulted in a resurgence of retrolental fibroplasia because of the more liberal use of oxygen to salvage profoundly ill babies. The great increase in the numbers of ocularly damaged babies since 1974 is caused in large part by the increasing survival rate of small preterm infants who seem to be particularly susceptible to oxygen therapy. Obviously, the problem posed in treating infants requiring oxygen therapy is how to avoid both dangers.

In administering oxygen to sick infants, the critical factor in preventing damage to both the brain and the eyes is the partial pressure of oxygen in the arterial blood. But as yet, the exact level above which damage to the eyes will occur, or below which brain damage will result, is not known. Cavanaugh suggests that it would probably be *ideal* to keep arterial oxygen concentrations between 65 to 85 mmHg.[9] This would require a method of constantly monitoring blood gases which has not been perfected as yet.

significance of arterial blood gases

In order to administer oxygen in proper dosage, measurements of the infant's arterial oxygen tension must be made. The differences in the partial pressures of gases determine the direction in which these gases move—flowing from a higher pressure to a lower one. The partial pressures of oxygen and carbon dioxide are expressed as P_{O_2} and P_{CO_2} respectively. Although the P_{O_2} measures only the oxygen in solution, it generally ac-

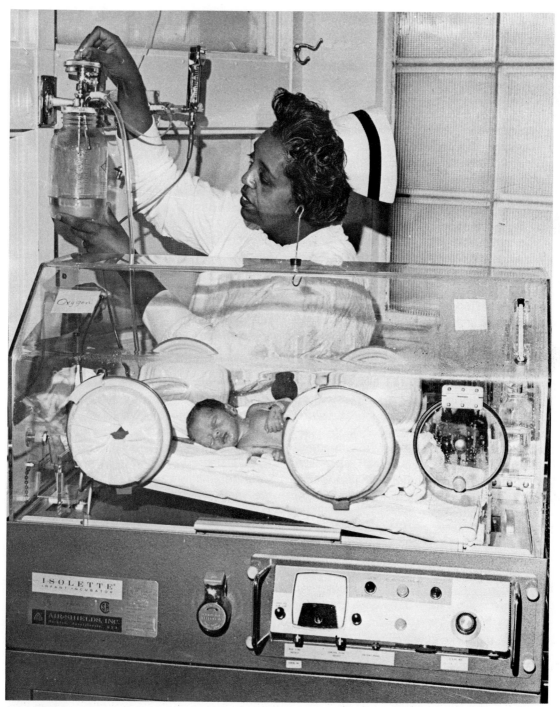

fig. 30-12 Setting up suction. Note high humidity level as indicated by condensation on the walls of the isolette. Note the infant's position. (*Photograph courtesy of the Long Island Jewish-Hillside Medical Center, New York.*)

curately reflects the oxygen saturation of hemoglobin. In the adult, blood is almost 100 percent saturated at a P_{O_2} of between 90 to 100 mmHg, whereas in the newborn the P_{O_2} ranges between 60 to 100 mmHg.

In the infant, cyanosis does not usually occur until the P_{O_2} falls below 50 mmHg, and in the very small baby it may not appear until it falls below 32 to 42 mmHg. Therefore, difficulties often exist before cyanosis is evident, because adverse physiologic changes occur in the infant when the arterial P_{O_2} falls below 50 mmHg. Recognizing that damage occurs when the P_{O_2} falls below 50 mmHg and that levels over 100 mmHg often result in blindness and damage to the lungs, it is currently considered safe and effective to give sufficient oxygen to maintain the infant's arterial P_{O_2} between 50 to 100 mmHg. Serial determinations of arterial P_{O_2} are made to accomplish this.

laboratory data The nurse must be able to interpret the results of the blood gas determinations made on the infant. Table 30-5 outlines the normal blood gas and pH values for the infant.

In severe respiratory distress resulting from hyaline membrane disease, the characteristic biochemical abnormalities are *hypoxemia, hypercapnia,* and *acidosis.* The arterial blood gases and pH determinations found in severely ill infants are as follows:

Hypoxemia P_{O_2} falls below 40 mmHg (normal lower limit: 50 mmHg)

Hypercapnia P_{CO_2} *rises over 65 mm Hg (normal upper limit: 45 mmHg)*

Acidosis pH generally below 7.15

sampling sites for blood gas determinations P_{O_2} determinations can be made only on arterial samples; capillary samples are useless for this purpose. During the first few days of life arterial blood is usually taken from an umbilical artery catheter. After the catheter is withdrawn the temporal, radial, or brachial arteries are used but separate punctures are required for each determination (Fig. 30-13).

Blood samples obtained from an indwelling umbilical *vein* catheter cannot be used to assess arterial oxygen tension but are useful for P_{CO_2} and pH determinations. The pH of central venous blood is 0.02 to 0.03 unit lower than arterial blood; the P_{CO_2} is 5 to 6 mmHg higher.

Many centers use umbilical artery catheters for parenteral fluid administration as well as for sampling arterial blood. Complications

table 30-5 Definitions of pH and blood gases and normal values

test		normal blood gas and pH values in infant
pH	A measure of the hydrogen ion concentration	7.35–7.45
P_{CO_2}	Represents the partial pressure of carbon dioxide dissolved in plasma	30–37 mmHg
P_{O_2}	Represents the partial pressure of oxygen	60–100 mmHg
HCO_3	A measure of plasma bicarbonate	20–25 meq/L

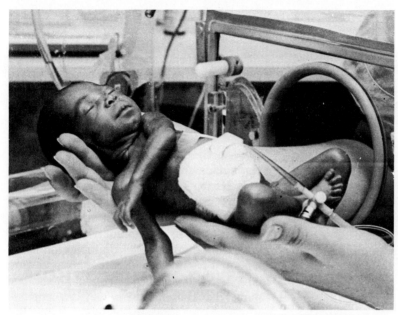

fig. 30-13 Umbilical line into one of the arteries for sequential blood gas determinations. (*Photograph by M. M. Miyato, courtesy of the Long Island Jewish-Hillside Medical Center, New York.*)

from indwelling catheters include thromboses, emboli, hemorrhage, and infection.

optimal oxygen therapy

Once the need for oxygen therapy has been established, frequent blood gas determinations should be used as a guide to ambient oxygen concentrations. Infants requiring continuous oxygen therapy for protracted periods of time should be cared for in a neonatal center equipped with adequate facilities and specially trained personnel. The American Academy of Pediatrics has revised its recommendations for the use of oxygen in treating newborns.[10]

Oxygen concentrations should be constantly monitored and aimed at maintaining the baby's arterial oxygen tension between 50 and 100 mmHg. The frequency of P_{O_2} determinations depends upon the condition of the infant. Samples may be required as often as every 15 min or every 6 to 8 h. Carbon dioxide tension and pH are always determined on the same blood sample.

Oxygen should always be ordered in percent concentration, not by flow rate. A variety of machines are in use which *constantly* monitor concentrations (Fig. 30-14). If such an analyzer is not available, the concentration of inspired oxygen must be measured with a conventional analyzer at least every 4 to 8 h, and at the time specimens are taken for blood gas determinations.

The nurse must keep a detailed record of the serial determinations made in reference to the percent of oxygen provided. Remember that the ultimate measure of optimal oxygen therapy is the arterial P_{O_2}.

It is generally understood and widely practiced that the infant who becomes cyanotic must be given enough oxygen to abolish the

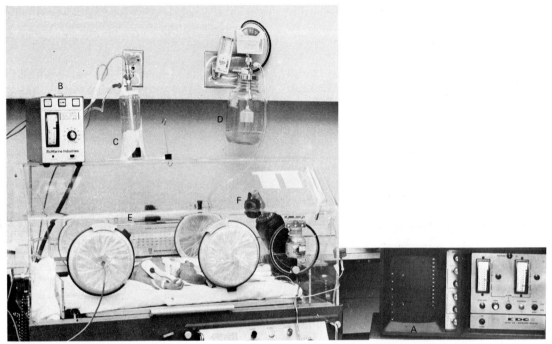

fig. 30-14 Infant with cardiac and respiratory monitoring. Attached are (a) respiratory and cardiac monitor; (b) oxygen regulator; (c) oxygen humidifier (nebulizer); (d) wall suction; (e) electric infusion pump; (f) Ambu bag. (*Photograph courtesy of the Long Island Jewish-Hillside Medical Center, New York.*)

cyanosis. If facilities are not available for blood gas determinations, the following method has been suggested as a practical clinical guide for estimating the appropriate concentrations of inspired oxygen. The intent here is to minimize the incidence of hyperoxemia. Oxygen concentration is gradually lowered by no more than 10 percent at a time—until the infant appears slightly cyanotic. The concentration is then maintained at a 10 percent higher level. For example, if cyanosis appears at 40 percent, the concentration is kept at a 50 percent level.

Except in cases where oxygen therapy is maintained for only a few hours, abruptly lowering concentrations is dangerous—often resulting in cyanosis and respiratory collapse. The longer the therapy, the longer the weaning period. Generally, a decrease of 10 percent every 3 to 4 h is well tolerated. However, a decrease of 3 to 5 percent every few hours may be necessary for infants who have received oxygen for over a week.

oxygen toxicity

As previously mentioned, retrolental fibroplasia is a disease directly related to excessive exposure to oxygen. It occurs mainly in preterm infants; the shorter the infant's gestational age, the greater his vulnerability. The only change observed during the period of oxygen therapy is retinal vasospasm. Within 1 month or more following the termination of treatment with oxygen, the retinal vessels dilate and proliferate, causing edema. Until this point, the process may cease, leaving slight or no resultant visual disturbance. However, if retinal detachment and scarring develop, blindness results.

Injury to the lungs may also result from hyperoxemia. The damage is characterized by thickening of the alveolar and vascular tissues, fibrosis, and atelectasis. As a result, diffusion of oxygen across the lungs is impaired. The abnormal radiologic appearance of the lungs does not disappear until several months after oxygen therapy has been discontinued.

methods of oxygen administration

1 *Incubator:* Constant delivery of concentrations beyond 60 to 70 percent cannot be ensured in incubators. Leakage often

occurs, and ambient concentrations drop rapidly when the portholes are open.

2 *Plastic head hood:* The hood should be used if concentrations must exceed 40 to 50 percent, or if the infant must be treated on an open table supplied with radiant heat from an overhead source (Fig. 30-15). The oxygen delivered to the hood must be humidified, and should be warmed to about 34°C (93.2°F).

3 *Intermittent mask and bag therapy:* This method may be used in situations of mild distress where prolonged assistance is not required. It has also been used as an alternate approach to respiratory distress. It is particularly appropriate for hospitals that do not have respirator programs which require special equipment and experienced personnel.

Therapy is given periodically, depend-

fig. 30-15 Infant with plastic hood for concentrated delivery of oxygen and humidity. The infant is under a light for treatment of bilirubin and therefore has bandaged eyes. Note restraints and intravenous infusion into an arm vein. (*Photograph by Mary Olsen Johnson, M.D.*)

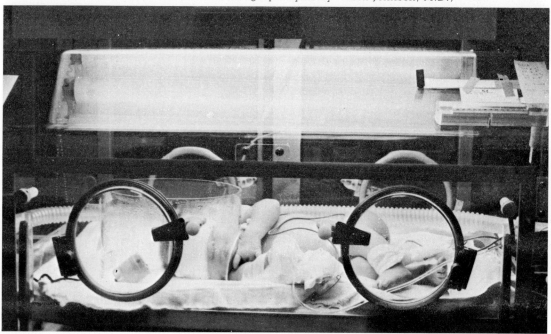

ing upon the needs of the infant—e.g., 10 min out of every 30. Blood gas determinations should be made before and after treatment, and are used as a guide to the frequency of baggings and oxygen requirements of the baby.

The mask must be held tightly over the face, avoiding the eyes as well as excessive pressure to prevent trauma. Gastric distension is prevented by passing a nasogastric tube with the free end left open. Nurses should be taught the procedure with the use of an infant simulator. The major complication is pneumothorax.

4 *Respirator therapy:* Mechanically assisted ventilation is reserved for babies in severe distress, especially those with hyaline membrane disease. Respiratory therapy is a formidable undertaking to be used only in properly manned and equipped centers. The technical problems encountered are numerous. With the exception of negative-pressure respirators, an endotracheal tube must be inserted and maintained in proper position. Should it slip forward into the trachea, it may enter the right main-stem bronchus and occlude the left one—leaving the left lung unaerated. Changes in lung compliance may necessitate adjustments in pressure and volume settings. The oxygen delivered to the baby must be humidified. It is essential that blood gases and pH be monitored at frequent intervals. Complications of respirator therapy include blockage of the endotracheal tube, pneumothorax, and infection (Fig. 30-16).

The care of a baby receiving such treatment is a challenge, and nursing responsibilities consist of regulating the respirator, observing the condition of the infant, maintaining bronchial toilet, suctioning the tracheal tube hourly or as frequently as is necessary, rotating the infant's position, and assisting with the collection of blood specimens.

The two major types of respirators used are:

a *Positive-pressure respirator.* A specific volume of tidal air is delivered to the lungs under restricted pressure via an endotracheal tube. The respirator is adjusted to permit the infant to trigger the machine even though his or her inspiratory efforts are very weak. If the infant fails to trigger it, automatic cycling occurs.

The controls on the respirator may set the end-expiratory pressure above zero, thereby preventing the lungs from completely collapsing at the end of the respiratory cycle. This achieves the same effect as the expiratory grunt, i.e., it increases arterial oxygen saturation. This type of respiratory therapy is termed positive end-expiratory pressure (PEEP).

b *Negative-pressure respirator* (tank respirator). The infant's body from the neck down is enclosed in a chamber intermittently surrounded by negative pressure, resulting in the movement of gas into and out of the lungs. A motor-driven vacuum connected to the body compartment produces the negative pressure. The body compartment is separated from the head compartment by an iris diaphragm that fits snugly around the baby's neck. The ambient oxygen concentration is controlled in the head chamber.

5 Continuous positive airway pressure (CPAP): This method of therapy requires that the infant be able to breathe spontaneously because it assists ventilation without the use of a mechanical respirator. The intent of CPAP is to maintain pressures above zero in the lungs even at the end of expiration, thereby forcing retention of air and preventing alveolar collapse. Stud-

ies indicate that arterial P_{O_2} increases with this type of therapy.

The treatment is carried out by delivering specific concentrations of oxygen through an apparatus attached to the nose, an endotracheal tube, or a face mask. The gas expired by the infant passes through an outflow system that is partially occluded by a screw clamp to maintain end-expiratory pressures above zero. The pressure can be regulated by the degree of occlusion exerted by the screw clamp. An aneroid manometer continuously registers the pressure within the system.

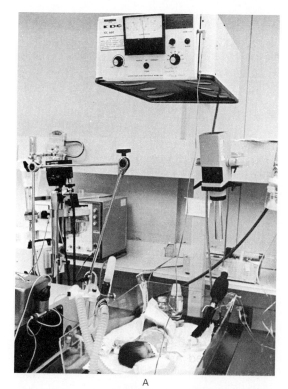

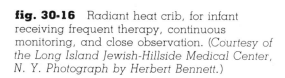

fig. 30-16 Radiant heat crib, for infant receiving frequent therapy, continuous monitoring, and close observation. (*Courtesy of the Long Island Jewish-Hillside Medical Center, N. Y. Photograph by Herbert Bennett.*)

A

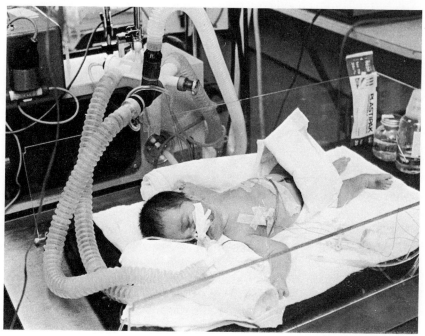

B

NUTRITIONAL REQUIREMENTS AND FEEDING

The optimal requirements of the low-birth-weight infant are not known precisely. Recent evidence indicates that there is a critical period of brain growth in the newborn, and studies suggest that early postnatal malnutrition may permanently impair this growth. Much controversy exists regarding all aspects of feeding premature infants; i.e., when to start, nutritive requirements, safest method, strength of formula, etc. At present, early feedings (oral or intravenous) are preferred by most practitioners.

The literature is replete with studies regarding the nutritional requirements of low-birth-weight infants. Most texts recommend at least 120 cal/kg per day, but recent studies support a wide range of 84 to 142 cal/kg per day.

Protein intake of 2.25 to 2.75 g/kg per day appears adequate, but the protein must be of such quality as to provide sufficient amounts of all essential amino acids, including those that are essential only for premature infants. For example, very small neonates lack enzymes to convert phenylalanine to tyrosine and methionine to cystine. Thus the quality of protein is most important in feeding low-birth-weight infants. Human milk or humanized cow milk protein appears to meet the needs of these infants to a greater extent than does untreated cow milk protein. Daily protein intakes of up to 4 g/kg per day appear to be well tolerated and generally safe for older, rapidly growing infants. But since no advantages of such high protein intake have been demonstrated, there is little reason to offer such high quantities. Protein in excess of actual requirements taxes the infant's metabolic machinery for disposing of the excess. If the infant's body is incapable of responding adequately, complications such as azotemia

and metabolic acidosis may occur. Also, studies have associated very high protein intake—6 g/kg per day—with poor neurological development.

The type and amount of fat to be given are also in question. Since the premature baby tends to absorb fats poorly, most formulas used have a low fat content. Yet, fatty acids are apparently essential and efficiently absorbed, and a deficiency may result in loose stools and skin lesions.

The premature's rapid growth and low antenatal storage of vitamins can result in significant deficiencies. The administration of multivitamin preparations is begun very early. These preparations usually contain vitamins A, C, D, E, and a number of the B group. Vitamins are given just before the bottle feeding. If the baby cannot suck on a dropper, or is being tube-fed, the vitamins are added to the formula. Some nurseries use formulas prepared with vitamins added so that additional supplements are not necessary. At about the third week of life, the infant is given iron to compensate for the depletion of fetal stores and to support rapid growth.

The physician prescribes the formula and the amount according to the baby's condition. At first, sterile water or a glucose solution is given. As the infant's condition permits, he or she progresses to diluted and then full-strength milk. The variety of recommended feedings include breast milk and proprietary formulas especially made up for prematures.

Because of the infant's small stomach capacity, overfeeding can result in regurgitation or vomiting followed by aspiration, abdominal distension, or respiratory distress. At first, the volume of formula ordered may be as small as 2 to 3 mL. Adjustments are made in accordance with the infant's ability to tolerate larger volumes. Babies who are able to suck on the nipple are fed every 3 h, and tube-fed babies every 1 to 2 h. As the infants mature and approach 4 lb, they are usually satisfied with feedings every 4 h. If distension is noted, the nurse should bubble the baby before the feeding.

Four basic principles which the nurse must adhere to when feeding the infant include (1) use of sterile equipment, (2) administering the correct amount of formula, (3) conserving the infant's energy, and (4) preventing aspiration of fluid. To avoid disturbing the baby after feeding, all necessary nursing care should be done beforehand.

methods of feeding

The nipple method is usually used for babies over 1500 g who can suck well without tiring. Bottle feeding should not exceed 20 min. A small, soft, cross-cut nipple is generally used. If a nipple with holes is used, the milk should drop slowly when the bottle is inverted. The

infant should be held in an upright position, bubbled during and after feeding, and then positioned on his or her abdomen. The baby may also be positioned on his or her side, with the head of the bed slightly elevated to facilitate bubbling and help prevent regurgitation.

gavage The infant is fed through a catheter passed via the mouth and esophagus into the cardiac end of the stomach (Fig. 30-17). Formula is passed through the barrel of a syringe attached to the catheter. Two methods are appropriate for measuring the distance the catheter should be passed. This can be accomplished by extending the tube from the tip of the ear to the tip of the nose to the xiphoid process, or simply by extending it from the bridge of the nose to the xiphoid process. The tube is then marked with tape to ensure that it will be inserted the correct

fig. 30-17 *Gavage feeding of the preterm infant. (Courtesy of the Long Island Jewish-Hillside Medical Center, New York.)*

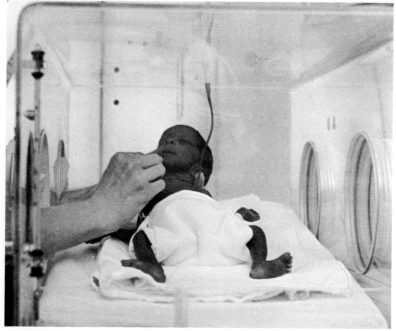

distance. The procedure for gavage feeding is outlined below:

1 Collect all equipment and measure the formula.
2 Place the baby in a dorsal recumbent position.
3 Restrain the infant.
4 Measure and mark the correct distance to pass the catheter. (A No. 8 or 10 French catheter is used, depending upon the size of the infant.)
5 Lubricate the end of the catheter with sterile water.
6 Insert the catheter through the infant's mouth. Although the possibility of passing the catheter into the larynx is slight, the nurse always verifies that the tube is properly positioned in the stomach by using one of the following methods:
   a Insert the end of the catheter into a medicine glass filled with sterile water. Watch for regular bubbling which indicates that the tube is in the trachea.
   b Flick the baby's heel to stimulate crying. If the baby cries, the tube is properly positioned.
   c Gently aspirate for gastric contents.
   d Insert 0.5 mL air through the tube while listening with a stethoscope for the rush of air as it enters the stomach.
7 Attach the barrel of the syringe to the catheter and administer the premeasured amount of formula by slow gravity flow.
8 Pinch the tube and withdraw it quickly. (This prevents dripping of the formula from the tube into the pharynx from where it could be easily aspirated.)
9 Hold the baby in a sitting position and bubble. (Avoid pressure on the stomach.)
10 The baby should be placed on it's side in a low Fowler's position for ½ h after feeding to encourage bubbling and hinder regurgitation, then placed in a prone position.

During the feeding, the nurse must observe the baby for rapid respirations, retractions, and cyanosis which could indicate the need for a rest period or interruption of the feeding. As the baby matures and the sucking ability improves, the child may be alternately gavage- and bottle-fed. If the infant repeatedly sucks on the tube, it may indicate that he or she is ready for nipple feedings.

indwelling nasogastric tube   A plastic tube is passed through the nostril into the stomach and left in place for a variable length of time. The formula is administered through a syringe attached to a catheter. The upper part of the catheter is taped to the infant's face. The tube should be changed at least every 3 to 5 days. The proximal end of the catheter is closed between feedings, either by a device fitted with a stopper or by clamping it.

The position of air in the stomachs of premature infants has been studied, resulting in the recommendation that small infants requiring tube feedings be fed while positioned on their stomachs. This is not possible if the infant is in respiratory distress; such an infant should be fed in a position halfway between the stomach and right side. A diaper roll can be used to support the infant in this position. The head of the mattress should be slightly elevated.

The nurse should open the tube for a few minutes before the feeding to permit escape of air from the stomach. Proper positioning of the tube must be assured by using the method described earlier of inserting air through the tube. Some practitioners recommend aspirating the stomach of air and fluid content before feeding. This permits expulsion of air from the stomach, and prevents overfeeding. The amount of material obtained is deducted from the total amount of feeding ordered. The substance (food and fluid) aspirated is returned to the stomach before the feeding, in order not to deplete electrolytes. The new feeding is injected at a slow, steady pace, or allowed to enter the tube by gravity flow. Afterwards 1 mL sterile water is administered to clear the tube of milk. If the baby evidences any signs of distress, the feeding is slowed or discontinued. After feeding, the infant should be placed on its abdomen. If the baby is dyspneic, the child is placed on his or her left side.

intravenous feeding This method of feeding provides the infant with fluids and calories via an umbilical venous or arterial catheter, or by peripheral intravenous routes.

naso-oral jejunal and naso-oral duodenal feedings These methods require passing an indwelling tube through either the nose or the mouth and stomach into the small intestine. Continuous feedings are then administered via an infusion pump or at intervals through a syringe attached to the catheter. An isotonic solution may be used to prevent dumping.

Studies show that these methods of feeding offer advantages over gastric gavage in that the infant is less fatigued and there is less gastric distension and aspiration. Also, these methods do not subject the neonate to any new portal of entry for infection. Researchers have reported excellent utilization of nutrients as measured by good weight gain in infants fed by the naso-oral jejunal method. Some of the difficulties encountered with naso-oral jejunal feedings include intestinal perforation, intussusception, necrotizing enterocolitis, catheter blockage, infection of the nasal passages, changes in intestinal flora, vomiting, and diarrhea. Because of these problems, some neonatal centers now use naso-oral duodenal feedings, which they consider to be a superior alternative to either gastric gavage or naso-oral jejunal feeding procedures.[11]

parenteral alimentation Infusions containing proteins and sugar are given to the infant via an umbilical venous or arterial catheter, or by peripheral intravenous routes. The catheter is attached to an infusion pump. This method is used when oral feedings must be delayed, or to supplement nipple or tube feedings which frequently cannot provide an adequate nutritive intake. Since most infants can be given a limited intake of nutrients via the oral route, supplemental alimentation is generally sufficient.

However, seriously ill neonates may require *total* intravenous alimentation. In such an instance, all nutrients required by the infant, including carbohydrates, protein hydrolysates, vitamins, and minerals, are administered intravenously. Generally, the catheter is fed into the superior vena cava via the external or internal jugular vein. This method of feeding is complex, requiring excellent personnel and facilities. It carries many hazards, and the use of this technique as the sole method of feeding should be reserved for very select high-risk infants.

DISORDERS REQUIRING INTRAVENOUS THERAPY

Biochemical equilibrium in the preterm infant is vital to the baby's life. The infant's fluid and electrolyte balance is so delicate that it is easily upset by immaturity or illness. The speed with which a small baby can become dehydrated, hypoglycemic, or acidotic is startling. Intravenous therapy is frequently lifesaving to these infants.

dehydration and electrolyte imbalance

If the infant does not receive fluids, he or she will become dehydrated within a few hours. Vomiting and diarrhea can result in a critical loss of fluid and electrolytes.

The infant's fluid requirements are extremely high because the very large surface area in proportion to body weight necessitates great heat production to maintain life. The heat produced by the infant consumes at least twice as much water per kilogram of body weight as the adult. The baby's rapid growth results in a high production of metabolites. Therefore, the infant has a greater *obligatory water loss*; i.e., the infant needs a large amount of water to rid the body of waste materials. In addition, the kidneys are immature and do not efficiently concentrate urine.

The preterm infant may not evidence typical signs of dehydration such as fever, reduced skin turgor, sunken eyeballs and fontanels, dryness of the tongue and mucous membranes, and reduced urinary output. The most obvious and significant indication of dehydration in very small infants is *weight loss*.

Depletion of electrolytes usually accompanies dehydration. Sodium and potassium imbalances are frequently encountered. Blood tests are done to determine fluid and electrolyte replacement needs.

At first, low-birth-weight infants are unable to take oral feedings in sufficient amounts to meet their fluid needs. In the first few days, their requirements are low because of edema, but they quickly increase to approximately 150 mL/kg/day. If these infants cannot take fluids or are unable to take sufficient amounts through the gastrointestinal tract, intravenous therapy will be given.

hypoglycemia

Very small infants are susceptible to hypoglycemia because of their low stores of glycogen. In addition, their metabolic response to cold stress, acidosis, and hypoxia results in the abnormal utilization of glucose. In the first three days of life, blood glucose ranges from 20 to 100 mg/100 mL with an average of 40 mg/100 mL. Two consecutive samples indicating a level below 20 mg/100 mL is diagnostic.

It is estimated that disturbed glucose homeostasis causes symptoms in about 5 to 10 percent of these babies. Signs and symptoms are confusing and overlapping with those of other conditions, e.g., apnea, cyanosis, dyspnea, tachypnea, tremors, irritability, upward rolling of the eyes, convulsions, coma, lethargy, weak cry, and refusal to feed. If the signs disappear within 5 min after intravenous glucose, no matter the blood glucose level, hypoglycemia is probably the etiologic factor.

In infants weighing less than 1250 g, low blood sugar levels are particularly common after birth and in the days following. Intravenous glucose solutions are given routinely to these small infants after birth and at variable periods thereafter. Blood glucose tests should be performed every 4 to 8 h for the first 2 days, and thereafter continued at less frequent intervals for about a week.

Early feeding of premature infants has been found in many studies to reduce the likelihood of hypoglycemic episodes. One critical factor noted by most researchers is that a sudden cessation of intravenous administration may cause marked hypoglycemia in otherwise normal infants. Intravenous fluids must be continued until oral intake is adequate.

If hypoglycemia is diagnosed, the infant is immediately treated with 25 percent glucose solution. Maintenance infusion of 15 percent glucose is continued for a period of 24 to 48 h, the concentration of glucose infused is then lowered to 10 percent and later to 5 percent. Untreated cases may result in death or brain damage.

Lilien has recently reported that as a result of treatment with continuous intravenous glucose infusion, the infants can develop hyperglycemia and consequently suffer from diuresis and dehydration.[12] It is therefore suggested that blood glucose determinations be done every 2 h when an infant is on such therapy.

acid-base disturbances

Acid-base disturbances frequently cause death in small infants. These problems occur in response to cold stress, respiratory difficulty, starvation, infection, and gastrointestinal disturbances. In order to give intelligent care and assess the patient's progress, the nurse must be able to correlate laboratory data with the infant's clinical course. This requires a basic understanding of the dynamics of acid-base balance.

The acidity of any fluid is expressed as pH—a value of 7 being considered neutral. However, the normal range of pH for arterial blood is slightly alkaline—7.35 to 7.45, and values under or over these are considered acidic or alkaline respectively. The majority of clinical deviations occur between a pH of 7.00 and 7.25, representing serious acidosis. Death ensues when the pH falls below 6.8 or rises above 7.8.

Acids—both *violatile* and *fixed*—are relentlessly produced in the body, and must be neutralized and eliminated in order to maintain the delicate pH balance.

Carbonic acid—which is volatile—is the major acid produced in the body. The carbon dioxide resulting from tissue metabolism goes into solution as carbonic acid, but the protein buffer system of the erythrocytes prevents the pH from falling below normal. The portion of carbonic acid which enters the erythrocytes is buffered by hemoglobin, where a series of chemical reactions converts it to bicarbonate. This bicarbonate is then released into plasma as sodium bicarbonate. Therefore, a large quantity of the carbon dioxide that originates in the tissues is carried in plasma as sodium bicarbonate. The carbonic acid remaining in the blood is eliminated through the lungs as carbon dioxide.

The principle fixed acids produced by normal metabolism are lactic, sulfuric, and phosphoric. These acids are neutralized while carried in the blood by the sodium bicarbonate/carbonic acid buffer system, and finally eliminated through the kidneys. For example, lactic acid is buffered by sodium bicarbonate and converted to sodium lactate plus carbonic acid. The salt (sodium lactate) is excreted through the kidneys, and the carbonic acid exhaled as carbon dioxide.

It is evident, therefore, that three principal mechanisms function to protect the body against excessive accumulation of acids:

1 Buffering activity of the erythrocytes and plasma.
   a Protein buffer system of hemoglobin for volatile carbonic acid
   b Sodium bicarbonate/carbonic acid buffer system for fixed acids—lactic, sulfuric, phosphoric
2 Elimination of carbon dioxide through the lungs (Blood levels of CO_2 are controlled by the lungs.)
3 Excretion of fixed acids through the kidneys (The concentration of bicarbonate is controlled by the kidneys.)

laboratory tests for measuring acid-base status Table 30-5 outlines the major tests performed to assess the infant's acid-base status; Table 30-6 indicates the variations in pH, P_{CO_2}, and HCO_3 expected in the major disturbances.

collection of samples The above tests are performed on arterial blood samples if an indwelling umbilical artery catheter is in place. If this route is not available, samples of capillary blood for P_{CO_2} and pH determinations can be obtained from a heel prick. In order to obtain an arterialized capillary sample, the heel of the infant must be warmed with a moist pack for 5 min before the sample

table 30-6 Blood gas and pH variations in the major disturbances

test	metabolic acidosis	metabolic alkalosis	respiratory acidosis	respiratory alkalosis
pH	↓	↑	↓	↑
P_{CO_2}	Ratio to HCO_3↑	Ratio to HCO_3↓	↑	↓
HCO_3	↓	↑	Ratio to P_{CO_2}	Ratio to P_{CO_2}↑

is taken. As mentioned previously, oxygen tension can be determined accurately only from arterial blood. Thus blood obtained from a heel prick is of no use in P_{O_2} testing.

To avoid inaccurate results, blood gas and pH determinations should be carried out immediately after the samples are collected. If necessary, the blood can be stored in the refrigerator for up to 2 h before testing without significant alterations in readings. Blood samples must never be kept at room temperature.

acidosis and alkalosis Acid-base balance is primarily dependent upon the relative quantities of bicarbonate and carbonic acid present in the extracellular fluid. The normal ratio of this buffer system is 20 parts bicarbonate (HCO_3) to 1 part carbonic acid (H_2CO_3). The chart shown in Table 30-6 demonstrates how a shift in the normal ratio can result in acidosis or alkalosis. Equilibrium will be affected by changes in the concentration on either side. If compensation is successful, a normal ratio *comparable* to 20 parts bicarbonate to 1 part carbonic acid is reestablished so that the pH remains normal. A decrease in bicarbonate or an increase in carbonic acid results in a lowered pH, or acidosis; an increase in bicarbonate or a decrease in carbonic acid results in a higher pH, or alkalosis.

metabolic acidosis Metabolic acidosis results from an increase in the concentration of nonvolatile acids. The major causes include

excessive accumulation of acids from impaired metabolism and infection, excessive loss of base from diarrhea, and impaired renal functioning preventing the adequate excretion of acids.

As fixed acids accumulate in the blood, the bicarbonate level drops in order to neutralize the acids. The normal 20:1 ratio of bicarbonate to carbonic acid is altered. *Hyperventilation* is the compensatory process. Through excess excretion of carbon dioxide, it may be possible to lower the carbonic acid concentration to match the lowered bicarbonate level, thereby restoring the normal ratio. Although the pH remains normal if the infant compensates, both the serum bicarbonate concentration and the P_{CO_2} are low.

metabolic alkalosis An increase in the concentration of bicarbonate results in metabolic alkalosis. In the infant, the primary causes are administering excessive doses of sodium bicarbonate intravenously, and the loss of large quantities of hydrochloric acid from persistent vomiting, causing an excessive accumulation of base.

In this disturbance, the infant *hypoventilates* in an effort to retain carbon dioxide and thus increase the carbonic acid concentration to match the increased level of bicarbonate. In this compensated state, the pH is normal, but both the serum bicarbonate concentration and the P_{CO_2} are elevated.

respiratory acidosis An increase in the concentration of carbonic acid caused by inadequate pulmonary gas exchange produces respiratory acidosis. Asphyxia and hyaline membrane disease are the primary causes.

As carbonic acid builds up in the blood, the kidneys retain bicarbonate in an effort to bring the buffer ratio back into balance. If the baby compensates, the pH remains normal, but both the P_{CO_2} and the serum bicarbonate concentration are elevated.

The respiratory attempt to hyperventilate and eliminate the excessive carbon dioxide is generally not successful because of the underlying pulmonary disease. *Tachypnea* is the result of this extraordinary effort.

respiratory alkalosis Respiratory alkalosis results from an increase in the concentration of base. The major cause is hyperventilation, which produces excessive elimination of carbon dioxide. In high-risk infants, it has been encountered in situations where mechanical respirators have been improperly set.

In an effort to offset the decrease in carbonic acid, the kidneys increase the excretion of bicarbonate. In this compensated condition, the pH remains normal, but the serum bicarbonate concentration and the P_{CO_2} are low.

Since most preterm infants tend to be slightly acidotic, with the pH falling as low as 7.25, pathologic problems may easily result in severe acidosis. The small infant's lungs and kidneys function with little reserve capacity to excrete excess acids, and therefore small babies are extremely liable to respiratoy and metabolic acidosis.

It is possible for the infant to suffer from both metabolic and respiratory disturbances simultaneously. Such a condition is termed *mixed acidosis* or *alkalosis.* Mixed acidosis is the most common problem found in preterm infants suffering from hyaline membrane disease and asphyxia. In this condition, the combination of retained carbon dioxide and diminished bicarbonate results in a serious decrease in pH, which is frequently lethal to the infant. The treatment of acidosis is administration of sodium bicarbonate intravenously. The exact quantity is ordered by the physician, and it is always diluted to avoid damage to the blood vessels from the extremely alkaline pH.

Recently, the use of sodium bicarbonate in treating acidemia in severely ill neonates has been linked with an increase in intracranial hemorrhage. The literature indicates that many of the solutions given were hypertonic and thus caused cerebral hemorrhage. Finberg asserts that the present controversy over the role of sodium bicarbonate in producing hemorrhage in neonates can be resolved by examining three specific factors of the solutions used—quantity, concentration, and rate of flow.[13]

INTRAVENOUS THERAPY

In the first few precarious days following the premature's birth, parenteral therapy is frequently used to administer water, electrolytes, glucose, sodium bicarbonate, nutrients, and drugs.

Small infants are given minute amounts of fluid because of their small blood volume. A baby weighing 1160 g (2½ lb) has a blood volume of approximately 116 mL. It is impressive to compare this small volume with that of 5000 to 6000 mL found in the adult. Babson states that in the first 3 days of life, the volume is about 70 to 80 mL/kg/24 h; then as tolerated the volume is gradually increased to 135 mL/kg/24 h.[14] Thus, in the first few days— depending upon age and condition— the preterm infant receives approximately 3 to 8 mL intravenous fluid per hour. (There appears to be a consensus among authorities that the water requirement is approximately

150 mL/kg/24 h from about the fourth day on.) Although the physician orders the specific solution and amount to be given, it is the nurse who ensures that the required therapy is precisely carried out.

The most accessible veins in which to start an infusion are in the scalp (Fig. 30-18). A scalp vein infusion may require use of a sand bag to hold the infant's head in position. The intravenous infusion may also be started in one of the peripheral veins of the extremities. If the site is in the arm or ankle, a small armboard will be necessary to immobilize the part. Various types of restraints are often necessary on an extremity to prevent movements which might result in dislodging the needle (Fig. 30-19).

Convenient but potentially dangerous sites of administration are the umbilical vein or artery. In intensive care units, umbilical catheterizations are now commonly performed to administer fluids to high-risk and sick infants. The cathether is marked with radiopaque material so that, after insertion, its proper position in the vessel can be assured through x-ray. The major complications include infection, thrombophlebitis, and liver damage.

The rate of administration is best controlled by using an electric infusion pump. Infusion pumps reduce the risks of dehydration and circulatory overload. However, infiltration does occur with these devices.

Infusion accidents can be prevented by careful observation and hourly charting of intake and output. Edema around the infusion site indicates infiltration; if this is noted, the nurse must immediately discontinue the infusion. An infiltrated intravenous infusion may

fig. 30-18 Starting an intravenous infusion in a scalp vein.

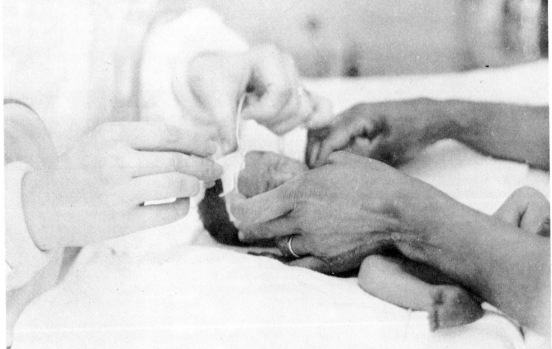

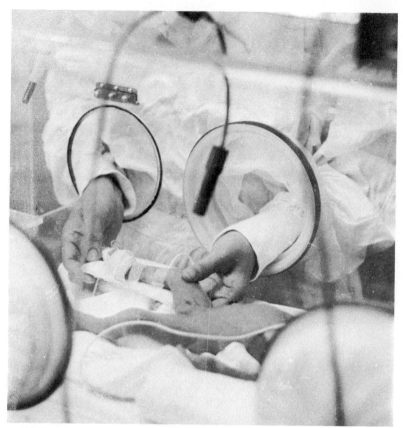

fig. 30-19 Note small board to which leg is attached for an infusion into an ankle vein.

interfere with circulation in the extremity. Signs of circulatory interference include pallor, cyanosis, and cool skin temperature below the affected area.

During therapy, the nurse must be alert for significant physiologic changes in the infant's condition. Dehydration or circulatory overload is best diagnosed by changes in weight. Infants should be weighed at least every 12 to 24 h. In order to avoid disconnecting monitors every time the baby is weighed, all the equipment attached to the infant should be included in the initial baseline weight. All intake and output must be measured, and specific gravity and glucose tests performed on each voided specimen. The nurse keeps a record of all serial pH and blood gas determinations made.

Very rarely, *hypodermoclysis* may be substituted for intravenous therapy if there is difficulty in using the veins, or proper equipment for an infusion is not available. Small amounts of isotonic fluid are injected into the subscapular area, either by continuous drip or by syringe.

PREVENTION OF INFECTION

Postnatal infection is acquired from personnel, from equipment, and from other infants in the nursery. Preterm infants are more vulnerable to infection than full-term infants. They have a poor defense against invasion by infectious agents because of a low level of antibodies circulating in the plasma (immunoglobins), immature phagocytosis, and inability to localize infection.

The *lack* of specific symptoms indicative of infection is unique in the preterm infant. Fever is often absent, and coughing is rare. Even in the presence of a fulminating infection, only vague symptoms may be observed, i.e., refusal to feed, lethargy, hyperirritability, vomiting, diarrhea, low-grade fever, cyanosis, irregular respirations, and apnea.

The three most common bacterial diseases found in premature infants are pneumonia, septicemia, and meningitis. Approximately 75 to 85 percent of these bacterial infections are caused by gram-negative rods—principally *Escherichia coli* and *Pseudomonas aeruginosa,* in that order. Gram-positive cocci—*streptococci* being the most common—are the major cause of the remaining 15 to 24 percent of these infections.

In the late 1950s and early 1960s, *staphylococci* were the primary etiologic factor in nursery epidemics. This resulted in the enforcement of stringent isolation and medical aseptic practices in the nursery. Whether or not these rigid policies influenced the subsequent decline of epidemiologic strains of staphylococci is uncertain and unproved. Some researchers have suggested that the main reason staphylococci epidemics have diminished may be the passing of a boom phase in the long-term natural life cycle of the organisms. With the present relaxation of rigid infection control techniques in many nurseries, it remains to be seen if an upsurge of epidemics will occur.

Many studies have been published regarding the spread of staphylococcal infections in newborns. Colonization occurs when the organisms settle on the tissue of the skin, nose, and throat without producing disease. There is a much higher incidence of disease in infants who have become colonized with the organisms. These infections may occur while the infant is in the nursery or after discharge. Many infants become ill at home. In some cases, the infant remains well but spreads the infection to other family members. The practice of good hand-washing technique by nursery personnel is considered the most crucial factor in preventing the spread of staphylococci in the nursery.

Following the decline of epidemics of staphylococcal infections, nurseries have experienced a rise in the incidence of infections due to gram-negative rods—*Pseudomonas* being one of the most prevalent. These bacteria are termed "water bugs" because they can thrive and proliferate in water alone. The introduction of a gamut of mechanical equipment in the care of infants is the principal cause of the high incidence of these infections. Gram-negative bacteria in the nursery are spread primarily by contaminated equipment, particularly those utilizing moisture of any kind, i.e., incubators, and plastic sleeves on portholes, resuscitative equipment, face masks, suction machines, wash basins, Zephiran solutions, soap dishes, etc. The surveillance and sterilization of equipment are essential in preventing spread of infection.

It is the nurse's responsibility to ensure that all equipment used is appropriately cleaned and sterilized. If the equipment permits, all potentially infectious objects should be autoclaved or gas-sterilized. When oxygen is in use, the humidifier must be changed daily and the water changed every 8 h. Plastic disposable tubes should be used from oxygen outlets and discarded every 24 h.

At present, the trend is to simplify infection control techniques used in the nursery, the rationale being that many of the rigid practices of the past proved useless when tested scientifically. The single most important factor in preventing spread of infection by any organism is handwashing. The principal mode of cross-infection is failure of personnel to wash hands between the handling of different infants. Personnel should perform a 2 min scrub to a level above the elbows when first entering the nursery, and wash for 30 to 60 s between caring for different babies. Both soaps and detergents are used. Heeding the warnings issued in 1971, many institutions have banned the use of hexachlorophene. However, because some nurseries have experienced a subsequent outbreak of staphylococcal infections, they have resumed limited use of hexachlorophene detergents for personnel caring for infants. Iodinated detergents are effective against gram-negative rods as well as gram-positive organisms, but such preparations are often irritating to the skin.

Personnel giving direct care to the infant in a crib or incubator should wear short-sleeved scrub dresses to facilitate washing. A long-sleeved gown should be worn by personnel when removing an infant from an incubator or bassinet, and must be changed between the handling of different infants. Some institutions do not require physicians and other personnel to wear gowns provided the infant is cared for in the incubator.

Nursing responsibility The majority of postnatally acquired infections are preventable if sensible hygienic practices of proved value are carried out. It is neither possible nor desirable to secure a germ-free environment in the nursery, and all practices are designed to minimize the risk of spreading infection by personnel, equipment, and cross-contamination of infants. The nurse is in a better position than other staff members to ensure the success of infection control procedures, because of close and continuous contact with the infants. The baby must be closely observed for redness at the base of the cord, discharge from the eyes, skin eruptions, changes in skin color, and signs of respiratory infection. Any suggestive symptom must be immediately reported to the physician. The nurse should be aware of the incidence of infections in the nursery and be alert to possible sources of contamination. The nurse must accept the responsibility of appraising and regulating the hygienic demeanor of the many specialists, technicians, and ancillary personnel involved in the infants' care. Sick personnel pose a serious threat to the infant and should not enter the nursery.

Studies have shown that the incidence of infectious disease does not increase when parents are allowed into the nursery, but the precautions regarding hand washing and gowning must be enforced.

"Suspect" and isolation nurseries are no longer considered essential except for infants with diarrhea and draining infections.

ROUTINE DAILY CARE

Throughout this chapter, the nurse's responsibilities have been described in detail in relation to the infant's specific problems and needs. Routine care procedures differ at various institutions, but the basics are summarized below:

The nurse gives total care to the infant at periodic intervals in order to avoid repeatedly disturbing the baby. All equipment is collected beforehand, and the nurse must work efficiently—giving complete care without tiring or exhausting the baby. If the infant's vital signs are not monitored, they are taken before the baby is handled.

When a baby is admitted to the nursery, a bath should not be given until the temperature has stabilized for at least 4 h. Studies carried out by Kopelman[15] and Powell[16] indicate that small premature infants are particularly susceptible to the toxic effects of hexachlorophene. Therefore, such preparations should not be used for bathing. Despite tradition, it is not necessary to bathe infants completely on a daily basis. In fact, it is important that the complete bath be omitted for small sick infants. Even if a bath is not given, the genitals and creases of the thighs and buttocks must be kept clean.

Small babies are weighed daily before feedings; larger ones less often. The small baby may lose 10 to 20 percent of the birth weight, and the larger infants from 5 to 10 percent in the first week of life. Very small infants often take 1 month or even longer to regain their birth weights.

In order to facilitate postural drainage from the lungs, the infant's position should be changed every 1 to 2 h. The incubator can be adjusted to provide a Fowler's or Trendelenburg position. If respiratory distress is observed, the infant should be placed in a low Fowler's position. In this position, the flexed neck may cause narrowing of the trachea so that a thin diaper roll may be needed under the shoulders to slightly hyperextend the infant's neck. Flexed and abducted arms will permit greater expansion of the thorax. When the baby is placed in a Fowler's position, a diaper roll inserted under the buttocks prevents the baby from slipping down in the incubator (Fig. 30-20). An infant in respiratory distress must never be positioned on the abdomen.

During the entire process of caring for the baby, the nurse closely observes the infant's respirations, skin condition, color, cry, activity, and muscle tone. It may be necessary to stimulate the infant by flicking the heel in order to test the quality of the cry. The times of the first voiding and defecation should be noted. In a study of 180 preterm infants, Mangurten reported that 80 percent of the infants passed the first stool by 24 h after birth.[17] It should be dark green and sticky. The nurse should be concerned if it appears pale and firm, since it then may be indicative of a meconium plug causing obstruction or

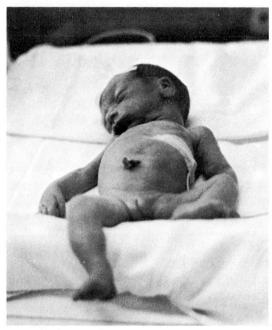

fig. 30-20 Infant in a slightly elevated position with a diaper roll to prevent slipping down.

Hirschsprung's disease. Abdominal distension must be detected immediately, since it may signify gastrointestinal disturbance and interferes with respiration. Below are listed critical observations which can be made only by nurses, not by monitors.

1 Respiratory distress characterized by grunting, retractions, flaring nares, pallor, or cyanosis
2 Detection of regurgitation and vomiting (to prevent aspiration)
3 Sucking ability and acceptance of feedings
4 Skin condition, color, and lesions
5 Changes in activity
6 Frequency and character of urine and stools

After morning care, the baby's condition is noted and recorded every 1 to 4 h, depending upon the condition. All efforts should be made to assign one nurse to a particular infant in order to ensure consistency of approach and valid comparative observations.

PSYCHOLOGIC NEEDS OF THE MOTHER OF A PRETERM INFANT

In recent decades we have come to understand the adverse and often devastating effects suffered by an infant separated from its mother. It has been well established that the infant requires a warm, intimate, and continuous relationship with its mother or mother surrogate in order to ensure normal psychologic and physical development. Knowing that early maternal deprivation affects the infant, it appears reasonable to conjecture that to some degree maternal behavior may be altered by isolation from the infant. The important—and as yet unanswered—question today is whether a critical or sensitive period exists for the mother in the immediate postnatal period in which physical contact is important for the development of normal mothering behavior.

Animal studies have repeatedly demonstrated that the development of normal mothering behavior for most species requires immediate physical contact with the young in the postnatal period. If the animal mother is separated from the infant during the critical period after delivery, deviant maternal behavior usually results. Infant deprivation in many species results in the actual rejection and/or destruction of the offspring.

Researchers suggest that bonds of affection begin to form before delivery, but that they are fragile and vulnerable in the early days of life. The human studies in this area focus on observing the mother/newborn relationship. Klaus and coworkers suggest that the human mother exhibits specific routine be-

havior patterns after delivery.[18] They have shown through filmed observations that "touch" and "eye-to-eye" contact appear to play an important role in establishing bonds of affection between the mother and her infant. They reported that when alert mothers of full-term infants were presented their nude newborns, each mother began touching her baby's extremities with her fingertips, and within a few minutes used her entire hand to stroke the infant's body. The expression of affection and love for the baby was repeatedly evidenced by the mother assuming an *en face* position in relation to her baby; i.e., the mother rotated the position of her face in such a way that her eyes and those of the infant directly met. During the first hour of life the baby's reaction was observed to coincide with the mother's natural response of eye-to-eye contact. The baby was then alert, attentive, and able to meet the intense gaze of the mother. Many great artists have been able to capture on canvas this moving expression of love and tenderness.

In the future, further investigation may reveal that alterations in current hospital policies are required for the ultimate good of mother and baby. Klaus contends that separation in the immediate newborn period may be a significant component in mothering disorders connected with failure to thrive, child abuse, and emotional and behavioral problems found in both natural and adopted children.[19]

Progressive neonatal centers are already attempting to alter procedures to decrease the effects of physical separation. The mother expects a perfect baby, and a preterm infant brings with it shock, grief, anxiety, fear, and a blow to her self-esteem as a mother. Her defenses are down and she requires support. The guilt and psychologic sense of separation felt by the mother are intense. She should be encouraged to see her infant at the earliest opportunity. It has been demonstrated that unless parents have a history of serious emotional disorders, their grief is not compounded by early and close contact with an infant who does not survive. As soon as the infant's condition permits, the mother should visit and fondle the baby while it is still in the incubator, and should repeatedly bathe and feed the baby before discharge from the hospital. The nurse should explain in detail all the equipment surrounding the infant, and all questions should be answered with simple, honest explanations and with great patience.

Throughout life, all human beings have the same basic needs and perform the same basic functions. It is the quality with which one moves through the experiences of day-to-day living that gives life meaning, value, and beauty. The need of the infant for uncompromising love, care, and affection is so crucial to future development and life that any effort made by the professional to secure a meaningful mother/infant relationship is a significant contribution to the human condition.

"UP, OUT OF THE VALLEY OF THE SHADOW OF DEATH"[20]

This is our ultimate hope and goal for all parents who must face the death of their infant. Psychological studies indicate that parents generally view the infant as an extension of themselves and that the loss of a baby is a devastating experience for the family. The attachment to the neonate is more emotional than social because of the short time permitted in the development of the relationship, as well as the limited contact with the baby resulting from hospitalization.

It is recognized that many factors influence an individual's reaction to death—age, past experiences, philosophy, religious conviction, culture, intelligence, emotional stability, etc. Dr. Kübler-Ross, a leader in the study of thanatology in this country, described five coping mechanisms used by dying patients at the time of terminal illness. An analogy has since been drawn between these mechanisms and the stages in the grieving process which include denial, anger, bargaining, depression, and acceptance. The nurse should be able to identify and accept the bereaved parents' behavior. But it is important to understand that the stages of grieving are guidelines, not dictums. For many, the first reaction to the death of an infant is that it is unreal, a nightmare, an error, a hallucination, but for some, it is very real and absurd.

The grieving of the family as a whole is of monumental importance in helping individual members come to terms with the tragedy. The mourning of all members together—whether in silence or weeping, laughing or talking or reminiscing, but always in some manner sharing their pain, anguish, grief, and humor—offers support and solidarity which can lead to insight and healing.

Just as it is important to grieve collectively as a family, it is equally important that we recognize that suffering is always individual and lonely, and we must allow time for it. Although suffering is a universal experience, it is the one barrier that shuts each of us away, alone. Besides mourning and suffering, the bereaved individual requires understanding, patience, and love from those closest to her or him. But most important, healing ultimately requires that the individual maintain a willingness to remain vulnerable—a determination to take another chance, recognizing full well that he or she may lose again.

The following guidelines are intended to assist nurses in their role as therapeutic agents in relating to bereaved family members.

1 Understand and attempt to come to terms with one's own feelings and philosophy regarding death.
2 Recognize that parents have the right to

have their questions answered frankly and honestly.

3 Be able to identify and accept the behavior of bereaved parents in relation to the various stages of grieving identified by Kübler-Ross.

4 Recognize that parents should be offered the opportunity of planning and taking part in the funeral and burial procedures. Such involvement may drive home the reality and finality of the loss, but it does not ensure it. Thus, if parents wish to handle the funeral activities in other ways, their right to do so must be respected.

5 Help the parents understand that the reactions so often seen in children after a death in the family—regression, acting out, insomnia, bad dreams, etc.—are normal coping mechanisms for children meeting such a crisis.

6 Recognizing the importance of having the family grieve together, collectively sharing their loss.

7 Suffering, although a universal experience, is always individual and lonely.

8 Recognize the importance of the understanding, patience, and love which only the family and very close loved ones can offer the bereaved.

9 Recognize that healing takes *time*—often much more time than anyone wishes to admit—and it differs with each individual.

Thus, the nurse working with parents of prematurely born infants must learn to be not only technically skilled but also deeply supportive of the parents during crises.

study questions

1 What differentiates a preterm infant from a SGA neonate? Why do the SGA babies account for a large proportion of perinatal mortality?

2 Before caring for a preterm infant, outline what information it would be essential for you to collect in order to have an adequate data base upon which to formulate a plan of care.

3 What are the major physiologic handicaps encountered by the preterm neonate?

4 Develop a profile of what you consider to be realistic personal and professional qualifications required by a nurse to work effectively in a neonatal intensive care center.

5 What are some of the major morbidity problems encountered in preterm infants who survive?

references

1 *Standards and Recommendations for Hospital Care of Newborn Infants,* American Academy of Pediatrics, Evanston, Ill., 1971, p. 11.

2 American College of Obstetrics and Gynecology, *Obstetric and Gynecologic Terminology,* Davis, Philadelphia, 1972, p. 402.

3 F. C. Battaglia and L. O. Lubchenko, "A Practical Classification of Newborn Infants by Weight and Gestational Age," *Journal of Pediatrics,* **71:**159, 1967.

4 D. Cavanagh and M. R. Talisman, *Prematurity and the Obstetrician,* Appleton-Century-Crofts, New York, 1969, p. 29.

5 L. O. Lubchenco, et al., "Sequelae of Premature Birth," *American Journal of Diseases of Children,* **106:**101, 1973.

6 G. Rawlings, et al., "Changing Prognosis for Infants of Very Low Birth Weight," *Lancet,* **1:**516, 1971.

7 L. M. Dubowitz, V. Dubowitz, and C. Goldberg, "Clinical Assessment of Gestational Age in the Newborn Infant," *Journal of Pediatrics,* **77:**1, 1970.

8 P. H. Perlstein, N. K. Edwards, and J. M. Sutherland, "Apnea in Premature Infants and Incubator-Air-Temperature," *New England Journal of Medicine,* **282:**461, 1970.

9 Cavanagh, op. cit., p. 456.

10 *Standards and Recommendations for Hospital Care of Newborn Infants,* op. cit., p. 12.

11 B. Rothfeder and M. Tiedeman, "Feeding the Low-Birth-Weight Neonate," *Nursing 77,* **7:**58, 1977.

12 L. Lilien, et al., "Treatment of Neonatal Hypoglycemia with Continuous Intravenous Glucose Infusion," *Journal of Pediatrics* **91:**779, 1977.

13 L. Finberg, "The Relationship of Intravenous Infusion and Intracranial Hemorrhage—a Commentary," *Journal of Pediatrics,* **91:**777, 1977.

14 S. G. Babson and R. C. Benson, *Management of the High-Risk Pregnancy and Intensive Care of the Neonate,* 2d ed., Mosby, St. Louis, 1971, p. 204.

15 A. E. Kopelman, "Cutaneous Absorption of Hexach-

lorophene in Low Birthweight Infants," *Journal of Pediatrics,* **82:**976, 1973.

16   H. Powell, et al., "Hexachlorophene Myelinopathy in Premature Infants," *Journal of Pediatrics,* **82:**976, 1973.

17   H. H. Mangurten, C. I. Slade, and C. J. Reidle, "First Stool in the Preterm, Low Birth-weight Infant," *Journal of Pediatrics,* **82:**1033, 1973.

18   M. Klaus, J. Kennell, N. Plumb, et al., "Human Maternal Behavior at the First Contact with Her Young," *Pediatrics,* **46:**187, 1970.

19   M. Klaus and J. Kennell, "Mothers Separated from Their Newborn Infants," *Pediatric Clinics of North America,* **17:**1015, 1970.

20   J. Higgins, "Up, Out of the Valley of the Shadow of Death," *The New York Times,* December 10, 1977.

bibliography

Auld, P. A. M.: "Oxygen Therapy for Premature Infants," *Journal of Pediatrics,* **78:**705, 1971.

Bedford, W., et al.: "Determination of Optimal Continuous Positive Airway Pressure for the Treatment of IRDS by Measurement of Esophageal Pressure," *Journal of Pediatrics,* **91:**449, 1977.

Bryan, M. H., et al.: "Supplemental Intravenous Alimentation in Low Birth-weight Infants," *Journal of Pediatrics,* **82:**940, 1973.

Corbet, J., et al.: "Controlled Trial of Bicarbonate Therapy in High-Risk Premature Newborn Infants," *Journal of Pediatrics,* **91:**771, 1977.

Davies, P. A.: "Bacterial Infection in the Fetus and Newborn," *Archives of Diseases of Children,* **46:**1, 1971.

Fanaroff, M. B., et al.: "Controlled Trial of Continuous Negative External Pressure in the Treatment of Severe Respiratory Distress Syndrome," *Journal of Pediatrics,* **82:**921, 1973.

Goldman, H. I., et al.: "Late Effects of Early Dietary Protein Intake on Low Birth Weight Infants," *Journal of Pediatrics,* **85:**764, 1974.

Goodman, M. B.: "Two Mothers' Reaction to the Deaths of Their Premature Infants," *Journal Obstetric, Gynecologic and Neonatal Nursing,* **4:**3:25, May/June, 1975.

Gutberlets, R. B., and M. Cornblath: "Neonatal Hypoglycemia Revisited, 1975," *Pediatrics,* **58:**10, 1976.

Harris, T. R., and M. Nugent: "Continuous Arterial Oxygen Tension Monitoring in the Newborn Infant," *Journal of Pediatrics,* **82:**929, 1973.

Heese, H. deV., et al.: "Intermittent Positive Pressure Ventilation in Hyaline Membrane Disease," *Journal of Pediatrics,* **76:**183, 1970.

Heird, C., and L. Anerson: "Requirements and Methods of Feeding Low Birth Weight Infants," *Current Problems in Pediatrics,* **7:**8, 1977.

———, and R. W. Winters: "Total Parenteral Nutrition: The State of the Art," *Journal of Pediatrics,* **86:**2, 1975.

Klaus, M., R. Jerauld, N. Kreger, et al.: "Maternal Attachment: Importance of the First Post-partum Days," *New England Journal of Medicine,* **286:**460, 1972.

Korones, B.: *High-Risk Newborn Infants,* Mosby, St. Louis, 1972.

Mann, L. I., et al.: "Antenatal Diagnosis of the Small-for-Gestational-Age Fetus," *American Journal Obstetrics and Gynecology,* **120:**995, 1974.

McCormick, Q.: "Retinopathy of Prematurity," *Current Problems in Pediatrics,* **7:**10, 1977.

Nalepka, C. D.: "Understanding Thermoregulation in Newborns," *Journal of Obstetric, Gynecologic and Neonatal Nursing,* **5:**6:17, Nov/Dec 1976.

Nelson, R. M., et al.: "Increased Hypoxemia in Neonates Secondary to the Use of Continuous Positive Airway Pressure," *Journal of Pediatrics,* **91:**87, 1977.

Patton, B. (ed.): "Neonatal Care," *Nursing Clinics of North America,* **13**(1), March 1978.

Raiha, N. C. R., et al.: "Milk Protein—Quantity and Quality in Low Birth Weight Infants," *Pediatrics,* **57:**659, 1976.

Richardson, C. P., et al.: "Effects of Continuous Positive Airway Pressure (CPAP) on Pulmonary Function in Early Stages of Respiratory Distress Syndrome (RDS)," *Pediatric Research,* **10:**993, 1976.

Schlesinger, E. R.: "Neonatal Intensive Care: Planning for Services and Outcomes Following Care," *Journal of Pediatrics,* **82:**916, 1973.

Shaw, J. C. L.: "Parenteral Nutrition in the Management of Sick Low Birthweight Infants," *Pediatrics Clinics of North America,* **20:**333, 1973.

Sinclair, J. C.: "Heat Production and Thermo-regulation in the Small-for-date Infant," *Pediatrics Clinics of North America,* **17:**147, 1970.

Stahlman, M., et al.: "A Six-Year Follow-up of Clinical Hyaline Membrane Disease," *Pediatrics Clinics of North America,* **20:**433, 1973.

———: "Negative Pressure Assisted Ventilation in Infants with Hyaline Membrane Disease," *Journal of Pediatrics,* **76:**174, 1970.

Stephenson, J. M, et al.: "The Effect of Cooling on Blood Gas Tensions in Newborn Infants," *Journal of Pediatrics,* **76:**848, 1970.

Stocker, J., et al.: "Ultrasonic Cephalometry: Its Use in Estimating Fetal Weight," *Obstetrics and Gynecology,* **45:**275, 1975.

Teberg, A. J., et al.: "Effect of Phototherapy on Growth of Low-Birth-Weight Infants—Two-Year Follow-up," *Journal of Pediatrics,* **91:**92, 1977.

Weight (mass) pounds and ounces to grams

Example: To obtain grams equivalent to 6 lb, 8 oz, read "6" on top scale, "8" on side scale; equivalent is 2948 g.

Ounces (oz)	Pounds (lb)														
	0	1	2	3	4	5	6	7	8	9	10	11	12	13	14
0	0	454	907	1361	1814	2268	2722	3175	3629	4082	4536	4990	5443	5897	6350
1	28	482	936	1389	1843	2296	2750	3203	3657	4111	4564	5018	5471	5925	6379
2	57	510	964	1417	1871	2325	2778	3232	3685	4139	4593	5046	5500	5953	6407
3	85	539	992	1446	1899	2353	2807	3260	3714	4167	4621	5075	5528	5982	6435
4	113	567	1021	1474	1928	2381	2835	3289	3742	4196	4649	5103	5557	6010	6464
5	142	595	1049	1503	1956	2410	2863	3317	3770	4224	4678	5131	5585	6038	6492
6	170	624	1077	1531	1984	2438	2892	3345	3799	4252	4706	5160	5613	6067	6520
7	198	652	1106	1559	2013	2466	2920	3374	3827	4281	4734	5188	5642	6095	6549
8	227	680	1134	1588	2041	2495	2948	3402	3856	4309	4763	5216	5670	6123	6577
9	255	709	1162	1616	2070	2523	2977	3430	3884	4337	4791	5245	5698	6152	6605
10	283	737	1191	1644	2098	2551	3005	3459	3912	4366	4819	5273	5727	6180	6634
11	312	765	1219	1673	2126	2580	3033	3487	3941	4394	4848	5301	5755	6209	6662
12	340	794	1247	1701	2155	2608	3062	3515	3969	4423	4876	5330	5783	6237	6690
13	369	822	1276	1729	2183	2637	3090	3544	3997	4451	4904	5358	5812	6265	6719
14	397	850	1304	1758	2211	2665	3118	3572	4026	4479	4933	5386	5840	6294	6747
15	425	879	1332	1786	2240	2693	3147	3600	4054	4508	4961	5415	5868	6322	6776

Note: 1 lb = 453.59237 g; 1 oz = 28.349523 g; 1000 g = 1 kg. Gram equivalents have been rounded to whole numbers by adding one when the first decimal place is 5 or greater.

Temperature, Fahrenheit (F) to Celsius* (C)

°F	°C	°F	°C	°F	°C	°F	°C
95.0	35.0	98.0	36.7	101.0	38.3	104.0	40.0
95.2	35.1	98.2	36.8	101.2	38.4	104.2	40.1
95.4	35.2	98.4	36.9	101.4	38.6	104.4	40.2
95.6	35.3	**98.6**	**37.0**	101.6	38.7	104.6	40.3
95.8	35.4	98.8	37.1	101.8	38.8	104.8	40.4
96.0	35.6	99.0	37.2	102.0	38.9	105.0	40.6
96.2	35.7	99.2	37.3	102.2	39.0	105.2	40.7
96.4	35.8	99.4	37.4	102.4	39.1	105.4	40.8
96.6	35.9	99.6	37.6	102.6	39.2	105.6	40.9
96.8	36.0	99.8	37.7	102.8	39.3	105.8	41.0
97.0	36.1	100.0	37.8	103.0	39.4	106.0	41.1
97.2	36.2	100.2	37.9	103.2	39.6	106.2	41.2
97.4	36.3	100.4	38.0	103.4	39.7	106.4	41.3
97.6	36.4	100.6	38.1	103.6	39.8	106.6	41.4
97.8	36.6	100.8	38.2	103.8	39.9	106.8	41.6

Note: $°C = (°F - 32) \times 5/9$. Celsius temperature equivalents rounded to one decimal place by adding 0.1 when second decimal place is 5 or greater.

* The metric system replaced the term "centigrade" with "Celsius" (the inventor of the scale).

Length, inches to centimeters

1-in increments   Example: To obtain the number of centimeters equivalent to 22 in, read "20" on top scale, "2" on side scale, equivalent is 55.9 cm.

Inches (in.)	0	10	20	30	40
0	0	25.4	50.8	76.2	101.6
1	2.5	27.9	53.3	78.7	104.1
2	5.1	30.5	55.9	81.3	106.7
3	7.6	33.0	58.4	83.8	109.2
4	10.2	35.6	61.0	86.4	111.8
5	12.7	38.1	63.5	88.9	114.3
6	15.2	40.6	66.0	91.4	116.8
7	17.8	43.2	68.6	94.0	119.4
8	20.3	45.7	71.1	96.5	121.9
9	22.9	48.3	73.7	99.1	124.5

One-quarter (¼)-in increments Example: To obtain centimeters equivalent to 14¾ in, read "14" on top scale, "1" on side scale, equivalent is 37.5 cm.

10 to 15 in.

	10	11	12	13	14	15
0	25.4	27.9	30.5	33.0	35.6	38.1
¼	26.0	28.6	31.1	33.7	36.2	38.7
½	26.7	29.2	31.8	34.3	36.8	39.4
¾	27.3	29.8	32.4	34.9	37.5	40.0

16 to 21 in.

	16	17	18	19	20	21
0	40.6	43.2	45.7	48.3	50.8	53.3
¼	41.3	43.8	46.4	48.9	51.4	54.0
½	41.9	44.5	47.0	49.5	52.1	54.6
¾	42.5	45.1	47.6	50.2	52.7	55.2

Note: 1 in = 2.540 cm. Centimeter equivalents rounded one decimal place by adding 0.1 when second decimal place is 5 or greater, for example, 33.48 becomes 33.5.

Source: Ross Inservice Nursing Aid No. 1. Ross Laboratories, Division of Abbott Laboratories, Columbus, Ohio.

APPENDIX 2

THE PREGNANT PATIENT's BILL OF RIGHTS*

The Pregnant Patient has the right to participate in decisions involving her well-being and that of her unborn child, unless there is a clearcut medical emergency that prevents her participation. In addition to the rights set forth in the American Hospital Association's "Patient's Bill of Rights," the Pregnant Patient, because she represents TWO patients rather than one, should be recognized as having the additional rights listed below.

1   *The Pregnant Patient has the right,* prior to the administration of any drug or procedure, to be informed by the health professional caring for her of any potential direct or indirect effects, risks or hazards to herself or her unborn or newborn infant which may result from the use of a drug or procedure prescribed for or administered to her during pregnancy, labor, birth or lactation.

* *Source:* Prepared by Doris Haire, Chair., Committee on Health Law and Regulation, International Childbirth Education Association, Inc., Rochester, N.Y.

2   *The Pregnant Patient has the right,* prior to the proposed therapy, to be informed, not only of the benefits, risks and hazards of the proposed therapy but also of known alternative therapy, such as available childbirth education classes which could help to prepare the Pregnant Patient physically and mentally to cope with the discomfort or stress of pregnancy and the experience of childbirth, thereby reducing or eliminating her need for drugs and obstetric intervention. She should be offered such information early in her pregnancy in order that she may make a reasoned decision.

3   *The Pregnant Patient has the right,* prior to the administration of any drug, to be informed by the health professional who is prescribing or administering the drug to her that any drug which she receives during pregnancy, labor and birth, no matter how or when the drug is taken or administered, may adversely affect her unborn baby, directly or indirectly, and

that there is no drug or chemical which has been proven safe for the unborn child.

4   *The Pregnant Patient has the right* if cesarean birth is anticipated, to be informed prior to the administration of any drug, and preferably prior to her hospitalization, that minimizing her and, in turn, her baby's intake of nonessential pre-operative medicine will benefit her baby.

5   *The Pregnant Patient has the right,* prior to the administration of a drug or procedure, to be informed of the areas of uncertainty if there is NO properly controlled follow-up research which has established the safety of the drug or procedure with regard to its direct and/or indirect effects on the physiological, mental and neurological development of the child exposed, via the mother, to the drug or procedure during pregnancy, labor, birth or lactation—(this would apply to virtually all drugs and the vast majority of obstetric procedures).

6   *The Pregnant Patient has the right,* prior to the administration of any drug, to be informed of the brand name and generic name of the drug in order that she may advise the health professional of any past adverse reaction to the drug.

7   *The Pregnant Patient has the right* to determine for herself, without pressure from her attendant, whether she will accept the risks inherent in the proposed therapy or refuse a drug or procedure.

8   *The Pregnant Patient has the right* to know the name and qualifications of the individual administering a medication or procedure to her during labor or birth.

9   *The Pregnant Patient has the right* to be informed, prior to the administration of any procedure, whether that procedure is being administered to her for her or her baby's benefit (medically indicated) or as an elective procedure (for convenience, teaching purposes or research).

10   *The Pregnant Patient has the right* to be accompanied during the stress of labor and birth by someone she cares for, and to whom she looks for emotional comfort and encouragement

11   *The Pregnant Patient has the right* after appropriate medical consultation to choose a position for labor and for birth which is least stressful to her baby and to herself.

12   *The Obstetric Patient has the right* to have her baby cared for at her bedside if her baby is normal, and to feed her baby according to her baby's needs rather than according to the hospital regimen.

13   *The Obstetric Patient has the right* to be informed in writing of the name of the person who actually delivered her baby and the professional qualifications of that person. This information should also be on the birth certificate.

14   *The Obstetric Patient has the right* to be informed if there is any known or indicated aspect of her or her baby's care or condition which may cause her or her baby later difficulty or problems.

15   *The Obstetric Patient has the right* to have her and her baby's hospital medical records complete, accurate and legible and to have their records, including Nurses' Notes, retained by the hospital until the child reaches at least the age of majority, or to have the records offered to her before they are destroyed.

16   *The Obstetric Patient,* both during and after her hospital stay, has the right to have access to her complete hospital medical records, including Nurses' Notes, and to receive a copy upon payment of a reasonable fee and without incurring the expense of retaining an attorney.

It is the obstetric patient and her baby, not the health professional, who must sustain any trauma or injury resulting from the use of a drug or obstetric procedure. The observation of the rights listed above will not only permit the obstetric patient to participate in the decisions involving her and her baby's health care, but will help to protect the health professional and the hospital against litigation arising from resentment or misunderstanding on the part of the mother.

GLOSSARY

abortion   termination of pregnancy of a fetus weighing less than 500 g or of a pregnancy of less than 19 completed weeks after conception
  spontaneous occurring without assistance; lay term, "miscarriage"
  induced brought on by external methods: D and C (dilation and curettage), vacuum aspiration, salinization

abruptio placentae   tearing away of the placenta from the wall of the uterus, accompanied by pain; there may be concealed bleeding or overt, visible bleeding

acini (pl.), acinus (sing.)   smallest, saccular division of a gland, occurring in grapelike clusters, as in the mammary gland

acrocyanosis   cyanotic or bluish discoloration of the hands and/or feet of the newborn as a result of inadequate circulation or coldness

afterbirth   the products of conception (excluding the baby) that are expelled during the delivery—placenta and membranes (sac) and umbilical cord. Syn., secundines

afterpains   discomfort caused by the contraction of the uterus postpartally as it returns to its prepregnant condition; usually occurring in the multipara

amenorrhea   cessation or absence of menstruation

amniocentesis   removal of some of the amniotic fluid from the amniotic sac by way of a needle inserted through the abdominal wall of the mother for the purpose of examining the fluid

amnion   inner layer of the fetal membranes or sac, which secretes amniotic fluid

amniotic fluid embolism   a rare postpartal occurrence, in which amniotic fluid enters the maternal circulation. The cells, debris and fluid form emboli, usually in the lungs.

amniotomy   rupturing of the amniotic sac by artificial means

androgenic hormone   a hormone that has the property of producing male secondary sexual characterics

anencephalus   a fetus born without a brain or cranial bones

anovulatory   associated with lack or absence of ovulation

anoxia   lack or absence of oxygen

antenatal   prenatal, before birth

antepartal   occurring before labor and delivery

antibody   substance produced by the body for protection against the specific antigen that triggered its production

antigen   any substance, usually of protein material, which triggers the production of antibodies, such as foreign blood cells, bacteria

apnea   absence or cessation of respirations

areola   pigmented area surrounding the nipple

asphyxia neonatorum   respiratory failure in the newborn, resulting from an insufficient oxygen-carbon dioxide exchange

ballottement rebounding movement of the fetus when uterus (or cervix) is tapped by the examiner. Syn., passive fetal movement

Bandl's ring retracted ring occurring between the lower and upper segments of the uterus and resulting from an obstructed labor; may be a sign of impending uterine rupture. Syn., pathologic retraction ring

basal body temperature (BBT) lowest usual temperature of the body taken before rising

bilirubin the red-orange pigment that results from the breakdown of hemoglobin and which can cause jaundice of the skin, when the level rises above 5 mg/ 100 mL in the newborn

Braxton Hicks contractions painless, intermittent contractions of the uterus which occur throughout pregnancy; often mistaken for labor contractions

Braxton Hicks version a maneuver to change the position of the fetus by external and internal manipulation

breech buttocks
breech presentation delivery in which the buttocks or feet of the fetus are presented at the outlet, instead of the vertex (head)
footling one or both feet present at the opening
frank buttocks are the presenting part
full or complete buttocks and feet present at the pelvic brim

Candida albicans a yeastlike fungus which produces monilial infection in the vaginal canal of the woman and may cause thrush in the infant

caput head

caput succedaneum swelling or edema on the head of the infant occurring during labor and/or delivery

cephalhematoma trauma of labor and delivery resulting in a collection of blood on the head of the fetus between the bone and the periosteum, defined by the suture lines

cephalic referring to the head

cerclage procedure procedure for the treatment of incompetent cervix

cholasma gravidarum brownish-yellow patches of pigmentation occurring during pregnancy, particularly on the face and neck. Syn., mask of pregnancy

choanal atresia blockage of the posterior nares present at birth

chorion the outermost membrane of the developing fetus, which gives rise to the fetal portion of the placenta and extends to form the outer layer of the amniotic sac

chorionic pertaining to the chorion

chorionic gonadotropin hormone produced by the chorion and excreted in the urine of the pregnant woman; its presence in the urine is a possible sign of pregnancy

chorionic villi fingerlike projections of the chorion which invade the decidua basalis and form the fetal portion of the placenta

cleft lip congenital/genetic opening of the upper lip extending from the nares; may involve one or both nares

cleft palate congenital/genetic opening of the roof of the mouth

colostrum yellowish white fluid expressed from the breast during pregnancy preceding the formation of milk; caloric and cathartic values of this substance are questioned

congenital laryngeal stridor a harsh, crowing, vibrating sound produced by the newborn of infant upon inspiration

Coombs' test blood test to determine the presence of antibodies
direct determination of antibodies attached to blood cells, particularly maternal (anti-Rh) antibodies attached to fetal blood cells
indirect determination of free-floating or unattached antibodies, particularly those (anti-Rh) in the maternal circulation (serum)

corpus luteum yellow body of material found in the site of the ruptured graafian follicle which persists for several months during pregnancy, secreting progesterone

crowning the appearance of the vertex, or head, at the external vaginal orifice

D and C dilation and curettage; a surgical procedure involving dilation of the cervix and removal of the uterine contents

decidua enriched endometrial lining of pregnancy shed after pregnancy terminates
basalis the portion of the endometrium underlying the embedded embryo and from which the maternal portion of the placenta is formed
capsularis that outer portion of the decidua enveloping the embryo
vera the remainder of the endometrium not containing the embedded embryo

dilation the act of stretching or opening

dilatation enlargement of an organ or orifice
of the cervix; the state of enlargement or opening of the cervix to allow for passage of the fetus

Doderlein's bacillus common vaginal gram-negative organism producing lactic acid which tends to inhibit the growth of pathogenic organisms

Down's syndrome formerly known as mongolism; a congenital/genetic abnormality in which 47 chromosomes are present in the fetus. Syn., trisomy 21

dystocia difficult, abnormal labor

eclampsia abnormal reaction of the body to pregnancy, resulting in convulsions and possible coma; usually preceded by hypertension, albuminuria, and edema

ectopic pregnancy pregnancy that occurs outside the uterine cavity

effacement thinning of the cervix to allow for passage of the fetus; in primigravidas, occurs prior to dilatation, and in multigravidas, occurs simultaneously with dilatation

engagement descent of the fetus into the pelvis until the presenting part reaches the level of the ischial spines

engorgement stasis of blood and lymph in the breast, causing tenderness, firmness, and discomfort prior to onset of lactation

episiotomy a surgical incision of the perineum to enlarge the external vaginal opening to prevent laceration of the vulva, perineum, and adjacent structures

Epstein's pearls tiny, white, beadlike ephithelial cysts on the roof of the mouth of the newborn on either side of the median ridge; not to be confused with thrush, which is patchy

erythroblastosis fetalis hemolytic disorder of the fetus or newborn in which maternal anti-Rh antibodies destroy fetal blood cells, causing jaundice and other symptoms

estriol a metabolite produced by the placenta, found in the urine of pregnant women and measured in an attempt to determine placental function or dysfunction

estrogenic hormone a hormone which has the property of producing female secondary sexual characteristics

fetal pertaining to fetus

fetus the offspring from the moment of conception until the pregnancy is terminated or completed

fontanel the space at the junction of three or more fetal and cranial bones, covered with a tough membrane
  anterior junction of sagittal, frontal, and coronal sutures, on anterior portion of skull. Syn., "soft spot," greater fontanel
  posterior junction of lambdoid and sagittal sutures. Syn., lesser fontanel

foramen ovale opening between the right and left atria of the heart in the fetus; closes after birth

fundus the upper portion of the uterus

G-6-PD Glucose-6-phosphate dehydrogenase deficiency is an inherited erythrocyte enzyme deficiency

gestation length of time necessary for intrauterine growth and development of the fetus

graafian follicle fluid-filled sac in the ovary housing the maturing ovum

gravid pregnant

gravida a pregnant woman
  primigravida woman pregnant for the first time
  multigravida woman pregnant for the second time or more

hemorrhage in obstetrics, loss of blood in excess of 500 mL after the third stage of labor

hyaline membrane disease see *idiopathic respiratory distress syndrome* (RDS)

hydatidiform mole grapelike, cystic masses of degenerated chorionic villi, usually benign

hydramnios "water"; excessive amniotic fluid. Syn., polyhydramnios

hyperemesis gravidarum excessive, severe vomiting during pregnancy

hypofibrinogenemia reduced amounts of fibrinogen in the blood

hypospadias congenital/genetic defect in which the urethra of the male opens on the underside of the penis

hypoxia deficient amount of oxygen

icterus jaundice

icterus gravis neonatorum see *erythroblastosis fetalis*

idiopathic respiratory distress syndrome a severe respiratory syndrome of the newborn or preterm infant resulting in the development of a hyaline membrane in the lungs; may be fatal. Syn., RDS, hyaline membrane disease

inertia (uterine) inefficient, weak, or absent uterine contractions
  primary occurring early in labor
  secondary occurring after labor is established. Syn., uterine dysfunction

involution returning of the pelvic organs and structures to resemble their prepregnant state or condition

ischemia reduction of blood supply to an area

jaundice yellowish color of skin, sclera, mucous membrane, and excretions. Syn., icterus

kernicterus excessive bilirubin deposits in the brain, causing neurologic changes; may cause permanent brain damage or death

lanugo soft, fine, downy hair found on preterm and newborn infants

lightening the tilting or dropping of the fetus forward and downward into the true pelvis; occurs 2 or 3 weeks before the end of gestation in the primigravida, or at the beginnning of labor in many multigravidas

linea nigra the darkening of the abdominal line between the umbilicus and the symphysis pubis during pregnancy, caused by hormonal changes

lochia uterine discharge after delivery which consists of the sloughing decidua, tissue, blood, and cells; lasts 2 or 3 weeks

mastalgia pain in the breast

mastitis inflammation of the breast

menarche first menstrual flow

menorrhagia abnormally long or excessive menstrual bleeding

menses menstruation

menstruation cyclic uterine discharge of blood, tissue, and cells as a result of hormonal changes in the body. Syn., menses

mentum chin

milia tiny, white or yellow beadlike sebaceous cysts found primarily on the face of the newborn

miscarriage lay term for spontaneous abortion

mittelschmerz lower abdominal pain generally associated with ovulation

molding temporary changes in the shape of the head of the newborn, as it accommodates to the birth canal during labor and delivery

multigravida a woman who has been pregnant more than once

multipara a woman who has delivered more than once

neonatal referring to the newborn infant

nephrotoxic any substance or material which exerts a poisonous effect on the kidney

newborn infant a living infant during the first 27 days, 23 h, and 59 min of its life

nidation embedding of the fertilized ovum into the lining of the uterus

nulligravida a woman who has never been pregnant

nullipara a woman who has never delivered a viable baby

occiput back of the head; occipital bone

ophthalmia neonatorum acute, purulent conjunctivitis of the eyes of the newborn, usually caused by gonococcus

organogenesis the growth of various tissues of the fetus into organs. Period of organogenesis—first 12 weeks

ototoxic any substance or material poisonous to the ear

ovum female reproductive cell

oxytocin synthetic or natural substance which stimulates the uterus to contract

parity the state of having given birth to one infant or more than one infant; multiple births are considered as one parous delivery

parturient a laboring woman

parturition the act of giving birth

phenylketonuria (PKU) a genetic disorder involving the deficiency of the enzyme phenylalanine hydroxylase

phlegmasia alba dolens phlebitis of the femoral or iliac vein, resulting in edema of the leg. Syn., milk leg

placenta previa abnormally low implantation of the placenta in the uterus

polyhydramnios excessive amniotic fluid. Syn., hydramnios

position the relationship of a designated point on the presenting part of the fetus to a designated point in the maternal pelvis which has been divided into four quardrants

postpartum the period of time following delivery

preeclampsia abnormal bodily reaction to pregnancy characterized by edema, hypertension, and proteinuria, and occurring after the twentieth week of pregnancy; often referred to as toxemia

premature infant an infant born up through 37 completed weeks of gestation. Syn., preterm infant

presentation relationship of the long axis of the fetus to the long axis of the mother. Syn., lie

presenting part that anatomic part of the fetus that is closest to the cervix and felt by the examiner on vaginal or rectal examination—usually the head or buttocks

primigravida woman pregnant for the first time

primipara woman who has delivered for the first time a viable infant (over 20 weeks' gestation)

pseudocyesis false pregnancy

puerperium the 42 days after delivery

quickening the first active movements of the fetus detectable by the mother, at approximately 16 to 18 weeks of gestation

respiratory distress syndrome (RDS) see *idiopathic respiratory distress syndrome*

resuscitation restoration of breathing, life, or consciousness of one who is apparently dead and whose respirations have ceased

retrolental fibroplasia (RLF) a fibrous membrane which may occur behind the lens in the eye as a result of high oxygen concentration administered to a preterm infant

rugae transverse folds of the vaginal mucous membrane

secundines placenta and fetal membranes

Shirodkar technique purse-string suturing procedure for an incompetent cervix

show blood-tinged mucous discharge occurring during labor as the cervix dilates. Syn., bloody show

souffle, fetal a blowing or whistling sound of the blood as it rushes through the fetal arteries in the umbilical cord. Syn., funic souffle, umbilical souffle, Kennedy's sign

souffle, uterine the blowing, blurred sound of the maternal blood as it rushes through the uterine arteries. Syn., Kergaradec's sign

spermatozoon male reproductive cell. Syn., sperm

spinnbarkheit changes in the stretchability of the cervical mucosa during ovulation

stillborn a fetus, over 20 weeks' gestation, born without life

subinvolution a delay in the return of the pelvic organs and structures to their prepregnant state

supine hypotensive syndrome hypotension resulting from the pressure of the enlarged uterus upon the vena cava, blocking venous return

syncope fainting or light-headedness, common in early pregnancy

teratogen any agent or substance which has the capacity to alter fetal growth and development

term infant a live baby born after 38 to 42 weeks of gestation (from time of last menstrual period). Syn., full-term infant

thrush white, patchy oral lesions of the newborn caused by *Candida albicans*

toxemia see *preeclampsia, eclampsia*

tracheoesophageal fistula (TEF) congenital/genetic disorder in which the esophagus and trachea are connected, or the esophagus ends in a blind pouch and there is a lower connection in the trachea to the esophagus

Trichomonas viginalis protozoan infection of the vagina; Skene's ducts and urinary tract may also be infected

trimester approximately one-third of the gestational period when using LMP

first trimester the first day of the last normal menstrual period through 14 weeks' gestation

second trimester fifteenth through twenty-eighth week of gestation

third trimester twenty-ninth through the forty-second completed week of gestation and birth

umbilical cord life line between the fetus and placenta through which nourishment and waste pass; contains two arteries and one vein surrounded by Wharton's jelly. Syn., funis

vernix caseosa cheeselike covering on the fetus which protects the skin from the drying and wrinkling properties of the amniotic fluid

viability capability of survival, over 20 weeks' gestation

Wharton's jelly gelatinous connective tissue which surrounds the umbilical vessels giving support to the umbilical cord

zona zone; belt or girdle

zygote the fertilized ovum

INDEX

747

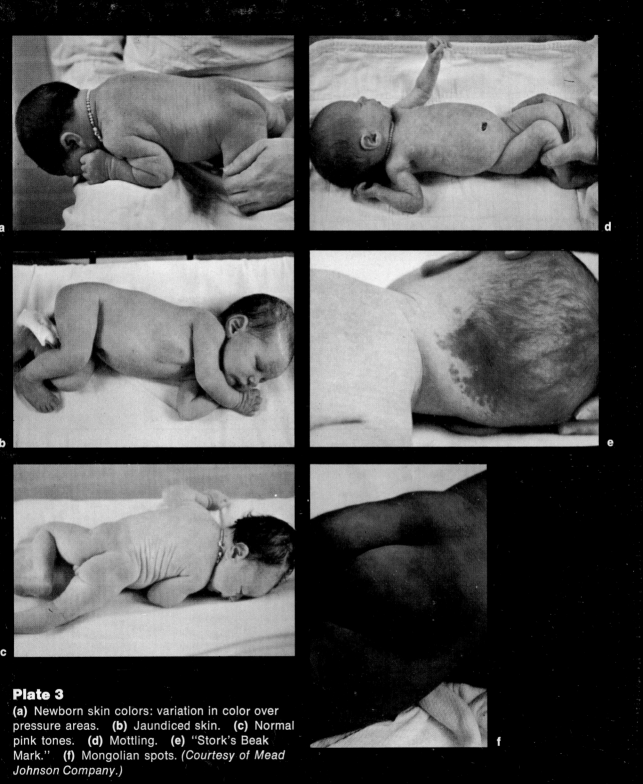

Plate 3

(a) Newborn skin colors: variation in color over pressure areas.   (b) Jaundiced skin.   (c) Normal pink tones.   (d) Mottling.   (e) "Stork's Beak Mark."   (f) Mongolian spots. *(Courtesy of Mead Johnson Company.)*